Advances in the Diagnosis and Management of Vasculitis

Advances in the Diagnosis and Management of Vasculitis

Guest Editor

Alicia Rodriguez-Pla

MDPI

Basel • Beijing • Wuhan • Barcelona • Belgrade • Novi Sad • Cluj • Manchester

Guest Editor
Alicia Rodriguez-Pla
Premier Rheumatology, P. C.
Fresno, CA
USA

Editorial Office
MDPI AG
Grosspeteranlage 5
4052 Basel, Switzerland

This is a reprint of the Special Issue, published open access by the journal *Diagnostics* (ISSN 2075-4418), freely accessible at: https://www.mdpi.com/journal/diagnostics/special_issues/MJE91FD2YN.

For citation purposes, cite each article independently as indicated on the article page online and as indicated below:

Lastname, A.A.; Lastname, B.B. Article Title. *Journal Name* **Year**, *Volume Number*, Page Range.

ISBN 978-3-7258-7500-9 (Hbk)
ISBN 978-3-7258-7501-6 (PDF)
https://doi.org/10.3390/books978-3-7258-7501-6

Contents

About the Editor

Alicia Rodriguez-Pla

Alicia Rodriguez-Pla earned her medical degree from the University of Navarra in Spain and completed rheumatology training in Barcelona (Spain). She obtained her Ph.D. from the Universitat Autonoma de Barcelona while working on giant cell arteritis. Her interest in vasculitis led her to pursue post-doctoral training in the U.S. from 2003 to 2007, where she worked as a visiting post-doctoral research fellow at Johns Hopkins University. During her last two years at Johns Hopkins, she was funded through a Vasculitis Clinical Research Consortium (VCRC)/Vasculitis Foundation (VF) fellowship. She also received a Master's in Public Health (MPH) at The Johns Hopkins Bloomberg School of Public Health. In addition, she worked on lupus research at the Baylor Institute for Immunology Research in Dallas before completing a clinical fellowship in rheumatology at Boston University, where her interest in scleroderma increased. She completed her residency in internal medicine at Lahey Hospital and Medical Center in Burlington, MA. She worked as an Assistant Professor in the Rheumatology Division at the University of Arizona in Tucson and at Mayo Clinic Arizona before becoming the Rheumatology Division Chief at UCSF Fresno in September 2022, where she was also an Assistant Professor of Clinical Medicine. While at the University of Arizona, she was the Director of the Vasculitis Center and the Co-Director of the Scleroderma Program. At Mayo Clinic Arizona, she was the Director of the Vasculitis Program. In May 2023, she joined Sierra Pacific Arthritis and Rheumatology Centers. At the end of 2025, she established her own private practice, Premier Rheumatology, P. C., in Fresno, California. She is a physician-scientist, and her main interests are vasculitis, scleroderma, and IgG4-related disease. She is interested in translational and clinical research. She is board-certified in internal medicine and rheumatology by the American Board of Internal Medicine (ABIM).

Preface

It is with immense pleasure that we present this Reprint, a curated collection of eleven significant articles originally published in the Special Issue "Advances in the Diagnosis and Management of Vasculitis" for the journal *Diagnostics*.

This compilation reflects the dynamic and rapidly advancing nature of research in the field of systemic vasculitis, bringing together diverse perspectives from leading research groups across Spain, Poland, the USA, Germany, Romania, and Turkey.

The primary subject of this Reprint is the multifaceted nature of primary systemic vasculitides—a group of rare but potentially life-threatening diseases characterized by blood vessel inflammation. The scope of the works is intentionally broad, covering large-vessel vasculitis, such as giant cell arteritis and Takayasu arteritis, as well as small-vessel involvements like ANCA-associated vasculitis and IgA vasculitis. By including original research, case reports, and comprehensive reviews, this Reprint addresses the entire clinical trajectory, from the initial diagnostic hurdle to long-term therapeutic management and the prevention of relapses.

The aim and purpose of this collection are to provide a centralized resource that highlights the most recent breakthroughs in the field. In recent years, the management of vasculitis has undergone a paradigm shift. We have moved from a heavy reliance on high-dose glucocorticoids toward a more nuanced "steroid-sparing" approach powered by targeted biological therapies. This Reprint serves to document these advances, focusing on the search for reliable biomarkers and the implementation of innovative imaging techniques—such as PET-CT and advanced neurosonography—that allow for earlier intervention and more precise monitoring of disease activity.

The motivation for assembling this scientific work stems from the inherent diagnostic challenges these diseases pose. Vasculitis often mimics other conditions, leading to delays that can result in irreversible organ damage or vision loss. Our goal was to bridge the gap between bench research and clinical practice, providing evidence-based insights that can immediately impact patient outcomes.

This Reprint is addressed to a wide audience of healthcare professionals and scientists. It is intended for rheumatologists, internists, radiologists, and immunologists who seek to refine their diagnostic accuracy and therapeutic strategies. Furthermore, it provides a robust foundation for students and early-career researchers looking to understand the current landscape and future directions of vasculitis research. We hope that the insights shared in these pages inspire further collaboration and innovation, ultimately leading to a brighter future for patients living with these complex conditions.

Alicia Rodriguez-Pla
Guest Editor

diagnostics

MDPI

Editorial

Advances in Diagnosing and Managing Primary Systemic Vasculitides: A Transforming Landscape

Alicia Rodriguez-Pla

Premier Rheumatology, P. C., 1189 E Herndon Avenue, Suite 101, Fresno, CA 93720, USA; arp@premierrheumatology.org

As we conclude this Special Issue of *Diagnostics*, "Advances in the Diagnosis and Management of Vasculitis," we reflect on a vibrant collection of eleven articles that span the globe from Spain and Poland to the USA, Germany, Romania, and Turkey. This international collaboration underscores a universal knowledge in rheumatology: while vasculitis remains a diagnostic "chameleon," our collective ability to understand it has never been stronger [1,2].

The primary systemic vasculitides occupy a unique space in medicine—rare enough to challenge timely recognition, and serious enough to demand urgent, evidence-based action. Despite the significant progress over the past two decades, the path from symptom onset to accurate diagnosis remains fraught with complexity, and therapeutic strategies continue to evolve at an unprecedented pace. The approval of avacopan for anti-neutrophil cytoplasmic antibody (ANCA)-associated vasculitis (AAV) in 2021 [3], the Food and Drug Administration (FDA) approval of upadacitinib for giant cell arteritis (GCA) in April 2025 [4], and the accelerating integration of advanced imaging modalities into clinical workflows have collectively reshaped how we conceptualize and manage these diseases [5]. This Special Issue of *Diagnostics* was conceived to capture this momentum—bringing together original research, reviews, and case reports that address diagnostic challenges, emerging biomarkers, novel imaging approaches, treatment strategies, and patient outcomes across the vasculitis spectrum.

1. Diagnostic Complexity of Giant Cell Arteritis

GCA remains the most common systemic vasculitis in adults over 50 years of age, yet its heterogeneous presentation continues to pose significant diagnostic hurdles [6]. Updated classification criteria, advances in imaging technologies, the evolving biomarker landscape, and emerging therapeutic strategies including the role of targeted therapies are rapidly transforming the management paradigm [7–9]. Importantly, no single pathognomonic feature defines GCA and that a multimodal approach integrating clinical assessment, laboratory evaluation, and imaging is essential to reduce the risk of complications such as irreversible vision loss [10].

The urgency of rapid diagnosis is illustrated by Stańska et al., who present a case report of a 74-year-old patient in whom diagnostic delays led to bilateral vision loss. Their work supports ultrasound as the first-line imaging tool for suspected GCA, in alignment with the 2023 European League Against Rheumatism (EULAR) recommendations that position color duplex sonography (PCDS) above temporal artery biopsy (TAB) for its sensitivity, non-invasiveness, and wide availability, while acknowledging that operator expertise remains a key limiting factor, and TAB remains a valuable tool in many clinical situations [11].

2. The Expanding Role of Imaging

Imaging has emerged as a central pillar in vasculitis diagnosis and monitoring. The role of positron emission tomography/computed tomography (PET/CT) in GCA has been established, especially in specific clinical scenarios—including atypical presentations, suspicion of large vessel involvement, and diagnostic uncertainty in the setting of mimickers—in which this imaging modality can provide decisive information [12]. Color duplex ultrasound and magnetic resonance imaging have also been found to be helpful tools for diagnosing GCA [13].

3. Rare Presentations and Diagnostic Mimickers

The vasculitis spectrum extends beyond GCA and AAV. In the arena of monogenic vasculopathies, [14] contributed an important case report on hepatic vascular involvement in deficiency of adenosine deaminase 2 (DADA2), describing large regenerative nodules with a focal nodular hyperplasia (FNH)-like appearance not previously reported in this setting. Notably, etanercept therapy resulted in sustained clinical stabilization and the marked regression of liver lesions over nine years of follow-up, expanding our understanding of the hepatic manifestations and treatment responsiveness in this rare condition.

4. ANCA-Associated Vasculitis: From Pathogenesis to Prognosis

Significant advances in biomarker research in AAV is helping to change the treatment paradigm [15,16]. In the context of the expanding therapeutic armamentarium—including avacopan, which was found to be superior to prednisone in sustained remission at 52 weeks in the ADVOCATE trial —the ability to stratify patients by relapse risk has direct implications for treatment selection and monitoring intensity [17].

5. Nephritis in IgA Vasculitis: Outcomes Under Immunosuppression

Yıldırım et al. contributed a prospective observational study of 49 adults with IgA vasculitis nephritis (IgAVN), an area with a notable absence of specific management guidelines. Their findings challenge the prevailing perception of uniformly poor renal outcomes in adults, demonstrating that ESRD occurred in only one patient (2%) when effective immunosuppressive therapy was employed. The identification of nephrotic-range proteinuria as an independent risk factor for unfavorable outcomes (OR: 17.18) provides a practical prognostic marker. Importantly, the study also highlights the infection risk associated with immunosuppression, particularly in older adult patients—a reminder that therapeutic gains must be weighed against treatment-related morbidity [18].

6. A Transformative Era

Collectively, these 11 contributions illustrate that the field of vasculitis is undergoing a transformation driven by converging advances in imaging, immunopathogenesis, targeted therapeutics, and clinical phenotyping. The expanding application of US, PET/CT, and contrast-enhanced ultrasound (CEUS) across the vasculitis spectrum enables earlier diagnosis, more precise disease monitoring, and better-informed therapeutic decision-making [19,20]. The common thread among these diverse papers, ranging from prospective studies in Turkey to retrospective cohorts in Spain, is the urgent need to reduce treatment toxicity without compromising efficacy. The approval of complement inhibitors such as avacopan for AAV [21] and JAK inhibitors such as upadacitinib for GCA [4] mark a paradigm shift toward mechanism-based, steroid-sparing strategies to offer a roadmap for improving long-term outcomes and quality of life.

However, many unresolved questions persist. The optimal duration and intensity of immunosuppression, the role of imaging in treatment de-escalation, the identification of

https://doi.org/10.3390/diagnostics16050788

validated biomarkers for disease activity and relapse prediction, and the development of tailored approaches for rare vasculitis phenotypes all require continued investigation. The diversity of contributions in this Special Issue—spanning LVV, small-vessel vasculitis, IgA vasculitis, IgG4-RD, and monogenic vasculopathy—reflects the breadth of the challenges and the vitality of the research community dedicated to addressing them.

I am deeply grateful to all contributing authors for their rigorous work and to the reviewers whose constructive assessments strengthened each manuscript. I hope that this collection serves as both a practical resource for clinicians and a catalyst for future study, advancing us closer to the ultimate goals: timely diagnosis, personalized treatment, and improved outcomes and quality of life for all patients with vasculitis.

Funding: This research received no external funding.

Conflicts of Interest: The author declares the following financial interests/personal relationships that may be considered as potential competing interests: Alicia Rodriguez-Pla (ARP) is the owner and founder of Premier Rheumatology. ARP also reports serving as a member of an independent Data Monitoring Committee for Bristol Myers Squibb and has served as a member of a scientific advisory board for AstraZeneca. These roles occurred within the 36 months prior to this submission. The companies and entities had no role in the design of this study; in the collection, analyses, or interpretation of data; in the writing of this manuscript; or in the decision to publish the results. ARP also previously served as a Principal Investigator for clinical trials involving Systemic Lupus Erythematosus and IgG4-Related Disease sponsored by Zenas BioPharma. These roles concluded in 2025 and were outside the scope of the submitted work on vasculitis diagnostics.

References

1. Casal Moura, M.; Merkel, P.A.; Jayne, D.; Cid, M.C.; Basu, N.; Hellmich, B.; Terrier, B.; Rutgers, A.; Gordon, J.; Verhoeven, P.; et al. Challenges in the diagnosis, classification and prognosis of ANCA-associated vasculitis. *Nat. Rev. Rheumatol.* **2025**, *21*, 719–736. [CrossRef]
2. Matza, M.A.; Arevalo, A.B.; Unizony, S. Imaging Challenges and Developments in Large-vessel Vasculitis. *Rheum. Dis. Clin. N. Am.* **2024**, *50*, 603–621. [CrossRef] [PubMed]
3. Jayne, D.R.W.; Merkel, P.A.; Schall, T.J.; Bekker, P.; Group, A.S. Avacopan for the Treatment of ANCA-Associated Vasculitis. *N. Engl. J. Med.* **2021**, *384*, 599–609. [CrossRef] [PubMed]
4. Upadacitinib (Rinvoq) for giant cell arteritis. *Med. Lett. Drugs Ther.* **2025**, *67*, 114–115. [CrossRef]
5. Aldasoro, V.; Betech-Antar, V.; Castaneda, S.; de Miguel, E.; Rosales, J.J.; Garcia-Velloso, M.J. Diagnosis of giant cell arteritis by 18F-FDG PET/CT in patients on glucocorticoid therapy: Importance of delayed imaging. *Clin. Exp. Rheumatol.* **2025**, *43*, 595–601. [CrossRef]
6. de Mornac, D.; Agard, C.; Hardouin, J.B.; Hamidou, M.; Connault, J.; Masseau, A.; Espitia-Thibault, A.; Artifoni, M.; Ngohou, C.; Perrin, F.; et al. Risk factors for symptomatic vascular events in giant cell arteritis: A study of 254 patients with large-vessel imaging at diagnosis. *Ther. Adv. Musculoskelet. Dis.* **2021**, *13*, 1–11. [CrossRef]
7. Ponte, C.; Grayson, P.C.; Robson, J.C.; Suppiah, R.; Gribbons, K.B.; Judge, A.; Craven, A.; Khalid, S.; Hutchings, A.; Watts, R.A.; et al. 2022 American College of Rheumatology/EULAR classification criteria for giant cell arteritis. *Ann. Rheum. Dis.* **2022**, *81*, 1647–1653. [CrossRef]
8. Tomoyose, R.; Miyata, T.; Shiraishi, W.; Ogura, T.; Koga, N.; Agawa, Y.; Umemura, T.; Tsujimoto, Y.; Nakajima, H.; Sakamoto, H.; et al. Gadolinium-enhanced MR improved motion sensitized driven equilibrium (iMSDE) for intracranial vessel imaging in giant cell arteritis. *J. Stroke Cerebrovasc. Dis.* **2022**, *31*, 106697. [CrossRef] [PubMed]
9. Rizzo, C.; La Barbera, L.; Miceli, G.; Tuttolomondo, A.; Guggino, G. The innate face of Giant Cell Arteritis: Insight into cellular and molecular innate immunity pathways to unravel new possible biomarkers of disease. *Front. Mol. Med.* **2022**, *2*, 933161. [CrossRef]
10. Marvisi, C.; Macaluso, F.; Ricordi, C.; Cavazza, A.; Muratore, F.; Salvarani, C. Diagnostic approach in giant cell arteritis. *Autoimmun. Rev.* **2025**, *24*, 103743. [CrossRef]
11. Stanska, W.; Kruszewski, R.; Juszkiewicz, A.; Bachta, A.; Tlustochowicz, W. Giant Cell Arteritis: Can Simple Ultrasound Examination Prevent Complex Consequences? *Diagnostics* **2024**, *14*, 2071. [CrossRef]
12. Yin, P.; Abikhzer, G.; Alberini, J.L.; Slart, R.H. [18F]FDG PET/CT imaging of giant cell arteritis: Contemporary practical guide to image acquisition and interpretation. *Q. J. Nucl. Med. Mol. Imaging* **2025**, *69*, 69–81. [CrossRef] [PubMed]

https://doi.org/10.3390/diagnostics16050788

13. van Nieuwland, M.; Colin, E.M.; Vermeer, M.; Wagenaar, N.R.L.; Vijlbrief, O.D.; van Zandwijk, J.K.; Slart, R.; Koffijberg, H.; Jebbink, E.G.; van der Geest, K.S.M.; et al. A direct comparison in diagnostic performance of CDUS, FDG-PET/CT and MRI in patients suspected of giant cell arteritis. *Rheumatology* **2025**, *64*, 1392–1399. [CrossRef] [PubMed]
14. Sparchez, M.; Damian, L.; Socaciu, M.A.; Fufezan, O.; Sparchez, Z. Hepatic Vascular Involvement in Adenosine Deaminase 2 Deficiency (DADA2): Case Reports and Literature Review. *Diagnostics* **2026**, *16*, 189. [CrossRef]
15. Trattner, R.; Iordanou, M.; Ohlsson, S.; Martin, M.; Segelmark, M.; Blom, A.M. Complement factors as biomarkers in ANCA-associated vasculitis in remission. *Clin. Exp. Immunol.* **2025**, *219*, uxaf037. [CrossRef] [PubMed]
16. Baas, L.; Krol, R.M.; Hagen, E.C.; Spierings, J.; Teng, Y.K.O.; Koelman, C.A.; Remmelts, H.H.F. Biomarkers Detecting the Activity of ANCA-Associated Vasculitis: A Systematic Literature Review. *Int. J. Nephrol.* **2025**, *2025*, 3133057. [CrossRef]
17. Wawrzycka-Adamczyk, K.; Korkosz, M.; Musial, J.; Wojcik, K. Relapse Predictors in Antineutrophil Cytoplasmic Antibody (ANCA)-Associated Vasculitis. *Diagnostics* **2024**, *14*, 1849. [CrossRef]
18. Yildirim, F.; Kutu, M.E.; Calik, Y.; Kalkan, K.; Akkuzu, G.; Ozgur, D.S.; Karaalioglu, B.; Deniz, R.; Guzelant Ozkose, G.; Ince, B.; et al. Disease Course and Long-Term Outcomes in Adult IgA Vasculitis Nephritis: A Prospective Observational Study. *Diagnostics* **2025**, *15*, 957. [CrossRef]
19. Molina-Collada, J.; Castrejon, I.; Rivera, J.; Martinez-Barrio, J.; Nieto-Gonzalez, J.C.; Lopez, K.; Montero, F.; Trives, L.; Gonzalez, C.; Alvaro-Gracia, J.M. The role of ultrasound and FDG-PET/CT to detect extracranial artery involvement in patients with suspected large vessel vasculitis. *Mod. Rheumatol.* **2023**, *33*, 549–556. [CrossRef]
20. Bosch, P.; Dejaco, C.; Schmidt, W.A.; Schluter, K.D.; Pregartner, G.; Schafer, V.S. Ultrasound for diagnosis and follow-up of chronic axillary vasculitis in patients with long-standing giant cell arteritis. *Ther. Adv. Musculoskelet. Dis.* **2021**, *13*, 1–9. [CrossRef]
21. Aldhuaina, K.; Alghanim, K. Efficacy and safety of avacopan in the treatment of ANCA-associated vasculitis: A systematic review and meta-analysis. *BMC Rheumatol.* **2025**, *9*, 115. [CrossRef] [PubMed]

https://doi.org/10.3390/diagnostics16050788

diagnostics

MDPI

Review

Diagnostic Challenges and Modern Therapeutic Strategies in Giant Cell Arteritis

Alicia Rodriguez-Pla

Premier Rheumatology, P. C., 1189 E Herndon Avenue, Suite 101, Fresno, CA 93720, USA;
arp@premierrheumatology.org; Tel.: +1-559-421-3768

Abstract

Giant cell arteritis (GCA) represents one of the most diagnostically challenging systemic vasculitides, characterized by its heterogeneous clinical presentation, lack of pathognomonic features, and potential for devastating complications, with a special concern for irreversible vision loss. This comprehensive review synthesizes current evidence regarding the multifaceted diagnostic challenges in GCA, incorporating recent advances in classification criteria, imaging technologies, biomarker research, and emerging therapeutic strategies.

Keywords: giant cell arteritis; temporal arteritis; vasculitis; diagnostic challenges; differential diagnosis; temporal artery biopsy

1. Introduction and Clinical Significance

GCA is an inflammatory disease of large and medium-sized vessels that predominantly affects individuals over 50 years of age, with peak incidence between 70 and 80 years [1], and it is specially concerning for visual loss [2]. The condition's clinical significance extends beyond its inflammatory nature, as delayed diagnosis can result in catastrophic complications, including permanent blindness, which occurs in 15–20% of untreated patients, stroke, aortic dissection, and aortic aneurysm formation [3–5].

The pathophysiology of GCA involves complex interactions between adaptive and innate immune systems, with granulomatous inflammation involving arterial walls and resulting in vessel occlusion and tissue ischemia [6]

The reason GCA is so difficult to manage is that different "pockets" of inflammation in the artery respond differently to therapy. The clinical manifestations of GCA are the direct result of a spatially organized inflammatory process within the temporal artery wall. Recent research using spatial transcriptomics has demonstrated that macrophages and T cells are not uniformly distributed; rather, they organize into three functionally distinct layers that dictate disease progression and treatment response [7,8]. The adventitia serves as the primary gateway for leukocyte entry and the epicenter of the systemic acute-phase response. Here, a cluster of differentiation (CD)64^{+} macrophages and Th17 cells forms a potent proinflammatory circuit. This layer is characterized by the high production of interleukin (IL)-6, IL-1β, and IL-23. This "adventitial signature" correlates strongly with elevated C-reactive protein (CRP), erythrocyte sedimentation rate (ESR), and constitutional symptoms such as fever and weight loss. Importantly, this pathway is highly sensitive to glucocorticoids and IL-6 receptor antagonists, e.g., tocilizumab, often resulting in a rapid normalization of systemic markers. Tissue injury is concentrated in the arterial media, where multinucleated giant cells and CD206^{+} macrophages orchestrate the degradation of the internal elastic lamina. This destructive phenotype is driven by the secretion of matrix metalloproteinase (MMP)-9, YKL-40/chitinase 3-like, and reactive oxygen species (ROS). Recent data highlight granulocyte macrophage colony-stimulating factor (GM-CSF) as the master regulator of this medial destruction, providing a rationale for the use of GM-CSF receptor blockers, e.g., mavrilimumab, to prevent permanent structural damage to the vessel wall. The most clinically catastrophic feature of GCA, luminal occlusion, occurs in the intima. This layer is dominated by CD163^{+} and folate receptor (FR)-β+ macrophages, which drive a "response-to-injury" program. These cells secrete vascular endothelial growth factor (VEGF) and platelet-derived growth factor (PDGF), triggering neoangiogenesis and the migration of myofibroblasts. Unlike the adventitial inflammatory markers, this intimal remodeling program is notably resistant to glucocorticoids. This explains the "vascular-systemic dissociation" frequently observed in GCA, where patients may develop ischemic complications, e.g., vision loss, despite having a normal CRP and an apparently suppressed systemic inflammatory response (Figure 1) [7–12].

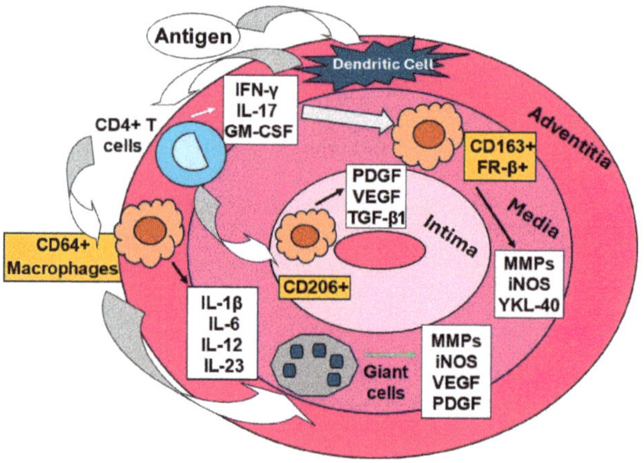

Figure 1. Compartmentalized macrophage and T cell effector functions in GCA: layer-specific immunopathology and steroid resistance mechanisms. The inflammatory landscape of GCA exhibits a functionally distinct "division of labor" across the arterial wall, with each compartment contributing to specific pathogenic outcomes. (A) Adventitia, systemic signaling hub: CD64^{+} macrophages and CD4^{+} Th17 cells orchestrate systemic inflammation through production of IL-6, IL-1β, and IL-23, which drive hepatic acute-phase protein synthesis, with elevated CRP and serum amyloid A (SAA), and constitutional symptoms like fever and malaise. This axis is highly glucocorticoid-responsive. (B) Media, zone of vascular wall destruction: multinucleated giant cells derived from macrophage fusion and CD206^{+} alternatively activate macrophages localize to the internal elastic lamina (IEL), where they secrete MMP-9, MMP-2, and the chitinase 3-like protein YKL-40. These proteases, combined with reactive oxygen species (ROS) by activated nicotinamide adenine dinucleotide phosphate (NADPH) oxidase, mediate degradation of elastin and collagen, resulting in focal wall thinning, medial necrosis, and aneurysmal dilatation. (C) Intima, zone of occlusive remodeling: CD163^{+}/FR-β^{+} alternatively activate macrophages, and resident myofibroblasts secrete platelet-derived growth factor (PDGF) and vascular endothelial growth factor (VEGF), promoting neoangiogenesis, intimal smooth muscle cell hyperplasia, and progressive luminal narrowing, leading to tissue ischemia. While the adventitial IL-6/Th17 axis responds dramatically to glucocorticoids, the medial giant-cell-driven matrix destruction and CD163^{+}-mediated intimal remodeling exhibit relative steroid resistance, perpetuating subclinical inflammation and late-stage ischemic complications even after initial clinical remission. Abbreviations: CD, cluster of differentiation; iNOS, inducible nitric oxide synthase; MMP: matrix metalloproteinases; PDGF, platelet-derived growth factor; IL: interleukin; GM-CSF: granulocyte macrophage colony-stimulating factor; TGF-β1, transforming growth factor-β1; IFN, interferon; FR, folate receptor.

https://doi.org/10.3390/diagnostics16030470

Despite significant advances in understanding pathogenic mechanisms, the etiology remains unknown, and diagnostic approaches continue to rely on combinations of clinical assessment, laboratory findings, imaging, and histopathological examination [13].

The diagnostic challenges of GCA can be divided into two major categories: (1) failure to diagnose the disease correctly and in a timely manner, which may be complicated due to its unspecific symptoms; (2) diagnosing GCA in patients who do not have the disease but a mimicker.

2. Material and Methods

This narrative review summarizes current evidence on diagnostic challenges, including evolving classification criteria and therapeutic strategies in GCA. We conducted a comprehensive literature search of PubMed/MEDLINE, Web of Science, and Scopus databases for articles published through December 2025. Search terms included combinations of MeSH terms and keywords: "giant cell arteritis", "temporal arteritis", "large vessel vasculitis", "diagnosis", "classification criteria", "imaging", "ultrasound", "temporal artery biopsy", "biomarkers", "treatment", "glucocorticoids", and "biologics".

We prioritized peer-reviewed original research articles, systematic reviews and meta-analyses, randomized controlled trials, large observational cohort studies, and evidence-based clinical guidelines. We primarily focused on publications from the last 10 years while including seminal earlier works that established foundational concepts. We focused on clinically relevant studies addressing diagnostic accuracy, classification criteria performance, imaging modality comparisons, biomarker validation, and therapeutic efficacy.

We emphasize that this is narrative and not a systematic review. Therefore, we did not conduct formal systematic quality assessments or meta-analysis, but we critically evaluated the strength and consistency of evidence throughout our synthesis. By "prioritization", we mean that when multiple sources addressed the same topic, we preferentially cited peer-reviewed original research, systematic reviews, meta-analyses, and randomized controlled trials over case reports, editorials, or lower-quality evidence. This is a narrative synthesis based on expert clinical judgment rather than a systematic review with predefined inclusion criteria and quality scoring. Throughout the manuscript, we explicitly note areas of conflicting evidence, methodological limitations of studies, and gaps in the current literature to provide appropriate critical appraisal while maintaining the narrative review format.

3. Risk Factors and Epidemiological Consideration

3.1. Genetic Factors

GCA is not considered a purely hereditary disease that is directly inherited. Research indicates that a genetic predisposition plays a role in increasing an individual's susceptibility to GCA. However, although certain genetic factors may raise the risk, they do not guarantee the development of the disease.

Genetic predisposition is suggested through familial clustering and association with specific human leukocyte antigen (HLA) alleles, though the specific genetic factors remain unidentified. The HLA-DRB1*04 alleles, especially HLA-DRB10*401 and HLA-DRB10*404, have been identified as significant genetic risk factors, particularly in Caucasian populations. The HLA-DRB1 molecules are involved in antigen presentation to CD4+ T cells, suggesting that specific HLA variants may present antigens that trigger pathogenic immune responses in genetically predisposed individuals. While there is a higher incidence of GCA in families with a history of the condition, familial cases are relatively rare, accounting for about 1% of all patients. This complex genetic landscape underscores that while genetics contribute to risk, there are other factors also at play [14,15].

https://doi.org/10.3390/diagnostics16030470

3.2. Geographic and Demographic Patterns

The incidence of GCA varies significantly worldwide, with North American estimates ranging from 15 to 30 cases per 100,000 individuals aged 50 and older [16]. Scandinavian countries report the highest incidence rates, suggesting that genetic, environmental, and/or geographic factors may play important roles in disease susceptibility [17]. A recent meta-analysis examining nine studies found an overall pooled prevalence of 51.74 cases per 100,000 people over 50 years, with prevalence remaining stable across publication years using linear fit modeling [18].

The female predominance is consistent across populations, with women affected 2–4 times more frequently than men [16]. This gender disparity likely reflects hormonal influences on immune system function, though the specific mechanisms remain incompletely understood [19]. Age represents the most significant risk factor, with the disease rarely occurring before age 50 and demonstrating an exponential increase in incidence with advancing age [1,20].

Some studies reported a seasonal variation with increased diagnostic frequency during fall and winter months, suggesting possible infectious triggers or environmental precipitants [21], although none of them has been yet demonstrated.

3.3. Pathophysiological Risk Factors

Several age-related biological processes contribute to GCA susceptibility. Immunosenescence, characterized by declining naïve T and regulatory T cell populations, accumulation of CD28-null T cells with enhanced cytotoxic potential, decreased thymic output reducing T cell receptor diversity, and increased proinflammatory cytokine production, including IL6-IL1β, and antitumor necrosis factor (TNF)α, which creates a proinflammatory state termed "inflammaging", and shifts in CD4/CD8 cell distributions, creates a proinflammatory milieu conducive to vasculitis development [10,22,23].

Concurrent vascular aging, marked by loss of arterial elasticity and increased wall stiffness, provides the structural substrate for inflammatory targeting. Age-related loss of adventitial *vasa vasorum* may create hypoxic conditions in the arterial wall, while accumulation of oxidative damage and advanced glycation end products in the elastic lamina may generate neoantigens that trigger autoimmune responses [24,25].

4. Clinical Presentation and Diagnostic Complexity

4.1. Cranial Manifestations

The classic cranial presentation of GCA encompasses a constellation of symptoms that, while characteristic, are not pathognomonic. New-onset headaches are often described as severe and different from previous headache patterns [26–28]. Temporal artery abnormalities, including tenderness, thickening, or reduced pulsation, provide important physical examination findings and are present in 40–60% of cases, making them one of the more common physical signs in GCA [13,29].

Jaw claudication due to ischemia of masticatory muscles during chewing demonstrates high specificity for GCA, approximately 90%, and occurs in 35–50% of patients [30–32]. While jaw claudication is less common than temporal artery abnormalities, its high specificity makes it a particularly valuable diagnostic clue when present [13,33,34]. The "chewing gum test", while not superior to clinical history alone, may provide additional diagnostic utility when pain onset occurs within two minutes of chewing [35].

Visual complications are also part of the cranial manifestations, but we will discuss them separately given their potentially devastating clinical consequences.

https://doi.org/10.3390/diagnostics16030470

4.2. Visual Complications

Visual manifestations represent the most feared complications of GCA, occurring in 15–20% of patients and potentially progressing to irreversible blindness [36–38]. Arteritic anterior ischemic optic neuropathy (AAION) constitutes the most common mechanism, characterized by acute monocular vision loss with "chalk-white" optic disc edema, often accompanied by retinal whitening or cotton wool spots [39,40].

The spectrum of visual involvement includes transient visual disturbances, diplopia from cranial nerve palsies, and various patterns of visual field defects [41,42]. Central retinal artery occlusion occurs in approximately 10% of cases [43,44], while posterior ischemic optic neuropathy and choroidal infarction represent less common but serious manifestations [45–48]. The irreversible nature of most visual complications underscores the critical importance of rapid diagnosis and treatment initiation [49,50].

4.3. Systemic and Constitutional Symptoms

Constitutional symptoms, including fatigue, fever, anorexia, and unintentional weight loss, occur in 40–60% of GCA patients [51–53]. These non-specific symptoms often precede more characteristic manifestations and may lead to diagnostic delays, particularly in patients presenting with isolated systemic features [53,54].

Polymyalgia rheumatica (PMR) coexists with GCA in approximately 40–50% of cases, manifesting as bilateral shoulder and pelvic girdle pain, weakness, and stiffness [55]. The relationship between PMR and GCA remains complex, with some experts considering them manifestations of the same disease spectrum [56]. PMR symptoms may precede, accompany, or follow GCA diagnosis, and their presence should prompt careful evaluation for underlying vasculitis [57].

4.4. Extracranial Large Vessel Disease

Recognition of extracranial large vessel involvement has expanded significantly with advanced imaging capabilities. Large vessel GCA (LV-GCA) affects the aorta and its major branches in 50–80% of patients, depending on imaging modality sensitivity [58]. This phenotype may be present without classic cranial symptoms, leading to diagnostic challenges and potential delays [59–61]. Patients with isolated extracranial disease often present with non-specific constitutional symptoms, refractory PMR, fever of unknown origin, or limb claudication. Specific presentations may include limb claudication, upper extremities more commonly than lower, blood pressure discrepancies > 10 mmHg between arms in cases of subclavian involvement, carotid or subclavian bruits, or absent pulses, especially radial pulses. Some patients report unexplained fever, night sweats, or refractory PMR that fails to respond adequately to moderate-dose glucocorticoids.

Characteristic imaging findings in LV-GCA include concentric mural thickening with fluorodeoxyglucose (FDG) uptake or contrast enhancement in a "macaroni sign" pattern, typically involving subclavian arteries (75–80%), thoracic aorta (40–60%), and abdominal aorta (30–40%). The axillary arteries show bilateral involvement in a majority of cases, which is highly specific for GCA versus atherosclerotic disease [62].

The absence of temporal artery abnormalities in these patients necessitates high clinical suspicion and appropriate imaging to establish diagnosis. Recognition of isolated LV-GCA is critical as these patients often do not meet traditional diagnostic criteria focused on cranial symptoms, potentially leading to diagnostic delay. The 2022 American College of Rheumatology (ACR)/European League Against Rheumatism (EULAR) criteria partially address this gap by incorporating imaging of large vessels and assigning points for bilateral axillary involvement [63,64].

https://doi.org/10.3390/diagnostics16030470

Patients with extensive large vessel involvement may require longer duration of glucocorticoid therapy and have higher relapse rates during tapering. Some evidence suggests that these patients may benefit from earlier introduction of steroid-sparing agents, though this remains an area requiring further study [65].

5. Laboratory Findings and Biomarkers

5.1. Traditional Inflammatory Markers

Erythrocyte sedimentation rate (ESR) and C-reactive protein (CRP) remain cornerstone laboratory tests in GCA evaluation, though their limitations are well recognized. ESR elevation (>50 mm/h using the Westergren method) occurs in approximately 76–84% of GCA patients, while CRP demonstrates slightly higher sensitivity, at 86–98%, depending on the study population [66–70]. However, normal inflammatory markers occur in approximately 4–20% of biopsy-proven cases (with most studies reporting 7–10%), representing a population enriched for atypical presentations such as early disease course, predominantly large vessel involvement without cranial manifestations, or concurrent use of medications that suppress inflammatory markers such as tocilizumab or glucocorticoids [59,71,72].

The combination of ESR and CRP provide enhanced diagnostic utility, with concordant elevation yielding 99% sensitivity for positive temporal artery biopsy. Conversely, both normal ESR and CRP confer high negative predictive value, though this cannot definitively exclude diagnosis in patients with high clinical suspicion [70].

5.2. Platelet Count and Hematological Parameter

Thrombocytosis (>400 × $10^3/\mu$L) occurs in 50–70% of GCA patients (range from multiple studies) and demonstrates comparable diagnostic performance to traditional inflammatory markers [73]. Platelet counts >400 × $10^3/\mu$L show specificity of 80–90% (95% confidence interval (CI): 75–92%) for positive temporal artery biopsy, though sensitivity remains moderate at 50–60% [74]. The combination of elevated CRP and platelet count may provide optimal diagnostic utility, with both positive tests yielding 77% positive predictive value [75].

Normochromic normocytic anemia affects approximately 60–80% of patients, with mean hemoglobin levels around 11.7 ± 1.6 g/dL [76]. Leukocytosis occurs less consistently but may accompany active disease phases [77].

5.3. Emerging Biomarkers

Research into novel biomarkers has identified several promising candidates that could potentially enhance diagnostic accuracy and disease monitoring. However, while numerous candidate biomarkers have been identified, most have been evaluated in single-center studies with limited sample sizes and lack independent validation in diverse populations. Furthermore, few studies have demonstrated that these biomarkers provide diagnostic or prognostic information beyond that available from ESR, CRP, and platelet count.

Among emerging biomarkers, SAA shows the most clinical potential because it strongly correlates with disease activity, it demonstrates elevation in GCA patients compared to healthy controls, and it demonstrates superior sensitivity to ESR for detecting active vasculitis (85–90% vs. 76–84%). SAA may decline more rapidly with effective treatment, potentially enabling earlier detection of inadequate response [78–80]. SAA assays are already available in many clinical laboratories, facilitating rapid translation. However, SAA lacks specificity for GCA vs. other inflammatory conditions, as in the case of ESR and CRP [78].

Cytokine profiling reveals elevated levels of interleukin-6 (IL-6), IL-23, and various chemokines in GCA patients [81–84]. IL-6 levels correlate with disease activity and form the rationale for tocilizumab therapy [81]. B-cell activating factor (BAFF) and chitinase 3-like protein (YKL-40) show promise as inflammatory markers with potential roles in disease pathogenesis [85,86].

Vascular remodeling biomarkers including matrix metalloproteinases (MMPs), especially MMP-2, MMP-9, and MMP12; vascular endothelial growth factor (VEGF); and angiopoietins may provide insights into vessel wall damage and repair processes [11,12,15,87]. These reflect vascular remodeling processes but are not GCA-specific, and require specialized assays not widely available. These may have greater utility as research tools for understanding pathogenesis than as clinical biomarkers.

The most promising future approach may be composite biomarker panels combining traditional markers (ESR, CRP, platelets) with selected novel markers (e.g., SAA, IL-6) and clinical parameters, potentially enhanced by machine learning algorithms. Such algorithms could improve diagnostic accuracy and predict relapse risk but require rigorous validation in prospective multicenter cohorts before clinical implementation. It is important to take into account that none of these novel biomarkers have achieved clinical implementation yet, and further validation studies are required.

6. Imaging Advances and Diagnostic Modalities

6.1. *Ultrasound as First-Line Imaging*

Color Doppler ultrasound (CDUS) has emerged as the preferred initial imaging modality for suspected GCA with cranial involvement, as supported by 2018 EULAR recommendations [88]. The pathognomonic "halo sign", representing hypoechoic vessel wall thickening, demonstrates sensitivity of 43–77% and specificity of 89–100% when compared to ACR 1990 criteria [89]. However, while the 2018 EULAR recommendations support CDUS as first-line imaging for suspected cranial GCA, implementation varies globally due to limited availability of trained operators experienced in vascular ultrasound, particularly in resource-limited settings, rural areas, and healthcare systems without dedicated rheumatology-based ultrasound programs [90]. Ultrasound advantages include non-invasiveness, immediate availability when integrated into rheumatology practice, cost-effectiveness, and ability to examine multiple vessel territories [91,92]. The technique allows assessment of both cranial arteries (temporal, occipital, facial) and extracranial vessels (axillary, subclavian, carotid) [93]. Bilateral halo signs increase diagnostic specificity to 100%, though sensitivity decreases with glucocorticoid treatment duration [94].

Technical considerations for optimal ultrasound performance include the use of high-frequency transducers (>15 MHz), experienced sonographers, and standardized examination protocols [95]. The addition of extracranial vessel assessment increases sensitivity from 70% to 89% while maintaining specificity at around 91% [89,92].

6.2. *Advanced Cross-Sectional Imaging*

Magnetic resonance imaging (MRI) with vessel wall imaging has demonstrated excellent diagnostic performance, with sensitivity of 94% and specificity of 85% for GCA diagnosis. High-resolution MRI can detect mural inflammation in temporal arteries, with grading systems distinguishing physiologic from pathologic enhancement. The technique shows utility in extracranial vessel assessment and may obviate need for temporal artery biopsy when clearly normal [96,97].

Computed tomography angiography (CTA) provides complementary structural information regarding vessel stenosis, occlusion, and aneurysm formation [98–100]. While less sensitive than MRI for early inflammatory changes, CTA offers superior assessment of calcification and luminal abnormalities [100].

https://doi.org/10.3390/diagnostics16030470

6.3. Nuclear Medicine Imaging

18F-fluorodeoxyglucose (FDG) positron emission tomography (PET)/computerized tomography (CT) demonstrates sensitivity of 80% and specificity of 91% for large vessel vasculitis diagnosis [101]. The technique excels in detecting aortic and major branch vessel involvement, with particular utility in extracranial disease phenotypes [102]. FDG uptake typically affects subclavian arteries (75%), thoracic and abdominal aorta (50%), and axillary arteries (40%) [103].

PET/CT limitations include reduced sensitivity in cranial vessels due to spatial resolution constraints and decreased uptake following glucocorticoid treatment initiation [104]. The technique requires careful timing, with optimal diagnostic yield within three days of treatment and declining sensitivity after 10 days [105].

6.4. Multimodal Imaging Approaches

Integration of multiple imaging modalities provides comprehensive vascular assessment and may optimize diagnostic accuracy [106]. Proposed algorithms suggest initiating with ultrasound for cranial assessment, followed by FDG-PET/CT or MRI for extracranial evaluation in appropriate clinical contexts. This approach maximizes detection of both cranial and large vessel involvement while maintaining cost-effectiveness [107,108].

6.5. Fast-Track Diagnostic Pathways

Fast-track clinics dedicated to rapid evaluation of suspected GCA have demonstrated significant improvements in patient outcomes. These pathways typically incorporate same-day or next-day assessment combining clinical evaluation, inflammatory marker testing, and vascular ultrasound, with treatment initiation based on this integrated assessment.

Evidence from multiple centers demonstrates that fast-track pathways reduce time to diagnosis from weeks to days (median 0–2 days vs. 9–24 days in traditional pathways), decrease rates of irreversible vision loss (0–5% vs. 13–20%), and reduce unnecessary temporal artery biopsies and prolonged glucocorticoid courses in patients without GCA [109,110]. Cost-effectiveness analyses suggest that these pathways are economically favorable due to prevention of vision loss and reduced diagnostic testing.

Critical elements of successful fast-track clinics include dedicated access for urgent referrals, availability of experienced vascular ultrasonographers, integrated rheumatology–ophthalmology care pathways for patients with visual symptoms, and standardized protocols for treatment initiation and follow-up. Implementation challenges include resource allocation, staff training, and establishing referral networks, but outcomes support wider adoption of this model.

6.6. Integration of 2023 EULAR Imaging Recommendations

The 2023 EULAR recommendations for imaging in large vessel vasculitis provide updated guidance emphasizing multimodal imaging approaches. Key recommendations include the following: (1) CDUS as first-line imaging for suspected cranial GCA when expertise is available; (2) FDG-PET/CT, MRA, or CTA for assessment of extracranial large vessel involvement; (3) systematic evaluation of both cranial and extracranial vessels in all GCA patients when feasible; (4) recognition that negative imaging does not exclude GCA in patients with high clinical suspicion; and (5) consideration of repeat imaging in patients with disease relapse or atypical features. These recommendations emphasize that imaging should complement, rather than replace, clinical judgment and that the choice of modality should consider local expertise, availability, and individual patient factors [107].

https://doi.org/10.3390/diagnostics16030470

7. Temporal Artery Biopsy: Evolving Role

7.1. Current Diagnostic Performance

The temporal artery biopsy (TAB) remains important as a diagnostic tool despite imaging advances, with specificity approaching 100% and sensitivity of 61–77% [111]. The Society for Cardiovascular Pathology guidelines emphasize standardized processing and interpretation protocols to optimize diagnostic yield [112] (Figure 2).

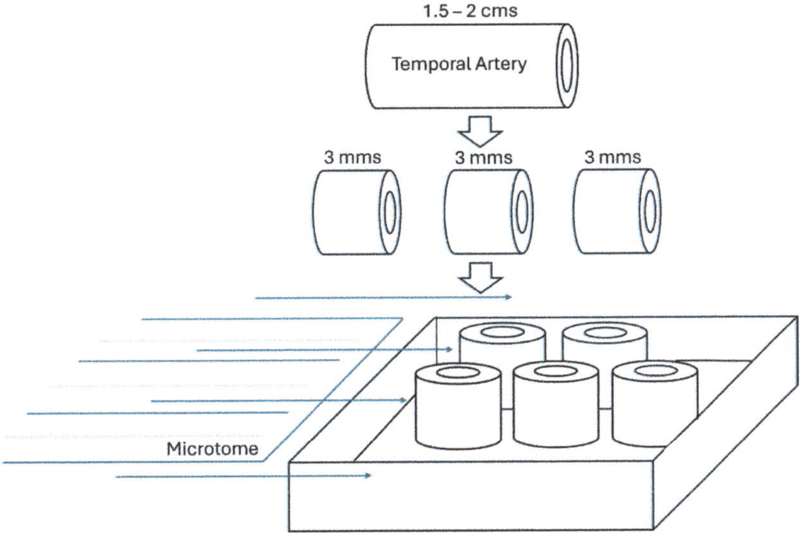

Figure 2. Schematic representation of pathological processing of temporal artery specimens. To minimize the high rate of false-negative results due to "skip lesions" (areas of inflammation interspersed with normal artery) or inadequate sampling, the guidelines standardize the handling of the specimen. (1) Optimal specimen length: the consensus recommends an adequate length (often cited as 1.5–2 cm to maximize the chance of capturing a skip lesion. (2) Complete submission: The entire segment of the biopsied artery should be submitted for processing. (3) Serial sectioning: Instead of only examining a few cuts, the specimen should be evaluated by serial sectioning at multiple levels. This means cutting the entire artery segment into numerous thin sections (e.g., in a specific interval) to examine the vessel at many different points along its length, drastically improving the chance of finding a focal lesion.

Factors affecting TAB sensitivity include specimen length (optimal >2 cm), number of examined sections, timing relative to glucocorticoid initiation, and disease segmental nature [113]. Bilateral biopsy may improve diagnostic yield in cases of high clinical suspicion with negative unilateral results [111].

7.2. Histopathological Considerations

Characteristic histopathological features include granulomatous inflammation with multinucleated giant cells, IEL destruction, and arterial wall thickening [112] (Figure 3). However, giant cells are present in only 50–60% of positive biopsies, and their absence does not exclude diagnosis [113]. Alternative inflammatory patterns, including lymphocytic infiltration without giant cells, may represent valid diagnostic findings [113,114].

The distinction between "healed arteritis" and age-related arteriosclerosis affecting the temporal artery remains challenging and lacks definitive criteria [115]. Recent guidelines recommend caution in diagnosing healed arteritis based solely on intimal thickening or medial fibrosis without clear inflammatory markers [112].

https://doi.org/10.3390/diagnostics16030470

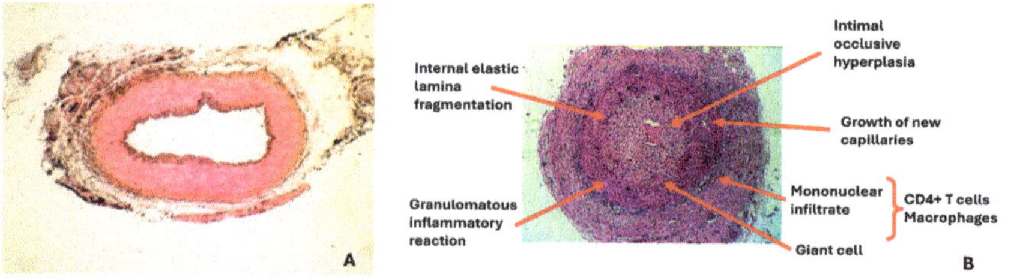

Figure 3. (**A**) **Image of a normal temporal artery biopsy without signs of inflammation/vasculitis.** Hematoxylin and eosin (H&E) stain, original magnification ×25. (**B**) **This image demonstrates findings consistent with vasculitis in a temporal artery biopsy, a common finding in GCA.** Key features shown include the following. (1) Panarteritis: A dense inflammatory infiltrate of mononuclear cells is visible throughout all layers of the vessel wall (tunica adventitia, media, and intima). (2) Intimal thickening and lumen occlusion: The inner layer (tunica intima) is markedly thickened and proliferative, leading to severe luminal stenosis and near-occlusion of the artery's central channel. (3) Thrombus formation: Fibrinoid material and inflammatory cells are seen within the center of the narrowed lumen. Hematoxylin and eosin (H&E) stain, original magnification ×25 (same magnification as panel A for direct comparison). Temporal artery biopsy specimens are from the personal collection of Dr. Rodriguez-Pla.

7.3. Integration with Clinical Assessment

TAB should be considered within comprehensive clinical context rather than as a standalone diagnostic test [116]. The procedure remains valuable when imaging results are inconclusive or contraindicated, and in research settings requiring histopathological confirmation [13,117]. Fast-track clinical pathways often initiate treatment based on clinical and imaging findings while awaiting biopsy results [109].

8. Classification Criteria Evolution

8.1. 1990 American College of Rheumatology (ACR) Criteria Limitations

The 1990 ACR classification criteria require three of five features: age > 50 years, new headache, temporal artery abnormality, ESR > 50 mm/h, and abnormal arterial biopsy [118]. These criteria demonstrate 93.5% sensitivity and 91.2% specificity when distinguishing GCA from other forms of vasculitis in patients already diagnosed with vasculitis (original ACR validation study [118]), but show significantly lower sensitivity (53–80%) when applied in broader clinical settings where the differential diagnosis included non-vasculitic conditions. These criteria show limitations in contemporary practice.

Recognized shortcomings include underrepresentation of patients with isolated ocular manifestations, lack of incorporation of imaging findings, absence of large vessel involvement criteria, and potential for missing cases with normal inflammatory markers [119]. The criteria were designed for classification purposes to include patients in clinical trials and not for diagnosis, limiting their clinical applicability [118].

8.2. 2022 ACR/EULAR Classification Criteria

The updated 2022 classification criteria address many limitations of previous versions while incorporating modern diagnostic modalities [64]. The new criteria require age $\geq$ 50 years as absolute requirement plus cumulative score $\geq$ 6 points from weighted clinical, laboratory, and imaging features [64].

Key innovations include incorporation of imaging findings (positive temporal artery biopsy or halo sign +5 points), recognition of large vessel involvement (bilateral axillary involvement +2 points, FDG-PET activity throughout aorta +2 points), and expanded clinical features, including morning stiffness and scalp tenderness [64]. Validation studies demonstrate an area under the curve of 0.91 with 87% sensitivity and 95% specificity [64].

Despite significant advances, the 2022 ACR/EULAR criteria have important limitations that affect clinical implementation. The criteria's incorporation of imaging findings, while improving sensitivity for large vessel disease, creates dependency on imaging availability and expertise that varies globally. In settings without access to vascular ultrasound or FDG-PET/CT, the criteria may perform less optimally than in resource-rich environments where they were primarily validated.

The weighted point-based system, while statistically more sophisticated than the simple 3-of-5 approach of the 1990 criteria, introduces practical challenges. Clinicians must calculate cumulative scores incorporating diverse elements with different point values, which may be cumbersome in busy clinical settings compared to dichotomous criteria. Furthermore, the requirement for age $\geq$ 50 years as an absolute inclusion criterion means that the criteria cannot classify younger patients with GCA-like presentations, though such cases, while rare, do occur.

An additional limitation is that classification criteria are designed to create homogeneous populations for clinical trials rather than to diagnose individual patients. The 2022 criteria were validated against final clinical diagnosis, but "gold standard" diagnostic criteria for GCA do not exist, potentially leading to circular reasoning. Patients with atypical presentations or early disease may not fulfill classification criteria, but, nonetheless, require treatment. This highlights the importance of not using them for diagnosis.

Finally, the criteria assign equal weight to halo sign and positive temporal artery biopsy (+5 points each), yet these tests have different performance characteristics depending on timing relative to glucocorticoid initiation, clinical phenotype, and technical quality. This simplified approach may not reflect the nuanced diagnostic reasoning required in complex cases.

8.3. Side-By Side Comparison of the 1990 ACR and the 2022 ACR/EULAR Classification Criteria for GCA

The 2022 ACR/EULAR classification criteria represent a major update to the 1990 criteria, primarily by integrating imaging studies and moving to a weighted point-based system. The new 2022 criteria aim to improve sensitivity and more accurately classify patients, particularly those with large vessel-GCA (LV-GCA) that do not involve the temporal arteries (Table 1).

The 1990 ACR criteria were validated against other forms of vasculitis, not against non-inflammatory conditions, which partially explains the performance differences in real-world clinical settings where the differential diagnosis is broader.

The new criteria were developed to address the limitations of the 1990 criteria, which had low sensitivity, especially for patients who primarily had large vessel involvement without typical cranial symptoms.

The key changes are listed below:

1. **Inclusion of imaging:** The most significant change is the incorporation of imaging—specifically ultrasound (halo sign) and FDG-PET/CT—allowing for the classification of patients based on objective non-invasive evidence.
2. **Increased weight for key findings:** Highly specific findings like a positive biopsy/halo sign (+5 points) and sudden visual loss (+3 points) are weighted more heavily, reflecting their high diagnostic value.
3. **Expanded clinical criteria:** Symptoms like PMR (morning stiffness) and scalp tenderness are formally included as weighted criteria, improving classification in the early or non-classic stages of the disease.

https://doi.org/10.3390/diagnostics16030470

Table 1. Comparison of 1990 ACR and 2022 ACR/EULAR criteria.

Criteria	1990 ACR Criteria	2022 ACR/EULAR Criteria
Number of items	5 items.	10 items.
Classification rule	$\geq$3 of 5 (equal weighting).	Score $\geq$ 6 points (weighted items).
Age requirement	One of 5 items.	Mandatory requirement.
New additions	N/A.	Morning stiffness, sudden vision loss, jaw claudication, CRP, temporal artery ultrasound, bilateral axillary involvement, FDG-PET.
Sensitivity	93.5% (vs. other vasculitides, original validation study); 53–80% (vs. non-vasculitic conditions, subsequent validation studies) *.	87%.
Specificity	80–91%.	95%.
Strengths	Simple, straightforward.	Better discrimination, incorporates imaging, improved large vessel detection.
Limitations	Poor for LV- GCA, no imaging criteria, outdated.	More complex, requires more investigations.
Imaging modalities	None (biopsy only).	Temporal artery ultrasound, FDG-PET.
Best application	Cranial GCA with systemic symptoms.	All GCA phenotypes (cranial, large vessel, constitutional).

* The original Hunder et al. 1990 [118] ACR validation study tested giant cell arteritis against other vasculitides only. The 53–80% specificity against non-vasculitic conditions is derived from subsequent validation studies [119, 120].

9. Differential Diagnostic Challenges

9.1. Mimicking Conditions

Different conditions share clinical features with GCA, and we call them mimickers. Most mimickers are infections, malignancies, atherosclerosis, and other vasculitides. Some of them can be easily distinguished through specific diagnostic tests, e.g., infectious etiologies identifiable through cultures or serology, or some malignancies that can be diagnosed by pathology, imaging, and/or laboratory testing. On occasions, the distinction is more challenging and requires a more comprehensive evaluation. A differential diagnosis should thoroughly rule out all the possible mimickers before diagnosing and treating GCA, especially in those patients without pathological confirmation.

The TAB, despite its limitations discussed in Section 7, maintains importance as a diagnostic tool, particularly when imaging results are inconclusive [120]. From my point of view, the importance of having a positive temporal artery biopsy lies in the confirmation of GCA avoiding the need for further evaluation. If the patient does not repond or relapses during treatment, we should pursue other treatment modalities for GCA or investigate the treatment compliance. In contrast, if the patient has had no biopsy done or if it has been negative, in case of lack of response to treatment, it may be necessary to perform additional testing to rule out other possible alternative diagnosis.

Infectious causes, including bacterial endocarditis, septicemia with mycotic aneurysms, syphilis, mycobacterial infections, and even viral infections, require exclusion through appropriate microbiological testing [121–123].

Malignancies may manifest with constitutional symptoms, elevated inflammatory markers, and vascular involvement, as in patients with GCA. Therefore, cases of suspected GCA necessitate comprehensive evaluation, including age-appropriate cancer screening [121,122].

https://doi.org/10.3390/diagnostics16030470

Primary central nervous system vasculitis can mimic GCA with headache and neurological symptoms but typically affects younger patients and involves smaller intracranial vessels [124,125]. Other systemic vasculitides, including antineutrophil cytoplasmic antibody (ANCA)-associated vasculitis [126], Takayasu arteritis [127], and secondary vasculitis associated with connective tissue diseases [128] or infections [123], require differentiation through specific serological testing, imaging patterns, demographic characteristics, additional clinical manifestations, and biopsy findings [129]. In addition, complicating the picture even more, GCA may coexist with other types of systemic vasculitis [130]. Atherosclerotic disease with secondary inflammation may simulate large vessel involvement but typically demonstrates different distribution patterns and risk factor profiles [59,129].

Misdiagnosing GCA may have severe consequences [131]. It is important to remember that diagnostic criteria do not exist, and the classification criteria have been developed to decide inclusion of the patients in clinical trials; they often fail to differentiate mimics from true GCA [64,118,119]. Clinician vigilance and expertise, biopsy for pathology confirmation whenever possible, and fast improving imaging tools are critical for ruling out or confirming GCA and should be used widely used in the setting of careful clinical judgement and consideration of all possible alternative diagnosis. Diagnostic delays may result in severe outcomes, and patients who are misdiagnosed with GCA are at serious risk of suffering severe adverse effects from high doses of prolonged glucocorticoids therapy. Reducing diagnostic delay is essential for improving patient survival in severe mimic cases [131].

A systematic approach to excluding mimickers includes the following. (1) Comprehensive infectious workup in patients with fever or atypical features (blood cultures, HIV, syphilis, tuberculosis screening, viral serologies based on exposure history, coccidiosis, histoplasmosis, or Lyme disease depending on geographical location). (2) ANCA serology and urinalysis in all suspected GCA cases. (3) Age-appropriate cancer screening and consideration of PET/CT (which can identify both GCA and malignancy). (4) Assessment for features atypical for GCA that should prompt consideration of alternative diagnoses (age < 50 years, lack of cranial symptoms with isolated systemic features, neurological deficits, renal involvement, pulmonary infiltrates). (5) Temporal artery biopsy in diagnostically uncertain cases, or biopsy of other affected organs, as specific histopathological patterns (infectious organisms, malignant cells) can identify mimickers (Table 2).

Table 2. Distinguishing features of major GCA mimickers.

Mimicker	Shared Features with GCA	Distinguishing Features
Infectious endocarditis	Fever, elevated inflammatory markers, headache, anemia.	Blood cultures positive, heart murmur, cardiac imaging abnormalities, absence of temporal artery or large vessel inflammation on imaging.
ANCA-associated vasculitis	Constitutional symptoms, elevated inflammatory markers, vascular involvement.	Positive ANCA serology (anti-PR3 or anti-MPO), smaller vessel involvement (glomerulonephritis, pulmonary hemorrhage), different demographic (younger patients), nasal/sinus involvement common.
Primary CNS vasculitis	Headache, neurological symptoms, elevated inflammatory markers.	Neurological deficits, abnormal brain MRI with multiple lesions, CSF pleocytosis, angiographic abnormalities of intracranial vessels, negative temporal artery biopsy and extracranial imaging.
Metastatic cancer	Constitutional symptoms, elevated inflammatory markers, anemia, weight loss.	Identification of primary tumor or metastases on imaging, abnormal tumor markers, absence of arterial inflammation, lymphadenopathy.
Atherosclerosis	Large vessel involvement on imaging, vascular stenosis, old age.	Calcified plaques, eccentric rather than concentric vessel wall thickening, traditional cardiovascular risk factors, lower inflammatory marker elevations.

Abbreviations: ANCA, antineutrophil cytoplasmic antibody; CNS, central nervous system; CSF, cerebrospinal fluid; GCA, giant cell arteritis; MRI, magnetic resonance imaging; MPO, myeloperoxidase; PR3, proteinase 3.

https://doi.org/10.3390/diagnostics16030470

9.2. Age-Related Diagnostic Considerations

The elderly population affected by GCA frequently presents diagnostic challenges due to multiple comorbidities and frequent atypical presentations [132]. Age-related changes, including presbyopia, cataracts, and chronic pain conditions, may mask or mimic GCA symptoms [133,134]. Polypharmacy and medication interactions may complicate laboratory interpretation and treatment decisions [135].

Cognitive impairment in elderly patients may limit symptom reporting accuracy and adherence to diagnostic procedures [136]. Healthcare providers must maintain a high index of suspicion while carefully evaluating competing diagnoses in this vulnerable population [137].

10. Treatment Implications and Monitoring

10.1. Glucocorticoid Therapy

High-dose glucocorticoids remain the cornerstone of GCA treatment. Optimal initial glucocorticoid dosing remains debated. Traditional regimens used prednisolone 40–60 mg daily for uncomplicated cranial disease, but recent evidence suggests that lower initial doses (30–40 mg daily) may provide equivalent efficacy with reduced toxicity in selected patients [138]. Patients with visual involvement require higher doses, with most guidelines recommending intravenous methylprednisolone 500–1000 mg daily for 3 days followed by high-dose oral therapy [139]. Treatment should be initiated immediately upon clinical suspicion without waiting for confirmatory testing, as delays beyond 48 h may result in irreversible complications, especially permanent visual loss [140].

Tapering strategies significantly impact outcomes. Rapid tapering (reaching 10 mg daily by 3 months) increases relapse risk compared to more gradual approaches. The GCA Actemra (GiACTA) trial's 26-week taper (from 40 mg to zero) demonstrated feasibility in tocilizumab-treated patients but resulted in high relapse rates (86%) in placebo-treated patients [141]. The optimal tapering schedule remains debated, with EULAR recommendations suggesting reduction to 15–20 mg daily within 2–3 months and <5 mg daily by one year [142,143]. Current evidence supports individualized tapering based on symptoms, inflammatory markers, and imaging findings, with slower tapers (maintaining 10–15 mg daily for 6–12 months) in high-risk patients, including those with large vessel involvement, cranial ischemic complications, or relapsing disease [144,145]. However, relapse rates of 40–75% during tapering necessitate careful monitoring and individualized approaches [146]. Prolonged glucocorticoid exposure results in significant toxicity in >80% of patients, including posterior subcapsular cataracts (41%), bone fractures (38%), infections (31%), and hypertension (22%), among others [147].

10.2. Steroid-Sparing Agents

Tocilizumab represents the first Food and Drug Administration (FDA)-approved steroid-sparing agent for GCA, demonstrating significant efficacy in the GiACTA trial with sustained remission rates of 56% (weekly dosing) and 53% (every other week) compared to 14–18% with placebo at 52 weeks [141]. The drug provides substantial glucocorticoid-sparing effects and improved health-related quality of life [141].

Long-term tocilizumab studies reveal relapse rates of approximately 50% following discontinuation, suggesting a potential need for extended treatment in selected patients [148]. Cost considerations, side effects such as liver damage, worsening hyperlipidemia or increased infection risks, and the lack of universal patient response limit widespread accessibility, highlighting need for additional therapeutic options [149].

Upadacitinib was FDA-approved for the treatment of GCA in November 2024 based on the results of the SELECT-GCA clinical trial. The trial demonstrated that 15 mg daily of upadacitinib in combination with a glucocorticoid taper achieved a sustained remission rate of 46% compared to 29% in the placebo group, with a safety profile consistent with other approved indications [150].

Meta-analysis of individual patient data suggests that methotrexate 15–25 mg weekly provides modest reduction in relapse risk (RR 0.65–0.85) and cumulative glucocorticoid exposure (mean reduction 842 mg over first year), though these benefits are substantially smaller than those seen with tocilizumab or upadacitinib [151–154].

Practical considerations for methotrexate use include dosing typically 15–20 mg weekly (oral or subcutaneous), mandatory folic acid supplementation, baseline assessment and monitoring of liver and renal function and blood counts, and awareness that beneficial effects may not become apparent until 12–16 weeks of therapy. The modest benefit–risk profile suggests that methotrexate may be most appropriate for patients unable to access or tolerate biologics, or as adjunctive therapy in refractory cases.

Leflunomide shows promise in recent studies, with relapse reduction in over 75% of patients and favorable safety profile [155].

Critical Appraisal of Biologic Evidence

Tocilizumab's efficacy is supported by the high-quality GiACTA trial (n = 251, randomized, double-blind) which demonstrated sustained remission in 56% (weekly dosing) vs. 14% (placebo) at 52 weeks. However, critical analysis reveals important limitations: (1) after tocilizumab discontinuation at 52 weeks, approximately 50% of patients relapsed within the subsequent year, raising questions about optimal treatment duration; (2) the trial excluded patients with recent visual loss, limiting generalizability to high-risk patients; (3) cost (approximately $30,000–40,000 USD annually) limits accessibility; and (4) while glucocorticoid-sparing effects are substantial, patients still received significant cumulative glucocorticoid exposure (1862 mg in weekly tocilizumab arm vs. 3296 mg in placebo arm) [141,156].

Upadacitinib approval is based on the SELECT-GCA trial (n = 428), which showed sustained remission in 46% vs. 29% (placebo) with similar safety to other indications [150]. Critical considerations include the following: (1) shorter follow-up (52 weeks) than available for tocilizumab (multiyear data available); (2) the 17-percentage-point difference, while statistically significant, represents modest absolute benefit; (3) the trial used a shorter glucocorticoid taper (26 weeks) compared to typical clinical practice; (4) as an oral medication, upadacitinib may offer convenience advantages over subcutaneous tocilizumab, but requires consideration of JAK-inhibitor class warnings (infections, malignancy, cardiovascular events) established in other diseases. While upadacitinib demonstrated a statistically significant benefit (46% vs. 29%, absolute difference 17 percentage points), this is notably more modest than tocilizumab's performance in GiACTA (56% vs. 14%, absolute difference 42 percentage points), suggesting that tocilizumab remains the preferred biologic agent when glucocorticoid-sparing therapy is indicated.

Head-to-head trials comparing tocilizumab and upadacitinib are lacking, and biomarkers to guide selection between these agents are not available. Treatment selection currently relies on factors including patient preference for administration route, comorbidities, cost/insurance coverage, and physician experience.

10.3. Emerging Therapeutic Targets

Multiple novel therapeutic approaches are under investigation, reflecting improved understanding of GCA pathophysiology [114,157] (Figure 4).

IL-17 inhibition with secukinumab demonstrated encouraging results in Phase II trials, with sustained remission rates of 59.3% compared to 8.0% with placebo [158]. However,

https://doi.org/10.3390/diagnostics16030470

The Phase III GCAptAIN study (NCT04930094), which evaluated secukinumab in adults with newly diagnosed or relapsing GCA did not meet its primary endpoint of sustained remission at week 52 according to results announced by Novartis in 2024 (full peer-reviewed results pending publication). The failure of the Phase III trial to confirm Phase II results suggests that the Phase II findings may represent a false positive, and IL-17 inhibition does not appear to be an effective therapeutic target for GCA based on current evidence. Publication of the complete Phase III dataset will be important for understanding why the promising Phase II results were not reproduced.

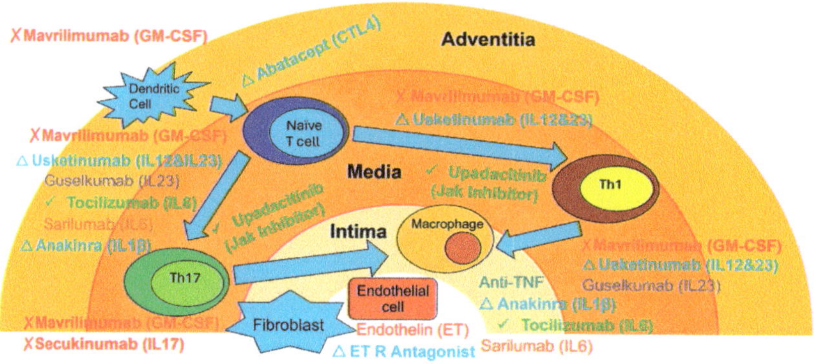

Figure 4. Therapeutic targets in GCA according to pathogenesis. This schematic illustrates the inflammatory cascade across the three layers of the arterial wall, the adventitia, media, and intima, and identifies the specific points of intervention for current and emerging biologic therapies. **In the adventitia,** the process is initiated by DCs which activate naïve T cells. This costimulation is targeted by abatacept (cytotoxic T-lymphocyte associated protein 4 [CTLA4]-Ig). **In the media,** activated T cells differentiate into Th1 and Th17 subsets. GM-CSF (targeted by mavrilimumab) and IL-12/23 (targeted by ustekinumab) drive this differentiation. JAK inhibitors act intracellularly to block these signaling pathways. **In the intima,** effector cells like macrophages and fibroblasts accumulate, leading to IL-6 production (targeted by tocilizumab/sarilumab) and TNF release. Endothelial cells release endothelin (ET), which promotes vascular remodeling and narrowing, countered by ET receptor antagonists. Agents are color-coded by regulatory/development status: green checkmark (✓)—FDA-approved agents (tocilizumab, upadacitinib); red X (✗)—Phase III failed (secukinumab) or development-terminated agents (mavrilimumab); blue triangle (△)—investigational agents (abatacept, ustekinumab, anakinra, endothelin receptor antagonists). **Abbreviations:** CTL4, Cytotoxic T-Lymphocyte Associated Protein 4; ET/ET R, endothelin/endothelin receptor, GM-CSF, Granulocyte-Macrophage Colony-Stimulating Factor; IL, interleukin; JAK, Janus Kinase; Th1, T Helper Type 1 cell; Th17, T Helper Type 17 cell; TNF, tumor necrosis factor.

GM-CSF receptor blockade with mavrilimumab targets multiple pathogenic pathways and showed significant flare reduction in Phase II studies [9]. In early 2024, Kiniksa terminated its licensing agreement for mavrilimumab and discontinued its development for GCA to pivot to a cardiovascular-focused pipeline, effectively halting the planned Phase III trial. This termination prevented definitive evaluation of the GM-CSF pathway in GCA and raises questions about the clinical translational potential of this mechanism in GCA management.

As some of these are recently completed trials, we note where information is derived from company announcements pending full peer-reviewed publication.

Additional investigational agents include IL-1 receptor antagonists (anakinra), IL-23 inhibitors (guselkumab), and T cell costimulation blockers (abatacept) [114]. These diverse mechanisms reflect the complex pathophysiology of GCA and potential for personalized therapeutic approaches based on individual disease phenotypes [159].

10.4. Long-Term Disease Management

Treatment duration varies considerably among patients, with meta-analysis revealing that 89.7% remain on glucocorticoids at one year, 75.2% at two years, and 44.3% at five years. Mean glucocorticoid doses at these timepoints are 9.1 mg/day and 7.8 mg/day, respectively [160].

10.5. Predictors of Disease Relapse

Disease relapse occurs in 30–50% of patients during treatment tapering, with higher rates in younger patients, females, and those with large vessel involvement [161].

Identifying patients at high relapse risk could enable personalized monitoring and treatment strategies. Established predictors of increased relapse risk include the following:

1. Clinical factors:
    - Large vessel involvement at diagnosis.
    - Younger age at diagnosis (<60–65 years).
    - Female sex (modest association.
    - PMR symptoms at diagnosis.
    - History of prior relapse.
    - Prolonged disease duration and treatment.
2. Laboratory/imaging markers:
    - Persistently elevated or slow-to-normalize inflammatory markers during initial treatment.
    - Persistent vascular inflammation on FDG-PET or ultrasound despite clinical remission.
    - Thrombocytosis at diagnosis or during follow-up.
3. Treatment-related factors:
    - Rapid glucocorticoid tapering (reduction >10 mg/month).
    - Glucocorticoid dose <10–15 mg daily at time of relapse consideration.
    - Non-adherence to treatment.

Machine learning algorithms incorporating multiple clinical and laboratory parameters have demonstrated 71–76% accuracy in predicting relapse, superior to individual risk factors, though these require prospective validation before clinical implementation. The development and validation of composite risk scores could enable stratified approaches with intensive monitoring and preemptive treatment adjustments for high-risk patients [161].

11. Prognosis and Long-Term Outcomes

11.1. Visual Outcomes

Visual recovery following GCA-related vision loss remains disappointingly limited, with only 15% of patients showing improvement in visual acuity within the first month, and 5% demonstrating corresponding visual field improvement [162]. Visual deterioration occurs in approximately 27% of eyes within the first week despite high-dose intravenous glucocorticoids, with greatest risk in the first six days [163].

The irreversible nature of most visual complications emphasizes the critical importance of prevention through early recognition and treatment [164]. Recent studies suggest that 13.7% of GCA patients experience vision loss, which rarely recovers and is statistically more likely with advancing age [36].

https://doi.org/10.3390/diagnostics16030470

11.2. Cardiovascular and Aortic Complications

GCA patients demonstrate significantly increased risk of aortic aneurysm development, with five-year risk of 3.6% compared to 1.8% in controls. Thoracic aortic aneurysms occur in 2.2% versus 1.0% of controls, while abdominal aortic aneurysms affect 1.8% versus 0.8% [4]. These complications may develop years after initial diagnosis and require long-term surveillance [165].

Aortic dissection represents a rare but life-threatening complication, occurring in approximately 1% of patients [166]. Symptomatic aortitis at diagnosis, characterized by chest or abdominal pain, identifies patients at particularly high risk for subsequent aortic complications with hazard ratio of 6.64 [167,168]. However, overall survival may not differ significantly from age-matched populations, particularly beyond the first five years following diagnosis [169].

11.3. Prevention and Mitigation of GCA-Related and Treatment-Related Complications

Given that >80% of GCA patients experience glucocorticoid-related toxicity, proactive prevention strategies are essential.

All patients initiating glucocorticoid therapy should undergo baseline bone density assessment and receive calcium (1200–1500 mg daily) and vitamin D (800–1000 IU daily) supplementation, with bisphosphonate therapy for those with osteoporosis or high fracture risk [170–172].

Baseline screening and regular monitoring for diabetes and hypertension are critical, with early intervention when indicated.

Vaccinations should be updated before initiating immunosuppression (pneumococcal, influenza, zoster), and *Pneumocystis jirovecii* pneumonia (PJP) prophylaxis considered in patients receiving >20 mg prednisone daily for >1 month [173,174].

Annual ophthalmologic examination for cataracts and glaucoma is recommended. Given the 5-year aortic aneurysm risk of 3.6% (nearly double that of controls), systematic vascular surveillance is warranted. Baseline chest imaging to assess the thoracic aorta and consideration of periodic imaging (every 2–3 years) with CTA, MRA, or ultrasound for aortic assessment is recommended [175–177]. More frequent monitoring (annually) should be considered in patients with symptomatic aortitis at diagnosis, extensive large vessel involvement, or persistent vascular inflammation on imaging [175–177].

Emergency treatment protocols should be established for any new visual symptoms, with patient education regarding warning signs (amaurosis fugax, diplopia, visual field defects) [178,179].

Aspirin therapy (81–100 mg daily) may reduce cranial ischemic event risk, though evidence is not definitive [178,179].

Regular assessment of quality of life, physical therapy to maintain function, early introduction of steroid-sparing agents in high-risk patients, and screening for depression (affecting 20–30% of GCA patients) optimize long-term outcomes [180,181].

These preventive strategies require systematic implementation through structured care pathways [182].

12. Future Directions and Emerging Technologies

12.1. Artificial Intelligence (AI) and Machine Learning

AI applications in GCA diagnosis and management represent rapidly evolving areas with significant potential [161,183,184]. Machine learning algorithms demonstrate effectiveness in predicting GCA diagnosis and relapse risk, with random forest models achieving 71–76% accuracy using clinical and laboratory data [185–187].

https://doi.org/10.3390/diagnostics16030470

Deep learning approaches for ultrasound image analysis show promise for automated halo sign detection and diagnostic support [183,184]. Convolutional neural networks applied to temporal artery biopsy specimens may enhance histopathological interpretation and reduce inter-observer variability [188].

Point-of-care ultrasound (POCUS) combined with AI-driven diagnostics could revolutionize GCA diagnosis, particularly in emergency and primary care settings [189]. Such systems could provide rapid, on-the-spot diagnosis and potentially prevent up to 500,000 cases of visual impairment projected by 2050 [190].

12.2. Advanced Imaging Technologies

Novel imaging techniques continue to expand diagnostic capabilities and disease understanding [191]. Contrast-enhanced ultrasound, shear wave elastography, and ultrasound biomicroscopy offer enhanced tissue characterization and may improve diagnostic accuracy [192].

PET-MRI integration combines the inflammatory detection capabilities of PET with superior anatomical resolution of MRI. Novel PET tracers beyond FDG may provide more specific inflammatory targeting and reduced background uptake [193].

Black blood MRI techniques and orbital MRI show particular promise for detecting cranial vessel involvement and ophthalmic complications. These advances may enable earlier detection of subclinical disease and better monitoring of treatment response [194].

12.3. Personalized Medicine Approaches

The recognition of distinct GCA phenotypes suggests potential for personalized diagnostic and therapeutic strategies. Evidence increasingly supports phenotype-based treatment stratification: (1) cranial-predominant GCA may be optimally managed with shorter treatment courses (18–24 months); (2) large vessel-predominant GCA likely requires longer treatment duration (>2–3 years) with routine imaging surveillance given higher relapse rates; and (3) PMR-overlap phenotype requires clarification regarding optimal management intensity [175,195].

Emerging evidence suggests that biomarker-guided therapeutic selection may improve outcomes. High IL-6 levels at diagnosis predict better tocilizumab response in some studies [196]. However, despite IL-6 having been detected in temporal arteritis, and the efficacy of IL-6-inbition treatments, the diagnostic value of serum IL-6 for GCA is limited. Although IL-6 measurement is increasingly available in many laboratories, it is likely to have similar limitations to the analysis of ESR and CRP despite much higher costs, which limits its use in clinical practice [197]. Imaging-detected persistent vascular inflammation during clinical remission identifies high relapse risk patients who may benefit from treatment intensification [198]. Pharmacogenomic applications show promise: polymorphisms in glucocorticoid receptor genes (NR3C1, HSD11B1, ABCB1) influence efficacy and toxicity [199], while variants in IL-6 pathway genes may predict tocilizumab response and [200,201].

Integration of clinical, laboratory, and imaging data into composite risk scores could enable precision medicine, including diagnostic risk scores, relapse risk scores, and complication risk scores [202]. Machine learning algorithms have demonstrated 71–76% accuracy in predicting relapse [187], though prospective validation is required before clinical implementation.

Translating personalized medicine to clinical reality requires validation of phenotype classifications in large multicenter cohorts, prospective biomarker validation studies with predefined treatment algorithms, clinical trials testing phenotype-specific protocols versus standard care, development of point-of-care assays, integration of prediction algorithms into electronic health records, and cost-effectiveness analyses [203,204].

https://doi.org/10.3390/diagnostics16030470

13. Conclusions

Giant cell arteritis exemplifies the challenges of diagnosing and managing heterogeneous systemic vasculitis in an aging population. Three key developments have transformed the GCA landscape, and they define the path forward.

First, the diagnostic paradigm has shifted from biopsy-centric, criteria-based classification toward multimodal, probabilistic assessment. The integration of vascular imaging with clinical evaluation enables earlier diagnosis, particularly of large-vessel-predominant disease. The 2022 ACR/EULAR classification criteria formalize this approach, though accessibility challenges and the classification-versus-diagnosis distinction remain important limitations.

Second, therapeutic advances, particularly tocilizumab and upadacitinib approval, provide evidence-based alternatives to prolonged glucocorticoid monotherapy, yet important questions remain. The modest absolute benefits (46–56% sustained remission versus 14–29% with placebo) highlight the need for more effective therapies and biomarkers to guide therapeutic selection, optimal treatment duration, and strategies for preventing late complications.

Third, the evolution toward personalized medicine, supported by phenotypic classification, imaging-based risk stratification, and emerging predictive algorithms, offers potential to match treatment intensity to individual patient risk, though this requires prospective validation.

Key priorities for advancing GCA care include development of composite biomarker panels, comparative effectiveness trials of biologics and combination strategies, standardized implementation of fast-track diagnostic pathways, systematic aortic surveillance protocols, integration of AI-assisted diagnostic tools, and investigation of treatment de-escalation strategies.

Important limitations remain in the GCA literature, including heterogeneity in diagnostic criteria across studies, limited head-to-head imaging comparisons, predominantly Caucasian study populations limiting generalizability, and paucity of data on optimal treatment duration and safe discontinuation predictors.

GCA management has evolved from diagnostic uncertainty and treatment limited to glucocorticoids to an era of sophisticated imaging, mechanistically targeted therapeutics, and emerging precision medicine approaches. The ultimate goal, i.e., preventing irreversible complications while minimizing treatment toxicity through early, accurate diagnosis and personalized management, is increasingly achievable but requires sustained research investment and systematic quality improvement efforts.

Funding: This research received no external funding.

Institutional Review Board Statement: Not applicable.

Informed Consent Statement: Not applicable.

Data Availability Statement: No new data were created or analyzed in this study. Data sharing is not applicable to this article.

Conflicts of Interest: Alicia Rodriguez-Pla (ARP) is the owner and founder of Premier Rheumatology, P. C. ARP also reports serving as a member of an independent Data Monitoring Committee for Bristol Myers Squibb and has served as a member of a scientific advisory board for AstraZeneca. These roles occurred within the 36 months prior to this submission. The companies and entities had no role in the design of the study; in the collection, analyses, or interpretation of data; in the writing of the manuscript; or in the decision to publish the results. ARP also formerly served as a Principal Investigator for clinical trialsinvolving systemic lupus erythematosus and IgG4-related

https://doi.org/10.3390/diagnostics16030470

diseasesponsored by Zenas BioPharma. Her involvement in those trials concludedin 2025. These past roles are outside the scope of the current review onvasculitis.

Abbreviations

The following abbreviations are used in this manuscript:

AAION	Arteritic anterior ischemic optic neuropathy
ACR	American College of Rheumatology
AI	Artificial intelligence
BAFF	B-cell activating factor
CD	Cluster of differentiation
CDUS	Color Doppler ultrasound
CTL4	Cytotoxic T-lymphocyte associated protein 4
CRP	C-reactive protein
CT	Computed tomography
CTA	Computed tomography angiography
DC	Dendritic Cell
ESR	Erythrocyte sedimentation rate
ET/ET R	Endothelin/Endothelin receptor
EULAR	European League Against Rheumatism
FDG	Fluorodeoxyglucose
FDG-PET	Fluorodeoxyglucose positron emission tomography
FR	Folate receptor
GiACTA	Giant cell arteritis Actemra trial
GM-CSF	Granulocyte macrophage colony-stimulating factor
HLA	Human leukocyte antigen
IL	Interleukin
i NOS	inducible nitric oxide synth2ase
JAK	Janus Kinase
IEL	Internal elastic lamina
IFN-γ	Interferon-γ
iNOS	inducible nitric oxide synthase
LV-GCA	Large vessel giant cell arteritis
MMP	Matrix metalloproteinase
MPO	Myeloperoxidase
MRA	Magnetic resonance angiography
MRI	Magnetic resonance imaging
PDGF	Platelet-derived growth factor
PET	Positron emission tomography
PMR	Polymyalgia rheumatica
POCUS	Point-of-care ultrasound
PR-3	Proteinase-3
SAA	Serum amyloid A
TAB	Temporal artery biopsy
TGF-β1	Transforming growth factor-β1
Th1	T Helper Type 1 cell
Th17	T Helper Type 17 cell
TNF	Tumor necrosis factor
VEGF	Vascular endothelial growth factor

References

1. Weyand, C.M.; Goronzy, J.J. Giant-cell arteritis and polymyalgia rheumatica. *N. Engl. J. Med.* **2014**, *371*, 1653. [CrossRef]
2. Do, T.; Gulati, G.; Lee, H.S.; Cord, B.; Ghiassi, M.; Hacein-Bey, L.; Liu, Y.A. Ocular Manifestations of Giant Cell Arteritis. *Adv. Ophthalmol. Optom.* **2025**, *10*, 297–311. [CrossRef]

https://doi.org/10.3390/diagnostics16030470

3. Lyne, S.A.; Ruediger, C.; Lester, S.; Kaur, G.; Stamp, L.; Shanahan, E.M.; Hill, C.L. Clinical phenotype and complications of large vessel giant cell arteritis: A systematic review and meta-analysis. *Jt. Bone Spine* **2023**, *90*, 105558. [CrossRef]
4. Chacko, J.A.; Chauhan, M.Z.; Phillips, P.H.; Ramakrishnaiah, R.H.; Chacko, J.G. Aortic and Carotid Complications in Patients with Giant Cell Arteritis. *Am. J. Ophthalmol.* **2025**, *278*, 65–72. [CrossRef] [PubMed]
5. Fein, A.S.; Ko, M.W. Neuro-Ophthalmologic Complications of Giant Cell Arteritis: Diagnosis and Treatment. *Semin. Neurol.* **2019**, *39*, 673–681. [CrossRef] [PubMed]
6. Akiyama, M.; Ohtsuki, S.; Berry, G.J.; Liang, D.H.; Goronzy, J.J.; Weyand, C.M. Innate and Adaptive Immunity in Giant Cell Arteritis. *Front. Immunol.* **2020**, *11*, 621098. [CrossRef] [PubMed]
7. van Sleen, Y.; Jiemy, W.F.; Pringle, S.; van der Geest, K.S.M.; Abdulahad, W.H.; Sandovici, M.; Brouwer, E.; Heeringa, P.; Boots, A.M.H. A Distinct Macrophage Subset Mediating Tissue Destruction and Neovascularization in Giant Cell Arteritis: Implication of the YKL-40/Interleukin-13 Receptor alpha2 Axis. *Arthritis Rheumatol.* **2021**, *73*, 2327–2337. [CrossRef]
8. Weyand, C.M.; Goronzy, J.J. Immunology of Giant Cell Arteritis. *Circ. Res.* **2023**, *132*, 238–250. [CrossRef]
9. Cid, M.C.; Unizony, S.H.; Blockmans, D.; Brouwer, E.; Dagna, L.; Dasgupta, B.; Hellmich, B.; Molloy, E.; Salvarani, C.; Trapnell, B.C.; et al. Efficacy and safety of mavrilimumab in giant cell arteritis: A phase 2, randomised, double-blind, placebo-controlled trial. *Ann. Rheum. Dis.* **2022**, *81*, 653–661. [CrossRef]
10. Rizzo, C.; La Barbera, L.; Miceli, G.; Tuttolomondo, A.; Guggino, G. The innate face of Giant Cell Arteritis: Insight into cellular and molecular innate immunity pathways to unravel new possible biomarkers of disease. *Front. Mol. Med.* **2022**, *2*, 933161. [CrossRef]
11. Rodriguez-Pla, A.; Martinez-Murillo, F.; Savino, P.J.; Eagle, R.C., Jr.; Seo, P.; Soloski, M.J. MMP-12, a novel matrix metalloproteinase associated with giant cell arteritis. *Rheumatology* **2009**, *48*, 1460–1461. [CrossRef]
12. Rodriguez-Pla, A.; Bosch-Gil, J.A.; Rossello-Urgell, J.; Huguet-Redecilla, P.; Stone, J.H.; Vilardell-Tarres, M. Metalloproteinase-2 and -9 in giant cell arteritis: Involvement in vascular remodeling. *Circulation* **2005**, *112*, 264–269. [CrossRef]
13. Rodriguez-Pla, A.; Rossello-Urgell, J.; Bosch-Gil, J.A.; Huguet-Redecilla, P.; Vilardell-Tarres, M. Proposal to decrease the number of negative temporal artery biopsies. *Scand. J. Rheumatol.* **2007**, *36*, 111–118. [CrossRef]
14. Marquez, A.; Solans, R.; Hernandez-Rodriguez, J.; Cid, M.C.; Castaneda, S.; Ramentol, M.; Rodriguez-Rodriguez, L.; Narvaez, J.; Blanco, R.; Ortego-Centeno, N.; et al. A candidate gene approach identifies an IL33 genetic variant as a novel genetic risk factor for GCA. *PLoS ONE* **2014**, *9*, e113476. [CrossRef]
15. Rodriguez-Pla, A.; Beaty, T.H.; Savino, P.J.; Eagle, R.C., Jr.; Seo, P.; Soloski, M.J. Association of a nonsynonymous single-nucleotide polymorphism of matrix metalloproteinase 9 with giant cell arteritis. *Arthritis Rheum.* **2008**, *58*, 1849–1853. [CrossRef] [PubMed]
16. Gonzalez-Gay, M.A.; Vazquez-Rodriguez, T.R.; Lopez-Diaz, M.J.; Miranda-Filloy, J.A.; Gonzalez-Juanatey, C.; Martin, J.; Llorca, J. Epidemiology of giant cell arteritis and polymyalgia rheumatica. *Arthritis Rheum.* **2009**, *61*, 1454–1461. [CrossRef] [PubMed]
17. De Smit, E.; Clarke, L.; Sanfilippo, P.G.; Merriman, T.R.; Brown, M.A.; Hill, C.L.; Hewitt, A.W. Geo-epidemiology of temporal artery biopsy-positive giant cell arteritis in Australia and New Zealand: Is there a seasonal influence? *RMD Open* **2017**, *3*, e000531. [CrossRef]
18. Li, K.J.; Semenov, D.; Turk, M.; Pope, J. A meta-analysis of the epidemiology of giant cell arteritis across time and space. *Arthritis Res. Ther.* **2021**, *23*, 82. [CrossRef]
19. Kim, H.I.; Lim, H.; Moon, A. Sex Differences in Cancer: Epidemiology, Genetics and Therapy. *Biomol. Ther.* **2018**, *26*, 335–342. [CrossRef]
20. Czihal, M.; Tschaidse, J.; Bernau, C.; Lottspeich, C.; Kohler, A.; Dechant, C.; Schulze-Koops, H.; Hoffmann, U.; Mackert, M.J.; Thurau, S. Ocular ischaemic complications in giant cell arteritis: CHADS2-score predicts risk of permanent visual impairment. *Clin. Exp. Rheumatol.* **2019**, *37*, 61–64. [PubMed]
21. Elling, P.; Olsson, A.T.; Elling, H. Synchronous variations of the incidence of temporal arteritis and polymyalgia rheumatica in different regions of Denmark; association with epidemics of Mycoplasma pneumoniae infection. *J. Rheumatol.* **1996**, *23*, 112–119.
22. Mohan, S.V.; Liao, Y.J.; Kim, J.W.; Goronzy, J.J.; Weyand, C.M. Giant cell arteritis: Immune and vascular aging as disease risk factors. *Arthritis Res. Ther.* **2011**, *13*, 231. [CrossRef] [PubMed]
23. Goronzy, J.J.; Lee, W.W.; Weyand, C.M. Aging and T-cell diversity. *Exp. Gerontol.* **2007**, *42*, 400–406. [CrossRef]
24. Lee, H.Y.; Oh, B.H. Aging and arterial stiffness. *Circ. J.* **2010**, *74*, 2257–2262. [CrossRef]
25. Weyand, C.M.; Hunder, N.N.; Hicok, K.C.; Hunder, G.G.; Goronzy, J.J. HLA-DRB1 alleles in polymyalgia rheumatica, giant cell arteritis, and rheumatoid arthritis. *Arthritis Rheum.* **1994**, *37*, 514–520. [CrossRef]
26. Osiowski, A.; Osiowski, M.; Stolarz, K.; Klepinowski, T.; Taterra, D. Headache as the most common manifestation of giant cell arteritis? A systematic review with meta-analysis. *Rheumatol. Int.* **2025**, *45*, 47. [CrossRef]
27. Ward, T.N.; Levin, M. Headache in giant cell arteritis and other arteritides. *Neurol. Sci.* **2005**, *26*, s134–s137. [CrossRef]
28. Baskar, S.; Etti, R.; Kitas, G.; Klocke, R. Cluster headache or giant cell arteritis? *BMJ Case Rep.* **2008**, *2008*, bcr0720080444. [CrossRef] [PubMed]

https://doi.org/10.3390/diagnostics16030470

29. Ihoriya, H.; Nakano, Y.; Otsuka, F. Temporal artery thickening in giant cell arteritis. *BMJ Case Rep.* **2021**, *14*, e247123. [CrossRef] [PubMed]
30. Lim, J.; Dures, E.; Bailey, L.F.; Almeida, C.; Ruediger, C.; Hill, C.L.; Robson, J.C.; Mackie, S.L. Jaw claudication and jaw stiffness in giant cell arteritis: Secondary analysis of a qualitative research dataset. *Rheumatol. Adv. Pract.* **2024**, *8*, rkad082. [CrossRef]
31. Francis, C.E.; Petersen, C.A. Jaw Claudication and Temporal Artery Abnormalities in Giant Cell Arteritis: Take Advantage of Clinical Clues: Response. *J. Neuroophthalmol.* **2017**, *37*, 458. [CrossRef]
32. Vitiello, G. Jaw Claudication and Temporal Artery Abnormalities in Giant Cell Arteritis: Take Advantage of Clinical Clues. *J. Neuroophthalmol.* **2017**, *37*, 458. [CrossRef] [PubMed]
33. Smetana, G.W.; Shmerling, R.H. Does this patient have temporal arteritis? *JAMA* **2002**, *287*, 92–101. [CrossRef]
34. van der Geest, K.S.M.; Sandovici, M.; Brouwer, E.; Mackie, S.L. Diagnostic Accuracy of Symptoms, Physical Signs, and Laboratory Tests for Giant Cell Arteritis: A Systematic Review and Meta-analysis. *JAMA Intern. Med.* **2020**, *180*, 1295–1304. [CrossRef]
35. Kuo, C.H.; McCluskey, P.; Fraser, C.L. Chewing Gum Test for Jaw Claudication in Giant-Cell Arteritis. *N. Engl. J. Med.* **2016**, *374*, 1794–1795. [CrossRef] [PubMed]
36. Smith, S.C.M.; Al-Hashimi, M.R.; Jones, C.D.; Mukhtyar, C.B. Frequency of visual involvement in a 10-year interdisciplinary cohort of patients with giant cell arteritis. *Clin. Med.* **2023**, *23*, 206–212. [CrossRef] [PubMed]
37. Chean, C.S.; Prior, J.A.; Helliwell, T.; Belcher, J.; Mackie, S.L.; Hider, S.L.; Liddle, J.; Mallen, C.D. Characteristics of patients with giant cell arteritis who experience visual symptoms. *Rheumatol. Int.* **2019**, *39*, 1789–1796. [CrossRef]
38. Curumthaullee, M.F.; Liozon, E.; Dumonteil, S.; Gondran, G.; Fauchais, A.L.; Ly, K.H.; Robert, P.Y.; Parreau, S. Features and risk factors for new (secondary) permanent visual involvement in giant cell arteritis. *Clin. Exp. Rheumatol.* **2022**, *40*, 734–740. [CrossRef]
39. Donaldson, L.; Margolin, E. Bilateral Anterior Ischemic Optic Neuropathy Due to Giant Cell Arteritis with Preservation of Central Visual Acuity. *J. Neuroophthalmol.* **2022**, *42*, e479–e481. [CrossRef]
40. Chopra, A.; Sharma, R.; Singla, K.; Saroya, A.S.; Verma, S.; Nagesha, C.K. Arteritic anterior ischemic optic neuropathy with hypotony, an alarming sign of severe form of giant cell arteritis. *Indian J. Ophthalmol.* **2022**, *70*, 3426–3427. [CrossRef]
41. Chazal, T.; Clavel, G.; Leturcq, T.; Philibert, M.; Lecler, A.; Vignal-Clermont, C. Characteristics and Prognosis of Binocular Diplopia in Patients with Giant Cell Arteritis. *J. Neuroophthalmol.* **2024**, *44*, 87–91. [CrossRef]
42. Castillejo Becerra, C.M.; Crowson, C.S.; Koster, M.J.; Warrington, K.J.; Bhatti, M.T.; Chen, J.J. Population-based Rate and Patterns of Diplopia in Giant Cell Arteritis. *Neuroophthalmology* **2022**, *46*, 75–79. [CrossRef]
43. Chaudhary, H.; Zachariah, S.; Schwartz, J. Central Retinal Artery Occlusion Secondary to Giant Cell Arteritis with Normal Inflammatory Markers. *J. Clin. Rheumatol.* **2021**, *27*, S335–S337. [CrossRef]
44. Charness, M.E.; Liu, G.T. Central retinal artery occlusion in giant cell arteritis: Treatment with nitroglycerin. *Neurology* **1991**, *41*, 1698–1699. [CrossRef] [PubMed]
45. Albarrak, A.M.; Mohammad, Y.; Hussain, S.; Husain, S.; Muayqil, T. Simultaneous bilateral posterior ischemic optic neuropathy secondary to giant cell arteritis: A case presentation and review of the literature. *BMC Ophthalmol.* **2018**, *18*, 317. [CrossRef] [PubMed]
46. Lopez, J.M.; Nazabal, E.R.; Muniz, A.M.; Rey del Corral, P. Detection of posterior ischemic optic neuropathy due to giant cell arteritis with magnetic resonance imaging. *Eur. Neurol.* **2001**, *46*, 109–110. [CrossRef] [PubMed]
47. Ness, S.D.; Butler, N.J.; Poulaki, V. Bilateral Macular Choroidal Infarction as a Manifestation of Giant Cell Arteritis. *Ophthalmic Surg. Lasers Imaging Retin.* **2018**, *49*, 540–543. [CrossRef]
48. Shinbashi, M.; Hakim, S.; Mechel, E.; Mehta, M.C.; Crow, R.W. An atypical presentation of giant cell arteritis: Fatigable signs to anterior ischemic optic neuropathy and choroidal infarction. *Clin. Case Rep.* **2023**, *11*, e7775. [CrossRef]
49. Tucker, S.M.; Haas, S.J.; Zaihra Rizvi, T. Predictors of Permanent Vision Loss in Giant Cell Arteritis. *Neuroophthalmology* **2025**, *49*, 60–68. [CrossRef]
50. Baalbaki, H.; Jalaledin, D.; Lachance, C.; Febrer, G.; Rheaume, M.; Makhzoum, J.P. Characterization of visual manifestations and identification of risk factors for permanent vision loss in patients with giant cell arteritis. *Clin. Rheumatol.* **2021**, *40*, 3207–3217. [CrossRef]
51. Gow, J.; Roofeh, D. An atypical manifestation of Giant cell arteritis (GCA): Constitutional symptoms & lingual ulcer in a 78-Year-Old male with negative temporal artery biopsies. *BMC Rheumatol.* **2025**, *9*, 53. [CrossRef] [PubMed]
52. Shukla, S.; Hull, R. Unintentional weight loss. Think of giant cell arteritis. *BMJ* **2011**, *342*, d2889. [CrossRef]
53. Schafer, V.S.; Warrington, K.J.; Williamson, E.E.; Kermani, T.A. Delayed diagnosis of biopsy-negative giant cell arteritis presenting as fever of unknown origin. *J. Gen. Intern. Med.* **2009**, *24*, 532–536. [CrossRef]
54. Gonzalez-Gay, M.A.; Garcia-Porrua, C.; Amor-Dorado, J.C.; Llorca, J. Fever in biopsy-proven giant cell arteritis: Clinical implications in a defined population. *Arthritis Rheum.* **2004**, *51*, 652–655. [CrossRef]
55. Sun, M.M.; Pope, J.E. Polymyalgia rheumatica and giant cell arteritis: Diagnosis and management. *Curr. Opin. Rheumatol.* **2025**, *37*, 32–38. [CrossRef]

https://doi.org/10.3390/diagnostics16030470

56. Lowe, M.; Sebastian, A. Polymyalgia rheumatica and giant cell arteritis: Are these two sides of the same coin? *Rheumatology* **2025**, *64*, 1583–1584. [CrossRef]
57. Blockmans, D. Why, how and when to look for occult giant cell arteritis in patients with polymyalgia rheumatica. *Rheumatology* **2025**, *64*, i55–i58. [CrossRef]
58. de Mornac, D.; Espitia, O.; Neel, A.; Connault, J.; Masseau, A.; Espitia-Thibault, A.; Artifoni, M.; Achille, A.; Wahbi, A.; Lacou, M.; et al. Large-vessel involvement is predictive of multiple relapses in giant cell arteritis. *Ther. Adv. Musculoskelet. Dis.* **2021**, *13*, 1759720X211009029. [CrossRef]
59. Rodriguez-Pla, A.; Naidu, S.G.; Butt, Y.M.; Davila, V.J. Normal inflammatory markers in giant cell arteritis with long-standing cranial and symptomatic large-vessel involvement. *BMJ Case Rep.* **2021**, *14*, e242602. [CrossRef] [PubMed]
60. de Boysson, H.; Liozon, E.; Lambert, M.; Dumont, A.; Boutemy, J.; Maigne, G.; Martin Silva, N.; Ly, K.H.; Manrique, A.; Bienvenu, B.; et al. Giant-Cell Arteritis: Do We Treat Patients with Large-Vessel Involvement Differently? *Am. J. Med.* **2017**, *130*, 992–995. [CrossRef] [PubMed]
61. de Boysson, H.; Dumont, A.; Liozon, E.; Lambert, M.; Boutemy, J.; Maigne, G.; Martin Silva, N.; Sultan, A.; Ly, K.H.; Aide, N.; et al. Giant-cell arteritis: Concordance study between aortic CT angiography and FDG-PET/CT in detection of large-vessel involvement. *Eur. J. Nucl. Med. Mol. Imaging* **2017**, *44*, 2274–2279. [CrossRef]
62. Lambert, M.; Weber, A.; Boland, B.; De Plaen, J.F.; Donckier, J. Large vessel vasculitis without temporal artery involvement: Isolated form of giant cell arteritis? *Clin. Rheumatol.* **1996**, *15*, 174–180. [CrossRef]
63. Hay, B.; Mariano-Goulart, D.; Bourdon, A.; Benkiran, M.; Vauchot, F.; De Verbizier, D.; Ben Bouallegue, F. Diagnostic performance of (18)F-FDG PET-CT for large vessel involvement assessment in patients with suspected giant cell arteritis and negative temporal artery biopsy. *Ann. Nucl. Med.* **2019**, *33*, 512–520. [CrossRef]
64. Ponte, C.; Grayson, P.C.; Robson, J.C.; Suppiah, R.; Gribbons, K.B.; Judge, A.; Craven, A.; Khalid, S.; Hutchings, A.; Watts, R.A.; et al. 2022 American College of Rheumatology/EULAR classification criteria for giant cell arteritis. *Ann. Rheum. Dis.* **2022**, *81*, 1647–1653. Erratum in *Ann. Rheum. Dis.* **2023**, *82*, e52. [CrossRef]
65. Palmowski, A.; Buttgereit, F. Reducing the Toxicity of Long-Term Glucocorticoid Treatment in Large Vessel Vasculitis. *Curr. Rheumatol. Rep.* **2020**, *22*, 85. [CrossRef]
66. Ellis, M.E.; Ralston, S. The ESR in the diagnosis and management of the polymyalgia rheumatica/giant cell arteritis syndrome. *Ann. Rheum. Dis.* **1983**, *42*, 168–170. [CrossRef]
67. Parikh, M.; Miller, N.R.; Lee, A.G.; Savino, P.J.; Vacarezza, M.N.; Cornblath, W.; Eggenberger, E.; Antonio-Santos, A.; Golnik, K.; Kardon, R.; et al. Prevalence of a normal C-reactive protein with an elevated erythrocyte sedimentation rate in biopsy-proven giant cell arteritis. *Ophthalmology* **2006**, *113*, 1842–1845. [CrossRef] [PubMed]
68. Lopez-Diaz, M.J.; Llorca, J.; Gonzalez-Juanatey, C.; Pena-Sagredo, J.L.; Martin, J.; Gonzalez-Gay, M.A. The erythrocyte sedimentation rate is associated with the development of visual complications in biopsy-proven giant cell arteritis. *Semin. Arthritis Rheum.* **2008**, *38*, 116–123. [CrossRef] [PubMed]
69. Kyle, V.; Cawston, T.E.; Hazleman, B.L. Erythrocyte sedimentation rate and C reactive protein in the assessment of polymyalgia rheumatica/giant cell arteritis on presentation and during follow up. *Ann. Rheum. Dis.* **1989**, *48*, 667–671. [CrossRef] [PubMed]
70. Kermani, T.A.; Schmidt, J.; Crowson, C.S.; Ytterberg, S.R.; Hunder, G.G.; Matteson, E.L.; Warrington, K.J. Utility of erythrocyte sedimentation rate and C-reactive protein for the diagnosis of giant cell arteritis. *Semin. Arthritis Rheum.* **2012**, *41*, 866–871. [CrossRef]
71. Currier, C.E.; Bays, A.M.; Thomason, J.L. Normal inflammatory markers in giant cell arteritis: A diagnostic blind spot. *Rheumatol. Int.* **2025**, *45*, 175. [CrossRef]
72. Martins, P.; Teixeira, V.; Teixeira, F.J.; Canastro, M.; Palha, A.; Fonseca, J.E.; Ponte, C. Giant cell arteritis with normal inflammatory markers: Case report and review of the literature. *Clin. Rheumatol.* **2020**, *39*, 3115–3125. [CrossRef]
73. Costello, F.; Zimmerman, M.B.; Podhajsky, P.A.; Hayreh, S.S. Role of thrombocytosis in diagnosis of giant cell arteritis and differentiation of arteritic from non-arteritic anterior ischemic optic neuropathy. *Eur. J. Ophthalmol.* **2004**, *14*, 245–257. [CrossRef] [PubMed]
74. Foroozan, R.; Danesh-Meyer, H.; Savino, P.J.; Gamble, G.; Mekari-Sabbagh, O.N.; Sergott, R.C. Thrombocytosis in patients with biopsy-proven giant cell arteritis. *Ophthalmology* **2002**, *109*, 1267–1271. [CrossRef] [PubMed]
75. Chan, F.L.Y.; Lester, S.; Whittle, S.L.; Hill, C.L. The utility of ESR, CRP and platelets in the diagnosis of GCA. *BMC Rheumatol.* **2019**, *3*, 14. [CrossRef] [PubMed]
76. Weiss, L.M.; Gonzalez, E.; Miller, S.B.; Agudelo, C.A. Severe anemia as the presenting manifestation of giant cell arteritis. *Arthritis Rheum.* **1995**, *38*, 434–436. [CrossRef]
77. Guggenberger, K.V.; Vogt, M.L.; Rowe, S.P.; Higuchi, T.; Schmalzing, M.; Tony, H.P.; Buck, A.K.; Bley, T.A.; Frohlich, M.; Werner, R.A. Clinical Utility of C-Reactive Protein and White Blood Cell Count for Scheduling an [18F]FDG PET/CT in Patients with Giant Cell Arteritis. *Nuklearmedizin* **2022**, *61*, 425–432. [CrossRef]

https://doi.org/10.3390/diagnostics16030470

78. Dartevel, A.; Toussaint, B.; Trocme, C.; Arnaud, M.; Simon, N.; Faure, P.; Bouillet, L. Serum amyloid A as a marker of disease activity in Giant cell arteritis. *Autoimmun. Rev.* **2020**, *19*, 102428. [CrossRef]
79. Hachulla, E.; Saile, R.; Parra, H.J.; Hatron, P.Y.; Gosset, D.; Fruchart, J.C.; Devulder, B. Serum amyloid A concentrations in giant-cell arteritis and polymyalgia rheumatica: A useful test in the management of the disease. *Clin. Exp. Rheumatol.* **1991**, *9*, 157–163.
80. O'Neill, L.; Rooney, P.; Molloy, D.; Connolly, M.; McCormick, J.; McCarthy, G.; Veale, D.J.; Murphy, C.C.; Fearon, U.; Molloy, E. Regulation of Inflammation and Angiogenesis in Giant Cell Arteritis by Acute-Phase Serum Amyloid A. *Arthritis Rheumatol.* **2015**, *67*, 2447–2456. [CrossRef]
81. Corbera-Bellalta, M.; Kamberovic, F.; Alba-Rovira, R.; Planas-Rigol, E.; Prieto-Gonzalez, S.; Farran-Centelles, N.; Tobias, E.; Jordan, A.; Alba, M.A.; Quintana, E.; et al. The IL-6 axis in vascular inflammation: Effects of IL-6 receptor blockade on vascular lesions from patients with giant-cell arteritis. *Ann. Rheum. Dis.* **2025**, *84*, 1387–1400. [CrossRef]
82. Pountain, G.; Hazleman, B.; Cawston, T.E. Circulating levels of IL-1beta, IL-6 and soluble IL-2 receptor in polymyalgia rheumatica and giant cell arteritis and rheumatoid arthritis. *Br. J. Rheumatol.* **1998**, *37*, 797–798. [CrossRef]
83. Conway, R.; O'Neill, L.; McCarthy, G.M.; Murphy, C.C.; Fabre, A.; Kennedy, S.; Veale, D.J.; Wade, S.M.; Fearon, U.; Molloy, E.S. Interleukin 12 and interleukin 23 play key pathogenic roles in inflammatory and proliferative pathways in giant cell arteritis. *Ann. Rheum. Dis.* **2018**, *77*, 1815–1824. [CrossRef]
84. Rodriguez-Pla, A.; Warner, R.L.; Cuthbertson, D.; Carette, S.; Khalidi, N.A.; Koening, C.L.; Langford, C.A.; McAlear, C.A.; Moreland, L.W.; Pagnoux, C.; et al. Evaluation of Potential Serum Biomarkers of Disease Activity in Diverse Forms of Vasculitis. *J. Rheumatol.* **2020**, *47*, 1001–1010. [CrossRef]
85. Johansen, J.S.; Baslund, B.; Garbarsch, C.; Hansen, M.; Stoltenberg, M.; Lorenzen, I.; Price, P.A. YKL-40 in giant cells and macrophages from patients with giant cell arteritis. *Arthritis Rheum.* **1999**, *42*, 2624–2630. [CrossRef] [PubMed]
86. van der Geest, K.S.; Abdulahad, W.H.; Rutgers, A.; Horst, G.; Bijzet, J.; Arends, S.; Roffel, M.P.; Boots, A.M.; Brouwer, E. Serum markers associated with disease activity in giant cell arteritis and polymyalgia rheumatica. *Rheumatology* **2015**, *54*, 1397–1402. [CrossRef] [PubMed]
87. Goodfellow, N.; Morlet, J.; Singh, S.; Sabokbar, A.; Hutchings, A.; Sharma, V.; Vaskova, J.; Masters, S.; Zarei, A.; Luqmani, R. Is vascular endothelial growth factor a useful biomarker in giant cell arteritis? *RMD Open* **2017**, *3*, e000353. [CrossRef] [PubMed]
88. Ehlers, L.; Askling, J.; Bijlsma, H.W.; Cid, M.C.; Cutolo, M.; Dasgupta, B.; Dejaco, C.; Dixon, W.G.; Feltelius, N.; Finckh, A.; et al. 2018 EULAR recommendations for a core data set to support observational research and clinical care in giant cell arteritis. *Ann. Rheum. Dis.* **2019**, *78*, 1160–1166. [CrossRef]
89. Bosch, P.; Bond, M.; Dejaco, C.; Ponte, C.; Mackie, S.L.; Falzon, L.; Schmidt, W.A.; Ramiro, S. Imaging in diagnosis, monitoring and outcome prediction of large vessel vasculitis: A systematic literature review and meta-analysis informing the 2023 update of the EULAR recommendations. *RMD Open* **2023**, *9*, e003379. [CrossRef]
90. Schmidt, W.A.; Schafer, V.S. Diagnosing vasculitis with ultrasound: Findings and pitfalls. *Ther. Adv. Musculoskelet. Dis.* **2024**, *16*, 1759720X241251742. [CrossRef]
91. Martins-Martinho, J.; Bandeira, M.; James, L.; Verdiyeva, A.; Fontes, T.; Lopes, A.R.; Naique, S.; Velho, I.; Khmelinskii, N.; Luqmani, R.; et al. The value of axillary, facial, occipital, subclavian and common carotid arteries ultrasound in the diagnosis of giant cell arteritis. *Rheumatology* **2025**, *64*, 1369–1376. [CrossRef]
92. Oshinsky, C.; Bays, A.M.; Sacksen, I.; Jernberg, E.; Zierler, R.E.; Pollock, P.S. The Usefullness of Subclavian Artery Ultrasound Assessment in Giant Cell Arteritis Evaluation. *J. Clin. Rheumatol.* **2023**, *29*, 43–46. [CrossRef]
93. Wojczal, J.; Kozera, G.; Luchowski, P.; Neubauer-Geryk, J. Advantages in diagnosis of giant cell arteritis by ultrasound. *Postep. Dermatol. Alergol.* **2019**, *36*, 25–28. [CrossRef]
94. Kirby, C.; Flood, R.; Mullan, R.; Murphy, G.; Kane, D. Evolution of ultrasound in giant cell arteritis. *Front. Med.* **2022**, *9*, 981659. [CrossRef]
95. Suzuki, T.; Ando, S.; Ohshima, M.; Suzuki, A. Clinical Images: Giant cell arteritis with positive temporal artery biopsy findings but without ultrasound halo sign. *Arthritis Rheumatol.* **2022**, *74*, 809. [CrossRef]
96. Rhee, R.L.; Bathla, G.; Rebello, R.; Kurtz, R.M.; Junek, M.; Warrington, K.J.; Khalidi, N.; Merkel, P.A.; Guggenberger, K.V.; Tamhankar, M.A.; et al. Vessel wall MRI in giant cell arteritis: Standardized protocol and scoring approach developed by an international working group. *Rheumatology* **2025**, *64*, 2910–2918. [CrossRef] [PubMed]
97. van Nieuwland, M.; Colin, E.M.; Vermeer, M.; Wagenaar, N.R.L.; Vijlbrief, O.D.; van Zandwijk, J.K.; Slart, R.; Koffijberg, H.; Jebbink, E.G.; van der Geest, K.S.M.; et al. A direct comparison in diagnostic performance of CDUS, FDG-PET/CT and MRI in patients suspected of giant cell arteritis. *Rheumatology* **2025**, *64*, 1392–1399. [CrossRef]
98. Hommada, M.; Mekinian, A.; Brillet, P.Y.; Abad, S.; Larroche, C.; Dhote, R.; Fain, O.; Soussan, M. Aortitis in giant cell arteritis: Diagnosis with FDG PET/CT and agreement with CT angiography. *Autoimmun. Rev.* **2017**, *16*, 1131–1137. [CrossRef] [PubMed]
99. Conway, R.; Smyth, A.E.; Kavanagh, R.G.; O'Donohoe, R.L.; Purcell, Y.; Heffernan, E.J.; Molloy, E.S.; McNeill, G.; Killeen, R.P. Diagnostic Utility of Computed Tomographic Angiography in Giant-Cell Arteritis. *Stroke* **2018**, *49*, 2233–2236. [CrossRef]

https://doi.org/10.3390/diagnostics16030470

100. Prieto-Pena, D.; Castaneda, S.; Martinez-Rodriguez, I.; Atienza-Mateo, B.; Blanco, R.; Gonzalez-Gay, M.A. Imaging Tests in the Early Diagnosis of Giant Cell Arteritis. *J. Clin. Med.* **2021**, *10*, 3704. [CrossRef] [PubMed]
101. Collada-Carrasco, J.; Gomez-Leon, N.; Castillo-Morales, V.; Lumbreras-Fernandez, B.; Castaneda, S.; Rodriguez-Laval, V. Role and potential of (18)F-fluorodeoxyglucose-positron emission tomography-computed tomography in large-vessel vasculitis: A comprehensive review. *Front. Med.* **2024**, *11*, 1432865. [CrossRef] [PubMed]
102. Imfeld, S.; Aschwanden, M.; Rottenburger, C.; Schegk, E.; Berger, C.T.; Staub, D.; Daikeler, T. [18F]FDG positron emission tomography and ultrasound in the diagnosis of giant cell arteritis: Congruent or complementary imaging methods? *Rheumatology* **2020**, *59*, 772–778. [CrossRef] [PubMed]
103. Ie, K.; Sakai, T.; Kurosu, E.; Motohashi, I.; Yagihashi, K.; Okuse, C.; Matsuda, T. A Long-term Persistent Vascular Fluorodeoxyglucose Uptake in a Patient with Large-vessel Vasculitis. *Intern. Med.* **2022**, *61*, 357–360. [CrossRef]
104. Tsai, Y.J.; Liu, C. Pitfalls on PET/CT Due to Artifacts and Instrumentation. *Semin. Nucl. Med.* **2021**, *51*, 646–656. [CrossRef] [PubMed]
105. Venables, M.; Taylor, A.; Murdoch, J.; De Sousa, J.L.; Keen, H. Use of fluorine-18-fluorodeoxyglucose positron emission tomography/computed tomography in diagnosing giant cell arteritis in a Western Australian tertiary centre: A 36-month analysis. *Intern. Med. J.* **2025**, *55*, 1308–1315. [CrossRef]
106. Allam, M.N.; Baba Ali, N.; Mahmoud, A.K.; Scalia, I.G.; Farina, J.M.; Abbas, M.T.; Pereyra, M.; Kamel, M.A.; Awad, K.A.; Wang, Y.; et al. Multi-Modality Imaging in Vasculitis. *Diagnostics* **2024**, *14*, 838. [CrossRef]
107. Ni, R.; Kohler, M.J. What is new in imaging to assist in the diagnosis of giant cell arteritis and Takayasu's arteritis since the EULAR and ACR/VF recommendations? *Front. Med.* **2024**, *11*, 1495644. [CrossRef]
108. Nadim, B.; Blassel, E.; Sheets, A.R.; Mitchell, R.N.; Aghayev, A. Multimodality imaging of pulmonary artery aneurysms due to giant cell arteritis: A case series. *Int. J. Cardiovasc. Imaging* **2025**, *41*, 631–638. [CrossRef]
109. Ludwig, D.R.; Voo, S.; Morris, V. Fast-track pathway for early diagnosis and management of giant cell arteritis: The combined role of vascular ultrasonography and [18F]-fluorodeoxyglucose PET-computed tomography imaging. *Nucl. Med. Commun.* **2023**, *44*, 339–344. [CrossRef]
110. Schmidt, W.A.; Czihal, M.; Gernert, M.; Hartung, W.; Hellmich, B.; Ohrndorf, S.; Riemekasten, G.; Schäfer, V.S.; Strunk, J.; Venhoff, N. Recommendations for defining giant cell arteritis fast-track clinics. English version. *Z. Rheumatol.* **2024**, *83*, 285–288. [CrossRef]
111. Parreau, S.; Liozon, E.; Chen, J.J.; Curumthaullee, M.F.; Fauchais, A.L.; Warrington, K.J.; Ly, K.H.; Weyand, C.M. Temporal artery biopsy: A technical guide and review of its importance and indications. *Surv. Ophthalmol.* **2023**, *68*, 104–112. [CrossRef]
112. Nair, V.; Fishbein, G.A.; Padera, R.; Seidman, M.A.; Castonguay, M.; Leduc, C.; Tan, C.D.; Rodriguez, E.R.; Maleszewski, J.J.; Miller, D.; et al. Consensus statement on the processing, interpretation and reporting of temporal artery biopsy for arteritis. *Cardiovasc. Pathol.* **2023**, *67*, 107574. [CrossRef]
113. Stamatis, P.; Turesson, C.; Mohammad, A.J. Temporal artery biopsy in giant cell arteritis: Clinical perspectives and histological patterns. *Front. Med.* **2024**, *11*, 1453462. [CrossRef]
114. Shiomi, M.; Watanabe, R.; Ishihara, R.; Tanaka, S.; Kageyama, G.; Hashimoto, M. Uncovering the New Biology of Giant Cell Arteritis to Guide Therapeutic Strategies. *J. Clin. Med.* **2025**, *14*, 6350. [CrossRef]
115. Lee, Y.C.; Padera, R.F.; Noss, E.H.; Fossel, A.H.; Bienfang, D.; Liang, M.H.; Docken, W.P. Clinical course and management of a consecutive series of patients with "healed temporal arteritis". *J. Rheumatol.* **2012**, *39*, 295–302. [CrossRef] [PubMed]
116. Fadoul, M.A.; McMackin, K.K.; Patel, R.; Daneshpooy, S.; Tjaden, B.L.; Batista, P.M.; Carpenter, J.P.; Lombardi, J.V. Validating the Clinical Value of Temporal Artery Biopsy. *Ann. Vasc. Surg.* **2023**, *92*, 82–86. [CrossRef] [PubMed]
117. Inayat, H.; Youn, S.; Bursztyn, L. Utility of online GCA risk models in predicting the result of temporal artery biopsy within a clinical setting: Study of diagnostic and screening tests. *Can. J. Ophthalmol.* **2024**, *59*, e483–e488. [CrossRef] [PubMed]
118. Hunder, G.G.; Bloch, D.A.; Michel, B.A.; Stevens, M.B.; Arend, W.P.; Calabrese, L.H.; Edworthy, S.M.; Fauci, A.S.; Leavitt, R.Y.; Lie, J.T.; et al. The American College of Rheumatology 1990 criteria for the classification of giant cell arteritis. *Arthritis Rheum.* **1990**, *33*, 1122–1128. [CrossRef]
119. Wiberg, F.; Naderi, N.; Mohammad, A.J.; Turesson, C. Evaluation of revised classification criteria for giant cell arteritis and its clinical phenotypes. *Rheumatology* **2021**, *61*, 383–387. [CrossRef]
120. Marvisi, C.; Macaluso, F.; Ricordi, C.; Cavazza, A.; Muratore, F.; Salvarani, C. Diagnostic approach in giant cell arteritis. *Autoimmun. Rev.* **2025**, *24*, 103743. [CrossRef]
121. Ramon, A.; Greigert, H.; Ornetti, P.; Bonnotte, B.; Samson, M. Mimickers of Large Vessel Giant Cell Arteritis. *J. Clin. Med.* **2022**, *11*, 495. [CrossRef] [PubMed]
122. Berti, A.; Moura, M.C.; Sechi, E.; Squizzato, F.; Costanzo, G.; Chen, J.J.; Warrington, K.J. Beyond Giant Cell Arteritis and Takayasu's Arteritis: Secondary Large Vessel Vasculitis and Vasculitis Mimickers. *Curr. Rheumatol. Rep.* **2020**, *22*, 88. [CrossRef]
123. Rodriguez-Pla, A.; Grill, M.F.; Fletcher, G.P.; Di Nome, M.A. Ischemic Optic Neuropathy Secondary to Varicella-Zoster Vasculitis Mimicking Giant Cell Arteritis: Case Report. *Case Rep. Neurol.* **2022**, *14*, 483–490. [CrossRef]

124. Younger, D.S. Primary central nervous system vasculitis and headache: Ten themes. *Curr. Opin. Neurol.* **2023**, *36*, 647–658. [CrossRef]
125. Rodriguez-Pla, A.; Monach, P.A. Primary angiitis of the central nervous system in adults and children. *Rheum. Dis. Clin. North. Am.* **2015**, *41*, 47–62, viii. [CrossRef] [PubMed]
126. Buhaescu, I.; Williams, A.; Yood, R. Rare manifestations of Churg-Strauss syndrome: Coronary artery vasospasm, temporal artery vasculitis, and reversible monocular blindness-a case report. *Clin. Rheumatol.* **2009**, *28*, 231–233. [CrossRef]
127. Stamatis, P. Giant Cell Arteritis versus Takayasu Arteritis: An Update. *Mediterr. J. Rheumatol.* **2020**, *31*, 174–182. [CrossRef] [PubMed]
128. Sharma, A.; Dhooria, A.; Aggarwal, A.; Rathi, M.; Chandran, V. Connective Tissue Disorder-Associated Vasculitis. *Curr. Rheumatol. Rep.* **2016**, *18*, 31. [CrossRef]
129. Evangelatos, G.; Grivas, A.; Pappa, M.; Kouna, K.; Iliopoulos, A.; Fragoulis, G.E. Cranial giant cell arteritis mimickers: A masquerade to unveil. *Autoimmun. Rev.* **2022**, *21*, 103083. [CrossRef]
130. Guardiola, J.M.; Rodriguez-Pla, A.; Lopez-Contreras, J.; Llobet, J.M.; Domingo, P.; Franco, M.; Diaz, C.; Vazquez, G. Simultaneous presence of C-ANCA and P-ANCA in a patient with concurrent Churg-Strauss syndrome and giant cell temporal arteritis. *Scand. J. Rheumatol.* **2000**, *29*, 68–69. [CrossRef]
131. Parreau, S.; Cayrou, C.; Dumonteil, S.; Laburthe, S.; Bosphore, G.; Desvaux, E.; Ratti, N.; Lopez, J.G.; Margotonne, M.; Couillard, F.; et al. Giant cell arteritis mimics with severe consequences: A long-term monocentric inception cohort. *Rheumatology* **2025**, *64*, 4726–4731. [CrossRef]
132. Stewart, C.; Asif, R.H.; Dakkak, T.; Singh, H.; Javaid, M.A.; Patel, N. Diagnostic Dilemmas in Giant Cell Arteritis: Overcoming Anchoring Bias. *Case Rep. Rheumatol.* **2025**, *2025*, 6632374. [CrossRef]
133. Hashemi, H.; Khabazkhoob, M.; Nabovati, P.; Ostadimoghaddam, H.; Shafaee, S.; Doostdar, A.; Yekta, A. The Prevalence of Age-Related Eye Disease in an Elderly Population. *Ophthalmic Epidemiol.* **2017**, *24*, 222–228. [CrossRef]
134. Presto, P.; Sehar, U.; Kopel, J.; Reddy, P.H. Mechanisms of pain in aging and age-related conditions: Focus on caregivers. *Ageing Res. Rev.* **2024**, *95*, 102249. [CrossRef] [PubMed]
135. Incir, S.; Bolayirli, M. Polypharmacy as a reason for misinterpreting laboratory results in the elderly. *Adv. Pharmacol.* **2025**, *104*, 515–581. [CrossRef] [PubMed]
136. Hallowell, E.S.; Van Patten, R. Clinical utility of self-reported and informant-reported cognitive complaints in older adults. *Int. Psychogeriatr.* **2022**, *34*, 1007–1010. [CrossRef] [PubMed]
137. Alharbi, T.A.F.; Rababa, M.; Alsuwayl, H.; Alsubail, A.; Alenizi, W.S. Diagnostic Challenges and Patient Safety: The Critical Role of Accuracy—A Systematic Review. *J. Multidiscip. Health* **2025**, *18*, 3051–3064. [CrossRef]
138. Walsh, M.; Merkel, P.A.; Peh, C.A.; Szpirt, W.; Guillevin, L.; Pusey, C.D.; De Zoysa, J.; Ives, N.; Clark, W.F.; Quillen, K.; et al. Plasma exchange and glucocorticoid dosing in the treatment of anti-neutrophil cytoplasm antibody associated vasculitis (PEXIVAS): Protocol for a randomized controlled trial. *Trials* **2013**, *14*, 73. [CrossRef]
139. Garvey, T.D.; Koster, M.J.; Warrington, K.J. My Treatment Approach to Giant Cell Arteritis. *Mayo Clin. Proc.* **2021**, *96*, 1530–1545. [CrossRef]
140. Hayreh, S.S. Giant cell arteritis: Its ophthalmic manifestations. *Indian J. Ophthalmol.* **2021**, *69*, 227–235. [CrossRef]
141. Stone, J.H.; Klearman, M.; Collinson, N. Trial of Tocilizumab in Giant-Cell Arteritis. *N. Engl. J. Med.* **2017**, *377*, 1494–1495. [CrossRef]
142. Collinson, N.; Tuckwell, K.; Habeck, F.; Chapman, M.; Klearman, M.; Stone, J.H. Development and implementation of a double-blind corticosteroid-tapering regimen for a clinical trial. *Int. J. Rheumatol.* **2015**, *2015*, 589841. [CrossRef]
143. Hellmich, B.; Agueda, A.; Monti, S.; Buttgereit, F.; de Boysson, H.; Brouwer, E.; Cassie, R.; Cid, M.C.; Dasgupta, B.; Dejaco, C.; et al. 2018 Update of the EULAR recommendations for the management of large vessel vasculitis. *Ann. Rheum. Dis.* **2020**, *79*, 19–30. [CrossRef]
144. Mensch, N.; Hemmig, A.K.; Aschwanden, M.; Imfeld, S.; Stegert, M.; Recher, M.; Staub, D.; Kyburz, D.; Berger, C.T.; Daikeler, T. Rapid glucocorticoid tapering regimen in patients with giant cell arteritis: A single centre cohort study. *RMD Open* **2023**, *9*, e003301. [CrossRef]
145. Gerard, A.L.; Simon-Tillaux, N.; Yordanov, Y.; Cacoub, P.; Tubach, F.; Saadoun, D.; Dechartres, A. Efficacy and safety of steroid-sparing treatments in giant cell arteritis according to the glucocorticoids tapering regimen: A systematic review and meta-analysis. *Eur. J. Intern. Med.* **2021**, *88*, 96–103. [CrossRef]
146. Alba, M.A.; Kermani, T.A.; Unizony, S.; Murgia, G.; Prieto-Gonzalez, S.; Salvarani, C.; Matteson, E.L. Relapses in giant cell arteritis: Updated review for clinical practice. *Autoimmun. Rev.* **2024**, *23*, 103580. [CrossRef]
147. Gale, S.; Wilson, J.C.; Chia, J.; Trinh, H.; Tuckwell, K.; Collinson, N.; Dimonaco, S.; Jick, S.; Meier, C.; Mohan, S.V.; et al. Risk Associated with Cumulative Oral Glucocorticoid Use in Patients with Giant Cell Arteritis in Real-World Databases from the USA and UK. *Rheumatol. Ther.* **2018**, *5*, 327–340. [CrossRef]

https://doi.org/10.3390/diagnostics16030470

148. Samec, M.J.; Rakholiya, J.; Langenfeld, H.; Crowson, C.S.; Abril, A.; Wang, B.; Mertz, L.; Rodriguez-Pla, A.; Bansal, P.; Burke, M.; et al. Relapse Risk and Safety of Long-Term Tocilizumab Use Among Patients with Giant Cell Arteritis: A Single-Enterprise Cohort Study. *J. Rheumatol.* **2023**, *50*, 1310–1317. [CrossRef] [PubMed]
149. Conway, R.; Putman, M.S.; Mackie, S.L. Benchmarking tocilizumab use for giant cell arteritis. *Rheumatol. Adv. Pract.* **2022**, *6*, rkac037. [CrossRef] [PubMed]
150. Blockmans, D.; Penn, S.K.; Setty, A.R.; Schmidt, W.A.; Rubbert-Roth, A.; Hauge, E.M.; Keen, H.I.; Ishii, T.; Khalidi, N.; Dejaco, C.; et al. A Phase 3 Trial of Upadacitinib for Giant-Cell Arteritis. *N. Engl. J. Med.* **2025**, *392*, 2013–2024. [CrossRef] [PubMed]
151. Jover, J.A.; Hernandez-Garcia, C.; Morado, I.C.; Vargas, E.; Banares, A.; Fernandez-Gutierrez, B. Combined treatment of giant-cell arteritis with methotrexate and prednisone. a randomized, double-blind, placebo-controlled trial. *Ann. Intern. Med.* **2001**, *134*, 106–114. [CrossRef]
152. Spiera, R.F.; Mitnick, H.J.; Kupersmith, M.; Richmond, M.; Spiera, H.; Peterson, M.G.; Paget, S.A. A prospective, double-blind, randomized, placebo controlled trial of methotrexate in the treatment of giant cell arteritis (GCA). *Clin. Exp. Rheumatol.* **2001**, *19*, 495–501.
153. Hoffman, G.S.; Cid, M.C.; Hellmann, D.B.; Guillevin, L.; Stone, J.H.; Schousboe, J.; Cohen, P.; Calabrese, L.H.; Dickler, H.; Merkel, P.A.; et al. A multicenter, randomized, double-blind, placebo-controlled trial of adjuvant methotrexate treatment for giant cell arteritis. *Arthritis Rheum.* **2002**, *46*, 1309–1318. [CrossRef]
154. Mahr, A.D.; Jover, J.A.; Spiera, R.F.; Hernandez-Garcia, C.; Fernandez-Gutierrez, B.; Lavalley, M.P.; Merkel, P.A. Adjunctive methotrexate for treatment of giant cell arteritis: An individual patient data meta-analysis. *Arthritis Rheum.* **2007**, *56*, 2789–2797. [CrossRef]
155. Tengesdal, S.; Diamantopoulos, A.P.; Myklebust, G. Leflunomide versus methotrexate in treatment of giant cell arteritis: Comparison of efficacy, safety, and drug survival. *Scand. J. Rheumatol.* **2019**, *48*, 333–335. [CrossRef]
156. Koster, M.J.; Warrington, K.J. Vasculitis syndromes: Tocilizumab—A new frontier for GCA therapy. *Nat. Rev. Rheumatol.* **2017**, *13*, 700–701. [CrossRef]
157. Thiel, J. Giant cell arteritis—New treatment targets at the horizon. *Semin. Arthritis Rheum.* **2025**, *72*, 152686. [CrossRef] [PubMed]
158. Venhoff, N.; Schmidt, W.A.; Bergner, R.; Rech, J.; Unger, L.; Tony, H.P.; Finzel, S.; Andreica, I.; Kofler, D.M.; Weiner, S.M.; et al. Safety and efficacy of secukinumab in patients with giant cell arteritis (TitAIN): A randomised, double-blind, placebo-controlled, phase 2 trial. *Lancet Rheumatol.* **2023**, *5*, e341–e350. [CrossRef] [PubMed]
159. Watanabe, R.; Goronzy, J.J.; Berry, G.; Liao, Y.J.; Weyand, C.M. Giant Cell Arteritis: From Pathogenesis to Therapeutic Management. *Curr. Treatm Opt. Rheumatol.* **2016**, *2*, 126–137. [CrossRef] [PubMed]
160. Moreel, L.; Betrains, A.; Molenberghs, G.; Blockmans, D.; Vanderschueren, S. Duration of Treatment with Glucocorticoids in Giant Cell Arteritis: A Systematic Review and Meta-analysis. *J. Clin. Rheumatol.* **2023**, *29*, 291–297. [CrossRef]
161. Moreel, L.; Betrains, A.; Molenberghs, G.; Vanderschueren, S.; Blockmans, D. Epidemiology and predictors of relapse in giant cell arteritis: A systematic review and meta-analysis. *Jt. Bone Spine* **2023**, *90*, 105494. [CrossRef]
162. Hayreh, S.S.; Zimmerman, B.; Kardon, R.H. Visual improvement with corticosteroid therapy in giant cell arteritis. Report of a large study and review of literature. *Acta Ophthalmol. Scand.* **2002**, *80*, 355–367. [CrossRef] [PubMed]
163. Danesh-Meyer, H.; Savino, P.J.; Gamble, G.G. Poor prognosis of visual outcome after visual loss from giant cell arteritis. *Ophthalmology* **2005**, *112*, 1098–1103. [CrossRef]
164. Ghaffar, M.T.; Ramachandran, D.; Makkuni, D. The Importance of Early Recognition of Rare Ischaemic Complications of GCA to Prevent Permanent Vision Loss. *Br. J. Hosp. Med.* **2024**, *85*, 1–6. [CrossRef]
165. de Boysson, H.; Aouba, A. An Updated Review of Cardiovascular Events in Giant Cell Arteritis. *J. Clin. Med.* **2022**, *11*, 1005. [CrossRef] [PubMed]
166. de Boysson, H.; Espitia, O.; Samson, M.; Tieulie, N.; Bachmeyer, C.; Moulinet, T.; Dumont, A.; Deshayes, S.; Bonnotte, B.; Agard, C.; et al. Giant cell arteritis-related aortic dissection: A multicenter retrospective study. *Semin. Arthritis Rheum.* **2021**, *51*, 430–435. [CrossRef] [PubMed]
167. Espitia, O.; Blonz, G.; Urbanski, G.; Landron, C.; Connault, J.; Lavigne, C.; Roblot, P.; Maillot, F.; Audemard-Verger, A.; Artifoni, M.; et al. Symptomatic aortitis at giant cell arteritis diagnosis: A prognostic factor of aortic event. *Arthritis Res. Ther.* **2021**, *23*, 14. [CrossRef]
168. Li, L.; Neogi, T.; Jick, S. Mortality in Patients with Giant Cell Arteritis: A Cohort Study in UK Primary Care. *Arthritis Care Res.* **2018**, *70*, 1251–1256. [CrossRef]
169. Brekke, L.K.; Fevang, B.S.; Diamantopoulos, A.P.; Assmus, J.; Espero, E.; Gjesdal, C.G. Survival and death causes of patients with giant cell arteritis in Western Norway 1972-2012: A retrospective cohort study. *Arthritis Res. Ther.* **2019**, *21*, 154. [CrossRef]
170. Buckley, L.; Guyatt, G.; Fink, H.A.; Cannon, M.; Grossman, J.; Hansen, K.E.; Humphrey, M.B.; Lane, N.E.; Magrey, M.; Miller, M.; et al. 2017 American College of Rheumatology Guideline for the Prevention and Treatment of Glucocorticoid-Induced Osteoporosis. *Arthritis Care Res.* **2017**, *69*, 1095–1110. [CrossRef]
171. Smith, A. An update on osteoporosis management and fracture prevention strategies. *JAAPA* **2025**, *38*, 15–21. [CrossRef]

https://doi.org/10.3390/diagnostics16030470

172. Humphrey, M.B.; Russell, L.; Danila, M.I.; Fink, H.A.; Guyatt, G.; Cannon, M.; Caplan, L.; Gore, S.; Grossman, J.; Hansen, K.E.; et al. 2022 American College of Rheumatology Guideline for the Prevention and Treatment of Glucocorticoid-Induced Osteoporosis. *Arthritis Care Res.* **2023**, *75*, 2405–2419. [CrossRef]
173. Cooley, L.; Dendle, C.; Wolf, J.; Teh, B.W.; Chen, S.C.; Boutlis, C.; Thursky, K.A. Consensus guidelines for diagnosis, prophylaxis and management of Pneumocystis jirovecii pneumonia in patients with haematological and solid malignancies, 2014. *Intern. Med. J.* **2014**, *44*, 1350–1363. [CrossRef]
174. Stern, A.; Green, H.; Paul, M.; Vidal, L.; Leibovici, L. Prophylaxis for Pneumocystis pneumonia (PCP) in non-HIV immunocompromised patients. *Cochrane Database Syst. Rev.* **2014**, *2014*, CD005590. [CrossRef] [PubMed]
175. Muratore, F.; Kermani, T.A.; Crowson, C.S.; Green, A.B.; Salvarani, C.; Matteson, E.L.; Warrington, K.J. Large-vessel giant cell arteritis: A cohort study. *Rheumatology* **2015**, *54*, 463–470. [CrossRef]
176. Garcia-Martinez, A.; Hernandez-Rodriguez, J.; Arguis, P.; Paredes, P.; Segarra, M.; Lozano, E.; Nicolau, C.; Ramirez, J.; Lomena, F.; Josa, M.; et al. Development of aortic aneurysm/dilatation during the followup of patients with giant cell arteritis: A cross-sectional screening of fifty-four prospectively followed patients. *Arthritis Rheum.* **2008**, *59*, 422–430. [CrossRef]
177. Owen, C.E.; Yates, M.; Liew, D.F.L.; Poon, A.M.T.; Keen, H.I.; Hill, C.L.; Mackie, S.L. Imaging of giant cell arteritis—Recent advances. *Best. Pract. Res. Clin. Rheumatol.* **2023**, *37*, 101827. [CrossRef] [PubMed]
178. Nesher, G.; Berkun, Y.; Mates, M.; Baras, M.; Rubinow, A.; Sonnenblick, M. Low-dose aspirin and prevention of cranial ischemic complications in giant cell arteritis. *Arthritis Rheum.* **2004**, *50*, 1332–1337. [CrossRef] [PubMed]
179. Qureshi, A.; Halilu, F.; Serafi, S.W.; Hauptman, H.; Flack, T. Evidence-based Role of Aspirin in Giant Cell Arteritis: A Literature Review. *J. Community Hosp. Intern. Med. Perspect.* **2022**, *12*, 11–16. [CrossRef]
180. Sattui, S.E.; Corral, M.; O'Donnell, D.C. Illness Burden and Unmet Patient Needs in Giant Cell Arteritis: Current State and Future Prospects. *Open Access Rheumatol.* **2025**, *17*, 117–134. [CrossRef]
181. Martins-Martinho, J.; Ponte, A.; Dourado, E.; Khmelinskii, N.; Barreira, S.C.; Cruz-Machado, A.R.; Macieira, C.; Teixeira, V.; Rodrigues, A.M.; Telles-Correia, D.; et al. Anxiety and depression in patients with giant cell arteritis. *Rheumatol. Adv. Pract.* **2024**, *8*, rkae013. [CrossRef]
182. Patil, P.; Williams, M.; Maw, W.W.; Achilleos, K.; Elsideeg, S.; Dejaco, C.; Borg, F.; Gupta, S.; Dasgupta, B. Fast track pathway reduces sight loss in giant cell arteritis: Results of a longitudinal observational cohort study. *Clin. Exp. Rheumatol.* **2015**, *33*, 103–106.
183. Avasarala, J.; Das, S.; Keshavamurthy, S. Point-of-Care Ultrasound with Artificial Intelligence-Driven Diagnostics in Giant Cell Arteritis: Blindness Prevention on a Global Scale. *J. Rheumatol.* **2024**, *51*, 1040–1041. [CrossRef] [PubMed]
184. Almadhoun, M.K.; Yadav, M.; Shah, S.D.; Mushtaq, L.; Farooq, M.; Eric, N.P.; Farooq, U.; Zahid, M.; Iftikhar, A. The Future of Giant Cell Arteritis Diagnosis and Management: A Systematic Review of Artificial Intelligence and Predictive Analytics. *Cureus* **2024**, *16*, e75181. [CrossRef]
185. Vries, H.S.; van Praagh, G.D.; Nienhuis, P.H.; Alic, L.; Slart, R. A Machine Learning Model Based on Radiomic Features as a Tool to Identify Active Giant Cell Arteritis on [(18)F]FDG-PET Images During Follow-Up. *Diagnostics* **2025**, *15*, 367. [CrossRef]
186. Chen, S.; Nie, R.; Shen, X.; Wang, Y.; Luan, H.; Zeng, X.; Chen, Y.; Yuan, H. Associations between age, red cell distribution width and 180-day and 1-year mortality in giant cell arteritis patients: Mediation analyses and machine learning in a cohort study. *Arthritis Res. Ther.* **2025**, *27*, 25. [CrossRef]
187. Venerito, V.; Emmi, G.; Cantarini, L.; Leccese, P.; Fornaro, M.; Fabiani, C.; Lascaro, N.; Coladonato, L.; Mattioli, I.; Righetti, G.; et al. Validity of Machine Learning in Predicting Giant Cell Arteritis Flare After Glucocorticoids Tapering. *Front. Immunol.* **2022**, *13*, 860877. [CrossRef]
188. Bourgade, R.; Elhannani, M.; Loussouarn, D.; Guedon, A.; Peteri, R.; Allix-Beguec, C.; Berthier, M.; Toquet, C.; Espitia, O.; Roncato, C.; et al. Deep learning for giant cell arteritis diagnosis on temporal artery biopsy. *Comput. Biol. Med.* **2025**, *196*, 110707. [CrossRef]
189. Kim, S.; Fischetti, C.; Guy, M.; Hsu, E.; Fox, J.; Young, S.D. Artificial Intelligence (AI) Applications for Point of Care Ultrasound (POCUS) in Low-Resource Settings: A Scoping Review. *Diagnostics* **2024**, *14*, 1669. [CrossRef]
190. Varma, R.; Vajaranant, T.S.; Burkemper, B.; Wu, S.; Torres, M.; Hsu, C.; Choudhury, F.; McKean-Cowdin, R. Visual Impairment and Blindness in Adults in the United States: Demographic and Geographic Variations From 2015 to 2050. *JAMA Ophthalmol.* **2016**, *134*, 802–809. [CrossRef] [PubMed]
191. Seo, J.; Kim, Y.S. Ultrasound imaging and beyond: Recent advances in medical ultrasound. *Biomed. Eng. Lett.* **2017**, *7*, 57–58. [CrossRef]
192. Chen, X.; Yu, H.; Wei, N.; Ozcan, B.B.; An, G.; Wu, Q.; Wang, N. Diagnostic performance of contrast-enhanced ultrasound combined with shear wave elastography in differentiating benign from malignant breast lesions: A systematic review and meta-analysis. *Gland Surg.* **2023**, *12*, 1610–1623. [CrossRef] [PubMed]
193. Sabbaghan, M.; Nigam, S.; Kasabasic, I.; Manepalli, M.; Wang, P.; Fan, J. The Development and Challenges of PET/MRI Dual-Modality Imaging Probes-An Update. *J. Magn. Reson. Imaging* **2025**, *62*, 1245–1259. [CrossRef]

https://doi.org/10.3390/diagnostics16030470

194. Chaganti, J.; Woodford, H.; Tomlinson, S.; Dunkerton, S.; Brew, B. Black blood imaging of intracranial vessel walls. *Pract. Neurol.* **2020**, *21*, 101–107. [CrossRef]
195. Estrada, P.; Narvaez, J.; Moya, P.; Roig-Vilaseca, D.; Camacho, O.; Navarro, V.; Heredia, S.; Cerda, D.; Reina, D.; Corominas, H. Clinical Phenotypes of Giant Cell Arteritis: Insights into Complications and Survival Outcomes. *Eur. J. Rheumatol.* **2024**, *11*, 33–38. [CrossRef] [PubMed]
196. Sun, X.; Fang, C.; Jin, S.; Li, J.; Yang, Y.; Zeng, X.; Tian, X. Serum IL-6 level trajectory for predicting the effectiveness and safety of tocilizumab in the treatment of refractory Takayasu arteritis. *Eur. J. Intern. Med.* **2024**, *126*, 77–82. [CrossRef]
197. Tombetti, E.; Hysa, E.; Mason, J.C.; Cimmino, M.A.; Camellino, D. Blood Biomarkers for Monitoring and Prognosis of Large Vessel Vasculitides. *Curr. Rheumatol. Rep.* **2021**, *23*, 17. [CrossRef]
198. de Boysson, H.; Liozon, E.; Lambert, M.; Parienti, J.J.; Artigues, N.; Geffray, L.; Boutemy, J.; Ollivier, Y.; Maigne, G.; Ly, K.; et al. 18F-fluorodeoxyglucose positron emission tomography and the risk of subsequent aortic complications in giant-cell arteritis: A multicenter cohort of 130 patients. *Medicine* **2016**, *95*, e3851. [CrossRef]
199. Niu, N.; Manickam, V.; Kalari, K.R.; Moon, I.; Pelleymounter, L.L.; Eckloff, B.W.; Wieben, E.D.; Schaid, D.J.; Wang, L. Human glucocorticoid receptor alpha gene (NR3C1) pharmacogenomics: Gene resequencing and functional genomics. *J. Clin. Endocrinol. Metab.* **2009**, *94*, 3072–3084. [CrossRef]
200. Traves, P.G.; Murray, B.; Campigotto, F.; Galien, R.; Meng, A.; Di Paolo, J.A. JAK selectivity and the implications for clinical inhibition of pharmacodynamic cytokine signalling by filgotinib, upadacitinib, tofacitinib and baricitinib. *Ann. Rheum. Dis.* **2021**, *80*, 865–875. [CrossRef] [PubMed]
201. Zorc, R.; Redmond, C.; Sylvester, M.; Maclean, M.; Yamamoto de Almeida, L.; Quinn, K.A.; Tomelleri, A.; Campochiaro, C.; Dagna, L.; Gutierrez-Rodrigues, F.; et al. A coding single nucleotide polymorphism in the interleukin-6 receptor enhances IL-6 signalling in CD4 T cells and predicts treatment response to tocilizumab in giant cell arteritis. *Ann. Rheum. Dis.* **2025**, *84*, 1401–1411. [CrossRef] [PubMed]
202. Sargi, C.; Ducharme-Benard, S.; Benard, V.; Meunier, R.S.; Ross, C.; Makhzoum, J.P. Assessment and comparison of probability scores to predict giant cell arteritis. *Clin. Rheumatol.* **2024**, *43*, 357–365. [CrossRef] [PubMed]
203. Primorac, D.; Ciechanover, A. Personalized medicine: The future is here. *Croat. Med. J.* **2024**, *65*, 169–173. [CrossRef] [PubMed]
204. Wurmann, P.; Karsulovic, C.; Sabugo, F.; Hernandez, C.; Zamorano Soto, P.; Mac-Namara, M. Cranial versus Extracranial Involvement in Giant Cell Arteritis: 15 Years Retrospective Cohort Analysis. *Open Access Rheumatol.* **2022**, *14*, 97–101. [CrossRef]

https://doi.org/10.3390/diagnostics16030470

diagnostics

Interesting Images

Central Retinal Artery Occlusion Associated with Takayasu Arteritis

Sehreen Mumtaz [1,*], Claire Wilson [2], Prasanna Vibhute [3], Eric R. Eggenberger [4], Florentina Berianu [1] and Andy Abril [1]

1 Department of Rheumatology, Mayo Clinic Florida, Jacksonville, FL 32224, USA; berianu.florentina@mayo.edu (F.B.); abril.andy@mayo.edu (A.A.)
2 Department of Internal Medicine, Mayo Clinic Florida, Jacksonville, FL 32224, USA; wilson.claire@mayo.edu
3 Department of Radiology, Mayo Clinic Florida, Jacksonville, FL 32224, USA; vibhute.prasanna@mayo.edu
4 Department of Ophthalmology, Mayo Clinic Florida, Jacksonville, FL 32224, USA; eggenberger.eric@mayo.edu
* Correspondence: mumtaz.sehreen@mayo.edu

Abstract: Takayasu arteritis is a chronic inflammatory vasculitis with granulomatous panarteritis particularly impacting large vessels including the aorta and its branches, especially the subclavian arteries, with clinical manifestation dependent on the involved artery. Sequelae of the active disease vary, including stenosis, occlusions, or aneurysmal dilatations of the large vessels. The prevalence of Takayasu arteritis is higher in the Asian population and in Japan, but quite low in the United States, varying from 0.9–8.4 per million people. Ocular manifestations are rare and lead to a delay in diagnosis and appropriate treatment. Ocular manifestations include Takayasu retinopathy, anterior ischemic optic neuropathy (AION), retinal artery occlusion (RAO) and retinal vein occlusion (RVO). We present two cases in which central retinal artery occlusion (CRAO) was associated with Takayasu arteritis. CRAO is an ophthalmic emergency with an incidence of 1.9 per 100,000 person years in the United States; only 5% of cases are arteritic, which can be observed with inflammatory vasculitides secondary to the formation of immune deposits.

Keywords: Takayasu arteritis; retinal artery occlusion; large-vessel vasculitis

A 35-year-old woman with a prior history of left central retinal artery occlusion and bilateral sensorineural hearing loss, initially concerning with respect to neurosarcoidosis (never histologically proven), presented for clinical follow-up. She had a complicated disease course dating back many years, involving different specialists, and including fluctuating hearing loss partially responsive to corticosteroids necessitating cochlear implants and developed central retinal occlusion of the left eye (Figures 1 and 2). This was concerning with respect to possible underlying inflammatory conditions such as neurosarcoidosis or Susac syndrome (MRI atypical sans corpus lesion), and she received IV immunoglobulin treatment. When she returned for follow-up, she had complaints of episodes of confusion, but quiescent symptoms without visual change, status post adalimumab and methotrexate addition. She sought emergency care for new transient arm numbness and confusion, and a neck CTA revealed carotid bulb circumferential thickening suggestive of vasculitis. A rind of soft tissue thickening involving the distal half of the common carotid artery, carotid bifurcation and the proximal internal and external carotid arteries was visualized. There was smooth narrowing of the encased carotid artery lumen, producing roughly 50% diameter stenosis of the distal common carotid artery. A small ulceration was noted on the left carotid bulb (Figures 3–5). The patient was initiated on infliximab with IV methylprednisolone and close follow-up with neurology and vascular medicine for management of Takayasu arteritis.

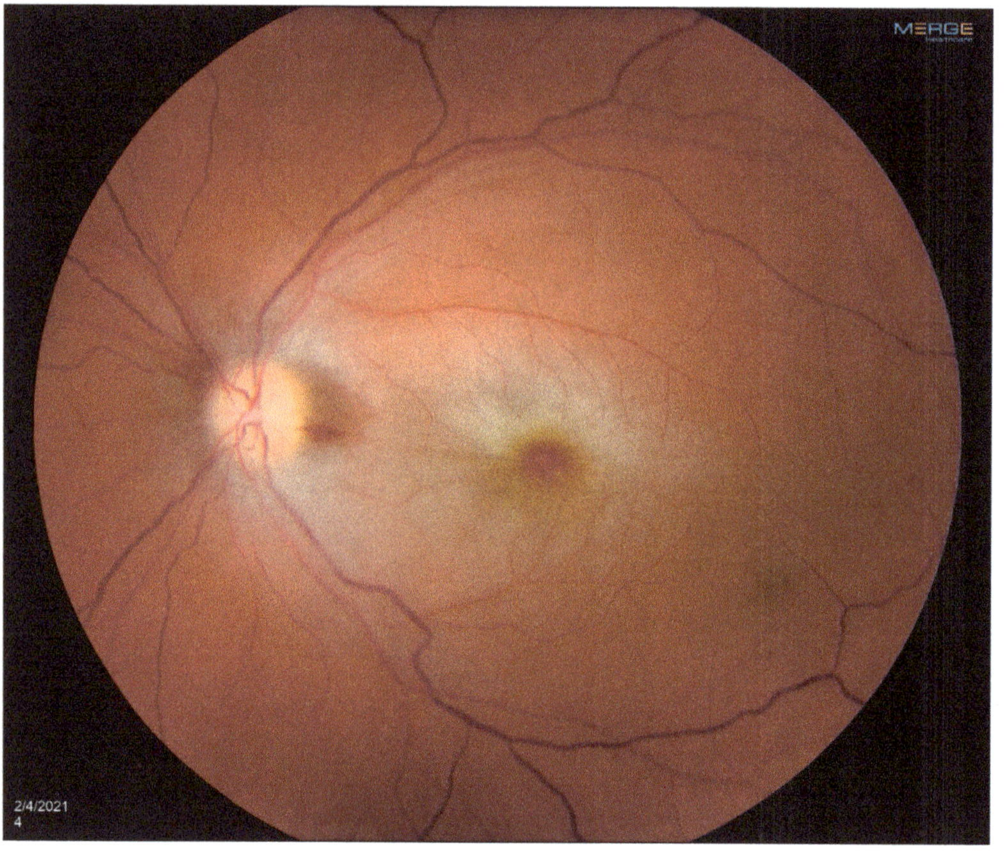

Figure 1. OS fundus photograph showing central retinal artery occlusion with characteristic cherry red spot and attenuated blood vessels. Patient developed left central retinal artery occlusion years prior to vasculitis diagnosis with loss of vision at a young age.

A 56-year-old woman was diagnosed with Takayasu arteritis in 1991, and initially treated with glucocorticoids for several years. Initial symptoms included constitutional symptoms and left-sided carotidynia. She had markedly elevated inflammatory markers and anemia at disease onset, and later developed erythema nodosum. Imaging studies in the early phase of her illness revealed moderate stenosis of the right subclavian artery and marked thickening of the left common carotid. She was subsequently treated with methotrexate and cyclosporine, and eventually her disease went into remission. In 2014, an MR angiogram of the chest showed radiographic evidence of vessel wall edema in the aorta, and at that time, the patient was started on mycophenolate mofetil. In November 2017, the patient developed blurry vision and there was leakage on her fluorescein angiogram, which was felt to be nonspecific. She was taken off mycophenolate due to no evidence of active vasculitis in clinical or laboratory findings. She was in remission; however, she required ascending aorta hemiarch repair and aortic valve replacement (and was subsequently on warfarin) for a dilated aortic root of 61 mm with histopathology showing healed arteritis. Two years later, she developed a paracentral scotoma in the left eye and was diagnosed by outside Ophthalmology as having branch retinal artery occlusion by retinal imaging, with suspected embolic disease in the context of subtherapeutic anticoagulation.

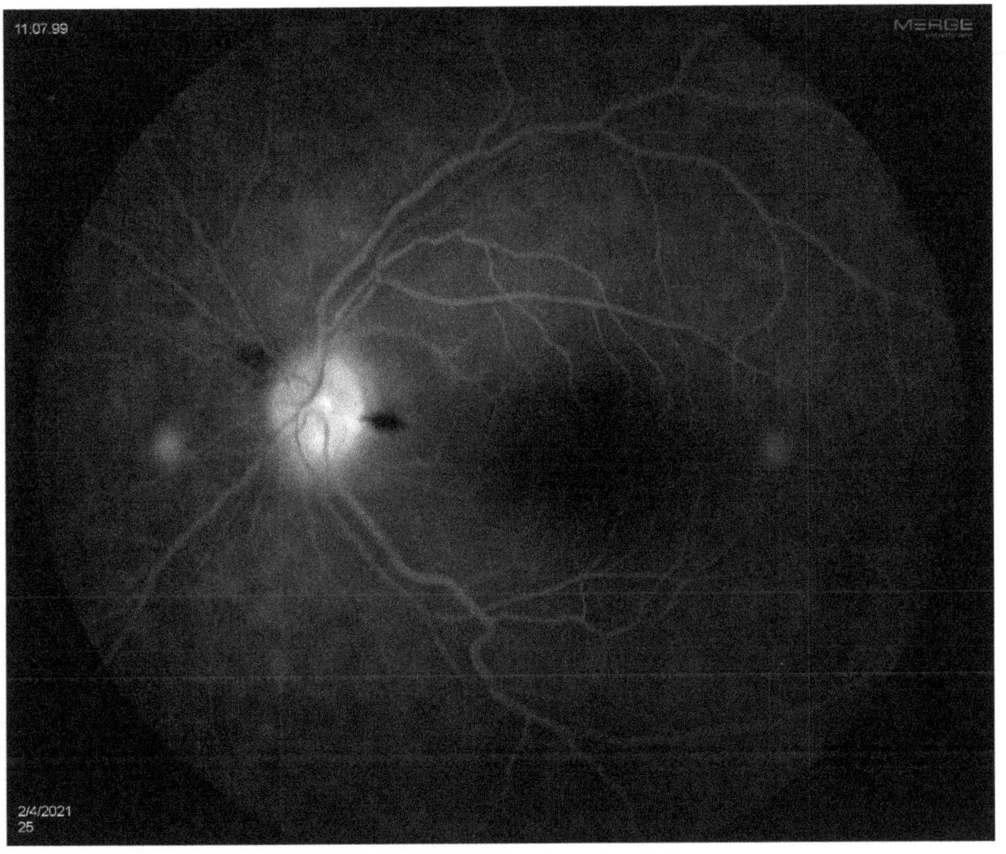

Figure 2. OS fluorescein angiogram showing arterial narrowing with some stain of vessels on the superior optic disc.

Clinical characteristics of patients with ocular manifestations and Takayasu's arteritis have been reported to be similar to those of patients without ocular manifestations with a mean age in the third decade of life and a majority of Asian origin. Ocular manifestations of Takayasu arteritis can be seen in a wide range (8.1–68%) of patients [1]. Apart from two case-based systematic reviews, the current literature is lacking in describing the extent of ocular involvement in Takayasu arteritis [1,2]. The current classification of Takayasu arteritis does not include visual changes, and consequently no ophthalmological examination is recommended, even after diagnosis, and ocular manifestations can go unnoticed.

A study by Pasko et al. noted ocular manifestations presenting prior to diagnosis of Takayasu arteritis in 74.6% of cases [3]. This may be explained by cases in which initial manifestations included constitutional symptoms that were non-specific. Limitation of flow in the carotid artery results in chronic ischemia and hypoperfusion retinopathy, and ocular ischemic syndrome may be of consequence [4]. It remains imperative to distinguish and categorize this ocular disorder and pursue retinal angiograms.

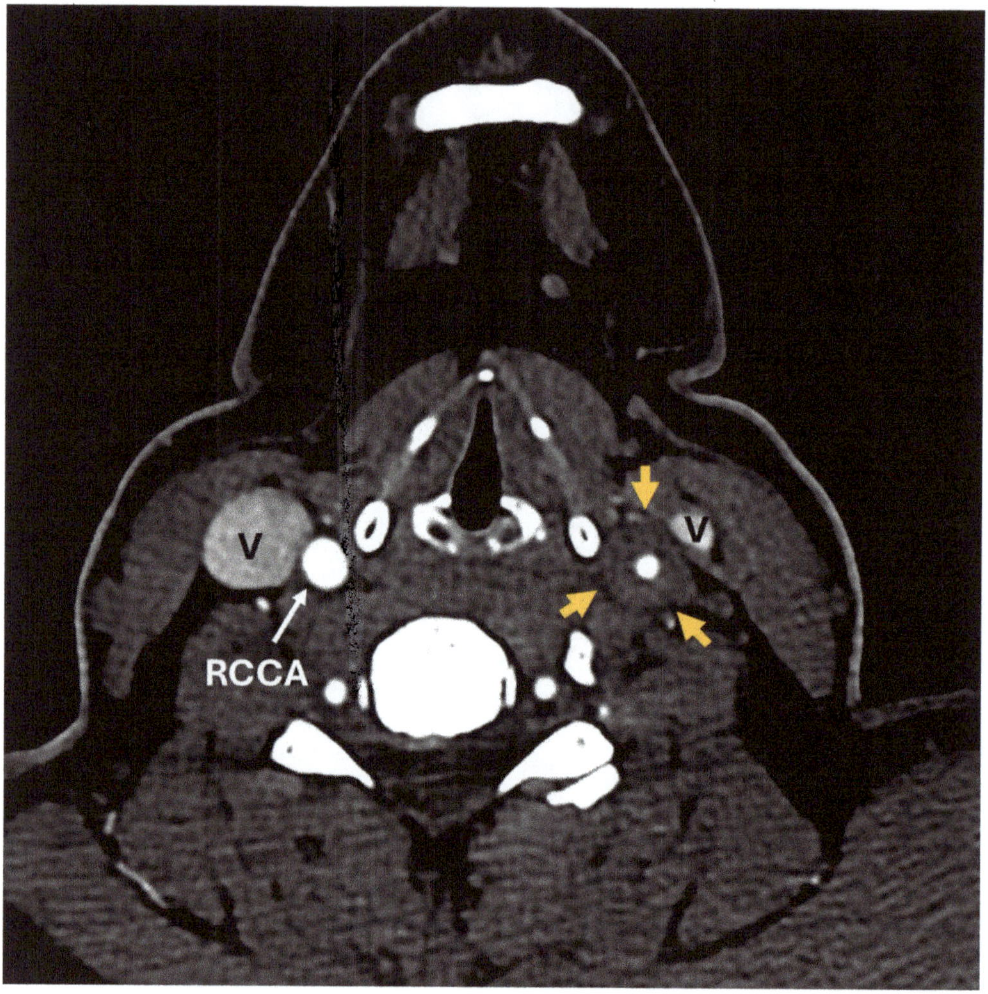

Figure 3. CT angiogram. Axial images below the level of carotid bifurcation show diffuse circumferential thickening of common carotid artery (CCA) and internal carotid artery (ICA) walls on the left side (orange arrows).

A study from 1994 pointed to the presence of Takayasu's retinopathy as a statistically significant poor prognostic factor [5]. Mirouse et al. associated Takayasu retinopathy independently with mortality and complication-free survival [6]. Reportedly, 64% of CRAO patients develop new vascular risk factors after a retinal occlusive event, implying this population of patients is prone to a secondary ischemic event and needs risk factor assessment [7]. Although medical management is the recommended initial management for Takayasu arteritis, patients who have vascular complications may require surgical interventions and endovascular procedures [8]. Medical management includes ocular massage, hyperbaric oxygen therapy, and intravenous tissue-type plasminogen activator; however, these are associated with risks, including mobilization of the embolus and exacerbating macular edema. Endovascular treatments, including intra-arterial thrombolysis, have shown promising results; however, they require exceptional skill to perform [9].

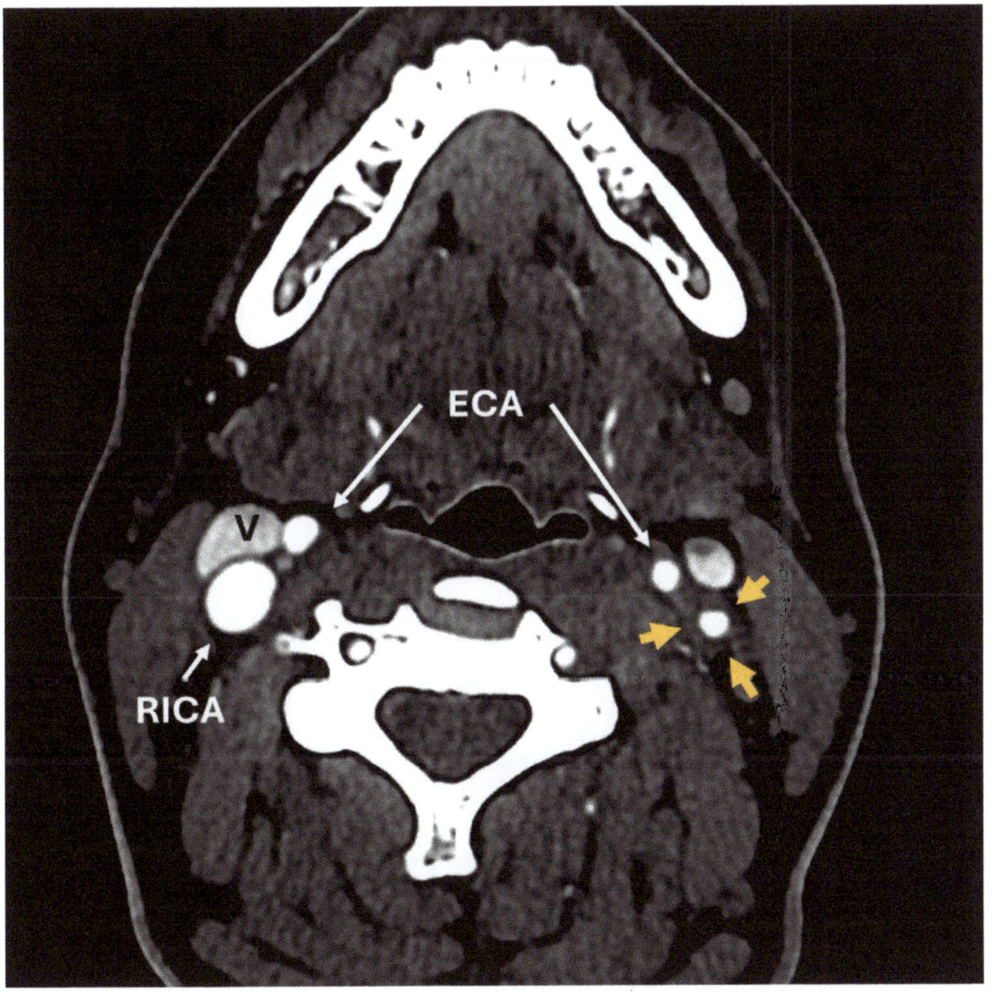

Figure 4. CT angiogram. Axial images above the level of carotid bifurcation show diffuse circumferential thickening of common carotid artery (CCA) and internal carotid artery (ICA) walls on the left side (orange arrows). Compare this to the normal wall thickness of the right carotid artery. White arrows point to the right common carotid artery (RCCA), right internal carotid artery (RICA) and bilateral external carotid arteries (ECAs). Internal jugular veins: (V). A repeat CT neck angiogram with contrast revealed a left-sided diffuse circumferential rim of soft tissue thickening involving the left carotid artery, which was concerning with respect to large-vessel vasculitis. It is unclear how long the carotid bulb thickening had been present.

Although information on ocular ischemia surgical management for Takayasu arteritis patients is limited, case series and case reports have demonstrated favorable results of balloon angioplasty and endovascular stenting in Takayasu retinopathy patients [1]. Adopting routine fundus fluorescein angiography for surveillance in patients with Takayasu arteritis may be beneficial. Newer diagnostic techniques, especially optical coherence tomography (OCT) angiography (OCTA), and novel diagnostics to assess retina perfusion must be investigated [1].

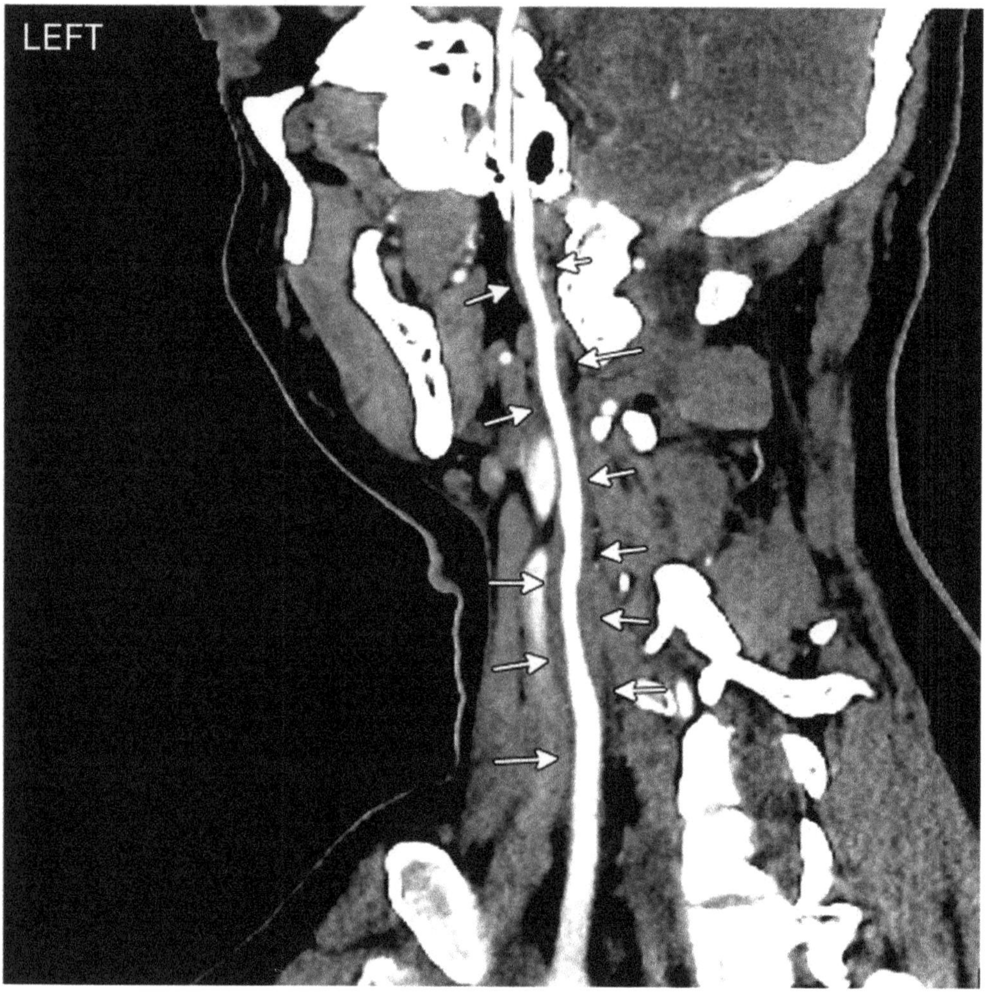

Figure 5. CT angiogram. Left carotid artery centerline reconstructions show diffuse arterial wall thickening (white arrows).

In young patients with visual loss and deficits, it is imperative to recall Takayasu arteritis as a potential suspect, even though such cases are rare, because it can translate into a meaningful difference in outcomes with proper management. Raising ophthalmological awareness of this association and increasing education regarding pursuing comprehensive diagnostic testing is crucial. Further investigation of arteritic CRAO in Takayasu arteritis patients is needed for the development and implementation of enhanced therapeutic techniques.

Author Contributions: Conceptualization, S.M., C.W. and A.A.; investigation, C.W. and S.M.; writing—original draft preparation, S.M. and C.W.; writing—review and editing, S.M. and C.W.; visualization, S.M., C.W., P.V., E.R.E. and A.A.; supervision, A.A. and F.B.; project administration, A.A. and F.B. All authors have read and agreed to the published version of the manuscript.

Funding: This study received no external funding.

Institutional Review Board Statement: This study was deemed exempt by the IRB at Mayo Clinic 1/31/24. IRB number 24-000157.

Informed Consent Statement: Informed consent was obtained from all subjects involved in this study.

Data Availability Statement: Written informed consent has been obtained from the patient to publish this paper.

Conflicts of Interest: The authors declare no conflicts of interest.

References

1. Zeng, Y.; Duan, J.; Ge, G.; Zhang, M. Therapeutic Management of Ocular Ischemia in Takayasu's Arteritis: A Case-Based Systematic Review. *Front. Immunol.* **2022**, *12*, 791278. [CrossRef] [PubMed]
2. Sanchez-Alvarez, C.; Crowson, C.S.; Koster, M.J.; Warrington, K.J. Prevalence of Takayasu Arteritis: A Population-based Study. *J. Rheumatol.* **2021**, *48*, 952. [CrossRef] [PubMed]
3. Szydełko-Paśko, U.; Przeździecka-Dołyk, J.; Nowak, Ł.; Małyszczak, A.; Misiuk-Hojło, M. Ocular Manifestations of Takayasu's Arteritis—A Case-Based Systematic Review and Meta-Analysis. *J. Clin. Med.* **2023**, *12*, 3745. [CrossRef] [PubMed]
4. Guclu, H.; Gurlu, V.P.; Ozal, S.A.; Guclu, O. Central Retinal Artery Occlusion in Takayasu's Arteritis as the First Presentation of the Disease. *Case Rep. Ophthalmol. Med.* **2016**, *2016*, 6492513. [CrossRef] [PubMed]
5. Ishikawa, K.; Maetani, S. Long-term outcome for 120 Japanese patients with Takayasu's disease. Clinical and statistical analyses of related prognostic factors. *Circulation* **1994**, *90*, 1855–1860. [CrossRef] [PubMed]
6. Mirouse, A.; Biard, L.; Comarmond, C.; Lambert, M.; Mekinian, A.; Ferfar, Y.; Kahn, J.-E.; Benhamou, Y.; Chiche, L.; Koskas, F.; et al. Overall survival and mortality risk factors in Takayasu's arteritis: A multicenter study of 318 patients. *J. Autoimmun.* **2018**, *96*, 35–39. [CrossRef] [PubMed]
7. Varma, D.D.; Cugati, S.; Lee, A.W.; Chen, C.S. A review of central retinal artery occlusion: Clinical presentation and management. *Eye* **2013**, *27*, 688–697. [CrossRef] [PubMed]
8. Maz, M.; Chung, S.A.; Abril, A.; Langford, C.A.; Gorelik, M.; Guyatt, G.; Archer, A.M.; Conn, D.L.; Full, K.A.; Grayson, P.C.; et al. 2021 American College of Rheumatology/Vasculitis Foundation Guideline for the Management of Giant Cell Arteritis and Takayasu Arteritis. *Arthritis Rheumatol.* **2021**, *73*, 1349–1365. [CrossRef] [PubMed]
9. Dagra, A.; Lucke-Wold, B.; McGrath, K.; Mehkri, I.; Mehkri, Y.; Davidson, C.G.; Gilberstadt, N.; Douglas, B.W.; Hoh, B. Central Retinal Artery Occlusion: A Review of Pathophysiological Features and Management. *Stroke Vasc. Interv. Neurol.* **2024**, *4*, e000977. [CrossRef]

diagnostics MDPI

Interesting Images

Giant Cell Arteritis: Can Simple Ultrasound Examination Prevent Complex Consequences?

Wiktoria Stańska *, Robert Kruszewski, Aleksandra Juszkiewicz, Artur Bachta and Witold Tłustochowicz

Department of Internal Medicine and Rheumatology, Military Institute of Medicine—National Research Institute, 04-141 Warsaw, Poland; rkruszewski@wim.mil.pl (R.K.); ajuszkiewicz@wim.mil.pl (A.J.); abachta@wim.mil.pl (A.B.); wtlustochowicz@wim.mil.pl (W.T.)
* Correspondence: wstanska@gmail.com

Abstract: Giant cell arteritis (GCA) is a rare disease of the arteries, occurring mainly in the elderly. Although the involvement of temporal arteries can be mostly symptomatic, the occlusion of ophthalmic arteries has severe consequences. GCA affecting temporal arteries is an emergency requiring quick commencement of treatment with glucocorticoids due to the serious consequences of neglect—blindness. According to the new guidelines released by EULAR, ultrasound is the tool of choice in support of the clinical diagnosis of giant cell arteritis, replacing temporal artery biopsy (TAB), as it is a sensitive and non-invasive method that is widely available. The main limitation is that the reliability of this imaging is based on the technical expertise of ultrasonographers. However, performing imaging should not delay commencing the treatment. In this work, we present ultrasound images from a case report of a 74-year-old female patient where difficulties in establishing a diagnosis led to vision loss in both eyes. In this example, we describe the ultrasound findings in giant cell arteritis, emphasizing its usefulness in supporting a diagnosis of GCA.

Keywords: GCA; vision loss; headache; ultrasonography; EULAR; OMERACT

Giant cell arteritis (GCA) is a rare disease of the arteries, affecting large and medium vessels, with cranial arteries—branches of carotid arteries—the most frequently involved. The condition occurs mainly in the elderly population, predominantly over 50 [1]. As the pathophysiology of GCA involves myointimal proliferation, it inevitably leads to ischemic events due to vessel occlusion [1]. Because of the involvement of cranial arteries in most cases, the signs and symptoms mainly include headaches of new onset in the temples and jaw claudication. Scalp tenderness and, importantly, visual disturbances are not uncommon [2]. That is why new-onset headaches, especially in the elderly population, should alert healthcare professionals. However, there are also general non-specific symptoms, such as weight loss, fatigue, and fever, with elevated inflammatory markers [3].

On physical examination, tender and thickened temporal arteries can be found. Giant cell arteritis, if left untreated, leads to blindness in 30% to 50% of patients, and vision loss is irreversible if the steroid treatment is not administered within a few hours [4]. The awareness of the doctors who consult the patient first is crucial as the patient requires rheumatology consultation immediately to shorten the diagnostic path and implement treatment without delay [1].

A 74-year-old female patient was consulted by a family medicine doctor several times because of neck pain radiating to the temporal areas of the head. The patient had a history of hypertension and was treated with lisinopril and hydrochlorothiazide (10 + 12.5 mg/day). The pain did not respond to a short course of dexibuprofen, and the painful sensation gradually increased. Moreover, she began having headaches, night sweats, edema of the submandibular area, and trismus also occurred. The condition was treated as a common cold with amoxicillin with clavulanic acid. However, the patient started experiencing light flashes two days after administering the antibiotic. The vision symptoms persisted, and additionally, nine days later, the patient's vision deteriorated in the right eye. The day after that, the patient reported difficulties with color vision. Eventually, the day after, blindness occurred.

Thus, the patient was urgently admitted to the local Ophthalmology Department. The patient presented with anisocoria (L > P), the pupillary light response was medium, and she denied having any sense of light. No pursuit movements of the eyes were observed. Eventually, fundus examination revealed papilledema of the left eye and right optic nerve atrophy.

In the Ophthalmology Department, imaging was performed, including CT of the face, MRI of the orbits, and head MRI. None of them showed any significant abnormalities. Laboratory blood tests revealed an elevated CRP level of 109.8 mg/L. Upon the findings mentioned above, giant cell arteritis was suspected.

Three intravenous pulses of 1000 mg of methylprednisolone were administered on three consecutive days, then switched to oral dexamethasone at a dose of 16 mg/day. As an adjuvant therapy, vinpocetine i.v. was added. Regardless of the treatment, the vision did not improve.

Therefore, the patient was referred to the Clinical Rheumatology Department to continue the evaluations and modify the treatment. On admission, she presented with vision loss in both eyes and swelling of both temporal arteries. The erythrocyte sedimentation rate (ESR) and CRP were back to normal after initial therapy in the Ophthalmology Department, with values of 11 mm/h and 1 mg/L, respectively. There were also no significant abnormalities in other laboratory tests at that point.

In the rheumatology ward, CT angiography was carried out, and it showed a lack of contrast filling in the ophthalmic arteries. An ultrasound examination showed thickened walls of the temporal and carotid arteries with a halo sign (Figure 1B–D) and positive compression sign (Figure 2). Upon analyzing the whole clinical picture and imaging studies, the primary diagnosis of giant cell arteritis was confirmed. Therapy with glucocorticoids was continued with a daily dose tapered to 45 mg of prednisone on the day of discharge. Methotrexate at an initial dose of 20 mg per week in subcutaneous injections was added, with a planned rapid escalation to a dose of 25 mg/week. As a standard approach in methotrexate therapy, the patient was advised to take folic acid once weekly at a dose of 15 mg. The patient was also consulted by an ophthalmologist once more. The eye specialist recommended a referral to rehabilitation, aiming to improve the quality of life with blindness and enable the patient to adapt to functioning in new conditions. The patient was discharged from the hospital in a general good condition and was further evaluated in an ambulatory mode.

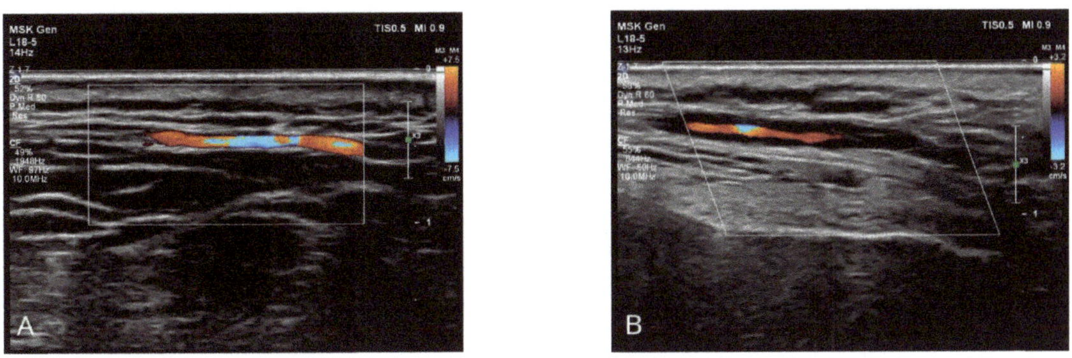

Figure 1. *Cont.*

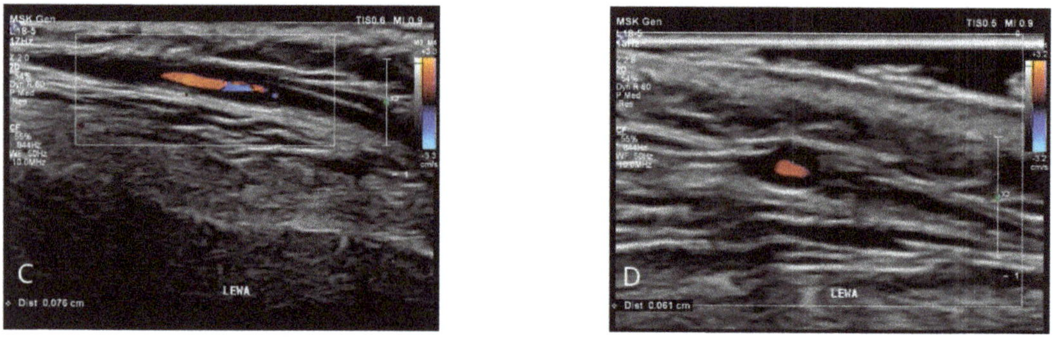

Figure 1. Ultrasonographic imaging of the temporal artery. Comparison of ultrasound images of an unchanged temporal artery (**A**) and inflammation of the temporal artery in giant cell arteritis (**B**). Both longitudinal (**C**) and transverse (**D**) views of the inflamed artery reveal the narrowing of the arterial lumen and homogenous, hypoechoic wall thickening (white markers), well delineated towards the luminal side, known as the "halo sign" [5].

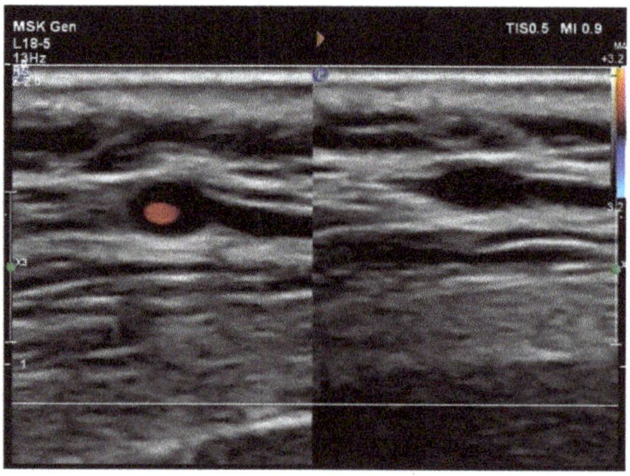

Figure 2. Detection of arterial inflammation by "compression sign". Pressure applied with an ultrasound probe collapses the artery. The resulting restriction of blood flow is confirmed by the absence or limitation of a Doppler signal in the arterial lumen. However, the thickened inflamed arterial wall remains visible as a hypoechoic area contrasting with the mid-echogenic to hyperechoic surrounding tissue [5].

The diagnostic process of GCA is challenging as some patients may present non-specific symptoms, mimicking other, less urgent conditions. Moreover, when a patient's clinical picture suggests GCA, it requires clinical experience and expertise to establish a prompt diagnosis, as a delay leads inevitably to serious consequences such as blindness [1]. Vision deterioration is often one of the first signs of GCA, as happened in the case of our patient. Recent registrations of patients with GCA showed the possible risk factors that are associated with visual involvement, which are older age and jaw claudication, while polymyalgia rheumatica, fever, a longer duration of symptoms, and a higher ESR lowered the risk of visual symptoms [6].

Imaging is recommended for every patient suspected of GCA. The "golden standard" for diagnosing giant cell arteritis has been performing temporal artery biopsy or conventional angiography for decades. However, according to the 2023 update of the EULAR [7] recommendations, ultrasound can be the first-line imaging test to be performed in cases of the suspicion of giant cell arteritis, thanks to its high diagnostic value (pooled sensitivity from studies with low RoB of 88% and a specificity of 96%). The imaging studies aim to investigate the mural inflammatory changes in the affected arteries [7].

Due to the overlap of intra- and extra-cranial phenotypes of giant cell arteritis, according to the guidelines, axillary arteries should also be included in the ultrasound examination. It broadens the diagnostic yield and provides higher sensitivities than checking temporal arteries only [8]. In cases where neither temporal nor axillary artery scans are diagnostic, additional vessels can be included in the examination, such as facial, occipital, carotid, vertebral, subclavian, and femoral arteries, as well as the aorta [7].

According to European guidelines, TAB is still an adequate option, especially when there is no access to imaging or the sonographer's expertise is insufficient [7]. The preponderance of any of these diagnostic tools is still contentious, as seen in discrepancies between European and American guidelines for giant cell arteritis [8,9]. While the EULAR guidelines are raising the predominance of ultrasound over temporal artery biopsy, the American College of Rheumatology and Vasculitis Foundation are still reserved towards comprehensive utilization of ultrasound [9]. TAB is put conditionally in the first place as an optimal diagnostic approach, with ultrasound imaging only as a complementary tool in centers with appropriate training and expertise. Such hesitancy towards ultrasound is explained by the lesser experience of rheumatologists and radiologists in the US in using ultrasound to diagnose the involvement of temporal arteries in GCA [8].

It is worth emphasizing that even though imaging is recommended as a support to establish a diagnosis, it should not delay commencing the treatment because of the severe consequences—permanent vision loss and other ischemic complications of GCA [7]. Treatment consisting of steroids should be implemented as soon as possible. It was shown that the delay in introducing steroids when visual disturbances/visual loss are already present is the strongest risk factor for permanent blindness [1]. It was shown that performing an ultrasound examination after introducing glucocorticoid treatment gives as reliable results as performing it before starting the treatment. Therefore, it is recommended that an ultrasound, if it cannot be performed before introducing treatment, should be carried out within 72 h of pharmacotherapy [7].

Ultrasound is a readily available non-invasive method for quickly diagnosing giant cell arteritis. This is compared to angio-CT, which has several drawbacks, such as it requires an imaging center in a hospital, the procedure takes more time, radiation exposure occurs, and the patient may exhibit contraindications for administering a contrast agent. Moreover, the waiting time for a CT scan may be too long for patients with conditions requiring rapid action, such as giant cell arteritis [7]. Regardless of the undisputable advantage of ultrasound over other imaging methods, it has some limitations. It requires trained and well-qualified practitioners whose experience in ultrasonography of head and neck vessels can diagnose the pathologies with confidence and a low risk of error [7].

All patients presenting typical signs and symptoms of GCA and raised inflammatory markers (C-reactive protein, Erythrocyte Sedimentation Rate) should be promptly sent to a specialistic center with state-of-the-art imaging and TAB for a work-up of a multidisciplinary team consisting of a rheumatologist, radiologist, ophthalmologist, and/or neurologist [1,7–9]. It is essential that the diagnostic process is prompt and without any unnecessary delay so the patient can receive the proper treatment on time by the appropriate team of healthcare professionals. Prolonged diagnosis, and thereby delayed treatment, results in irreversible consequences [1]. That is why the awareness and proper training of doctors who consult the patient first—at a low level of the healthcare ladder—is important, so they can refer patients to fast-track clinics that are properly prepared for such emergencies [1,7–9].

Due to the non-specific nature of the symptoms, the diagnosis of GCA is difficult. That is why this pathology is considered to be underdiagnosed, because of the low degree of clinical suspicion [9]. Moreover, as patients with GCA are referred to the hospital from Primary Care or out-of-hospital emergencies, it implies the need for comprehensive protocols that enable bidirectional communication channels guaranteeing referrals between specialists and the continuity of the care between the facilities. This could coordinate the services involved in the diagnostic and treatment process [9]. Another solution for improving the quality of care of patients with GCA is developing training sessions to continue the clinical education for healthcare professionals, at all levels of care involved in the process of the management of GCA [9].

The diagnosis of GCA is established upon the clinical picture and high inflammatory markers, supported by imaging or temporal artery biopsy. Giant cell arteritis with affected temporal arteries is an emergency, requiring immediate intervention and prompt administration of high doses of glucocorticosteroids. In these cases, the prognosis depends on the healthcare professionals, as a quick response and proper management can save many lives every year [1].

Author Contributions: Conceptualization, W.S. and R.K.; investigation, W.S., R.K. and A.J.; resources, R.K. and A.J.; writing—original draft preparation, W.S.; writing—review and editing, W.S. and R.K.; visualization, W.S.; supervision, R.K., A.B. and W.T.; funding acquisition, R.K., A.B. and W.T. All authors have read and agreed to the published version of the manuscript.

Funding: This research received no external funding.

Institutional Review Board Statement: Not applicable.

Informed Consent Statement: Informed consent was obtained from all subjects involved in the study. Due to the patient's vision loss, we could not obtain written informed consent. However, the patient verbally provided consent.

Data Availability Statement: No new data were created or analyzed in this study.

Conflicts of Interest: The authors declare no conflicts of interest.

References

1. Hellmich, B.; Agueda, A.; Monti, S.; Buttgereit, F.; Boysson, H.d.; Brouwer, E.; Cassie, R.; Cid, M.C.; Dasgupta, B.; Dejaco, C.; et al. 2018 Update of the EULAR recommendations for the management of large vessel vasculitis. *Ann. Rheum. Dis.* **2020**, *79*, 19–30. [CrossRef]
2. Ponte, C.; Martins-Martinho, J.; Luqmani, R.A. Diagnosis of giant cell arteritis. *Rheumatology* **2020**, *59*, iii5–iii16. [CrossRef] [PubMed]
3. Chen, J.J.; Leavitt, J.A.; Fang, C.; Crowson, C.S.; Matteson, E.L.; Warrington, K.J. Evaluating the incidence of arteritic ischemic optic neuropathy and other causes of vision loss from giant cell arteritis. *Ophthalmology* **2016**, *123*, 1999–2003. [CrossRef] [PubMed]
4. Hemmig, A.K.; Aschwanden, M.; Seiler, S.; Berger, C.T.; Köhn, P.; Kyburz, D.; Mensch, N.; Staub, D.; Stegert, M.; Imfeld, S.; et al. Long delay from symptom onset to first consultation contributes to permanent vision loss in patients with giant cell arteritis: A cohort study. *RMD Open* **2023**, *9*, e002866. [CrossRef] [PubMed]
5. Bruyn, G.A.; Iagnocco, A.; Naredo, E.; Balint, P.V.; Gutierrez, M.; Hammer, H.B.; Collado, P.; Filippou, G.; Schmidt, W.A.; Joulin, S.J.; et al. OMERACT definitions for ultrasonographic pathologies and elementary lesions of rheumatic disorders 15 years on. *J. Rheumatol.* **2019**, *46*, 1388–1393. [CrossRef] [PubMed]
6. Molina-Collada, J.; Domínguez-Álvaro, M.; Melero-González, R.B.; Fernández-Fernández, E.; Silva-Díaz, M.; Valero, J.A.; González, I.; Martín, J.S.; Narváez, J.; Calvo, I.; et al. Visual manifestations in giant cell arteritis: Identification of risk factors from the ARTESER Registry. *Rheumatology* **2024**, *10*, keae042. [CrossRef] [PubMed]
7. Dejaco, C.; Ramiro, S.; Bond, M.; Bosch, P.; Ponte, C.; Mackie, S.L.; Bley, T.A.; Blockmans, D.; Brolin, S.; Bolek, E.C.; et al. EULAR recommendations for the use of imaging in large vessel vasculitis in clinical practice: 2023 update. *Ann. Rheum. Dis.* **2024**, *83*, 741–751. [CrossRef] [PubMed]
8. Maz, M.; Chung, S.A.; Abril, A.; Langford, C.A.; Gorelik, M.; Guyatt, G.; Archer, A.M.; Conn, D.L.; Full, K.A.; Grayson, P.C.; et al. 2021 American College of Rheumatology/Vasculitis Foundation Guideline for the Management of Giant Cell Arteritis and Takayasu Arteritis. *Arthritis Rheumatol.* **2021**, *73*, 1349–1365. [CrossRef] [PubMed]
9. González García, A.; Del Arco, C.; Lucas Fernández, D.; Frías-Vargas, M.; Guillán, M.; Méndez-Bailón, M.; Ruiz Grinspan, M.; Aguado-Castaño, A.C.; Fraile Maya, J.; Latorre González, G.; et al. Executive summary on the optimization of the multidisciplinary and integrated approach to polymyalgia rheumatica and giant cell arteritis in Madrid region. *Rev. Clin. Esp.* **2024**, *224*, 48–56. [CrossRef] [PubMed]

diagnostics

MDPI

Article

Long-Term Follow-Up in Patients with Large-Vessel Vasculitis Applying Extracranial and Transcranial Duplex Sonography

Johanna Härtl, Sebastian Lambrecht, Felix Hess, Achim Berthele, Silke Wunderlich and Enayatullah Baki *

Department of Neurology, TUM Universitätsklinikum Klinikum Rechts der Isar, School of Medicine and Health, Technical University of Munich, Ismaningerstr. 22, 81675 München, Germany
* Correspondence: enayatullah.baki@mri.tum.de

Abstract

Background: Although large-vessel vasculitis (LVV) can affect both the anterior and posterior intracranial circulation, routine neurosonographic follow-up, including transcranial duplex sonography, has not been established. We aimed to characterize patients with giant cell arteritis (GCA) and Takayasu arteritis (TAK) regarding the detection of progressive or new-onset inflammatory vessel changes by using neurosonography, and to assess the impact on medical or interventional treatment strategies. **Methods:** We retrospectively identified all patients with LVV treated at our neurological department between January 2015 and October 2025 with at least one neurosonographic follow-up examination. Baseline and follow-up sonographic data, clinical characteristics, medical therapy, and interventional treatments were analyzed. **Results:** In total, 21 LVV patients (GCA, n = 16; TAK, n = 5) underwent sonographic follow-up (GCA: median 28 (2–106) months, 4.5 (2–33) sonographic assessments; TAK: 75 (33–255) months, 14 (4–60) sonographic assessments). Isolated or combined, progressive or new-onset intra- and extracranial arterial disease was detected in seven of the 16 GCA patients (43.8%), of whom three (18.8%) presented with ischemic stroke. Medical treatment was adapted in four progressive cases. In two patients, additional interventional treatment was performed. Among TAK, two of five (40%) patients showed progressive sonographic changes, with one patient experiencing an ischemic stroke requiring endovascular treatment for progressive common carotid artery stenosis and one patient showing asymptomatic intracranial ICA involvement. **Conclusions:** Progressive and symptomatic involvement of intracranial carotid and vertebral arteries is a frequent finding in patients with LVV. These changes can be effectively detected through comprehensive neurosonographic follow-up, including transcranial ultrasound assessment.

Keywords: giant cell arteritis; Takayasu arteritis; duplex sonography follow-up

1. Introduction

In addition to its diagnostic value, vascular ultrasound is increasingly used to monitor disease activity and the treatment response in large-vessel vasculitis (LVV) [1–6]. For giant cell arteritis (GCA), ultrasound examination of the extracranial arteries is routinely considered to monitor treatment and to detect disease relapses since IL-6 antibody therapy obscures laboratory markers of inflammation. The Outcome Measures in Rheumatology (OMERACT) Large Vessel Vasculitis Ultrasound Working Group recently developed a standardized ultrasound score (OGUS) for GCA, designed to quantify disease activity and enable longitudinal monitoring [7]. The OGUS includes intima-media thickness (IMT)

 https://doi.org/10.3390/diagnostics16030455

quotient measurements of the main branch of the superficial temporal artery, its frontal and parietal branches, and the axillary arteries, normalized to established reference values. Higher OGUS values may reflect greater inflammatory activity, potentially hold prognostic relevance, and indicate treatment failure [8]. Most current sonographic follow-up protocols for GCA rely on the OGUS or related IMT-based assessments, while only a few studies have additionally evaluated the extracranial carotid and vertebral arteries [1–3,9–11], and none have evaluated sonographic measurements of intracranial arteries. More recently, transorbital sonography measuring peak systolic velocity (PSV) of the central retinal artery has been applied, which may complement ophthalmologic evaluation and aid in the detection of ischemic complications in GCA [12,13].

Similarly, for Takayasu disease, the sonographic follow-up of brachiocephalic artery changes, with a focus on IMT measurements, neovascularization, and assessment of echogenicity, has proven valuable for long-term follow-up and monitoring of inflammatory vascular changes [14–19].

Neurosonographic follow-up examinations of intracranial arteries have not been systematically implemented in current monitoring protocols for either TAK or GCA. This gap persists despite intracranial arterial involvement being a recognized manifestation in both GCA and TAK. Intracranial vasculitis has been reported in approximately 7% of TAK patients. The cumulative risk of embolic or hemodynamic ischemic stroke in TAK with extra- and intracranial artery involvement is reported as 15–20% of patients [20–23]. In GCA, ischemic stroke occurs in about 3–7%, with emerging evidence suggesting that intracranial artery involvement may be more common than previously assumed: high-resolution black-blood magnetic resonance imaging (MRI) identified intracranial vessel wall alterations in 14.5% of GCA patients [24], and a recent systematic literature review of 102 studies summarized a total of 340 patients with reported intracranial vasculitis [25].

Currently, data on the frequency, temporal evolution, and potential therapeutic implications of intracranial vascular involvement as assessed by transcranial sonography remain scarce. Therefore, we conducted a retrospective analysis of patients with large-vessel vasculitis and serial sonographic follow-up at our comprehensive stroke center to evaluate the prevalence of neurosonographic changes and their impact on therapeutic decision-making in LVV.

2. Materials and Methods

2.1. Data Source, Patient Selection, and Cohort Development

In a retrospective approach, we identified all patients who were treated at our neurological department for giant cell arteritis or Takayasu arteritis and underwent at least one clinical and sonographic follow-up examination after baseline assessment between January 2015 and October 2025. All diagnoses were made in accordance with the ACR/EULAR criteria and confirmed by expert neurologists [26,27]. Sonographic follow-up was scheduled as indicated by clinical assessment. Clinical and sonographic data were retrieved from medical records.

2.2. Demographic, Clinical, and Sonographic Characteristics

Patient demographic and clinical characteristics included age at diagnosis and sex. We assessed the follow-up period and the number of sonographic examinations performed. Sonographic results were characterized at baseline by the presence of a halo sign in the temporal arteries (TA) and inflammatory involvement of the vertebral artery (VA), the subclavian artery (SA), the common carotid artery (CCA), the extracranial internal carotid artery (ICA), and intracranial arteries. New-onset inflammatory changes at follow-up sonography were assessed according to the anatomic site and time course of the disease. Medication

https://doi.org/10.3390/diagnostics16030455

and changes in treatment strategies, including medical and interventional procedures, were analyzed in patients with new-onset or progressive inflammatory vessel changes.

2.3. Sonographic Outcome Definitions

New-onset inflammatory artery disease was defined as the diagnosis of any newly detected vascular involvement during sonographic follow-up that was not reported at baseline sonographic assessment.

Progressive inflammatory arterial disease was defined as any significant deterioration of a previously documented vascular abnormality identified at baseline sonographic assessment, as demonstrated by increased severity at follow-up, such as progression of arterial stenosis.

2.4. Statistical Analysis

All statistical analyses were performed using "R" (version 1.4.1717; R Foundation for Statistical Computing, Vienna, Austria). Descriptive statistics were presented as frequencies with percentages for categorical variables, as means with standard deviations for normally distributed continuous variables, and as medians with ranges for ordinal or non-normally distributed variables as appropriate.

3. Results

3.1. Patient Cohort

Overall, 43 patients were treated in our neurological department for GCA or TAK between January 2015 and October 2025. Twenty-two patients did not present for sonographic follow-up evaluation and were therefore excluded from the study. In total, we identified 21 patients who met the above-defined criteria. Of these, 16 patients were diagnosed with GCA and five patients with TAK. The follow-up period was a median of 28 (2–106) months, with a median of 4.5 (2–33) sonographic assessments for GCA and 75 (33–255) months with 14 (4–60) sonographic assessments for TAK. At the baseline sonographic assessment, three patients with GCA (18.8%) and two patients with TAK (40%) had intracranial involvement of vasculitis. The study flow chart is depicted in Figure 1. A comparison of baseline characteristics (age, sex, diagnosis) between the 22 patients excluded from the final analysis due to loss to follow-up and the 21 patients included in the final analysis is depicted in Supplementary Table S1.

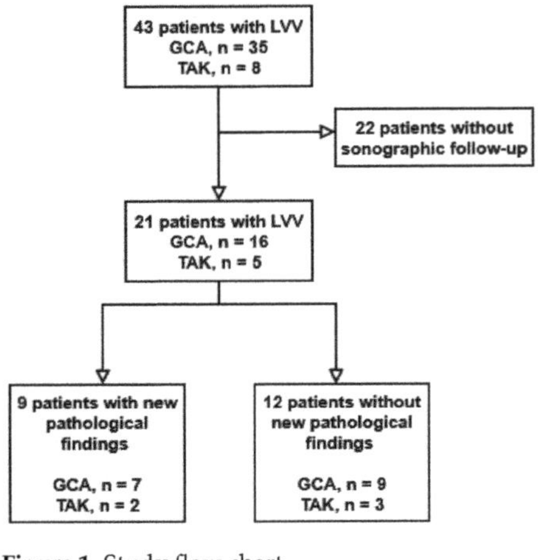

Figure 1. Study flow chart.

https://doi.org/10.3390/diagnostics16030455

3.2. Patients with New-Onset or Progressive Inflammatory Artery Disease in GCA

In total, we detected new-onset or progressive inflammatory artery disease in seven of the 16 (43.8%) GCA patients. Patient characteristics are depicted in Tables 1 and 2. Three patients (18.8%) presented with progressive halo sign in the TA; however, only one of these was symptomatic with headaches, and medical treatment was hence adjusted. We further observed one case of symptomatic new-onset intracranial anterior circulation disease, and two cases of combined symptomatic intracranial anterior and posterior artery disease, with one of these having combined extra- and intracranial VA involvement. All patients with new-onset or progressive intracranial inflammatory artery disease suffered ischemic complications and required adjustment of medical therapy. In two patients, additional interventional treatment of the anterior intracranial circulation was performed (stent angioplasty of the intracranial ICA, balloon dilatation of the intracranial ICA). Lastly, we observed one case of asymptomatic progressive extracranial VA involvement, which slightly regressed over a total follow-up of four months. Figure 2 illustrates the case of a 72-year-old GCA patient with intracranial VA involvement 4 months after the first diagnosis and bilateral cerebellar infarctions in the MRI scan. Figure 3 shows the case of a 64-year-old GCA patient with progression of bilateral, distal ICA stenosis.

Table 1. Baseline demographic, clinical, and sonographic characteristics. SD = standard deviation, n = number of patients, IA = intracranial arteries, VA = vertebral artery, CCA = common carotid artery, ICA = internal carotid artery, SA = subclavian artery.

Patient Characteristics			
		GCA	TAK
Patients	Number of patients included	16	5
	Age (years), mean (±SD)	72.8 ± 7.4	37.6 ± 8.4
	Gender		
	Female *n* (%)	9 (56.3%)	3 (60%)
	Male *n* (%)	7 (43.8%)	2 (40%)
	Follow-up period (months), median (range)	28 (2–106)	75 (33–255)
	Number of sonographic assessments during follow-up, median (range)	4.5 (2–33)	14 (4–60)
Baseline sonography	Halo sign TA, *n* (%)	13 (81.3%)	-
	Involvement of VA, *n* (%)	8 (50.0%)	2 (40%)
	Involvement of SA, *n* (%)	-	5 (100%)
	Involvement of CCA, *n* (%)	-	2 (40%)
	Involvement of extracranial ICA, *n* (%)	-	2 (40%)
	Involvement of anterior circulation IA, *n* (%)	3 (18.8%)	2 (40%)
New or progressive artery involvement detected in follow-up sonography	Total, *n* (%)	7 (43.8%)	2 (40%)
	Symptomatic progress, *n* (%)	4 (25.0%)	1 (20%)
	Progress or new-onset involvement of VA, *n* (%)	3 (18.8%)	-
	Progress or new-onset involvement of anterior circulation IA, *n* (%)	3 (18.8%)	1 (20%)
	Progress or new-onset involvement of CCA, *n* (%)	-	1 (20%)
	Change of medical treatment following progress, *n* (%)	4 (25.0%)	-
	Interventional treatment following progress, *n* (%)	2 (12.5%)	1 (20%)

https://doi.org/10.3390/diagnostics16030455

Table 2. Clinical and sonographical findings in patients with progressive inflammatory artery disease and their medical impact. GCA = giant cell arteritis, TAK = Takayasu arteritis, f = female, m = male, TA = temporal artery, VA = vertebral artery, ICA = internal carotid artery, CCA = common carotid artery, SA = subclavian artery, MTX = methotrexate, CYC = cyclophosphamide, TOC = tocilizumab, MPS = methylprednisolone.

Clinical and Sonographic Findings in Patients with Progressive Inflammatory Artery Involvement in LVV and Their Therapeutic Impact											
Clinical Information						**Progressive Inflammatory Artery Disease During Sonographic Follow-Up**			**Medical and Interventional Treatment Following Progress**		
	Age	**Sex**	**Follow-up Period (Months)**	**Number of Sonographic Examinations**	**Baseline Pathology**	**Time from First Diagnosis (Months)**	**Symptomatic Progress**	**Sonographic Findings**	**Baseline**	**Change**	**Interventional Treatment**
GCA	68	m	105	20	Halo TA Extracranial VA stenosis	36	-	Progressive halo sign TA	Prednisolone + MTX	-	-
GCA	67	f	55	19	Occlusion intracranial right VA	3	Recurrent left-hemispheric strokes	High-grade stenosis of both ICAs (petrous segment) Stenosis MCA left	Prednisolone	MPS pulse (1000 mg for 5 days), MTX	Stent angioplasty of the left intracranial ICA
GCA	64	m	30	33	Halo TA Intracranial right VA stenosis Intracranial, bilateral ICA stenosis	1	Recurrent bihemispheric strokes	Progressive stenosis ICA and MCA left Progressive stenosis VA right extracranial and both intracranial VA	Prednisolone	MTX, TOC, CYC	Balloon dilatation of both ICAs
GCA	83	m	60	3	Halo TA	41	-	Progressive halo TA	Prednisolone + TOC	-	-
GCA	80	f	4	4	Halo TA Extracranial VA stenosis	1	-	Progressive extracranial, right-side VA stenosis	Prednisolone + MTX	-	-
GCA	72	m	23	6	Halo TA Intracranial VA stenosis	4	Recurrent vertebro-basilar strokes	Intracranial, bilateral VA occlusion Intracranial, bilateral ICA stenosis	Prednisolone + TOC	MPS pulse (1000 mg for 5 days), CYC, MTX	-
GCA	80	m	12	2	Halo TA	5	Headache	Progressive halo TA	Prednisolone + TOC	Prednisolone dose increase	-
TAK	26	f	75	14	VA, SA, CCA, ICA (extracranial)	57	-	Intracranial left-side ICA stenosis	Prednisolone + Certolizumab	-	-
TAK	33	f	254	60	SA, ACC	95	Right-hemispheric stroke	Progressive right-side CCA stenosis	Prednisolone + MTX	-	Stent angioplasty right CCA

https://doi.org/10.3390/diagnostics16030455

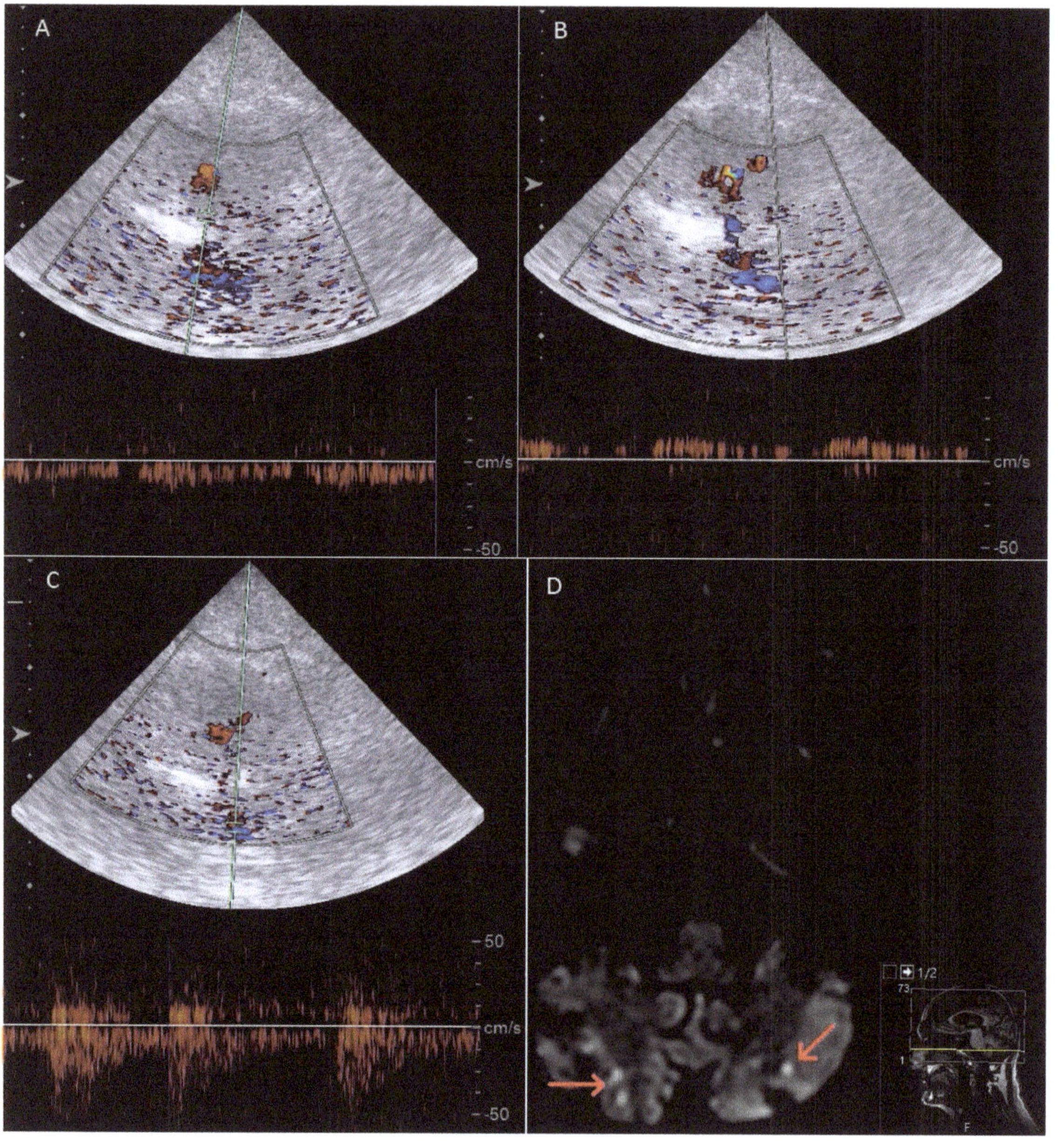

Figure 2. Exemplary case of a 72−year-old patient with GCA and images of a follow-up examination 4 months after the first diagnosis showing bilateral vertebral involvement. (**A**) Transnuchal duplex sonography showing highly reduced pulsatility of the right distal VA. (**B**) Retrograde perfused left distal VA. (**C**) Decreased blood flow in the basilar artery. (**D**) MRI scan (Diffusion Weighted Imaging sequence) showing new bilateral cerebellar infarctions (red arrows).

https://doi.org/10.3390/diagnostics16030455

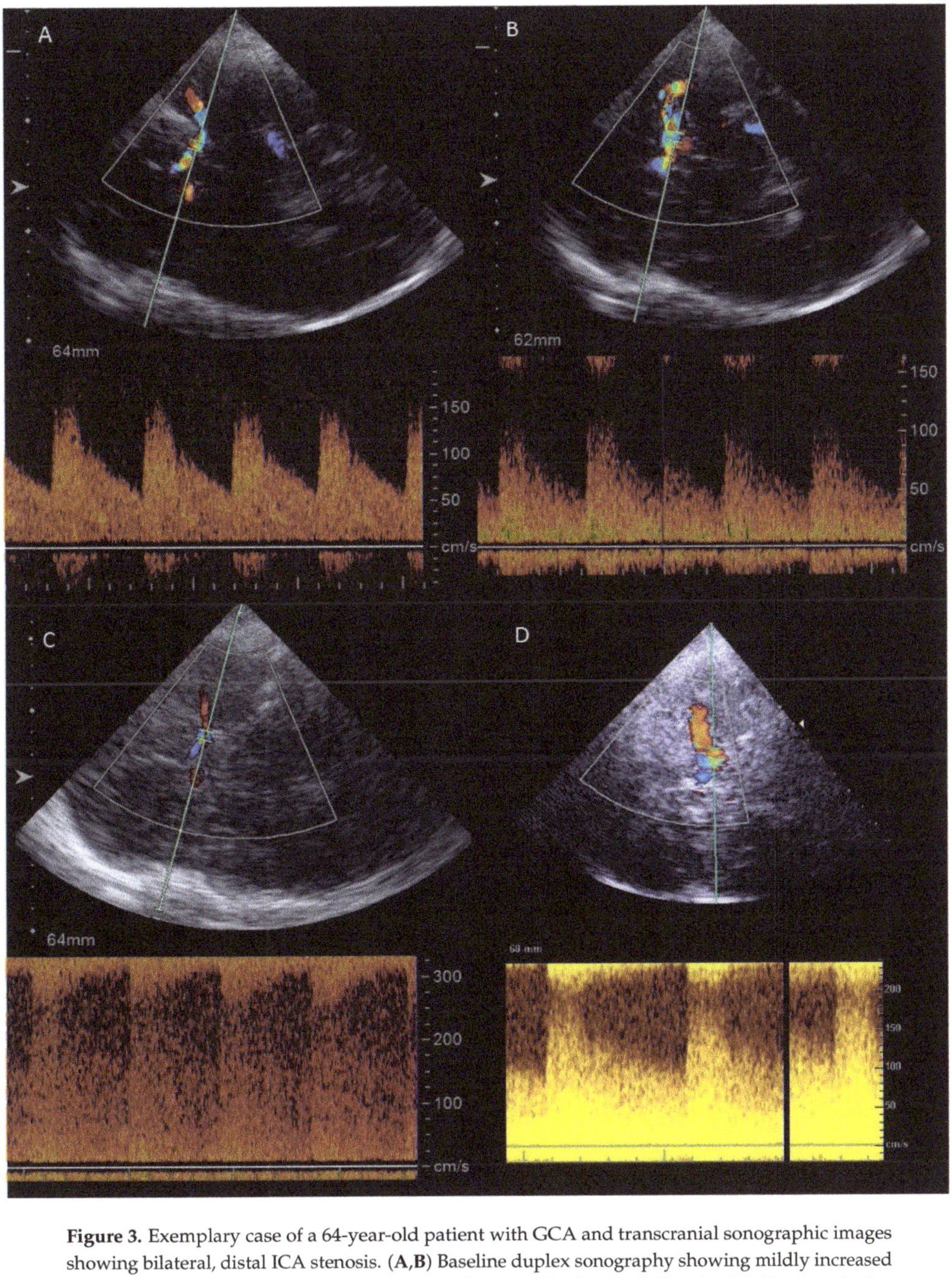

Figure 3. Exemplary case of a 64-year-old patient with GCA and transcranial sonographic images showing bilateral, distal ICA stenosis. (**A**,**B**) Baseline duplex sonography showing mildly increased blood flow velocity of the left (**A**) distal ICA and of the right (**B**) distal ICA. (**C**,**D**) Follow-up duplex sonography one month after baseline assessment showing highly increased blood flow velocity of the left (**C**) distal ICA and of the right (**D**) distal ICA.

3.3. Patients with New-Onset or Progressive Inflammatory Artery Disease in TAK

In total, we detected new-onset or progressive inflammatory artery disease in two of five TAK patients. Patient characteristics are depicted in Tables 1 and 2. One patient

https://doi.org/10.3390/diagnostics16030455

presented with asymptomatic intracranial involvement of the ICA, but we refrained from adjusting medical therapy. The sonographic and MR images of this patient are depicted in Figure 4. One patient presented with ischemic stroke due to progressive CCA involvement, and stent angioplasty of the CCA was performed.

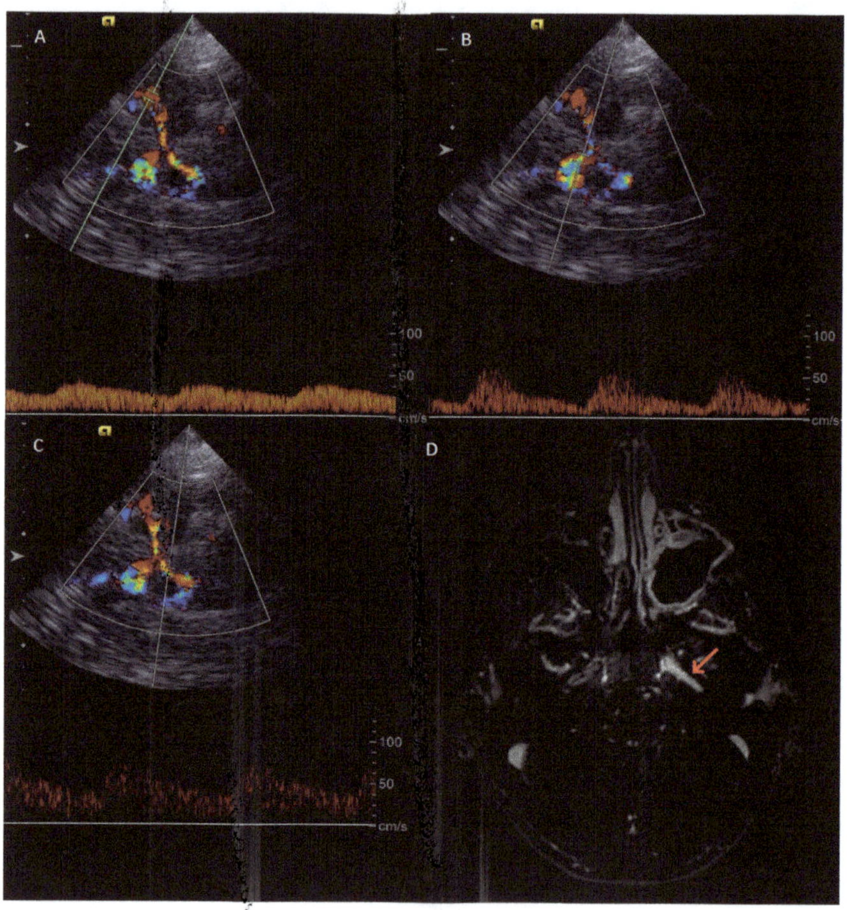

Figure 4. Exemplary case of a patient with TAK and images of a follow-up examination 5 years after the first diagnosis showing signs of high-grade stenosis of the left distal ICA. (**A**) Transcranial duplex sonography showing reduced pulsatility of the left distal MCA. (**B**) Retrograde perfused left ACA. (**C**) Cross-flow circulation from the left PCA to the left MCA through the posterior communicating artery (**D**) MRI scan (subtraction T1-weighted 3D TRA sequence) confirming high-grade stenosis and vascular inflammation of the left distal ICA (red arrow).

4. Discussion

We present the first study to demonstrate the value of transcranial neurosonography for detecting new-onset or progressive intracranial inflammatory vessel involvement during routine baseline and follow-up visits for LVV. To date, a comprehensive neurosonographic approach, including both transcranial and transnuchal sonography, has not been integrated into proposed study designs for sonographic follow-up or disease monitoring in GCA or TAK.

In GCA, current sonographic follow-up protocols primarily emphasize the measurement of IMT of the temporal and axillary arteries, as captured by composite scoring

https://doi.org/10.3390/diagnostics16030455

systems such as the OGUS, the halo count, the halo score, and the Southend halo score [2,3]. The clinical utility of these standardized ultrasound-based scoring systems in follow-up sonographic assessment has been supported by several studies. Inter alia, Kirby et al. demonstrated that the use of the OGUS, halo score, and halo count facilitated reproducible and standardized disease monitoring in clinical practice [9]. Ponte et al. reported that sonographic changes in the temporal and axillary arteries—particularly regression of the halo sign and a reduction in IMT—can occur rapidly in response to effective glucocorticoid therapy [28].

The assessment of further supraaortic branches—including the VA, SA, brachial artery, CCA, and ICA—has been incorporated into sonographic follow-up protocols, in addition to the scoring systems described above. Thus far, the examined arteries and their reported treatment responses vary between study protocols. For example, Seitz et al. reported a decline in the IMT of the SA, in addition to reductions in the axillary arteries and TA, after treatment induction with methylprednisolone pulse therapy followed by tocilizumab [29]. The treatment effect of tocilizumab, as assessed by sonographic IMT measurements, appeared later in the axillary and subclavian arteries than in the temporal artery. Hansen et al., in a prospective study of 48 therapy-naïve GCA patients, noted a rapid decrease in IMT in the temporal and axillary arteries within ten days of glucocorticoid initiation, in contrast to the slower changes in other supraaortic arteries, including the CCA and brachial arteries [10]. Similarly, Ford et al. demonstrated a rapid regression of inflammatory changes in the TA, whereas involvement of the SA and axillary arteries tended to persist on sonographic follow-up in a retrospective evaluation of 42 patients with a median follow-up of 5.1 months [30]. Haaversen et al. prospectively evaluated 132 GCA patients for halo signs in the temporal and facial arteries as well as for IMT changes in supraaortic vessels, including the CCA, VA, and SA, and reported moderate sensitivity and specificity for detecting clinical relapse as defined by the EULAR definitions of key symptoms and clinical findings suggestive of active disease [11]. Nielsen et al. performed a prospective clinical and sonographic follow-up of 47 patients at 8 weeks, 24 weeks, and 15 months, demonstrating that IMT measurements of the TA—particularly those included in the OGUS score—showed a moderate-to-strong correlation with disease activity. In contrast, large-vessel involvement, as assessed by IMT of the CCA, was associated with a poor treatment response [31]. Aschwanden et al. conducted a 24-month longitudinal follow-up of 42 patients, with a median of two sonographic examinations per patient. They found that regression of IMT in large arteries—specifically the CCA, ICA, external carotid artery, VA, SA, axillary artery, popliteal artery, and superficial femoral artery—was substantially less common than IMT reduction in the TA [32]. Schäfer et al. confirmed significant decreases in the total number of affected arteries, i.e., the CCA and VA, and in OGUS values, in 36 newly diagnosed patients who completed a 12-month follow-up period with regular sonographic assessments after treatment initiation [1]. In contrast to some of the previously described studies, in these patients, the mean IMT of the axillary artery normalized before the common TA.

For TAK, sonographic follow-up protocols mostly include IMT measurement of the CCA, SA, and VA, with an additional focus on vessel wall echogenicity. It has been reported that hypoechogenic vessel walls are commonly more prevalent in acute or new-onset inflammatory diseases, with possible long-term progression to hyperechogenic vessel wall changes accompanied by fibrotic stripes [14,18,33,34]. Thus far, various scores, including the above-mentioned parameters, have been proposed for differentiating active disease. Firstly, combining echogenicity and IMT measurements of the CCA, SA, and axillary artery, the Takayasu Ultrasound Index has been validated in the follow-up assessment of TAK [18]. Similarly, the ultrasonographic activity score (ULTRAS) has recently been

https://doi.org/10.3390/diagnostics16030455

proposed, which includes wall thickness and semi-quantitative echogenicity scores in patients with CCA involvement. Additionally, neovascularization, as detected by contrast-enhanced ultrasound and the presence of intramural arteries, has been described, indicating secondary inflammatory changes in TAK, which may be sonographically detectable in follow-up assessments [15,16,18]. Nevertheless, sonography has not been established for routine diagnostic follow-up in TAK [17,19]. If performed, the frequency of imaging follow-up in TAK has not been specified. A recent retrospective multicenter study favors patient-specific and individualized periods, as radiological progress was unlikely in the absence of clinical activity, but in the case of its detection, seemed highly relevant for medical treatment [19].

Collectively, these findings highlight the potential value of sonographic parameters as biomarkers of disease activity and treatment response in LVV. Since the pattern of vessels is highly variable, we propose adding transcranial sonography to the standard LVV work-up. Although inflammatory involvement of intracranial arteries has been described in both TAK and GCA [20–25], transcranial sonography has not been implemented in sonographic protocols thus far. In our patient population, baseline as well as new-onset or progressive intracranial artery involvement was relatively common in both GCA and TAK, and was well detected by a complete sonographic examination. Hence, we argue that the expansion of sonographic protocols, incorporating transcranial and transnuchal approaches in addition to a complete assessment of VA, CCA, and ICA, provides a more comprehensive evaluation of vascular inflammation in both baseline and follow-up assessments, and may identify patients at risk of ischemic complications.

Recent evidence suggests that transorbital sonography, with measurement of the peak systolic velocity (PSV) of the central retinal artery, may provide a tool for the assessment of intracranial vascular involvement in GCA [12,13]. Since the PSV of the central retinal artery can be directly affected by intracranial ICA pathology, this finding highlights the clinical relevance and frequency of intracranial artery involvement in GCA, and thereby the importance of additionally performing a comprehensive neurosonographic work-up that includes a complete transcranial assessment.

Data on the prevalence of extra- and intracranial involvement of the VA in GCA remain heterogeneous. Reported frequencies vary considerably depending on the characteristics of the studied cohort, particularly in patients presenting with GCA-associated stroke, and on the imaging modality employed [19–21]. For example, Penet et al. identified VA involvement in 2.4% of patients when assessed by sonography, whereas positron emission tomography (PET) revealed involvement in 22% [22]. Intracranial VA involvement has been reported in 83.9% of patients with intracranial GCA and GCA-related stroke, predominantly affecting the V3 and V4 segments before the origin of the posterior inferior cerebellar artery (PICA), and typically exhibiting the characteristic "slope sign" [19]. At baseline, we detected extra- or intracranial involvement of the VA in 50% of patients within our neurological cohort.

In our study, intracranial ICA involvement at baseline was identified in 18.8% of GCA patients. More recent evidence suggests that intracranial large-vessel anterior arteritis may be more common than previously recognized, predominantly detected by high-resolution MR imaging. Guggenberger et al. reported intracranial ICA involvement in 10.9% of patients using MR imaging with black-blood sequences and MR angiography [24]. Other MR-based studies have demonstrated intracranial ICA involvement in up to 50% of patients with GCA [35]. While vessel wall imaging is not feasible in transcranial ultrasound, the resulting hemodynamic ICA stenoses can be reliably identified, which may thus serve as a practical modality for longitudinal follow-up.

https://doi.org/10.3390/diagnostics16030455

The incidence of GCA-related stroke remains controversial, with reported rates ranging from 1.5% to 16%. Strokes have been reported to predominantly affect the vertebrobasilar circulation and are more frequently observed in male patients [36–39]. In our cohort, GCA-related stroke occurred in 18.8% of patients, all of whom exhibited sonographically detected new-onset or progressive inflammatory involvement of intracranial arteries and presented with intracranial VA stenosis at baseline as a possible risk factor for GCA-related stroke [39]. Of note, and contrary to the previously discussed literature, there was, even though limited by the restricted patient numbers, no evident increase in the occurrence of vertebro-basilar ischemic stroke in our patient cohort.

The finding of a progressive halo sign without clinical relevance in two GCA patients strengthens the importance of a standardized assessment using the proposed OGUS score, which was not routinely assessed during the study period [1,7,8].

The key limitation of our study is the relatively small sample size, which restricts the extent to which the findings can be generalized. However, our findings provide valuable clinical insights into a rare disease for which data are overall scarce, helping to expand the limited evidence base and create a potential blueprint for future prospective multicenter studies. Secondly, the retrospective design of the study represents another important limitation, as our analyses depend on clinical data from medical records that were not primarily collected for research purposes. For GCA, the above-described therapeutic uncertainties regarding both the localization and duration of inflammatory vessel wall changes following treatment initiation have thus far prevented sonography from being included in international EULAR recommendations on the clinical follow-up of patients without suspected disease relapse [5]. This lack of consensus on a standardized sonographic follow-up may account for the high rate of patients without sonographic follow-up, resulting in the discussed restricted numbers of included patients and possible selection and attrition bias. In our study, approximately half of the patients did not return for sonographic follow-up, representing a relatively high dropout rate. Due to the retrospective design, the reasons for non-attendance are unknown, and the resulting attrition bias limits the interpretation of the true prevalence of newly identified pathologies. One possible explanation for non-attendance at follow-up could be that some patients were clinically stable and asymptomatic, and therefore did not perceive a need for further evaluation. Thus, the pathological findings observed in the remaining cohort may appear more pronounced, giving a misleading impression of the true prevalence of pathological findings in sonographic follow-up of LVV patients.

Overall, this study demonstrates the feasibility and potential diagnostic yield of transcranial sonographic monitoring. However, it is not suitable to define a standardized monitoring protocol, mainly owing to its retrospective design and limited sample size. Notably, this is the first study to highlight these considerations, delineating the primary motivation for a prospective, multicenter trial with clear, protocol-defined time points and parameters for clinical and sonographic assessments. A large prospective trial would enable systematic evaluation of disease progression and the utility of sonographic monitoring, while minimizing bias and enhancing generalizability.

5. Conclusions

In conclusion, this study highlights the potential medical implications of comprehensive neurosonographic assessment in the follow-up of patients with GCA and TAK. The addition of transcranial and transnuchal sonography to the established protocols may help to detect progressive or new-onset inflammatory artery disease in known LVV, thereby influencing medical and interventional decision-making. Incorporating these modalities into routine follow-up examinations of patients with LVV could facilitate earlier recognition

https://doi.org/10.3390/diagnostics16030455

of clinically silent progression and hence identify patients at risk for ischemic complications. The central innovative aspect of this study lies in the inclusion of transcranial sonography, representing, to the best of our knowledge, the first systematic evaluation of this modality in patients with large-vessel vasculitis. By extending ultrasound assessment beyond extracranial vessels, this approach supports a more comprehensive, non-invasive diagnostic strategy that may contribute to future updates and refinements of EULAR recommendations for the imaging-based diagnosis and monitoring of LVV. Further prospective studies are warranted to validate these observations and to clarify their impact on patient outcomes.

Supplementary Materials: The following supporting information can be downloaded at: https://www.mdpi.com/article/10.3390/diagnostics16030455/s1, Table S1: Comparison of baseline characteristics of patients with GCA and TAK included and excluded from final analysis.

Author Contributions: Conceptualization: J.H. and E.B.; methodology: J.H. and E.B.; validation: S.W. and A.B.; formal analysis: J.H. and E.B.; investigation: J.H. and E.B.; data curation: J.H., E.B., S.L. and F.H.; writing—original draft preparation: J.H. and E.B.; writing—review and editing: J.H., E.B., S.L., F.H., A.B. and S.W.; visualization: J.H. and E.B.; supervision: S.W. and A.B. All authors have read and agreed to the published version of the manuscript.

Funding: This research received no external funding.

Institutional Review Board Statement: The study was conducted in accordance with the Declaration of Helsinki. Ethical approval was granted by the Ethics Committee of the Technical University of Munich, ID: 2025-647-S-SF, approval date: 3 December 2025.

Informed Consent Statement: Patient consent was waived due to the retrospective study design and data anonymization.

Data Availability Statement: The data that support the findings of this study are available upon reasonable request from the corresponding author.

Acknowledgments: We thank Beate Eckenweber, Maria Kassil, Christina Leonhard, and Rebecca Husel for their work at the local sonography laboratory and data acquisition.

Conflicts of Interest: The authors declare no conflicts of interest.

Abbreviations

The following abbreviations are used in this manuscript:

ACA	anterior cerebral artery
BA	basilar artery
CCA	common carotid artery
GCA	giant cell arteritis
ICA	internal carotid artery
IMT	intima-media thickness
LVV	large-vessel vasculitis
MCA	middle cerebral artery
MRI	magnetic resonance imaging
OGUS	giant cell arteritis ultrasonography score
PCA	posterior cerebral artery
PSV	peak systolic velocity
SA	subclavian artery
TA	temporal artery
TAK	Takayasu arteritis
TCD	transcranial duplex sonography
VA	vertebral artery

https://doi.org/10.3390/diagnostics16030455

References

1. Schäfer, V.S.; Dejaco, C.; Karakostas, P.; Behning, C.; Brossart, P.; Burg, L.C. Follow-up ultrasound examination in patients with newly diagnosed giant cell arteritis. *Rheumatology* **2025**, *64*, 732–739. [CrossRef] [PubMed]
2. Schmidt, W.A.; Schäfer, V.S. Diagnosing vasculitis with ultrasound: Findings and pitfalls. *Ther. Adv. Musculoskelet. Dis.* **2024**, *16*, 1759720x241251742. [CrossRef] [PubMed]
3. Kirby, C.; Flood, R.; Mullan, R.; Murphy, G.; Kane, D. Evolution of ultrasound in giant cell arteritis. *Front. Med.* **2022**, *9*, 981659. [CrossRef] [PubMed]
4. Luqmani, R.; Lee, E.; Singh, S.; Gillett, M.; Schmidt, W.A.; Bradburn, M.; Dasgupta, B.; Diamantopoulos, A.P.; Forrester-Barker, W.; Hamilton, W.; et al. The Role of Ultrasound Compared to Biopsy of Temporal Arteries in the Diagnosis and Treatment of Giant Cell Arteritis (TABUL): A diagnostic accuracy and cost-effectiveness study. *Health Technol. Assess.* **2016**, *20*, 1–238. [CrossRef]
5. Dejaco, C.; Ramiro, S.; Duftner, C.; Besson, F.L.; Bley, T.A.; Blockmans, D.; Brouwer, E.; Cimmino, M.A.; Clark, E.; Dasgupta, B.; et al. EULAR recommendations for the use of imaging in large vessel vasculitis in clinical practice. *Ann. Rheum. Dis.* **2018**, *77*, 636–643. [CrossRef]
6. Martins-Martinho, J.; Sopa, I.; Ponte, C. The value of ultrasound for monitoring disease activity in giant cell arteritis. *Vessel. Plus* **2024**, *8*, 34. [CrossRef]
7. Dejaco, C.; Ponte, C.; Monti, S.; Rozza, D.; Scirè, C.A.; Terslev, L.; Bruyn, G.A.W.; Boumans, D.; Hartung, W.; Hočevar, A.; et al. The provisional OMERACT ultrasonography score for giant cell arteritis. *Ann. Rheum. Dis.* **2023**, *82*, 556–564. [CrossRef]
8. Monti, S.; Ponte, C.; Schäfer, V.S.; Rozza, D.; Scirè, C.; Franchi, G.; Milanesi, A.; Khmelinskii, N.; Petzinna, S.M.; Carrara, G.; et al. The giant cell arteritis (GCA) ultrasound score (OGUS) at diagnosis and after initial treatment predicts future relapses in GCA patients: Results of a multicentre prospective study. *Ann. Rheum. Dis.* **2025**, *84*, 823–832. [CrossRef]
9. Kirby, C.; Molloy, D.; Cowley, S.; Flood, R.; Gheta, D.; Mullan, R.; Murphy, G.; Kane, D. A prospective cohort study evaluating the role of quantifying sonographic inflammatory changes in GCA. *Rheumatol. Adv. Pract.* **2025**, *9*, rkaf085. [CrossRef]
10. Hansen, M.; Hansen, I.T.; Keller, K.K.; Therkildsen, P.; Hauge, E.M.; Nielsen, B.D. Serial assessment of ultrasound sensitivity and scores in patients with giant cell arteritis before and 3 and 10 days after treatment. *Rheumatology* **2025**, *64*, 3895–3899. [CrossRef]
11. Haaversen, A.C.B.; Brekke, L.K.; Kermani, T.A.; Molberg, Ø.; Diamantopoulos, A.P. Vascular ultrasound as a follow-up tool in patients with giant cell arteritis: A prospective observational cohort study. *Front. Med.* **2024**, *11*, 1436707. [CrossRef]
12. Petzinna, S.M.; Burg, L.C.; Terheyden, J.H.; Bauer, C.J.; Karakostas, P.; Behning, C.; Holz, F.G.; Finger, R.P.; Schäfer, V.S. Transorbital ultrasonography reveals persistent decrease in retinal artery flow and optic nerve diameter in treated giant cell arteritis. *Rheumatology* **2025**, *65*, keaf456. [CrossRef] [PubMed]
13. Petzinna, S.M.; Terheyden, J.H.; Burg, L.C.; Bauer, C.J.; Karakostas, P.; Behning, C.; Holz, F.G.; Finger, R.P.; Schäfer, V.S. Imaging of ophthalmic manifestations: Optical coherence tomography angiography and transorbital ultrasound in giant cell arteritis. *Rheumatol. Int.* **2025**, *45*, 48. [CrossRef] [PubMed]
14. Sun, Y.; Yip, P.-K.; Jeng, J.-S.; Hwang, B.-S.; Lin, W.-H. Ultrasonographic Study and Long-term Follow-up of Takayasu's Arteritis. *Stroke* **1996**, *27*, 2178–2182. [CrossRef] [PubMed]
15. Dong, Y.; Wang, Y.; Wang, Y.; Tian, X.; Li, J.; Yang, Y.; Ge, Z.; Zhang, L.; Zou, M.; Wang, H.; et al. Ultrasonography and contrast-enhanced ultrasound for activity assessment in 115 patients with carotid involvement of Takayasu arteritis. *Mod. Rheumatol.* **2023**, *33*, 1007–1015. [CrossRef]
16. Herlin, B.; Baud, J.M.; Chadenat, M.L.; Pico, F. Contrast-enhanced ultrasonography in Takayasu arteritis: Watching and monitoring the arterial inflammation. *BMJ Case Rep.* **2015**, *2015*, 211094. [CrossRef]
17. Keleşoğlu Dinçer, A.B.; Kılıç, L.; Erden, A.; Kalyoncu, U.; Hazirolan, T.; Kiraz, S.; KaradaĞ, Ö. Imaging modalities used in diagnosis and follow-up of patients with Takayasu's arteritis. *Turk. J. Med. Sci.* **2021**, *51*, 224–230. [CrossRef]
18. Svensson, C.; Eriksson, P.; Zachrisson, H. Vascular ultrasound for monitoring of inflammatory activity in Takayasu arteritis. *Clin. Physiol. Funct. Imaging* **2020**, *40*, 37–45. [CrossRef]
19. Yıldırım, F.; Tastekin, F.; Bakkal, S.; Kutu, M.E.; Ocak, T.; San, S.; Avcu, A.; Kocaayan, H.; Işık, S.; Uludogan, B.C.; et al. Prognostic significance and rationality of regular non-invasive imaging follow-up in Takayasu arteritis: A large multicenter cohort study. *Semin. Arthritis Rheum.* **2025**, *74*, 152813. [CrossRef]
20. Johnson, A.; Emery, D.; Clifford, A. Intracranial Involvement in Takayasu's Arteritis. *Diagnostics* **2021**, *11*, 1997. [CrossRef]
21. Bond, K.M.; Nasr, D.; Lehman, V.; Lanzino, G.; Cloft, H.J.; Brinjikji, W. Intracranial and Extracranial Neurovascular Manifestations of Takayasu Arteritis. *AJNR Am. J. Neuroradiol.* **2017**, *38*, 766–772. [CrossRef] [PubMed]
22. Samaan, M.; Abramyan, A.; Sundararajan, S.; Nourollah-Zadeh, E.; Sun, H.; Nanda, A.; Roychowdhury, S.; Gupta, G. Cerebrovascular implications of takayasu arteritis: A review. *Neuroradiology* **2025**, *67*, 125–136. [CrossRef] [PubMed]
23. Huo, J.; Wang, B.; Yu, L.; Gao, D.; Cheng, R.; Wang, J.; Zhou, X.; Tian, T.; Gao, L. Clinical characteristics and outcomes in patients with Takayasu arteritis coexisting with myocardial ischemia and neurological symptoms: A multicenter, long-term, follow-up study. *Front. Cardiovasc. Med.* **2022**, *9*, 948124. [CrossRef] [PubMed]

https://doi.org/10.3390/diagnostics16030455

24. Guggenberger, K.V.; Vogt, M.L.; Song, J.W.; Fröhlich, M.; Schmalzing, M.; Venhoff, N.; Werner, R.A.; Hillenkamp, J.; Pham, M.; Meckel, S.; et al. High-resolution magnetic resonance imaging visualizes intracranial large artery involvement in giant cell arteritis. *Rheumatology* **2024**, *64*, 842–848. [CrossRef]
25. Patel, S.; Okaj, I.; Scott, J.; Atwal, S.; Stark, C.; Tahir, R.; Khalidi, N.; Junek, M. Intracranial GCA: A comprehensive systematic review. *Rheumatology* **2025**, *64*, 4517–4524. [CrossRef]
26. Grayson, P.C.; Ponte, C.; Suppiah, R.; Robson, J.C.; Gribbons, K.B.; Judge, A.; Craven, A.; Khalid, S.; Hutchings, A.; Danda, D.; et al. 2022 American College of Rheumatology/EULAR Classification Criteria for Takayasu Arteritis. *Arthritis Rheumatol.* **2022**, *74*, 1872–1880. [CrossRef]
27. Ponte, C.; Grayson, P.C.; Robson, J.C.; Suppiah, R.; Gribbons, K.B.; Judge, A.; Craven, A.; Khalid, S.; Hutchings, A.; Watts, R.A.; et al. 2022 American College of Rheumatology/EULAR Classification Criteria for Giant Cell Arteritis. *Arthritis Rheumatol.* **2022**, *74*, 1881–1889. [CrossRef]
28. Ponte, C.; Serafim, A.S.; Monti, S.; Fernandes, E.; Lee, E.; Singh, S.; Piper, J.; Hutchings, A.; McNally, E.; Diamantopoulos, A.P.; et al. Early variation of ultrasound halo sign with treatment and relation with clinical features in patients with giant cell arteritis. *Rheumatology* **2020**, *59*, 3717–3726. [CrossRef]
29. Seitz, L.; Christ, L.; Lötscher, F.; Scholz, G.; Sarbu, A.C.; Bütikofer, L.; Kollert, F.; Schmidt, W.A.; Reichenbach, S.; Villiger, P.M. Quantitative ultrasound to monitor the vascular response to tocilizumab in giant cell arteritis. *Rheumatology* **2021**, *60*, 5052–5059. [CrossRef]
30. Ford, J.A.; DiIorio, M.A.; Huang, W.; Sobiesczcyk, P.; Docken, W.P.; Tedeschi, S.K. Follow-up vascular ultrasounds in patients with giant cell arteritis. *Clin. Exp. Rheumatol.* **2020**, *38*, 107–111.
31. Nielsen, B.D.; Therkildsen, P.; Keller, K.K.; Gormsen, L.C.; Hansen, I.T.; Hauge, E.M. Ultrasonography in the assessment of disease activity in cranial and large-vessel giant cell arteritis: A prospective follow-up study. *Rheumatology* **2023**, *62*, 3084–3094. [CrossRef] [PubMed]
32. Aschwanden, M.; Schegk, E.; Imfeld, S.; Staub, D.; Rottenburger, C.; Berger, C.T.; Daikeler, T. Vessel wall plasticity in large vessel giant cell arteritis: An ultrasound follow-up study. *Rheumatology* **2018**, *58*, 792–797. [CrossRef] [PubMed]
33. Zachrisson, H.; Svensson, C.; Dremetsika, A.; Eriksson, P. An extended high-frequency ultrasound protocol for detection of vessel wall inflammation. *Clin. Physiol. Funct. Imaging* **2018**, *38*, 586–594. [CrossRef] [PubMed]
34. Schmidt, W.A. Role of ultrasound in the understanding and management of vasculitis. *Ther. Adv. Musculoskelet. Dis.* **2014**, *6*, 39–47. [CrossRef]
35. Siemonsen, S.; Brekenfeld, C.; Holst, B.; Kaufmann-Buehler, A.K.; Fiehler, J.; Bley, T.A. 3T MRI reveals extra- and intracranial involvement in giant cell arteritis. *AJNR Am. J. Neuroradiol.* **2015**, *36*, 91–97. [CrossRef]
36. Samson, M.; Jacquin, A.; Audia, S.; Daubail, B.; Devilliers, H.; Petrella, T.; Martin, L.; Durier, J.; Besancenot, J.F.; Lorcerie, B.; et al. Stroke associated with giant cell arteritis: A population-based study. *J. Neurol. Neurosurg. Psychiatry* **2015**, *86*, 216–221. [CrossRef]
37. Larivière, D.; Sacre, K.; Klein, I.; Hyafil, F.; Choudat, L.; Chauveheid, M.P.; Papo, T. Extra- and intracranial cerebral vasculitis in giant cell arteritis: An observational study. *Medicine* **2014**, *93*, e265. [CrossRef]
38. Pariente, A.; Guédon, A.; Alamowitch, S.; Thietart, S.; Carrat, F.; Delorme, S.; Capron, J.; Cacciatore, C.; Soussan, M.; Dellal, A.; et al. Ischemic stroke in giant-cell arteritis: French retrospective study. *J. Autoimmun.* **2019**, *99*, 48–51. [CrossRef]
39. Penet, T.; Lambert, M.; Baillet, C.; Outteryck, O.; Hénon, H.; Morell-Dubois, S.; Hachulla, E.; Launay, D.; Pokeerbux, M.R. Giant cell arteritis-related cerebrovascular ischemic events: A French retrospective study of 271 patients, systematic review of the literature and meta-analysis. *Arthritis Res. Ther.* **2023**, *25*, 116. [CrossRef]

https://doi.org/10.3390/diagnostics16030455

diagnostics MDPI

Review

Positron Emission Tomography/Computed Tomography in Polymyalgia Rheumatica: When and for What—A Critical Review

Elena Heras-Recuero [1], Teresa Blázquez-Sánchez [1], Laura Cristina Landaeta-Kancev [2], Marta Martínez de Bourio-Allona [2], Arantxa Torres-Roselló [1], Fernando Rengifo-García [1], Claritza Caraballo-Salazar [1], Raquel Largo [1], Santos Castañeda [3] and Miguel Ángel González-Gay [1,4,*]

[1] Division of Rheumatology, IIS-Fundación Jiménez Díaz, 28040 Madrid, Spain; elena.herasr@fjd.es (E.H.-R.); teresa.blazquezs@quironsalud.es (T.B.-S.); arantxa.torres@quironsalud.es (A.T.-R.); fernando.rengifo@quironsalud.es (F.R.-G.); claritza.caraballo@quironsalud.es (C.C.-S.); rlargo@fjd.es (R.L.)
[2] Department of Nuclear Medicine, Fundación Jiménez Díaz University Hospital, 28040 Madrid, Spain; laura.landaeta@quironsalud.es (L.C.L.-K.); marta.martinezb@quironsalud.es (M.M.d.B.-A.)
[3] Division of Rheumatology, Hospital Universitario de La Princesa, IIS-Princesa, 28006 Madrid, Spain; scastas@gmail.com
[4] Medicine and Psychiatry Department, University of Cantabria, 39008 Santander, Spain
* Correspondence: miguelaggay@hotmail.com

Abstract: Polymyalgia rheumatica (PMR) is an inflammatory disease common in people aged 50 years and older. This condition is characterized by the presence of pain and stiffness involving mainly the shoulder and pelvic girdle. Besides the frequent association with giant cell arteritis (GCA), several conditions may mimic PMR or present with PMR features. Since the diagnosis is basically clinical, an adequate diagnosis of this condition is usually required. Positron emission tomography/computed tomography (PET-CT) has proved to be a useful tool for the diagnosis of PMR. The use of 18F-FDG-PET imaging appears promising as it provides detailed information on inflammatory activity that may not be evident with traditional methods. However, since PET-CT is not strictly necessary for the diagnosis of PMR, clinicians should consider several situations in which this imaging technique can be used in patients with suspected PMR.

Keywords: FDG uptake; polymyalgia rheumatica; giant cell arteritis; positron emission tomography/computed tomography (PET-CT) with 18F-fluorodeoxyglucose (FDG)

1. Introduction

Polymyalgia rheumatica (PMR) is a common condition in individuals over 50 years in Western countries. PMR predominantly affects people aged 50 years and older, with an average age of onset of around 70 years [1–3]. It is rare in people under 50 years of age. PMR is more common in women than men, with a female/male ratio of approximately 2:1 [1–3].

The incidence of PMR varies geographically. In northern Europe and North America, the incidence is higher than in the other parts of the world. In this regard, in Sweden, the incidence of PMR ranges from 34 to 50 per 100,000 people aged 50 years and older per year [4,5]. In Norway, the annual incidence of PMR among residents aged 50 years and older was 112.6 per 100,000, with 137.7 per 100,000 in women and 83.2 per 100,000 in men [6]. In Olmsted County, Minnesota (USA), where the population is predominantly of Scandinavian descent, the incidence has been reported at 63.9 per 100,000 per year, with a prevalence of 701 per 100,000 [7,8]. A lower incidence was reported in southern Europe and other regions. In this regard, in Northern Spain, the incidence was 18.67 cases per 100,000 people aged 50 years and older per year between January 1987 and December 1996 [9]. In Reggio-Emilia (Italy), the average annual incidence rate of PMR was 12.8 per 100,000 population aged 50 years or older [10].

A genetic predisposition contributes to the development of PMR [11]. Certain types of human leukocyte antigens have been linked to an increased risk [12]. Moreover, an association with gene polymorphisms located outside the HLA region has also been described [13,14].

Environmental triggers, such as infections, may precipitate the onset of PMR in genetically predisposed individuals [1,3]. The exact nature of these triggers remains unclear. Some studies have suggested seasonal variations in the incidence of PMR, with higher rates of diagnosis in the winter months. This could be related to environmental factors like infections. PMR has been reported following influenza B infection and, more recently, after SARS-CoV-2 infection [15,16].

PMR is characterized by pain and stiffness in the shoulders and proximal parts of the arms, the hip girdles and proximal parts of the thighs, and the neck [17,18]. Diagnosing PMR is usually straightforward in typical patients who exhibit hip and shoulder involvement, along with elevated levels of erythrocyte sedimentation rate (ESR) or C-reactive protein (CRP). However, besides the frequent association with giant cell arteritis (GCA), several conditions may mimic PMR or present with PMR features [19]. On the other hand, in some cases, PMR can present with normal levels or with a slight increase in acute phase reactants, which makes diagnosis difficult [20]. Therefore, an adequate diagnosis of this condition is usually required.

2. PMR, a Condition Associated with Bursal Involvement

Arthroscopic examinations have revealed mild synovitis in the proximal joints of people with PMR. The inflammatory infiltration observed in the synovial membranes of the shoulder and other affected joints mainly consisted of macrophages and CD4 T lymphocytes [21]. However, this mild synovitis does not fully account for the musculoskeletal manifestations and diffuse pain involving the periarticular structures in patients with PMR. In this context, magnetic resonance imaging (MRI) and ultrasonography (US) investigations have identified subacromial/subdeltoid bursitis and biceps tenosynovitis, along with the synovitis of the glenohumeral joints in these individuals [17]. These observations support the idea that the involvement of extra-articular structures may contribute to the development of PMR [21–24].

In this sense, in addition to subacromial bursitis, both hip joint effusion and pelvic bursitis can also occur in PMR. Trochanteric bursitis, as well as the less common iliopsoas and ischiogluteal bursitis, have also been observed as part of the disease spectrum. [25]. In this regard, ischiogluteal bursitis is quite specific for PMR. Interspinous bursitis affecting the cervical and lower lumbar spine has been documented in patients with PMR and could potentially contribute to the neck and back pain reported by these individuals [26–28].

The 2012 EULAR/ACR preliminary classification criteria for PMR have included, for the first time, the use of US data whenever this information is available.

They highlight the importance of ultrasound findings showing bilateral subacromial/subdeltoid bursitis and trochanteric bursitis in diagnosing PMR in patients experiencing inflammatory pain in the shoulder or pelvic girdle [29]. The use of US enhanced the specificity of the updated 2012 EULAR and ACR criteria [30]. However, if there are no other suggestive clinical features present, isolated US abnormalities should not be sufficient to support a diagnosis of PMR [31].

3. Is PET-CT Useful for the Diagnosis of PMR?

For the purposes of this review, a literature search was conducted in PubMed through May 2024. The terms used for this search included "PET" or "positron emission tomography" or "FDG" or "fluorodeoxyglucose", combined with "PMR" or "polymyalgia".

Taking into account that the inflammation of large joints and periarticular structures is common in PMR, the visualization of inflammation in periarticular structures is of great help for diagnosis. Because of that, positron emission tomography/computed tomography (PET-CT) has proved to be a useful tool for the diagnosis of PMR [32,33]. In this regard, PET-CT uses the radioactive tracer fluorodeoxyglucose (18F-FDG), which accumulates in areas with high glucose metabolism, such as inflamed tissues. PET allows the identification of augmented metabolism in peripheral cells involved in inflammation, such as neutrophils, lymphocytes, monocytes, and macrophages. As discussed before, inflammation in PMR primarily affects the bursae, synovial joints, and tendons, and PET-CT can clearly visualize the areas of increased metabolic activity [34,35]. PET-CT can detect inflammatory changes before structural changes become apparent in conventional imaging like X-ray or magnetic resonance imaging. This early detection is crucial for initiating prompt treatment and managing symptoms effectively [36–38].

An important point to be kept in mind is that a wide spectrum of conditions can mimic PMR [17,39–41]. Among them, inflammatory arthritis, particularly late-elderly-onset rheumatoid arthritis that often presents with a polymyalgic phenotype, as well as other rheumatic conditions such as spondyloarthropathies, crystal-induced arthropathies, connective tissue diseases, or the remittent seronegative symmetrical synovitis with pitting edema (RS3PE) syndrome as well as infections and malignancies, may resemble isolated PMR [17]. Unlike these conditions, PMR presents with a well-defined periarticular inflammatory pattern that corresponds largely to the inflammation of bursal structures, which we will discuss below. PET-CT may also disclose the coexistence between PMR and GCA [40].

A few years ago, van der Geest et al. performed an extremely interesting systemic review on the diagnostic value of 18F-FDG-PET-CT in PMR. The review article included a meta-analysis that encompassed 20 studies [42]. Nine studies, encompassing 636 patients, were deemed eligible for inclusion in the meta-analysis [42]. The study confirmed a high prevalence of 18F-FDG uptake in several sites, including the interspinous bursae, hips, ischial tuberosities, shoulders, and sternoclavicular joints. The likelihood ratios for positive uptake in these areas were statistically significant, indicating their diagnostic value. The interspinous bursae showed the highest positive likelihood ratio, followed by uptake in the hips, ischial tuberosities, and shoulders [42]. However, the authors highlighted the moderate to high heterogeneity of these studies, which was attributed to variations in patient selection, scanning procedures, and interpretation criteria. Because of that, van der Geest et al. emphasized the need for standardized protocols in using 18F-FDG-PET/CT for diagnosing PMR [42].

Camellino et al. assessed the relationship between clinical symptoms and findings from FDG-PET-CT scans in patients with PMR [43]. These authors found a significant correlation between the clinical symptoms of PMR and increased FDG uptake in specific regions, such as the shoulder and hip girdles, indicating inflammation. Increased FDG uptake in vascular structures was also observed, suggesting a potential overlap with GCA, which often coexists with PMR.

The study reinforced the role of FDG-PET-CT in diagnosing and managing PMR by highlighting its ability to detect metabolic changes consistent with the disease's clinical manifestations [43].

Kim and Kim analyzed the diagnostic accuracy of FDG-PET-CT for PMR by synthesizing data from multiple studies [44]. To investigate this, the authors conducted a systematic review and meta-analysis of the studies employing FDG-PET-CT for diagnosing PMR. Their findings indicated that FDG-PET-CT demonstrated high sensitivity and specificity in detecting PMR [44]. These results advocate for incorporating this imaging technique into PMR diagnostic protocols. [44].

4. How Can We Detect the Presence of Inflammation in PMR Using PET?

There are two main methods for evaluating PET scans: visual evaluation and semi-quantitative evaluation. Here are the key differences between these methods:

Visual evaluation is based on the interpretation of PET images by a radiologist or nuclear medicine physician. This method is inherently subjective, as it depends on the experience and judgment of the observer. It involves visually inspecting the PET images for areas of increased uptake, which indicate inflammation. The intensity and pattern of uptake are assessed qualitatively, often using standardized criteria or scoring systems. It provides information on the number of sites with significant uptake equal to or greater than hepatic uptake [45]. Because of that, this method is relatively easy to evaluate and does not require complex software or extensive processing. It can be performed immediately after examination and often allows visual findings to be effectively correlated with clinical symptoms and other diagnostic information, making this method valuable in routine clinical practice.

The alternative method to PET evaluation in PMR is the semi-quantitative method that involves measuring standardized absorption/uptake values (SUVs) in specific regions of interest. In this semi-quantitative analysis, the mean maximum standardized uptake value (SUVmax) is determined. Receiver operating characteristic curves are used to establish optimal cutoffs for both the visual score and SUVmax in diagnosing PMR [45]. This provides a more objective measure of inflammation by quantifying the amount of radiotracer uptake. The semi-quantitative evaluation is more reproducible than visual assessment because it is based on standardized measurements rather than subjective interpretation. This reduces variability between observers. However, it requires additional time and resources, including specialized software and expertise in quantitative image analysis. It may not be immediately available in all clinical settings. Semi-quantitative methods can provide detailed information on the extent and intensity of inflammation, which may be particularly useful in research settings or for tracking disease progression over time. In clinical practice, these methods are often used complementarily. Visual assessment can quickly identify areas of concern, while semi-quantitative analysis can provide detailed information to confirm findings and track changes. In certain scenarios, such as ambiguous cases or research studies, a semi-quantitative assessment may offer additional value by providing precise data that can influence clinical decision-making. The choice between visual or semi-quantitative assessment depends on the clinical context, available resources, and the specific needs of the patient and healthcare provider. Integrating both methods can enhance diagnostic accuracy and provide a comprehensive evaluation of disease activity. Amat et al. confirmed that both methods are useful to identify PMR among patients presenting with rheumatic conditions [45]. In this regard, these authors assessed 222 18F-FDG PET-CT scans from two hundred and fifteen patients, of which 161 scans were performed on patients diagnosed with inflammatory rheumatic diseases, fifty-seven of them with PMR. The identification of PMR based on the presence of significant uptake in at least three sites showed a sensitivity of 86% and a specificity of 85.5%. The mean SUV max cutoff for diagnosing PMR was 2.168, with a sensitivity of 77.2% and a specificity of 77.6% [45].

5. PET-Scores: Useful to Differentiate PMR from Other Conditions

To improve the accuracy of 18F-FDG-PET-CT in distinguishing PMR from conditions that resemble PMR, various composite scores and algorithms have been proposed based on FDG uptake at specific sites. Typically, these scores evaluate the FDG uptake at targeted regions relative to liver uptake, with uptake equal to or higher than the liver uptake considered positive. The Leuven score evaluates twelve predefined anatomical sites (cervical spinous processes, lumbar spinous processes, left and right sternoclavicular joints, left and right ischial tuberosities, left and right greater trochanters, left and right hips, and left and right shoulders) using a three-point system: 0 (no elevated FDG uptake), 1 (moderately elevated FDG uptake, but less than the average liver uptake), or 2 (intense FDG uptake, equal to or greater than the average liver uptake) [46]. A modified version, the Leuven/Groningen score, showed similar accuracy with a simplified analysis focusing on four regions (sternoclavicular joints, interspinous lumbar processes, hips, and ischial tuberosity) [47]. The Leuven/Groningen score aggregates values, resulting in a total score that spans from 0 to 14 [47].

The Besançon index is another scoring system used in the assessment of inflammatory activity in patients suspected of having PMR. It evaluates inflammation in a wider range of anatomical sites compared to the Leuven score. Unlike the Leuven score, which evaluates twelve anatomical sites, the Besançon index assesses seventeen anatomical sites. It includes regions commonly affected by PMR, such as the shoulders, hips, spine, and other large joints, which are visually graded from 0 to 3 (0: no inflammation observed; 1: mild inflammation; 2: moderate inflammation; 3: severe inflammation). A grade of two or higher at any site indicates the presence of inflammation. This scoring system assists healthcare providers in diagnosing and managing PMR effectively. The Besançon score helps clinicians quantify the extent of inflammation in patients with PMR, aiding in the diagnosis and monitoring of disease activity. A higher total score indicates more widespread inflammation, potentially guiding treatment decisions [48].

The Saint-Étienne algorithm is another diagnostic tool used for assessing inflammatory activity in patients suspected of having PMR. This algorithm focuses on only two anatomical sites: the interspinous bursa and the trochanteric bursa. The presence of inflammation is typically assessed visually [47,49,50]. Another diagnostic tool used for evaluating inflammatory activity in patients with suspected PMR is the Heidelberg. Unlike the Saint-Étienne algorithm, it assesses five anatomical sites (interspinous bursa, trochanteric bursa, glenohumeral joint, hip joint, and ischial tuberosity). Similar to the Saint-Étienne algorithm, a grade of two or more at any of the assessed anatomical sites is considered positive for inflammation [47,49,50]. Both the Heidelberg and the Saint-Étienne algorithms provide a simplified approach to diagnosing PMR based on the presence of inflammation at specific anatomical sites. They offer a standardized method for clinicians to assess inflammatory activity, aiding in diagnosis and treatment decision making. Van der Geest et al. conducted a comparison of these scores and algorithms, revealing that the Leuven score exhibited the highest diagnostic utility [47]. Furthermore, the Leuven/Groningen score, which targets four predefined regions (sternoclavicular joints, interspinous lumbar bursae, hips, and ischial tuberosities), showed similar diagnostic accuracy with the added advantage of simplified analysis [47].

Recently, Brinth et al. evaluated the established scoring systems alongside a novel simplified scoring system called the Copenhagen score. This system employs either the visual or semi-quantitative analysis of periarticular FDG uptake in the shoulders and at the ischial tuberosities [51]. For the semi-quantitative analysis, the SUV peak at the target site was compared to the mean SUV of the superior vena cava and liver, and then converted into a three-point scoring system. As previously noted by Van der Geest et al. [47], all the scoring systems, including the simplest ones focusing on a few anatomical regions, exhibited good diagnostic performance for PMR in patients not treated with glucocorticoids [51].

Ikuma et al. conducted a study to identify key sites for distinguishing PMR from rheumatoid arthritis (RA) using 18F-FDG-PET-CT. The study involved 35 patients with PMR and 46 patients with RA. Their findings indicated that FDG uptake in the shoulder joints, lumbar vertebrae spinous processes, pubic symphysis, sternoclavicular joints, ischial tuberosities, greater trochanters, and hip joints helped differentiate PMR from RA. Specifically, FDG uptake in at least one of the ischial tuberosities showed the highest diagnostic value for distinguishing between the two conditions [52].

6. What about Other Clinical Studies?

Several clinical studies have assessed the role of PET in patients with PMR. In this regard, Casadepax-Soulet et al. conducted a retrospective study with 85 patients with new-onset PMR and 75 controls who underwent 18F-FDG PET-CT [53]. They performed both the quantitative and semi-quantitative analyses of FDG uptake at sixteen sites. They found that the patients with new-onset PMR had a higher mean number of sites with significant FDG uptake than the controls, particularly in the hips, shoulders, and ischial tuberosity [53].

Shoulder involvement is a hallmark of PMR as confirmed by Sondag et al. [48], Henckaerts et al. [54], and Yamashita et al. [55].

We investigated the effectiveness of 18F-FDG-PET-CT in detecting PMR in patients with large vessel GCA [56]. To explore this and identify the best predictors for diagnosing PMR using 18F-FDG-PET-CT in patients with large vessel GCA, we analyzed a cohort of 54 patients diagnosed with large vessel GCA at our hospital [56,57]. We assessed nine extravascular areas, encompassing 16 potential sites: acromioclavicular and sternoclavicular joints (2 each), hips (2), shoulders (2), greater trochanters (2), ischial tuberosities (2), symphysis pubis entheses (2), and cervical and lumbar interspinous processes. Each patient was assigned a total score ranging from 0 to 16, based on the sum of all the sites demonstrating significant FDG uptake [57]. Twenty-one of the fifty four patients with large vessel GCA had been clinically diagnosed as having PMR [56]. The patients with a clinical diagnosis of PMR more commonly exhibited significant extravascular FDG uptake at the sites examined. This was particularly evident in the shoulders, where 76.2% of the patients with PMR showed significant FDG uptake compared to 24.2% of those without PMR. Other areas, such as the cervical and lumbar interspinous processes, hips, and greater trochanters, also exhibited a higher frequency of significant FDG uptake in the patients with PMR ($p < 0.05$ for all the comparisons). Consequently, the total score of significant FDG uptake (SCORE 16) was higher in the patients with large vessel vasculitis-GCA and PMR compared to those without PMR (5.10 ± 4.05 vs. 1.73 ± 2.31; $p < 0.001$). These findings indicate that the number of affected extravascular sites was greater in patients with PMR [57]. According to our data, significant 18F-FDG-PET-CT uptake in the shoulder, greater trochanter, and lumbar interspinous areas may facilitate the identification of PMR in patients with large-vessel GCA. All of these observations are in line with the recommendations put forward by van der Geest et al., who highlight the importance of evaluating multiple anatomic sites, including the shoulders, sternoclavicular joints, interspinous bursae, ischial tuberosities, hips, and greater trochanters using 18F-FDG PET-CT to detect suspected PMR. As these authors concluded, the significant FDG uptake at multiple anatomic sites is a strong indication of PMR [42,58]. In this regard, Slart et al. confirmed that 18F-FDG PET-CT is highly effective to identify inflammation in large vessels, offering precise imaging that correlates well with clinical and histopathological findings [58]. Moreover, this imaging technique was also found to be very useful for detecting inflammation in characteristic areas such as the shoulders, hips, and ischial tuberosities. Therefore, this approach is highly valuable for distinguishing PMR from other inflammatory or degenerative conditions and for assessing the extent of the disease [58].

7. When Do We Have to Perform 18F-FDG PET-CT?

A potential limitation of the use of 18F-FDG-PET-CT in patients with suspected PMR is that this is an expensive technique not available in many centers yet. Moreover, some authors have emphasized that the routine use of 18F-FDG-PET/CT should not be recommended in the typical cases of PMR [41]. However, these authors suggest considering 18F-FDG-PET-CT in cases where patients with PMR present atypical features, lack elevated laboratory markers of inflammation, or have a history of cancer [58]. In this regard, a diagnosis of PMR in patients presenting with normal acute-phase reactants may be a challenge [20]. This is also the case for patients with a previous history of cancer [39,40]. With respect to this, it is true that patients with cancer often present with atypical features such as a lack of morning stiffness; more widespread pain, not only located in the shoulder and hip girdles; and poor response to glucocorticoids [39]. However, there are situations where a patient previously treated for cancer may genuinely have PMR. In such cases, it is crucial to rule out cancer relapse and accurately diagnose new-onset PMR.

Figure 1 shows the results of 18F-FDG PET-CT of an 82 year old woman diagnosed with PMR. Ten years earlier she had been diagnosed with breast cancer, treated with surgery, chemotherapy, and radiotherapy, currently in remission. PET-CT revealed increased FDG uptake in the shoulders, cervical and lumbar spine, and hips. These findings were consistent with PMR.

Interestingly, in a recent study that included 220 patients with suspected PMR and/or GCA over a two-year period, malignancy was only confirmed in seven patients (3.2%). Three of them were diagnosed with PMR concurrently with malignancy. These findings suggest that not all the patients suspected of having PMR/GCA need to undergo FDG-PET-CT systematically to rule out malignancy [59].

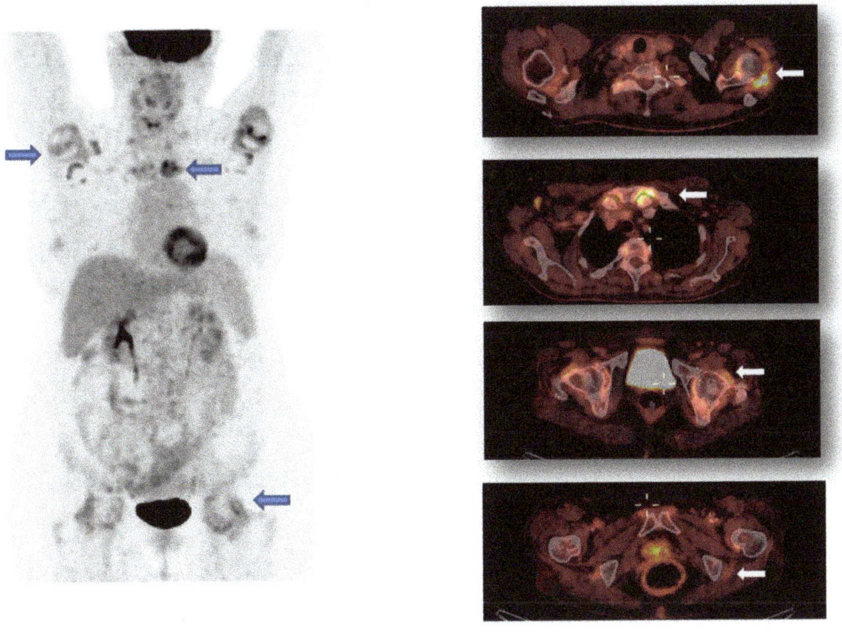

Figure 1. 82 year old woman with significant FDG uptake around the glenohumeral, sternoclavicular, costovertebral joints, lumbar interapophyseal spaces, coxofemoral joints, ischial tuberosities, and pubis, suggestive of diffuse osteoarticular pathology with an inflammatory component, in the context associated with PMR. Blue arrows: FDG uptake around glenohumeral, sternoclavicular and coxofemoral joint. White arrows: FDG upatake around glenomeral, esternoclavicular, coxofemoral and ischial tuberosities.

At this point, it is interesting to remark that the immune checkpoint inhibitors (ICIs) used in cancer patients can cause the appearance of a wide spectrum of musculoskeletal symptoms, sometimes indistinguishable from primary PMR (PMR-like syndrome) [60,61]. In these patients, PET may be useful to discriminate between primary PMR and those associated with ICI treatment. With respect to this, Vermeulen et al. suggest that ICI-PMR may show a milder course with less inflammation than primary PMR on 18F-FDG-PET-CT. As a result, patients with ICI-mediated PMR may be managed with a relatively low glucocorticoid dose, less than what is typically needed for patients with primary PMR [62].

18F-FDG PET-CT has proven valuable in identifying patients with a predominantly extracranial pattern of GCA [63–65]. More than 80% of the patients with GCA demonstrate increased FDG uptake on PET imaging, particularly affecting the thoracic and abdominal aorta. Additionally, this technique can detect vascular inflammation in the lower extremity arteries of GCA patients [65,66]. GCA may initially manifest as PMR, and imaging techniques, especially PET-CT, can reveal large vessel vasculitis in at least one-third of the patients initially diagnosed with isolated PMR [17]. Figure 2 illustrates increased FDG uptake in the aorta, indicating the presence of large vessel vasculitis in a patient with PMR who did not exhibit the ischemic manifestations of GCA.

EULAR experts also suggest that FDG-PET and MRI are effective tests for detecting large vessel involvement in patients presenting with PMR or systemic symptoms where GCA is a potential diagnosis [67]. However, further research is needed to determine whether PET-CT should be routinely performed in patients with PMR. Based on our clinical experience, we recommend considering PET-CT for patients with PMR who are resistant to prednisone doses of 15–20 mg/day or who present with atypical manifestations such as predominant symptoms in the pelvic girdle [68]. In some of these cases, an extracranial large-vessel GCA may be found.

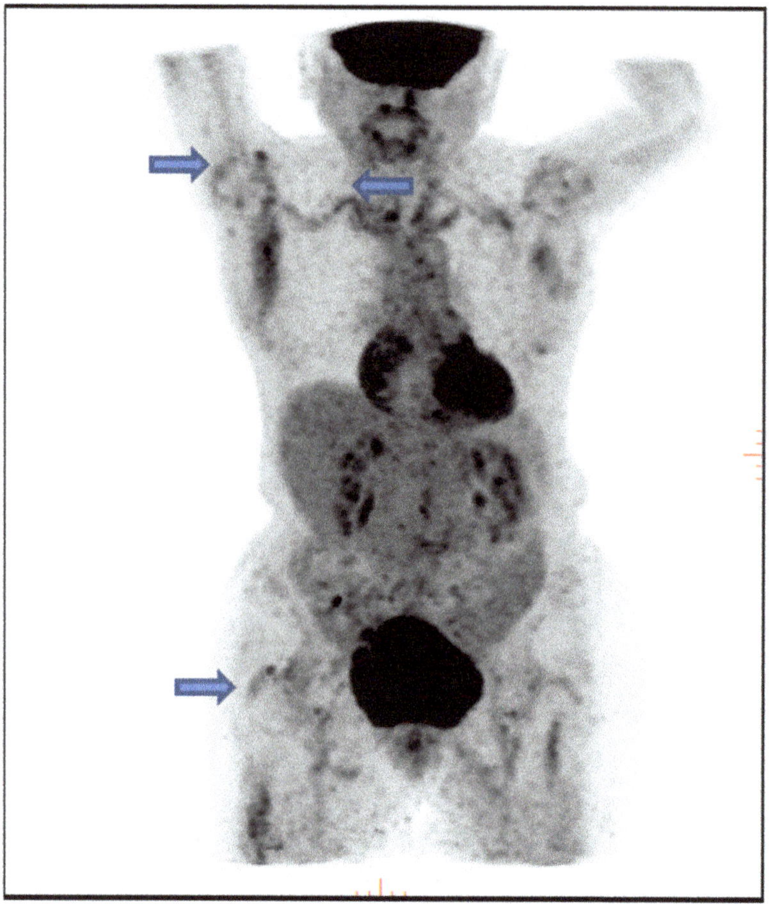

Figure 2. 65 year old woman with significant FDG uptake around the glenohumeral and coxofemoral joints (arrows) along with large vessel vasculitis.

8. Strengths and Weaknesses of PET-CT in Patients with PMR

18F-FDG PET-CT has been shown to be highly sensitive in detecting metabolic activity associated with inflammation, allowing for the early identification of inflammatory processes in PMR. Furthermore, this imaging technique can often identify "silent" extracranial large-vessel GCA, which is particularly useful for patients with PMR with atypical symptoms such as severe inflammatory low back pain or limb claudication. In these cases, PET-CT can reveal underlying vascular problems that might not be apparent by clinical examination alone [56,68].

Since FDG-PET-CT in the typical cases of PMR shows characteristic FDG uptake patterns in areas such as the ischial tuberosity, greater trochanter, lumbar or cervical spinous processes, and scapulohumeral joints [69,70], these findings help differentiate PMR from other conditions, particularly RA [70].

Pean de Ponfilly Sotier et al. assessed the effectiveness of 18F FDG PET CT imaging in distinguishing between PMR and atypical spondyloarthritis [71]. These authors found that PET-CT images provide distinctive uptake patterns that help differentiate these two conditions, which often present with overlapping symptoms. This diagnostic tool may help clinicians make more accurate diagnoses and ultimately improve patient management and treatment outcomes.

However, there are limitations to the use of PET-CT in patients with PMR. One of them is the cost and accessibility of the technique. Furthermore, PET-CT involves exposure to ionizing radiation, which constitutes a risk, especially with repeated use. This is a crucial consideration for patients who require multiple scans over time. Furthermore, while PET-CT is sensitive to inflammation, it is not specific to PMR. Increased FDG uptake can be seen in several other conditions, including infections, malignancies, and other inflammatory diseases, which may lead to false positives and unnecessary additional testing [72].

Another limitation is the use of glucocorticoids prior to performing FDG-PET-CT. In this sense, the use of glucocorticoids may reduce the sensitivity of this imaging technique [48,73]. With respect to this, it has been found that within 3 days of high-dose glucocorticoid treatment, FDG-PET-CT can diagnose large-vessel GCA with high sensitivity [74]. However, the degree of 18-FDG uptake is reduced in patients with large-vessel GCA after 72 h of treatment with high doses of glucocorticoids, and the results may be falsely negative if the PET-CT is performed ten days after the initiation of glucocorticoids [38]. Regarding isolated PMR, some experts consider that if FDG-PET-CT is performed for diagnostic purposes, glucocorticoids should be discontinued to improve diagnostic accuracy [75]. However, other experts consider that although the effect of prednisone/prednisolone at a dose of 15 mg/day, which is the average initial dose generally used in patients with isolated PMR, may lead to a reduction in FDG uptake, the distribution of uptake on PET-CT remains consistent with that observed in patients with PMR without prior glucocorticoid therapy [38].

Another point of debate is whether PET-CT should be used in the management of PMR. There are inconclusive results regarding its correlation with relapse risk or treatment response, and changes in FDG uptakes following corticosteroid treatment have been observed, indicating challenges in its utility for long-term management. In this regard, studies on repetitive 18-FDG-PET-CT in patients with isolated PMR before treatment with glucocorticoids was initiated, and then at 3 and 6 months it was indicated that the results of FDG-PET scans in patients with PMR did not correlate with their risk of relapse [76]. In addition, current guidelines do not universally recommend its use for all patients with PMR, especially in the absence of atypical symptoms or refractory disease, due to the aforementioned factors. Further research is needed to establish clear guidelines for its use in patients with PMR.

9. Potential Correlation between PET-CT and Ultrasonography (US) in PMR

PET-CT is highly sensitive in detecting inflammatory changes and, as previously discussed, can help differentiate PMR from other conditions such as GCA, which often coexists with PMR. However, it has limitations due to its high cost, limited availability, and radiation exposure. In contrast, musculoskeletal US is a non-invasive imaging technique that can visualize inflammation in joints and soft tissues. In PMR, US can detect bursitis, tenosynovitis, and synovitis, particularly in the shoulders and hips. Unlike PET-CT, US is cost-effective, widely available, and does not involve radiation exposure. It can provide real-time images and is useful for guiding joint aspirations or injections. However, US also has limitations, such as being operator-dependent and less effective at assessing deeper structures compared to PET-CT.

PET-CT and US can have complementary roles in managing patients with PMR. Both techniques can identify similar inflammatory changes, though through different ways. PET-CT provides a comprehensive overview of metabolic activity, while US offers a detailed structural imaging of superficial joints and tissues. Their combined use can increase diagnostic accuracy. Both PET-CT and US can detect bursitis in the shoulders and hips, which are the key diagnostic features of PMR. While PET-CT is highly sensitive, US is more practical for routine follow-up and monitoring.

In an interesting pictorial review on PET-CT in PMR, Rehak et al. reported on the use of 18F-FDG-PET-CT in a 55-year-old woman evaluated during a relapse of PMR to rule out co-incidental malignancy. PET-CT disclosed active inflammation in the shoulders, hips, and sternoclavicular joints, as well as near the ischial tuberosities and lumbar spinous interspaces. US confirmed these inflammatory changes. These findings support a good correlation between PET-CT and US [69].

10. Conclusions

In daily clinical practice, most patients with PMR are managed without the need of using PET-CT. In these cases, an appropriate clinical assessment and the routine laboratory markers of inflammation can help establish a diagnosis of PMR. However, PET-CT may be useful to establish a comprehensive evaluation of PMR [77].

Since PET-CT is not required for the diagnosis of PMR, clinicians must consider several situations in which this imaging technique may be used in patients with suspected PMR.

These situations are described below (Table 1):

Table 1. Situations in which we recommend performing PET-CT for identification of PMR.

Situations
Typical clinical manifestations but normal markers of inflammation
Patients with typical clinical features who do not experience adequate response to glucocorticoids
Patients with suspected PMR with atypical presentation
Suspected large vessel vasculitis indicative of extracranial GCA
To exclude other conditions that can mimic PMR (i.e., malignancies, infections, rheumatoid arthritis, and atypical spondyloarthritis)
PMR-like syndrome in cancer patients treated with immune checkpoint inhibitors (ICIs)

Abbreviations: PET-CT: positron emission tomography/computed tomography; PMR: polymyalgia rheumatica; GCA: giant cell arteritis.

Patients with typical clinical manifestations in which there is a shoulder inflammatory involvement associated with other clinical manifestations such as hip involvement but who have normal markers of inflammation [20,58].

An initial dose of prednisone/prednisolone ranging between 12.5 and 25 mg/day is recommended for the management of isolated PMR [78]. Following this procedure, most patients should improve. Consequently, FDG-PET-CT may be used in a patient with typical clinical features who does not experience adequate response (a remarkable improvement of symptoms within a week) after the onset of 15–25 mg of prednisone per day.

PET-CT may be also used in patients with suspected PMR with atypical presentations. It may also be the case in patients in whom the clinical picture is confusing and does not match common diagnostic criteria [39,58].

PET-CT may help us to exclude other conditions that present with similar symptoms, such as RA, malignancies, infections, or other inflammatory diseases [35,36].

Another indication may also be patients with suspected GCA as PMR and GCA are often overlapping conditions [38,79,80]. In this regard, PET-CT can be useful in detecting large-vessel inflammation in large vessels indicative of GCA [81,82]. With respect to this, a recent study that included a meta-analysis confirmed that 18F-FDG-PET-CT is a highly effective diagnostic tool for detecting extracranial large vessel vasculitis in patients with PMR. Its high sensitivity and specificity, coupled with its ability to provide a detailed visualization of vascular inflammation, make it a valuable addition to the diagnostic of conditions [83].

In summary, the search for a reliable diagnostic test is critical in patients with PMR, in particular in those who are not well-defined. As discussed by experts in the field [84], the use of 18F-FDG-PET imaging appears promising, offering detailed insights into inflammatory activity that may not be evident through traditional methods. However, while PET imaging shows potential, it is essential to weigh its cost, accessibility, and feasibility against its diagnostic benefits. Further research and clinical validation are necessary to determine whether PET can become a standard diagnostic approach for PMR.

Author Contributions: Conception, design, and interpretation of the data: E.H.-R., T.B.-S., R.L., S.C. and M.Á.G.-G. Acquisition of the data:E.H.-R., T.B.-S., L.C.L.-K., M.M.d.B.-A., A.T.-R., F.R.-G., C.C.-S., R.L., S.C. and M.Á.G.-G. All the authors have agreed to be personally accountable for their own contributions and to ensure that questions related to the accuracy or integrity of any part of the work, even ones in which the author was not personally involved, are appropriately investigated, resolved, and the resolution documented in the literature. All authors have read and agreed to the published version of the manuscript.

Funding: Miguel Ángel González-Gay research was supported by the Spanish Red de Investigación RICORS RD21/0002/0025 of the Instituto de Salud Carlos III, Spain.

Institutional Review Board Statement: The study was a review article and ethical review and approval was not needed.

Informed Consent Statement: Informed consent was obtained from all the subjects involved in the study.

Data Availability Statement: The data sets used and/or analyzed in the present study are available from the corresponding author upon request.

Conflicts of Interest: The authors declare no conflicts of interest.

References

1. Gonzalez-Gay, M.A.; Vazquez-Rodriguez, T.R.; Lopez-Diaz, M.J.; Miranda-Filloy, J.A.; Gonzalez-Juanatey, C.; Martin, J.; Llorca, J. Epidemiology of giant cell arteritis and polymyalgia rheumatica. *Arthritis Rheum.* **2009**, *61*, 1454–1461. [CrossRef] [PubMed]
2. González-Gay, M.A.; Pina, T. Giant cell arteritis and polymyalgia rheumatica: An update. *Curr. Rheumatol. Rep.* **2015**, *17*, 6. [CrossRef] [PubMed]
3. Lundberg, I.E.; Sharma, A.; Turesson, C.; Mohammad, A.J. An update on polymyalgia rheumatica. *J. Intern. Med.* **2022**, *292*, 717–732. [CrossRef] [PubMed] [PubMed Central]
4. Noltorp, S.; Svensson, B. High incidence of polymyalgia rheumatica and giant cell arteritis in a Swedish community. *Clin. Exp. Rheumatol.* **1991**, *9*, 351–355. [PubMed]
5. Schaufelberger, C.; Bengtsson, B.; Andersson, R. Epidemiology and mortality in 220 patients with polymyalgia rheumatica. *Br. J. Rheumatol.* **1995**, *34*, 261–264. [CrossRef] [PubMed]
6. Gran, J.T.; Myklebust, G. The incidence of polymyalgia rheumatica and temporal arteritis in the county of Aust Agder, south Norway: A prospective study 1987–1994. *J. Rheumatol.* **1997**, *24*, 1739–1743. [PubMed]
7. Doran, M.F.; Crowson, C.S.; O'Fallon, W.M.; Hunder, G.G.; Gabriel, S.E. Trends in the incidence of polymyalgia rheumatica over a 30 year period in Olmsted County, Minnesota, USA. *J. Rheumatol.* **2002**, *29*, 1694–1697. [PubMed]
8. Crowson, C.S.; Matteson, E.L. Contemporary prevalence estimates for giant cell arteritis and polymyalgia rheumatica, 2015. *Semin. Arthritis Rheum.* **2017**, *47*, 253–256. [CrossRef]
9. González-Gay, M.A.; García-Porrúa, C.; Vázquez-Caruncho, M.; Dababneh, A.; Hajeer, A.; Ollier, W.E. The spectrum of polymyalgia rheumatica in northwestern Spain: Incidence and analysis of variables associated with relapse in a 10 year study. *J. Rheumatol.* **1999**, *26*, 1326–1332. [PubMed]
10. Salvarani, C.; Macchioni, P.L.; Tartoni, P.L.; Rossi, F.; Baricchi, R.; Castri, C.; Chiaravalloti, F.; Portioli, I. Polymyalgia rheumatica and giant cell arteritis: A 5-year epidemiologic and clinical study in Reggio Emilia, Italy. *Clin. Exp. Rheumatol.* **1987**, *5*, 205–215. [PubMed]
11. Mattey, D.L.; Hajeer, A.H.; Dababneh, A.; Thomson, W.; González-Gay, M.A.; García-Porrúa, C.; Ollier, W.E.R. Association of giant cell arteritis and polymyalgia rheumatica with different tumor necrosis factor microsatellite polymorphisms. *Arthritis Rheum.* **2000**, *43*, 1749–1755. [CrossRef] [PubMed]
12. Dababneh, A.; Gonzalez-Gay, M.A.; Garcia-Porrua, C.; Hajeer, A.; Thomson, W.; Ollier, W. Giant cell arteritis and polymyalgia rheumatica can be differentiated by distinct patterns of HLA class II association. *J. Rheumatol.* **1998**, *25*, 2140–2145. [PubMed]
13. Gonzalez-Gay, M.A.; Hajeer, A.H.; Dababneh, A.; Garcia-Porrua, C.; Amoli, M.M.; Llorca, J.; Ollier, W.E. Interferon-gamma gene mi-crosatellite polymorphisms in patients with biopsy-proven giant cell arteritis and isolated polymyalgia rheumatica. *Clin. Exp. Rheumatol.* **2004**, *22* (Suppl. 36), S18–S20. [PubMed]
14. Zhao, S.S.; Mackie, S.L.; Larsson, S.C.; Burgess, S.; Yuan, S. Modifiable risk factors and inflammation-related proteins in polymyalgia rheumatica: Genome-wide meta-analysis and Mendelian randomisation. *Rheumatology* **2024**, keae308. [CrossRef] [PubMed]

15. Liozon, E.; Parreau, S.; Filloux, M.; Dumonteil, S.; Gondran, G.; Bezanahary, H.; Ly, K.H.; Fauchais, A.L. Giant cell arteritis or polymyalgia rheumatica after influenza vaccination: A study of 12 patients and a literature review. *Autoimmun. Rev.* **2021**, *20*, 102732. [CrossRef] [PubMed]
16. Manzo, C.; Castagna, A.; Ruotolo, G. Can SARS-CoV-2 trigger relapse of polymyalgia rheumatica? *Jt. Bone Spine* **2021**, *88*, 105150. [CrossRef] [PubMed] [PubMed Central]
17. González-Gay, M.A.; Matteson, E.L.; Castañeda, S. Polymyalgia rheumatica. *Lancet* **2017**, *390*, 1700–1712. [CrossRef] [PubMed]
18. Espígol-Frigolé, G.; Dejaco, C.; Mackie, S.L.; Salvarani, C.; Matteson, E.L.; Cid, M.C. Polymyalgia rheumatica. *Lancet* **2023**, *402*, 1459–1472. [CrossRef] [PubMed]
19. González-Gay, M.A.; García-Porrúa, C.; Salvarani, C.; Olivieri, I.; Hunder, G.G. Polymyalgia manifestations in different conditions mimicking polymyalgia rheumatica. *Clin. Exp. Rheumatol.* **2000**, *18*, 755–759. [PubMed]
20. González-Gay, M.A.; Rodríiguez-Valverde, V.; Blanco, R.; Fernández-Sueiro, J.L.; Armona, J.; Figueroa, M.; Martínez-Taboada, V.M. Polymyalgia rheumatica without significantly increased erythrocyte sedimentation rate: A more benign syndrome. *Arch. Intern. Med.* **1997**, *157*, 317–320. [CrossRef]
21. Meliconi, R.; Pulsatelli, L.; Uguccioni, M.; Salvarani, C.; Macchioni, P.; Melchiorri, C.; Focherini, M.C.; Frizziero, L.; Facchini, A. Leukocyte infiltration in synovial tissue from the shoulder of patients with polymyalgia rheumatica. Quantitative analysis and influence of corticosteroid treatment. *Arthritis Rheum.* **1996**, *39*, 1199–1207. [CrossRef] [PubMed]
22. Salvarani, C.; Cantini, F.; Olivieri, I.; Hunder, G.S. Polymyalgia rheumatica: A disorder of extraarticular synovial structures? *J. Rheumatol.* **1999**, *26*, 517–521.
23. Salvarani, C.; Cantini, F.; Olivieri, I.; Barozzi, L.; Macchioni, L.; Niccoli, L.; Padula, A.; De Matteis, M.; Pavlica, P. Proximal bursitis in active polymyalgia rheumatica. *Ann. Intern. Med.* **1997**, *127*, 27–31. [CrossRef] [PubMed]
24. Cantini, F.; Salvarani, C.; Olivieri, I.; Niccoli, L.; Padula, A.; Macchioni, L.; Boiardi, L.; Ciancio, G.; Mastrorosato, M.; Rubini, F.; et al. Shoulder ultrasonography in the diagnosis of polymyalgia rheumatica: A case-control study. *J. Rheumatol.* **2001**, *28*, 1049–1055. [PubMed]
25. Cantini, F.; Niccoli, L.; Nannini, C.; Padula, A.; Olivieri, I.; Boiardi, L.; Salvarani, C. Inflammatory changes of hip synovial structures in polymyalgia rheumatica. *Clin. Exp. Rheumatol.* **2005**, *23*, 462–468. [PubMed]
26. Salvarani, C.; Barozzi, L.; Cantini, F.; Niccoli, L.; Boiardi, L.; Valentino, M.; Pipitone, N.; Bajocchi, G.; Macchioni, P.; Catanoso, M.G.; et al. Cervical interspinous bursitis in active polymyalgia rheumatica. *Ann. Rheum. Dis.* **2008**, *67*, 758–761. [CrossRef] [PubMed]
27. Salvarani, C.; Barozzi, L.; Boiardi, L.; Pipitone, N.; Bajocchi, G.L.; Macchioni, P.L.; Catanoso, M.; Pazzola, G.; Valentino, M.; De Luca, C.; et al. Lumbar interspinous bursitis in active polymyalgia rheumatica. *Clin. Exp. Rheumatol.* **2013**, *31*, 526–531. [CrossRef] [PubMed]
28. Gonzalez-Gay, M.A. The clinical implication of cervical interspinous bursitis inthe diagnosis of polymyalgia rheumatica. *Ann. Rheum. Dis.* **2008**, *67*, 733–734. [CrossRef]
29. Dasgupta, B.; Cimmino, M.A.; Kremers, H.M.; Schmidt, W.A.; Schirmer, M.; Salvarani, C.; Bachta, A.; Dejaco, C.; Duftner, C.; Jensen, H.S.; et al. 2012 Provisional classification criteria for polymyalgia rheumatica: A European League against Rheumatism/American College of Rheumatology collaborative initiative. *Arthritis Rheum.* **2012**, *64*, 943–954. [CrossRef]
30. Macchioni, P.; Boiardi, L.; Catanoso, M.; Pazzola, G.; Salvarani, C. Performance of the new 2012 EULAR/ACR classification criteria for polymyalgia rheumatica: Comparison with the previous criteria in a single-centre study. *Ann. Rheum. Dis.* **2014**, *73*, 1190–1193. [CrossRef]
31. Sakellariou, G.; Iagnocco, A.; Riente, L.; Ceccarelli, F.; Carli, L.; Di Geso, L.; Sedie, A.D.; Filippucci, E.; Montecucco, C. Ultrasound imaging for the rheumatologist XLIII. Ultrasonographic evaluation of shoulders and hips in patients with polymyalgia rheumatica: A systematic literature review. *Clin. Exp. Rheumatol.* **2013**, *31*, 1–7. [PubMed]
32. Betrains, A.; Blockmans, D. Use of 18F-Fluorodeoxyglucose PET in the Diagnosis and Follow-up of Polymyalgia Rheumatica. *PET Clin.* **2020**, *15*, 147–152. [CrossRef] [PubMed]
33. Possemato, N.; Salvarani, C.; Pipitone, N. Imaging in polymyalgia rheumatica. *Reumatismo* **2018**, *70*, 51–58. [CrossRef] [PubMed]
34. Yuge, S.; Nakatani, K.; Yoshino, K.; Koyama, T. Diagnosing polymyalgia rheumatica on 18F-FDG PET/CT: Typical uptake patterns. *Ann. Nucl. Med.* **2018**, *32*, 573–577. [CrossRef]
35. González-Gay, M.Á.; Heras-Recuero, E.; Blázquez-Sánchez, T.; Caraballo-Salazar, C.; Rengifo-García, F.; Castañeda, S.; Largo, R. Broadening the clinical spectrum of giant cell arteritis: From the classic cranial to the predominantly extracranial pattern of the disease. *Expert. Rev. Clin. Immunol.* 2024, 1–12, *epub ahead of print*. [CrossRef] [PubMed]
36. Jamar, F.; van derLaken, C.J.; Panagiotidis, E.; Steinz, M.M.; van derGeest, K.S.M.; Graham, R.N.J.; Gheysens, O. Update on Imaging of In-flammatory Arthritis and Related Disorders. *Semin. Nucl. Med.* **2023**, *53*, 287–300. [CrossRef]
37. Mekenyan, L.; Karalilova, R.; Todorov, P.; Tepeliev, N.; Batalov, A. Imaging methods in polymyalgia rheumatica: A systematic review. *Rheumatol. Int.* **2023**, *43*, 825–840. [CrossRef]
38. Owen, C.E.; Poon, A.M.T.; Liu, B.; Liew, D.F.L.; Yap, L.P.; Yang, V.; Leung, J.L.; McMaster, C.R.; Scott, A.M.; Buchanan, R.R.C. Characterising polymyalgia rheumatica on whole-body 18F-FDG PET/CT: An atlas. *Rheumatol. Adv. Pract.* **2024**, *8*, rkae003. [CrossRef]
39. Gonzalez-Gay, M.A.; Garcia-Porrua, C.; Salvarani, C.; Olivieri, I.; Hunder, G.G. The spectrum of conditions mimicking polymyalgia rheumatica in Northwestern Spain. *J. Rheumatol.* **2000**, *27*, 2179–2184. [PubMed]

40. Paltta, J.; Suuronen, S.; Pirilä, L.; Palomäki, A. Differential diagnostics of polymyalgia rheumatica in a university hospital in Finland. *Scand. J. Rheumatol.* **2023**, *52*, 689–695. [CrossRef]
41. Gheysens, O.; de Ponfilly, M.P.; Nocturne, G.; Seror, R.; Besson, F.L.; Jamar, F. [18F]FDG-PET/CT in Polymyalgia Rheumatica: An Update and Future Aspects. *Semin. Nucl. Med.* **2023**, *54*, 371–378. [CrossRef] [PubMed]
42. van der Geest, K.S.M.; Treglia, G.; Glaudemans, A.W.J.M.; Brouwer, E.; Jamar, F.; Slart, R.H.J.A.; Gheysens, O. Diagnostic value of [18F]FDG-PET/CT in polymyalgia rheumatica: A systematic review and meta-analysis. *Eur. J. Nucl. Med. Mol. Imaging* **2021**, *48*, 1876–1889. [CrossRef] [PubMed]
43. Camellino, D.; Paparo, F.; Morbelli, S.D.; Pesce, G.; Bauckneht, M.; Bagnasco, M.; Cutolo, M.; Sambuceti, G.; Cimmino, M.A. Clinical and FDG-PET/CT correlates in patients with polymyalgia rheumatica. *Clin. Exp. Rheumatol.* **2022**, *40*, 78–85. [CrossRef] [PubMed]
44. Kim, K.; Kim, S.-J. Diagnostic performance of F-18 fluorodeoxyglucose PET/computed tomography for diagnosis of polymyalgia rheumatica: A meta-analysis. *Nucl. Med. Commun.* **2020**, *41*, 1313–1321. [CrossRef] [PubMed]
45. Amat, J.; Chanchou, M.; Olagne, L.; Descamps, L.; Flaus, A.; Bouvet, C.; Barres, B.; Valla, C.; Molnar, L.; Cougoul, A.; et al. Utility of 18F-Fluorodeoxyglucose Positron Emission Tomography in Inflammatory Rheumatism, Particularly Polymyalgia Rheumatica: A Retrospective Study of 222 PET/CT. *Front. Med.* **2020**, *7*, 394. [CrossRef] [PubMed]
46. Moreel, L.; Boeckxstaens, L.; Betrains, A.; Van Hemelen, M.; Vanderschueren, S.; Van Laere, K.; Blockmans, D. Diagnostic accuracy and validation of 18F-fluorodeoxyglucose positron emission tomography scores in a large cohort of patients with polymyalgia rheumatica. *Front. Med.* **2022**, *9*, 1026944. [CrossRef] [PubMed] [PubMed Central]
47. van der Geest, K.S.M.; van Sleen, Y.; Nienhuis, P.; Sandovici, M.; Westerdijk, N.; Glaudemans, A.W.J.M.; Brouwer, E.; Slart, R.H.J.A. Comparison and validation of FDG-PET/CT scores for polymyalgia rheumatica. *Rheumatology* **2022**, *61*, 1072–1082. [CrossRef] [PubMed] [PubMed Central]
48. Sondag, M.; Guillot, X.; Verhoeven, F.; Blagosklonov, O.; Prati, C.; Boulahdour, H.; Wendling, D. Utility of 18F-fluoro-dexoxyglucose positron emission tomography for the diagnosis of polymyalgia rheumatica: A controlled study. *Rheumatology* **2016**, *55*, 1452–1457. [CrossRef]
49. Flaus, A.; Amat, J.; Prevot, N.; Olagne, L.; Descamps, L.; Bouvet, C.; Barres, B.; Valla, C.; Mathieu, S.; Andre, M.; et al. Decision Tree with Only Two Musculoskeletal Sites to Diagnose Polymyalgia Rheumatica Using [18F]FDG PET-CT. *Front. Med.* **2021**, *8*, 646974. [CrossRef] [PubMed] [PubMed Central]
50. Owen, C.E.; Poon, A.M.T.; Yang, V.; McMaster, C.; Lee, S.T.; Liew, D.F.L.; Leung, J.L.; Scott, A.M.; Buchanan, R.R.C. Abnormalities at three musculoskeletal sites on whole-body positron emission tomography/computed tomography can diagnose polymyalgia rheumatica with high sensitivity and specificity. *Eur. J. Nucl. Med. Mol. Imaging* **2020**, *47*, 2461–2468. [CrossRef] [PubMed]
51. Brinth, L.S.; Hansen, A.; Jensen, D.V.; Madsen, O.R.; Broholm, R.; Krakauer, M. Diagnostic Value of Composite and Simplified FDG-PET/CT Scores in Polymyalgia Rheumatica and the Influence of Recent Glucocorticoid Treatment—A Retrospective Diagnostic Cohort Study. *Diagnostics* **2023**, *13*, 514. [CrossRef] [PubMed] [PubMed Central]
52. Ikuma, D.; Sawa, N.; Yamanouchi, M.; Oba, Y.; Mizuno, H.; Suwabe, T.; Hoshino, J.; Ubara, Y. Diagnostic value of 18F-fluorodeoxyglucose positron emission tomography and computed tomography for differentiating polymyalgia rheumatica and rheumatoid arthritis: Using classification and regression tree analysis. *Mod. Rheumatol.* **2024**, *34*, 474–478. [CrossRef] [PubMed]
53. Casadepax-Soulet, C.; Benali, K.; Crestani, B.; Piekarski, E.; Mahida, B.; Ebstein, E.; Juge, P.-A.; Forien, M.; Dieudé, P.; Ottaviani, S. Fluorine-18 fluorodeoxyglucose positron emission tomography/computed tomography in polymyalgia rheumatica: An observational study. *Clin. Exp. Rheumatol.* **2023**, *41*, 1456–1462. [CrossRef] [PubMed]
54. Henckaerts, L.; Gheysens, O.; Vanderschueren, S.; Goffin, K.; Blockmans, D. Use of 18F-fluorodeoxyglucose positron emission tomography in the diagnosis of polymyalgia rheumatica—A prospective study of 99 patients. *Rheumatology* **2018**, *57*, 1908–1916. [CrossRef] [PubMed]
55. Yamashita, H.; Kubota, K.; Takahashi, Y.; Minaminoto, R.; Morooka, M.; Ito, K.; Kano, T.; Kaneko, H.; Takashima, H.; Mimoiri, A. Whole-body fluorodeoxyglucose positron emission tomography/computed tomography in patients with active polymyalgia rheumatica: Evidence for distinctive bursitis and large-vessel vasculitis. *Mod. Rheumatol.* **2012**, *22*, 705–711. [CrossRef] [PubMed]
56. Heras-Recuero, E.; Landaeta-Kancev, L.C.; de Bourio-Allona, M.M.; Torres-Rosello, A.; Blázquez-Sánchez, T.; Ferraz-Amaro, I.; Castañeda, S.; Martínez-López, J.A.; Martínez-Dhier, L.; Largo, R.; et al. Positron Emission Computed Tomography Spectrum of Large Vessel Vasculitis in a Tertiary Center: Differences in 18F-fluorodeoxyglucose Uptake between Large Vessel Vasculitis with Predominant Cranial and Extracranial Giant Cell Arteritis Phenotypes. *J. Clin. Med.* **2023**, *12*, 6164. [CrossRef] [PubMed] [PubMed Central]
57. Heras-Recuero, E.; de Bourio-Allona, M.M.; Landaeta-Kancev, L.C.; Blázquez-Sánchez, T.; Torres-Roselló, A.; Álvarez-Rubio, M.; Belhaj-Gandar, M.; Martínez-López, J.A.; Martínez-Dhier, L.; Llorca, J.; et al. 18F-Fluorodeoxyglucose Positron Emission Tomography–Computed Tomography Findings of Polymyalgia Rheumatica in Patients with Giant Cell Arteritis. *J. Clin. Med.* **2023**, *12*, 6983. [CrossRef] [PubMed] [PubMed Central]
58. Slart, R.H.J.A.; Nienhuis, P.H.; Glaudemans, A.W.J.M.; Brouwer, E.; Gheysens, O.; van der Geest, K.S.M. Role of ^{18}F-FDG PET/CT in Large Vessel Vasculitis and Polymyalgia Rheumatica. *J. Nucl. Med.* **2023**, *64*, 515–521. [CrossRef] [PubMed]
59. Gorlen, T.F.; Brittain, J.M.; Østergaard, M.; Fischer, B.M.; Døhn, U.M.; Terslev, L. Low incidence of malignancy in patients with suspected polymyalgia rheumatica or giant cell arteritis, examined with FDG-PET/CT. *Front. Med.* **2024**, *11*, 1309905. [CrossRef] [PubMed] [PubMed Central]

60. Abdel-Wahab, N.; Suarez-Almazor, M.E. Rheumatic adverse events of immune checkpoint inhibitors in cancer immunotherapy. *Expert Rev. Clin. Immunol.* **2024**, 1–21. [CrossRef] [PubMed]
61. Liew, D.F.L.; Mackie, S.L.; Tison, A.; Sattui, S.E.; Yates, M.; Buchanan, R.R.C.; Owen, C.E.; Liew, D.F.; Mackie, S.L.; Tison, A.; et al. Immune Checkpoint Inhibitor-induced Polymyalgia Rheumatica. *Rheum. Dis. Clin. N. Am.* **2024**, *50*, 255–267. [CrossRef] [PubMed]
62. Vermeulen, O.C.B.; Brouwer, E.; Slart, R.H.J.A.; Sandovici, M.; Rutgers, A.; Hilterman, T.J.; Hiddinga, B.; Oosting, S.F.; Jalving, M.; de Heij, A.H.; et al. Immune checkpoint inhibitor-mediated polymyalgia rheumatica versus primary polymyalgia rheumatica: Comparison of disease characteristics and treatment requirement. *Rheumatology* **2024**, keae099. [CrossRef] [PubMed]
63. Desvages, A.; Hives, F.; Deprez, X.; Pierache, A.; Béhal, H.; Flipo, R.-M.; Paccou, J. Usefulness of 18F-Fluorodeoxyglucose Positron Emission Tomography in Diagnosing Polymyalgia Rheumatica and Large-Vessel Vasculitis: A Case-Control Study. *J. Clin. Med.* **2023**, *12*, 2844. [CrossRef] [PubMed] [PubMed Central]
64. Ponte, C.; Martins-Martinho, J.; Luqmani, R.A. Diagnosis of giant cell arteritis. *Rheumatology* **2020**, *59* (Suppl. 3), iii5–iii16. [CrossRef] [PubMed]
65. van der Geest, K.S.M.; Slijkhuis, B.G.C.; Tomelleri, A.; Gheysens, O.; Jiemy, W.F.; Piccolo, C.; Nienhuis, P.; Sandovici, M.; Brouwer, E.; Glaudemans, A.W.; et al. Positron Emission Tomography Imaging in Vasculitis. *Cardiol. Clin.* **2023**, *41*, 251–265. [CrossRef] [PubMed]
66. Germanò, G.; Versari, A.; Muratore, F.; Pipitone, N.; Bajocchi, G.L.; Catanoso, M.G.; Salvarani, C. Isolated vasculitis of the lower extremities in a patient with polymyalgia rheumatica and giant cell arteritis. *Clin. Exp. Rheumatol.* **2011**, *29* (Suppl. 64), S138–S139. [PubMed]
67. Dejaco, C.; Ramiro, S.; Bond, M.; Bosch, P.; Ponte, C.; Mackie, S.L.; Bley, T.A.; Blockmans, D.; Brolin, S.; Bolek, E.C.; et al. EULAR recommendations for the use of imaging in large vessel vasculitis in clinical practice: 2023 update. *Ann. Rheum. Dis.* **2023**, *83*, 741–751. [CrossRef] [PubMed]
68. Prieto-Peña, D.; Martínez-Rodríguez, I.; Loricera, J.; Banzo, I.; Calderón-Goercke, M.; Calvo-Río, V.; González-Vela, C.; Corrales, A.; Castañeda, S.; Blanco, R.; et al. Predictors of positive 18F-FDG PET/CT-scan for large vessel vasculitis in patients with persistent polymyalgia rheumatica. *Semin. Arthritis Rheum.* **2019**, *48*, 720–727. [CrossRef] [PubMed]
69. Rehak, Z.; Sprlakova-Pukova, A.; Kazda, T.; Fojtik, Z.; Vargova, L.; Nemec, P. ^{18}F-FDG PET/CT in polymyalgia rheumatica—A pictorial review. *Br. J. Radiol.* **2017**, *90*, 20170198. [CrossRef] [PubMed] [PubMed Central]
70. Kubota, K.; Yamashita, H.; Mimori, A. Clinical Value of FDG-PET/CT for the Evaluation of Rheumatic Diseases: Rheumatoid Arthritis, Polymyalgia Rheumatica, and Relapsing Polychondritis. *Semin. Nucl. Med.* **2017**, *47*, 408–424. [CrossRef] [PubMed]
71. Pean de Ponfilly-Sotier, M.; Besson, F.L.; Gomez, L.; Ottaviani, S.; Dieudé, P.; Pavy, S.; Mariette, X.; Seror, R.; Nocturne, G. Use of 18F FDG PET-CT to discriminate polymyalgia rheumatica and atypical spondylarthritis in clinical practice. *Jt. Bone Spine* **2022**, *89*, 105325. [CrossRef] [PubMed]
72. Emamifar, A.; Hess, S.; Gerke, O.; Hermann, A.P.; Laustrup, H.; Hansen, P.S.; Thye-Rønn, P.; Marcussen, N.; Svendstrup, F.; Gildberg-Mortensen, R.; et al. Polymyalgia rheumatica and giant cell arteritis—Three challenges—Consequences of the vasculitis process, osteoporosis, and malignancy: A prospective cohort study protocol. *Medicine* **2017**, *96*, e7297. [CrossRef] [PubMed] [PubMed Central]
73. Stellingwerff, M.D.; Brouwer, E.; Lensen, K.D.F.; Rutgers, A.; Arends, S.; van der Geest, K.S.M.; Glaudemans, A.W.J.M.; Slart, R.H.J.A. Different Scoring Methods of FDG PET/CT in Giant Cell Arteritis: Need for Standardization. *Medicine* **2015**, *94*, e1542. [CrossRef] [PubMed] [PubMed Central]
74. Nielsen, B.D.; Gormsen, L.C.; Hansen, I.T.; Keller, K.K.; Therkildsen, P.; Hauge, E.-M. Three days of high-dose glucocorticoid treatment attenuates large-vessel 18F-FDG uptake in large-vessel giant cell arteritis but with a limited impact on diagnostic accuracy. *Eur. J. Nucl. Med. Mol. Imaging* **2018**, *45*, 1119–1128. [CrossRef] [PubMed]
75. Nielsen, A.W.; Hansen, I.T.; Nielsen, B.D.; Kjær, S.G.; Blegvad-Nissen, J.; Rewers, K.; Sørensen, C.M.; Hauge, E.-M.; Gormsen, L.C.; Keller, K.K. The effect of prednisolone and a short-term prednisolone discontinuation for the diagnostic accuracy of FDG-PET/CT in polymyalgia rheumatica—A prospective study of 101 patients. *Eur. J. Nucl. Med. Mol. Imaging* **2024**, *51*, 2614–2624. [CrossRef] [PubMed]
76. Blockmans, D.; De Ceuninck, L.; Vanderschueren, S.; Knockaert, D.; Mortelmans, L.; Bobbaers, H. Repetitive 18-fluorodeoxyglucose positron emission tomography in isolated polymyalgia rheumatica: A prospective study in 35 patients. *Rheumatology* **2007**, *46*, 672–677. [CrossRef] [PubMed]
77. Camellino, D.; Cimmino, M.A. Imaging of polymyalgia rheumatica: Indications on its pathogenesis, diagnosis and prognosis. *Rheumatology* **2012**, *51*, 77–86. [CrossRef] [PubMed]
78. Dejaco, C.; Singh, Y.P.; Perel, P.; Hutchings, A.; Camellino, D.; Mackie, S.; Abril, A.; Bachta, A.; Balint, P.; Barraclough, K.; et al. 2015 Recommendations for the management of polymyalgia rheumatica: A European League against Rheumatism/American College of Rheumatology collaborative initiative. *Ann. Rheum. Dis.* **2015**, *74*, 1799–1807. [CrossRef] [PubMed]
79. Emamifar, A.; Ellingsen, T.; Hess, S.; Gerke, O.; Hviid Larsen, R.; Ahangarani Farahani, Z.; Syrak Hansen, P.; Jensen Hansen, I.M.; Petersen, H.; Marcussen, N.; et al. The Utility of 18F-FDG PET/CT in Patients with Clinical Suspicion of Polymyalgia Rheumatica and Giant Cell Arteritis: A Prospective, Observational, and Cross-sectional Study. *ACR Open Rheumatol.* **2020**, *2*, 478–490. [CrossRef] [PubMed] [PubMed Central]

80. Salvarani, C.; Padoan, R.; Iorio, L.; Tomelleri, A.; Terrier, B.; Muratore, F.; Dasgupta, B. Subclinical giant cell arteritis in polymyalgia rheumatica: Concurrent conditions or a common spectrum of inflammatory diseases? *Autoimmun. Rev.* **2024**, *23*, 103415. [CrossRef] [PubMed]
81. Galli, E.; Muratore, F.; Mancuso, P.; Boiardi, L.; Marvisi, C.; Besutti, G.; Spaggiari, L.; Casali, M.; Versari, A.; Rossi, P.G.; et al. The role of PET/CT in disease activity assessment in patients with large vessel vasculitis. *Rheumatology* **2022**, *61*, 4809–4816. [CrossRef] [PubMed]
82. Noriega-Álvarez, E.; Rodríguez-Alfonso, B.; Merino Argumánez, C.; Domínguez Gadea, L.; Peiró-Valgañón, V. Decoding polymyalgia rheumatica, the role of Nuclear Medicine Imaging. *Rev. Esp. Med. Nucl. Imagen. Mol. (Engl. Ed.)* **2024**, *43*, 63–72. [CrossRef] [PubMed]
83. García, A.G.; Fabregate, M.; Serralta, G.; de Miguel Campo, B.; Mozo, A.N.; Robles-Marhuenda, Á. The utility of 18F-FDG-PET/CT in detecting extracranial large vessel vasculitis in rheumatic polymyalgia or giant cell arteritis: A systematic review and meta-analysis. *Rev. Clin. Esp.* 2024, *in press*. [CrossRef]
84. Clifford, A.H.; Cimmino, M.A. In search of a diagnostic test for polymyalgia rheumatica: Is positron emission tomography the answer? *Rheumatology* **2018**, *57*, 1881–1882. [CrossRef] [PubMed]

diagnostics MDPI

Review

Relapse Predictors in Antineutrophil Cytoplasmic Antibody (ANCA)-Associated Vasculitis

Katarzyna Wawrzycka-Adamczyk [1,*], Mariusz Korkosz [1,2], Jacek Musiał [2] and Krzysztof Wójcik [1,2]

1 Rheumatology, Immunology and Internal Medicine Department, Kraków University Hospital, ul Jakubowskiego 2, 30-688 Kraków, Poland; mariusz.korkosz@uj.edu.pl (M.K.); krzysztof.wojcik@uj.edu.pl (K.W.)

2 Faculty of Medicine, Jagiellonian University Medical College, 31-008 Kraków, Poland; jacek.musial@uj.edu.pl

* Correspondence: kwawrzycka@su.krakow.pl; Tel.: +48-664-330-889

Abstract: Antineutrophil cytoplasmic antibody (ANCA)-associated vasculitides (AAVs) are a group of rare diseases with a chronic and relapsing course. Recent treatment guidelines offer many therapeutic options depending mainly on the type of diagnosis and disease manifestations. Areas that remain under discussion include whether all patients diagnosed with AAV belong to a homogeneous group with a similar prognosis at baseline or if the type and duration of remission-inducing treatment should depend on factors other than just diagnosis and disease severity. The aim of this review is to present the recent literature on the tools available to use while evaluating the risk of relapse in patients upon presentation as well as potential biomarkers of proceeding flare in patients upon remission.

Keywords: vasculitis; relapse; predictors

1. Introduction

Antineutrophil cytoplasmic antibody (ANCA)-associated vasculitides (AAVs) are a group of rare diseases with an incidence of 13–20 cases per million per year worldwide, including granulomatosis with polyangiitis (GPA), microscopic polyangiitis (MPA) and eosinophilic GPA (EGPA) [1–4]. The incidence of AAV has grown markedly over the last 30 years, which might be explained by the availability of ANCA testing, growing awareness of the diseases and evolution of classification criteria [5]. AAV clinical manifestations mostly reflect the fact that inflammation affects small and medium vessels and includes mostly upper and lower respiratory tract involvement, glomerulonephritis, and skin, eye and neurological symptoms. Since their first description in the 1930s, advancements in research on the diagnosis and treatment of these diseases have transformed them from rapidly progressing fatal conditions into chronic ones [6,7]. The latest treatment guidelines offer many therapeutic options depending on the type of diagnosis, disease manifestations, and other clinical variables. The intensity of the initial immunosuppressive remission induction depends mainly on the initial diagnosis of limited or generalized form of the disease, while maintenance therapy intensity and duration is rather uniform [8]. The treatment recommendations provide guidance for therapeutic decisions but do not address all questions regarding the care of patients with AAV. Areas that remain under discussion include whether all patients diagnosed with AAV belong to a homogeneous group with a similar prognosis at baseline or if the type and duration of remission-inducing treatment should depend on factors other than just diagnosis and the differentiation between limited and generalized forms. Given that AAV exacerbations lead to the accrual of organ damage, another research aim is to create a set of diagnostic tools that, along with the form of the disease, could predict the long-term efficacy of the applied treatment or the likelihood and timing of relapse [9]. Another challenge in AAV management is the outpatient monitoring of those who have achieved remission. Commonly used disease activity assessment tools, which guide immunosuppressive treatment intensification, rely on a set of results, including imaging, laboratory tests, and consultation outcomes. To obtain these results, it is necessary to repeat them regularly in asymptomatic patients or in an accelerated manner for patients reporting symptoms. The fact that some clinical manifestations, such as hematuria, may present with few symptoms can delay the recognition of disease relapse, thereby predisposing patients to persistent changes and the accumulation of irreversible organ damage. Some simple sets of laboratory tests are proposed to perform on a regular basis for an early relapse detection in patients upon remission, but other sensitive and specific tools are still under investigation [10,11].

It is worth emphasizing that EGPA is both pathogenetic and clinically different from other AAVs. Patients of this entity are rarely participants of the same clinical trials or other scientific studies assessing the course of exacerbations, so EGPA is not included in the study below.

2. Methodology

The methodology of this review was based on the literature search for the MEDLINE database including studies published before 30 May 2024. Only studies written in English were analyzed. The main search strategy included adult GPA, MPA and AAV cohorts combined with relapse terminology.

3. Baseline Relapse Risk Evaluation

The clinical manifestation at flare of AAV seems to play a role in predicting future exacerbation. Single-center experiences most commonly pointed at proteinase 3 (PR3) ANCA presence and lung involvement as factors predictive of relapse [12,13]. Large multicenter clinical trials have delivered further data to analyze the set of basic risk factors of relapse in AAV. In 2008, a group of patients in the Glomerular Disease Collaborative Network (GDCN, $n = 350$) in the southeastern US was compared with a group of patients in the French Vasculitis Study Group (FVSG, n = 434). During a mean follow-up of 45 months, the risk of exacerbation in the GDCN group was shown to coexist with the presence of anti-PR3 antibodies (HR 1.68), lung involvement (HR 1.68), and upper respiratory tract involvement (HR 1.58) [14]. Pooled results from NORAM, CYCAZAREM, CYCLOPS and MEPEX (>500 patients) (pooled trials cohort) showed that 38% of patients experienced relapse during the observation period (between 36 and 132 months). Anti-proteinase 3 antibodies and cardiovascular involvement were found to be independently associated with a higher risk of relapse, while a creatinine level more than 200 μmol/L at baseline was strongly associated with a reduced risk of flare [15]. A meta-analysis of 16 trials published in 2021 confirmed that significant risk factors for relapse include the presence of anti-PR3 ANCA positivity [HR 1.69], cardiovascular involvement [HR 1.78], creatinine >200 μmol/L [HR 0.39] and creatinine 101–200 μmol/L [HR 0.81] [16].

Similar observations were made in a meta-analysis searching for relapse predictors in cyclophosphamide-treated patients by He et al. A lower level of baseline serum creatine, proteinase 3 (PR3)-ANCA positivity at diagnosis and extrarenal organ involvement (lung, cardiovascular, upper respiratory, and gastrointestinal involvement), were found risk factors for an exacerbation at baseline [17]. A significant role of creatinine level on relapse risk was also confirmed in a big Polish cohort analysis. Also, skin, ENT and eye involvement were found to increase the risk of flare [18].

3.1. ANCA Testing

ANCA antibodies are an important pathogenetic element in the development of vasculitis with high sensitivity and specificity for AAV diagnosis [19,20]. Actual guidelines suggest using one-step antibody testing as a rapid, non-invasive tool in the diagnosis of patients with suspected vasculitis, based on the EUVAS study comparing the performance of ANCA IF and immunoassays and the subsequent changes introduced by the revised 2017 international consensus on the testing of ANCAs in granulomatosis with polyangiitis and microscopic polyangiitis [21,22]. Their identification is important in the process of classifying patients with a histopathological diagnosis of small vessel vasculitis [23–25]. However, it should be noticed, on the one hand, that some patients diagnosed with GPA, MPA and EGPA remain seronegative, and on the other hand, ANCA positivity is observed also in other diseases such as inflammatory bowel disease or drug-induced [26–28]. It is also worth emphasizing that racial differences are observed in the distribution of AAV serotypes in various populations, e.g., Caucasian patients diagnosed with GPA are mainly anti-ANCA-PR3-positive (65–75%), while in the Chinese population, the majority of patients with GPA show myeloperoxidase (MPO) positivity (71%) [29,30]. Overall, it should be concluded that while ANCA testing is an indispensable diagnostic tool in suspected AAV and has an important role in the classification process, it also has some limitations [31]. The performance of ANCA testing, its type and titer in predicting the recurrence of relapsing AAV patients remains debatable. The first reports regarding the potential role of ANCA titer in predicting exacerbations date back to the 1990s. The Kyndt team monitored disease status over 22 months in groups of patients completing remission-inducing treatment for GPA (then Wegener's granulomatosis, n = 21) and MPA (n = 17). They observed that the baseline ANCA pattern (IF) did not differentiate relapsers from non-relapsers; however, relapses occurred more frequently in patients with initial lung involvement [16 of 23 (70%) vs. 6 of 20 (30%)] and persisting ANCA presence (86% vs. 20% in the ANCA-negative group) [32]. The following years brought further evidence of the usefulness of dividing patients with AAV in terms of antibody specificity in stratifying the risk of exacerbations [33–36]. Lionaki's group compared this stratification system to the disease classification criteria and Chapel Hill Consensus Conference (CHCC) definitions, indicating that ANCA's specificity had the best relapse predictive model fit of all the tested methods [37]. Similar observations were provided by the first large clinical trials comparing different treatment regimens to induce and maintain remission in AAV. A cluster analysis of the results of five such studies (n = 673) selected the following clusters: 'renal AAV with PR3-ANCA positivity (40% of subjects), 'renal AAV without PR3-ANCA' (32%), 'non-renal AAV' (12%), 'cardiovascular AAV' (9%) and 'gastrointestinal AAV' (7%), differing from each other in both overall survival and the percentage of patients experiencing disease relapse, indicating the first subgroup as having the highest risk of recurrence [38]. In 2013, a retrospective analysis was conducted on factors responsible for not achieving disease remission within 6 months in the RAVE study (CYC/AZA vs. RTX in AAV). Among the study participants, 19% experienced disease relapse after initial improvement but before the 6-month mark of induction treatment. Among those who had severe flares, 92% were PR3-ANCA-positive, and 83% had GPA. A history of disease exacerbations prior to starting induction therapy was also considered an additional risk factor for early disease relapse at that time [39]. Not all analyses regarding the relationship between antibody type and disease relapse have been consistent. In a Japanese study from 2015, it was shown that both ANCA-PR3+ GPA and ANCA-MPO+GPA patient groups relapsed more frequently than MPA patients. It is worth noting, however, that this study involved a smaller group of patients compared to other studies on this topic and focused on a Japanese population characterized by significant differences in the type of antibodies present in GPA compared to Caucasian populations [40]. A pooled analysis from two large RCTs, RAVE and WGENT, found in 2016 that the risk of exacerbations in the MPO-ANCA-positive GPA and PR3-positive GPA groups did not differ from each other, but in the former group, it was higher than in the MPO-positive MPA group at both 12 and 18 months of follow-up. The risk of relapse in this cohort study was associated more closely with disease type rather than ANCA type [41]. A similar observation was made from a retrospective analysis of patients from Caen University Hospital (n = 150). Relapse-free survival was shorter in the group of patients with GPA than for patients with MPA; however, no differences in the risk of exacerbation were observed between patients with PR3+ and MPO+ [42]. The differences between the findings of these studies and earlier reports may stem from several factors. Firstly, the analyzed groups differ demographically and clinically. Some study populations include participants from clinical trials, which could impact the generalizability of findings to broader patient populations. Additionally, there are significant differences in cohort creation methodologies, such as the proportion of patients with new diagnoses versus those experiencing disease exacerbations. Moreover, variations exist in the speciality of medical centers recruiting patients (e.g., nephrology vs. rheumatology). These factors collectively contribute to the variability in study outcomes observed across different research efforts. Important answers to questions about the prognostic value of ANCA's baseline status were eventually provided by an analysis of a large population from the French Vasculitis Study Group registry. The study unequivocally demonstrated that while the group of patients with seronegative AAV did not differ in terms of 5- or 10-year relapse-free rates from the group of GPA and MPA patients with antibodies, a detailed analysis of PR3-ANCA-positive patients showed a higher frequency of vasculitis exacerbations compared to the rest of the AAV population. It is important to note, however, that this relationship did not impact differences in overall survival [43]. Summarizing, it can therefore be concluded that not the presence of ANCA antibodies but their specificity may be helpful in stratifying the risk of relapse in patients who achieve AAV remission. Together with phenotypic analysis, it may in the future be a tool for classifying patients with individual clusters in terms of the risk of recurrence and be the basis for differentiating the treatment model in individual groups. The impact of such changes on overall survival would need to be verified but could be helpful in reducing the immunosuppressant's exposure.

3.2. *Cell Count, Genetics, Infections, Histopathology and Other Predictors at Baseline*

Flow cytometry studies also allowed us to identify cell populations that may predict resistance to induction treatment. These include the population of CD27+CD38hi B cells, an increased percentage of which in the relapsers group was observed in both peripheral blood and urine. Their presence in the study material was interpreted as the result of migration from the kidneys, as these cells were also observed in the kidney biopsies of patients in the active phase of the disease [44]. In 2015, Graysson et al. conducted a trial focusing on the hypothesis that low-density granulocytes (LDGs) contribute to gene expression signatures in AAV. The RNA sequencing of whole blood in patients with AAV was compared. Differential expression between responders (n = 77) and nonresponders (n = 35) was detected in 2346 transcripts at the baseline visit. The increased expression of a granulocyte gene signature was associated with disease activity and decreased response to treatment. The source of this signature was likely LDGs [45].

Genome-wide association studies in AAV have led to the identification of the genetic background of AAV susceptibility such as *CTLA-4*, *PTPN22*, *FCGR2A*, *SERPINA1* (an endogenous inhibitor of PR3), and TLR9 genetic variations. It was also proven that GPA is associated with *HLA-DP1*, MPA with *HLA-DQ*, and EGPA with *HLA-DRB4* [46]. This discovery aroused questions about potential treatment resistance predictors among genetic factors. The carriers of *TNFSF13B rs3759467* (a single-nucleotide polymorphism) and homozygous carriers of *HLA-DPB1*04:01* were found to relapse earlier than non-carriers [47–49]. As genetic testing is not available in every clinical center and is also relatively complex and expensive, these research results seem to be more informative than have presently a practical impact.

The role of infectious factors on AAV development and course was debated for a long time. Thirty years ago, it was proven that the chronic nasal carriage of *S. aureus* identifies a subgroup of GPA patients who are at risk of relapses of the disease, suggesting a role for *S. aureus* in its pathophysiology and a possible clue for treatment [50,51]. This early observations were also supported by the fact that treating GPA patients with trimethoptim–sulfamethoxazole reduced the incidence of relapses [52]. An explanation of this phenomenon is complex and still not well described, but it is worth noting that GPA exhibits molecular features that allow its differentiation from other inflammatory disorders with nasal involvement and that a mucosal disbalance might orchestrate primary inflammation on site [53,54]. It has also been shown that in mice models, staphylococcus aureus plasmid-encoded 6-phosphogluconate dehydrogenase can induce anti-MPO autoimmunity, pointing at a possible molecular mimicry mechanism [55].

Most studies validating the histopathological classification of ANCA-associated glomerulonephritis focused on renal survival, although renal relapse probability was separately analyzed in a pooled cohort of patients from MEPEX and CYCAZAREM trials. Both clinical and histological parameters were taken under investigation. In this trial, sclerotic class ANCA-associated glomerulonephritis and the lack of interstitial infiltrates in baseline renal biopsies increased the instantaneous risk of renal relapse [56–59].

Some other relapse predictors at AAV flare have also been proposed: CCL18 serum levels, calprotectin at month 2 and 6 after RTX administration and a low number of circulating endothelial progenitor cells (EPCs) [60–62].

4. Relapse Predictors on Remission

Although cheap and easy to obtain, simple biomarkers of inflammation, like ESR, CRP, IL-6, IL-8, IL-15, IL-18BP, and matrix metalloproteinase-3 [MMP-3], seem to have a correlation with AAV activity and fail to predict relapse in longitudinal observations [63,64]. It raises questions about other possible tools for monitoring remission in order to early detect upcoming relapse.

4.1. ANCA Testing

Antibodies against PR3 most probably induce inflammation by directing the cells they bind to towards apoptosis, whereas antibodies against MPO stimulate cells to produce reactive oxygen species [65]. In vivo experiments have subsequently demonstrated that anti-MPO antibodies alone have the ability to induce full-blown vasculitis, whereas anti-PR3 antibodies have this potential only under specific conditions and typically induce milder forms of the disease [66–70]. These observations led to the hypothesis that an increase in ANCA titer may herald impending vasculitis exacerbations in patients who have achieved clinical remission, particularly in those with dominant capillaritis rather than granulomatous inflammation. Such measurements are cost-effective and non-invasive tools for monitoring patients in outpatient settings [71]. The initial reports on the predictive role of serial ANCA measurements in patients in remission suggested their high specificity. In a study by Tervaert et al., all exacerbations observed in the cohort of patients were preceded by a significant rise in ANCA titers [72]. In 1999, a serial analysis of ANCA levels in a group of patients with AAV showed that a significant titer increase was observed in 73% of exacerbations in patients with anti-MPO antibodies but only in 33% of exacerbations in those with anti-PR3 antibodies. This supports the hypothesis that the role of ANCA in monitoring remission in patients with AAV may vary depending on the disease phenotype [32]. Such observations were confirmed by subsequent studies. In a cohort of 166 patients with AAV, serial measurements of ANCA antibodies over a mean follow-up time of 49 $\pm$ 33 months revealed that a significant titer increase predicted vasculitis exacerbation primarily in patients with renal involvement (hazard ratio [HR], 11.09) and to a much lesser extent in patients with the involvement of other organs (HR, 2.79]) [73]. Additional information came from an extended analysis of the RAVE study (rituximab versus cyclophosphamide for remission induction), in which a rise in anti-PR3 antibodies was monitored. An increase measured by direct ELISA was associated with subsequent severe flare, especially in cases with renal involvement (HR, 7.94) and alveolar hemorrhage (HR, 24.19). This observation occurred only in the group of patients treated with rituximab, indicating that monitoring anti-PR3 levels may be applicable in a selected group of patients. It is also worth noting that a better predictive value was observed using the ELISA direct method than ELISA capture [74].

4.2. B-Cell Reconstitution

Over the past 15 years, rituximab has been increasingly playing a significant role in the treatment of AAV. As an antibody targeting B lymphocytes, it has not only proven to be non-inferior to conventional remission-inducing therapies but has also solidified its advantage as a maintenance therapy for sustaining remission [75–78]. It brought attention to B lymphocyte count as a predictive tool on remission. In the analysis of disease relapse during the first 6 months of remission induction therapy in the RAVE study, no correlation was observed between an increase in B cell count and subsequent exacerbation. None of the patients experiencing disease relapse within the first 6 months in the RTX-treated group had detectable B cells. Conversely, 47 out of 197 (24%) patients in the study had peripheral B cells present for up to 6 months of remission induction therapy but did not experience vasculitis relapse [39]. However, this observation changed from 6 months to 18 months of treatment where disease relapses were rare in the group of patients with B cell depletion [79]. In a long follow-up of RTX treatment, 71% of patients experienced B cell return at the time of relapse [80]. These observations were continued in the MAINRITSAN2 study. It compared two maintenance treatment regimens using rituximab for sustaining remission: fixed-dose maintenance (500 mg every 6 months) versus personalized dosing based on ANCA seroconversion, a 2-fold increase in ANCA titers, or the return of the peripheral B lymphocyte population. Both groups did not differ significantly in terms of relapse rates, but the personalized rituximab dosing group had reduced exposure to immunosuppression. Therefore, it can be inferred that these markers are useful for monitoring patients in remission to optimize treatment outcomes and cost-effectiveness [81]. Rituximab causes depletion not only of effector B lymphocytes but also of regulatory B cells. In a 2015 study by Bunch et al., the immunophenotypic profile of this cell lineage was observed, indicating that patients in remission of AAV who experienced a decrease in CD5+ regulatory B cells to less than 30% of all B lymphocytes tended to experience vasculitis exacerbations more quickly compared to those with CD5+ above 30% (median = 16 months versus 23 months, respectively) [82]. Other interesting observations focused on different B cell subtypes during remission. Naïve B cell repopulation appears to play a protective role against exacerbations, while an increase in PR3+ plasmablast populations signals exacerbation in patients treated with rituximab for remission induction [83]. Therefore, the immunophenotypic analysis of total B cell numbers appears to be an alternative or complementary approach to measuring ANCA levels as a potential predictor of exacerbation.

4.3. Other Potential Markers

Another proposed relapse predictor upon remission was a myelopoiesis gene signature in circulating leukocytes. In fact, PR3/MPO mRNA levels were not associated with future relapses in the analyzed cohort, but the authors hypothesized that undergoing steroid therapy might have affected the results [84]. Among other potential mechanisms in AAV etiopathogenesis, altered IgG glyco- and galactosialylation levels have also been debated. Those changes in the Fc region have been found to have an impact on IgG effector functions [85]. It was first described that in mass spectroscopy, low galactosylation and sialyation in total IgG1 but not PR3-ANCA IgG1 predicts disease reactivation in patients with GPA [86]. It was later shown by Wojcik et al. in a longitudinal observation that PR3-ANCA patients who experienced an ANCA rise and relapsed shortly thereafter presented lower IgG Fc-fucosylation levels compared to non-relapsing patients already 9 months before relapse [87]. Although the cost of such testing is relatively high, it is worth noting that the test was only performed as the second step in patients who experienced ANCA rise during follow-up. All these above mentioned methods are difficult to perform in the setting of everyday clinical practice.

Among other possible markers of upcoming flare, it is worth mentioning some simple and relatively cheap ones like urinary CD4+ count and persisting hematuria [88,89].

There are some combined relapse-predicting scores used to evaluate the treatment failures proposed, with the REACT score as the most recent one, and it is worth discussing the possibility of adding it to the baseline evaluation while starting treatment [90,91].

5. Discussion

All discussed markers are presented in Table 1.

Table 1. AAV relapse predictors.

Relapse Predictors	Well Described	Proposed
At baseline	antiPR3 presence respiratory tract and cardiovascular involvement *S. aureus* carriage	CD27+CD38hi B cells low-density granulocytes TNFSF13B rs3759467 (snp) HLA-DPB1*04:01 CCL18 calprotectin endothelial progenitor cells (EPCs) sclerotic class glomerulonephritis lack of interstitial infiltrates on renal biopsy
Upon remission	ANCA reappearance B cell reconstitution	galactosylation and sialyation in IgG1 IgG Fc-fucosylation urinary CD4+ count persisting hematuria

A series of analyses of potential relapse predictors in remission patients discussed in the literature prompts a consideration of whether using any of these predictors individually or in combination could justify intensifying treatment or if the optimal practice relies on an observation of clinical symptoms of disease relapse followed by implementing more aggressive therapy. It remains unclear how frequently follow-up visits should occur for patients exhibiting only serologic markers indicating impending exacerbation and whether the delayed recognition of subtly symptomatic disease recurrence may lead to increased chronic organ damage and consequently poorer outcomes. Additionally, it is unclear how often such markers should be measured and how to establish a cutoff for significant increases without raising false-positive prediction rates. It is worth noting that none of the analyzed potential relapse predictors demonstrate 100% specificity, and certainly, not every patient showing changes in these markers will develop vasculitis exacerbation or will do so with significant delay. It is also reasonable to evaluate potential differential diagnoses, like IgG4-related disease or malignancy, and overlapping syndromes, mainly treatment complications when early relapse occurs, especially in seronegative patients. The most challenging symptoms are those of the respiratory tract in patients with ENT involvement as infections might mimic disease progression or they coexist. It is still not well explored which of the discussed tools are disease-specific and distinguish between these two conditions.

6. Conclusions

Taking into consideration the heterogeneity of AAV, we can define, on the one hand, a subgroup with a low risk of relapse (female, anti-PR3-negative, high creatinine, no ENT involvement) who will be candidates for withdrawing the maintenance treatment, and on the other hand, the phenotype requiring probably lifelong maintenance therapy (male, PR3+, ENT, skin, eye involvement, low creatinine). But the majority of patients' risk will be in between and will require real-time monitoring using a clinical observation, self-reporting and laboratory parameters monitoring to decide about maintenance therapy duration or intensification. Patients for whom the search for potential relapse markers has yielded less significant results so far include seronegative patients, the EGPA group, those with non-renal forms, and those treated with medications other than anti-CD19. There are several potential biomarkers proposed in the literature to evaluate relapse potential both at flare and upon the remission of AAV and they will need additional validation.

Author Contributions: Conceptualization, K.W.-A. and K.W.; methodology, K.W.-A.; formal analysis, K.W.; investigation, K.W.-A.; resources, K.W.-A.; writing—original draft preparation, K.W.-A.; writing—review and editing, K.W.-A. and K.W.; visualization, K.W.-A.; supervision, K.W., J.M. and M.K. All authors have read and agreed to the published version of the manuscript.

Funding: This research received no external funding.

Conflicts of Interest: The authors declare no conflicts of interest.

References

1. Gonzalez-Gay, M.A.; Garcia-Porrua, C.; Guerrero, J.; Rodriguez-Ledo, P.; Llorca, J. The Epidemiology of the Primary Systemic Vasculitides in Northwest Spain: Implications of the Chapel Hill Consensus Conference Definitions. *Arthritis Rheum.* **2003**, *49*, 388–393. [CrossRef] [PubMed]
2. Watts, R.A.; Lane, S.E.; Bentham, G.; Scott, D.G. Epidemiology of Systemic Vasculitis: A Ten-Year Study in the United Kingdom. *Arthritis Rheum.* **2000**, *43*, 414–419. [CrossRef]
3. Mohammad, A.J.; Jacobsson, L.T.; Westman, K.W.; Sturfelt, G.; Segelmark, M. Incidence and Survival Rates in Wegener's Granulomatosis, Microscopic Polyangiitis, Churg-Strauss Syndrome, and Polyarteritis Nodosa. *Rheumatology* **2009**, *48*, 1560–1565. [CrossRef] [PubMed]
4. Jennette, J.C.; Falk, R.J.; Bacon, P.A.; Basu, N.; Cid, M.C.; Ferrario, F.; Flores-Suarez, L.F.; Gross, W.L.; Guillevin, L.; Hagen, E.C.; et al. 2012 Revised International Chapel Hill Consensus Conference Nomenclature of Vasculitides. *Arthritis Rheum.* **2013**, *65*, 1–11. [CrossRef]
5. Mohammad, A.J. An Update on the Epidemiology of ANCA-Associated Vasculitis. *Rheumatology* **2020**, *59* (Suppl. S3), 42–50. [CrossRef]
6. Walton, E.W. Giant-Cell Granuloma of the Respiratory Tract (Wegener's Granulomatosis). *Br. Med. J.* **1958**, *2*, 265–270. [CrossRef]
7. Tan, J.A.; Dehghan, N.; Chen, W.; Xie, H.; Esdaile, J.M.; Avina-Zubieta, J.A. Mortality in ANCA-Associated Vasculitis: A Meta-Analysis of Observational Studies. *Ann. Rheum. Dis.* **2017**, *76*, 1566–1574. [CrossRef]
8. Hellmich, B.; Sanchez-Alamo, B.; Schirmer, J.H.; Berti, A.; Blockmans, D.; Cid, M.C.; Holle, J.U.; Hollinger, N.; Karadag, O.; Kronbichler, A.; et al. EULAR Recommendations for the Management of ANCA-Associated Vasculitis: 2022 Update. *Ann. Rheum. Dis.* **2024**, *83*, 30–47. [CrossRef] [PubMed]
9. Robson, J.; Doll, H.; Suppiah, R.; Flossmann, O.; Harper, L.; Höglund, P.; Jayne, D.; Mahr, A.; Westman, K.; Luqmani, R.; et al. Damage in the ANCA-Associated Vasculitides: Long-Term Data from the European Vasculitis Study Group (EUVAS) Therapeutic Trials. *Ann. Rheum. Dis.* **2015**, *74*, 177–184. [CrossRef]
10. Terrier, B.; Darbon, R.; Durel, C.A.; Hachulla, E.; Karras, A.; Maillard, H.; Papo, T.; Puechal, X.; Pugnet, G.; Quemeneur, T.; et al. French Recommendations for the Management of Systemic Necrotizing Vasculitides (Polyarteritis Nodosa and ANCA-Associated Vasculitides). *Orphanet J. Rare Dis.* **2020**, *15*, 351. [CrossRef]
11. Yates, M.; Watts, R.A.; Bajema, I.M.; Cid, M.C.; Crestani, B.; Hauser, T.; Hellmich, B.; Holle, J.U.; Laudien, M.; Little, M.A.; et al. EULAR/ERA-EDTA Recommendations for the Management of ANCA-Associated Vasculitis. *Ann. Rheum. Dis.* **2016**, *75*, 1583–1594. [CrossRef] [PubMed]
12. Cao, Y.; Tian, Z.; Li, W.; Ma, L.; Yu, Y.; Ren, W. Predictors of Treatment Resistance and Relapse in Chinese Patients with Antineutrophil Cytoplasmic Antibody-Associated Disease. *J. Rheumatol.* **2014**, *41*, 916–922. [CrossRef]
13. Hassan, T.M.; Hassan, A.S.; Igoe, A.; Logan, M.; Gunaratnam, C.; McElvaney, N.G.; O'Neill, S.J. Lung Involvement at Presentation Predicts Disease Activity and Permanent Organ Damage at 6, 12 and 24 Months Follow-Up in ANCA-Associated Vasculitis. *BMC Immunol.* **2014**, *15*, 20. [CrossRef] [PubMed]
14. Pagnoux, C.; Hogan, S.L.; Chin, H.; Jennette, J.C.; Falk, R.J.; Guillevin, L.; Nachman, P.H. Predictors of Treatment Resistance and Relapse in Antineutrophil Cytoplasmic Antibody-Associated Small-Vessel Vasculitis: Comparison of Two Independent Cohorts. *Arthritis Rheum.* **2008**, *58*, 2908–2918. [CrossRef] [PubMed]
15. Walsh, M.; Flossmann, O.; Berden, A.; Westman, K.; Höglund, P.; Stegeman, C.; Jayne, D.; European Vasculitis Study Group. Risk Factors for Relapse of Antineutrophil Cytoplasmic Antibody-Associated Vasculitis. *Arthritis Rheum.* **2012**, *64*, 542–548. [CrossRef] [PubMed]
16. King, C.; Druce, K.L.; Nightingale, P.; Kay, E.; Basu, N.; Salama, A.D.; Harper, L. Predicting Relapse in Anti-Neutrophil Cytoplasmic Antibody-Associated Vasculitis: A Systematic Review and Meta-Analysis. *Rheumatol. Adv. Pract.* **2021**, *5*, rkab018. [CrossRef]
17. He, P.; Hu, J.P.; Tian, X.J.; He, L.J.; Sun, S.R.; Huang, C. Prevalence and risk factors of relapse in patients with ANCA-associated vasculitis receiving cyclophosphamide induction: A systematic review and meta-analysis of large observational studies. *Rheumatology* **2021**, *60*, 1067–1079. [CrossRef] [PubMed]
18. Wójcik, K.; Ćmiel, B.; Kułakowski, P.; Janowski, L.; Wawrzycka-Adamczyk, K.; Korkosz, M.; Masiak, A.; Zdrojewski, Z.; Bułło-Piontecka, B.; Dębska-Ślizień, A.; et al. Identification of ANCA-Associated Vasculitis Relapse Risk Factors for Building a Personalized Maintenance Therapy Scheme Model. *Ann. Rheum. Dis.* **2024**, *83*, 184.
19. Jennette, J.C.; Falk, R.J. Pathogenesis of Antineutrophil Cytoplasmic Autoantibody-Mediated Disease. *Nat. Rev. Rheumatol.* **2014**, *10*, 463–473. [CrossRef]

20. Bossuyt, X.; Rasmussen, N.; van Paassen, P.; Hellmich, B.; Baslund, B.; Vermeersch, P.; Blockmans, D.; Cohen Tervaert, J.W.; Csernok, E.; Damoiseaux, J. A Multicentre Study to Improve Clinical Interpretation of Proteinase-3 and Myeloperoxidase Anti-Neutrophil Cytoplasmic Antibodies. *Rheumatology* **2017**, *56*, 1533–1541. [CrossRef]
21. Damoiseaux, J.; Csernok, E.; Rasmussen, N.; Moosig, F.; van Paassen, P.; Baslund, B.; Vermeersch, P.; Blockmans, D.; Cohen Tervaert, J.W.; Bossuyt, X. Detection of Antineutrophil Cytoplasmic Antibodies (ANCAs): A Multicentre European Vasculitis Study Group (EUVAS) Evaluation of the Value of Indirect Immunofluorescence (IIF) versus Antigen-Specific Immunoassays. *Ann. Rheum. Dis.* **2017**, *76*, 647–653. [CrossRef] [PubMed]
22. Bossuyt, X.; Cohen Tervaert, J.W.; Arimura, Y.; Blockmans, D.; Flores-Suárez, L.F.; Guillevin, L.; Hellmich, B.; Jayne, D.; Jennette, J.C.; Kallenberg, C.G.M.; et al. Position Paper: Revised 2017 International Consensus on Testing of ANCAs in Granulomatosis with Polyangiitis and Microscopic Polyangiitis. *Nat. Rev. Rheumatol.* **2017**, *13*, 683–692. [CrossRef] [PubMed]
23. Suppiah, R.; Robson, J.C.; Grayson, P.C.; Ponte, C.; Craven, A.; Khalid, S.; Judge, A.; Hutchings, A.; Merkel, P.A.; Luqmani, R.A.; et al. American College of Rheumatology/European Alliance of Associations for Rheumatology Classification Criteria for Microscopic Polyangiitis. *Arthritis Rheumatol.* **2022**, *74*, 400–406. [CrossRef] [PubMed]
24. Robson, J.C.; Grayson, P.C.; Ponte, C.; Suppiah, R.; Craven, A.; Judge, A.; Khalid, S.; Hutchings, A.; Watts, R.A.; Merkel, P.A.; et al. 2022 American College of Rheumatology/European Alliance of Associations for Rheumatology classification criteria for granulomatosis with polyangiitis. *Ann. Rheum. Dis.* **2022**, *81*, 315–320. [CrossRef]
25. Grayson, P.C.; Ponte, C.; Suppiah, R.; Robson, J.C.; Craven, A.; Judge, A.; Khalid, S.; Hutchings, A.; Luqmani, R.A.; Watts, R.A.; et al. 2022 American College of Rheumatology/European Alliance of Associations for Rheumatology Classification Criteria for Eosinophilic Granulomatosis with Polyangiitis. *Ann. Rheum. Dis.* **2022**, *81*, 309–314. [CrossRef]
26. Holle, J.U.; Gross, W.L.; Holl-Ulrich, K.; Ambrosch, P.; Noelle, B.; Both, M.; Csernok, E.; Moosig, F.; Schinke, S.; Reinhold-Keller, E. Prospective long-term follow-up of patients with localised Wegener's granulomatosis: Does it occur as persistent disease stage? *Ann. Rheum. Dis.* **2010**, *69*, 1934–1939. [CrossRef]
27. Bossuyt, X. Serologic markers in inflammatory bowel disease. *Clin. Chem.* **2006**, *52*, 171–181. [CrossRef]
28. Pendergraft, W.F.; Niles, J.L. Trojan horses: Drug culprits associated with antineutrophil cytoplasmic autoantibody (ANCA) vasculitis. *Curr. Opin. Rheumatol.* **2014**, *26*, 42–49. [CrossRef]
29. Kitching, A.R.; Anders, H.J.; Basu, N.; Brouwer, E.; Gordon, J.; Jayne, D.R.; Kullman, J.; Lyons, P.A.; Merkel, P.A.; Savage, C.O.S.; et al. ANCA-associated vasculitis. *Nat. Rev. Dis. Primers* **2020**, *6*, 71. [CrossRef]
30. Chang, D.-Y.; Li, Z.-Y.; Chen, M.; Zhao, M.H. Myeloperoxidase-ANCA-positive granulomatosis with polyangiitis is a distinct subset of ANCA-associated vasculitis: A retrospective analysis of 455 patients from a single center in China. *Semin. Arthritis Rheum.* **2019**, *48*, 701–706. [CrossRef]
31. Moiseev, S.; Cohen Tervaert, J.W.; Arimura, Y.; Bogdanos, D.P.; Csernok, E.; Damoiseaux, J.; Ferrante, M.; Flores-Suárez, L.F.; Fritzler, M.J.; Invernizzi, P.; et al. 2020 international consensus on ANCA testing beyond systemic vasculitis. *Autoimmun. Rev.* **2020**, *19*, 102618. [CrossRef]
32. Kyndt, X.; Reumaux, D.; Bridoux, F.; Tribout, B.; Bataille, P.; Hachulla, E.; Hatron, P.Y.; Duthilleul, P.; Vanhille, P. Serial measurements of antineutrophil cytoplasmic autoantibodies in patients with systemic vasculitis. *Am. J. Med.* **1999**, *106*, 527–533. [CrossRef] [PubMed]
33. Hogan, S.L.; Falk, R.J.; Chin, H.; Cai, J.; Jennette, C.E.; Jennette, J.C.; Nachman, P.H. Predictors of relapse and treatment resistance in antineutrophil cytoplasmic antibody-associated small-vessel vasculitis. *Ann. Intern. Med.* **2005**, *143*, 621–631. [CrossRef] [PubMed]
34. Schirmer, J.H.; Wright, M.N.; Herrmann, K.; Laudien, M.; Nölle, B.; Reinhold-Keller, E.; Bremer, J.P.; Moosig, F.; Holle, J.U. Myeloperoxidase-Antineutrophil Cytoplasmic Antibody (ANCA)-Positive Granulomatosis With Polyangiitis (Wegener's) Is a Clinically Distinct Subset of ANCA-Associated Vasculitis: A Retrospective Analysis of 315 Patients From a German Vasculitis Referral Center. *Arthritis Rheumatol.* **2016**, *68*, 2953–2963.
35. Puéchal, X.; Pagnoux, C.; Perrodeau, É.; Hamidou, M.; Boffa, J.J.; Kyndt, X.; Lifermann, F.; Papo, T.; Merrien, D.; Smail, A.; et al. Long-Term Outcomes Among Participants in the WEGENT Trial of Remission-Maintenance Therapy for Granulomatosis With Polyangiitis (Wegener's) or Microscopic Polyangiitis. *Arthritis Rheumatol.* **2016**, *68*, 690–701. [CrossRef] [PubMed]
36. Iudici, M.; Pagnoux, C.; Courvoisier, D.S.; Cohen, P.; Hamidou, M.; Aouba, A.; Lifermann, F.; Ruivard, M.; Aumaître, O.; Bonnotte, B.; et al. Granulomatosis with polyangiitis: Study of 795 patients from the French Vasculitis Study Group registry. *Semin. Arthritis Rheum.* **2021**, *51*, 339–346. [CrossRef]
37. Lionaki, S.; Blyth, E.R.; Hogan, S.L.; Hu, Y.; Senior, B.A.; Jennette, C.E.; Nachman, P.H.; Jennette, J.C.; Falk, R.J. Classification of antineutrophil cytoplasmic autoantibody vasculitides: The role of antineutrophil cytoplasmic autoantibody specificity for myeloperoxidase or proteinase 3 in disease recognition and prognosis. *Arthritis Rheum.* **2012**, *64*, 3452–3462. [CrossRef]
38. Mahr, A.; Katsahian, S.; Varet, H.; Guillevin, L.; Hagen, E.C.; Höglund, P.; Merkel, P.A.; Pagnoux, C.; Rasmussen, N.; Westman, K.; et al. Revisiting the classification of clinical phenotypes of anti-neutrophil cytoplasmic antibody-associated vasculitis: A cluster analysis. *Ann. Rheum. Dis.* **2013**, *72*, 1003–1010. [CrossRef]
39. Miloslavsky, E.M.; Specks, U.; Merkel, P.A.; Seo, P.; Spiera, R.; Langford, C.A.; Hoffman, G.S.; Kallenberg, C.G.; St Clair, E.W.; Tchao, N.K.; et al. Clinical outcomes of remission induction therapy for severe antineutrophil cytoplasmic antibody-associated vasculitis. *Arthritis Rheum.* **2013**, *65*, 2441–2449. [CrossRef]

40. Ono, N.; Niiro, H.; Ueda, A.; Sawabe, T.; Nishizaka, H.; Furugo, I.; Yoshizawa, S.; Yoshizawa, S.; Tsukamoto, H.; Kiyohara, C.; et al. Characteristics of MPO-ANCA-positive granulomatosis with polyangiitis: A retrospective multi-center study in Japan. *Rheumatol. Int.* **2015**, *35*, 555–559. [CrossRef]
41. Miloslavsky, E.M.; Lu, N.; Unizony, S.; Choi, H.K.; Merkel, P.A.; Seo, P.; Spiera, R.; Langford, C.A.; Hoffman, G.S.; Kallenberg, C.G.; et al. Myeloperoxidase-Antineutrophil Cytoplasmic Antibody (ANCA)-Positive and ANCA-Negative Patients With Granulomatosis With Polyangiitis (Wegener's): Distinct Patient Subsets. *Arthritis Rheumatol.* **2016**, *68*, 2945–2952. [CrossRef] [PubMed]
42. Deshayes, S.; Martin Silva, N.; Khoy, K.; Yameogo, S.; Mariotte, D.; Lobbedez, T.; Aouba, A. Clinical impact of subgrouping ANCA-associated vasculitis according to antibody specificity beyond the clinicopathological classification. *Rheumatology* **2019**, *58*, 1731–1739. [CrossRef]
43. Puéchal, X.; Iudici, M.; Pagnoux, C.; Cohen, P.; Hamidou, M.; Aouba, A.; Lifermann, F.; Ruivard, M.; Aumaître, O.; Bonnotte, B.; et al. Comparative study of granulomatosis with polyangiitis subsets according to ANCA status: Data from the French Vasculitis Study Group Registry. *RMD Open.* **2022**, *8*, e002160. [CrossRef] [PubMed]
44. von Borstel, A.; Land, J.; Abdulahad, W.H.; Rutgers, A.; Stegeman, C.A.; Diepstra, A.; Heeringa, P.; Sanders, J.S. CD27+CD38hi B Cell Frequency During Remission Predicts Relapsing Disease in Granulomatosis With Polyangiitis Patients. *Front. Immunol.* **2019**, *10*, 2221. [CrossRef] [PubMed]
45. Grayson, P.C.; Carmona-Rivera, C.; Xu, L.; Lim, N.; Gao, Z.; Asare, A.L.; Specks, U.; Stone, J.H.; Seo, P.; Spiera, R.F.; et al. Neutrophil-Related Gene Expression and Low-Density Granulocytes Associated With Disease Activity and Response to Treatment in Antineutrophil Cytoplasmic Antibody-Associated Vasculitis. *Arthritis Rheumatol.* **2015**, *67*, 1922–1932. [CrossRef]
46. Li, W.; Huang, H.; Cai, M.; Yuan, T.; Sheng, Y. Antineutrophil Cytoplasmic Antibody-Associated Vasculitis Update: Genetic Pathogenesis. *Front. Immunol.* **2021**, *12*, 624848. [CrossRef]
47. Alberici, F.; Smith, R.M.; Fonseca, M.; Willcocks, L.C.; Jones, R.B.; Holle, J.U.; Wieczorek, S.; Neumann, T.; Martorana, D.; Gregorini, G.; et al. Association of a TNFSF13B (BAFF) Regulatory Region Single Nucleotide Polymorphism with Response to Rituximab in Antineutrophil Cytoplasmic Antibody-Associated Vasculitis. *J. Allergy Clin. Immunol.* **2017**, *139*, 1684–1687. [CrossRef]
48. Chang, D.Y.; Luo, H.; Zhou, X.J.; Chen, M.; Zhao, M.H. Association of HLA Genes with Clinical Outcomes of ANCA-Associated Vasculitis. *Clin. J. Am. Soc. Nephrol.* **2012**, *7*, 1293–1299. [CrossRef]
49. Hilhorst, M.; Arndt, F.; Joseph Kemna, M.; Wieczorek, S.; Donner, Y.; Wilde, B.; Thomas Epplen, J.; van Paassen, P.; Cohen Tervaert, J.W. HLA-DPB1 as a Risk Factor for Relapse in Antineutrophil Cytoplasmic Antibody-Associated Vasculitis: A Cohort Study. *Arthritis Rheumatol.* **2016**, *68*, 1721–1730. [CrossRef]
50. Stegeman, C.A.; Tervaert, J.W.; Sluiter, W.J.; Manson, W.L.; de Jong, P.E.; Kallenberg, C.G. Association of Chronic Nasal Carriage of Staphylococcus aureus and Higher Relapse Rates in Wegener Granulomatosis. *Ann. Intern. Med.* **1994**, *120*, 12–17. [CrossRef]
51. Popa, E.R.; Stegeman, C.A.; Abdulahad, W.H.; van der Meer, B.; Arends, J.; Manson, W.M.; Bos, N.A.; Kallenberg, C.G.; Tervaert, J.W. Staphylococcal Toxic-Shock-Syndrome-Toxin-1 as a Risk Factor for Disease Relapse in Wegener's Granulomatosis. *Rheumatology* **2007**, *46*, 1029–1033. [CrossRef]
52. Stegeman, C.A.; Cohen Tervaert, J.W.; de Jong, P.E.; Kallenberg, C.G. Trimethoprim–Sulfamethoxazole for the Prevention of Relapses of Wegener's Granulomatosis. *N. Engl. J. Med.* **1996**, *335*, 16–20. [CrossRef] [PubMed]
53. Laudien, M.; Häsler, R.; Wohlers, J.; Böck, J.; Lipinski, S.; Bremer, L.; Podschun, R.; Ambrosch, P.; Lamprecht, P.; Rosenstiel, P.; et al. Molecular signatures of a disturbed nasal barrier function in the primary tissue of Wegener's granulomatosis. *Mucosal Immunol.* **2011**, *4*, 564–573. [CrossRef]
54. Grayson, P.C.; Steiling, K.; Platt, M.; Berman, J.S.; Zhang, X.; Xiao, J.; Alekseyev, Y.O.; Liu, G.; Monach, P.A.; Kaplan, M.J.; et al. Defining the Nasal Transcriptome in Granulomatosis with Polyangiitis (Wegener's). *Arthritis Rheumatol.* **2015**, *67*, 2233–2239. [CrossRef]
55. Ooi, J.D.; Jiang, J.H.; Eggenhuizen, P.J.; Chua, L.L.; Van Timmeren, M.; Loh, K.L.; O'Sullivan, K.M.; Gan, P.Y.; Zhong, Y.; Tsyganov, K.; et al. A Plasmid-Encoded Peptide from Staphylococcus aureus Induces Anti-Myeloperoxidase Nephritogenic Autoimmunity. *Nat. Commun.* **2019**, *10*, 3392. [CrossRef]
56. Berden, A.E.; Ferrario, F.; Hagen, E.C.; Jayne, D.R.; Jennette, J.C.; Joh, K.; Neumann, I.; Noël, L.H.; Pusey, C.D.; Waldherr, R.; et al. Histopathologic classification of ANCA-associated glomerulonephritis. *J. Am. Soc. Nephrol.* **2010**, *21*, 1628–1636. [CrossRef] [PubMed]
57. Chang, D.Y.; Wu, L.H.; Liu, G.; Chen, M.; Kallenberg, C.G.M.; Zhao, M.H. Re-evaluation of the Histopathologic Classification of ANCA-Associated Glomerulonephritis: A Study of 121 Patients in a Single Center. *Nephrol. Dial. Transplant.* **2012**, *27*, 2343–2349. [CrossRef] [PubMed]
58. Muso, E.; Endo, T.; Itabashi, M.; Kakita, H.; Iwasaki, Y.; Tateishi, Y.; Komiya, T.; Ihara, T.; Yumura, W.; Sugiyama, T.; et al. Evaluation of the newly proposed simplified histological classification in Japanese cohorts of myeloperoxidase-anti-neutrophil cytoplasmic antibody-associated glomerulonephritis in comparison with other Asian and European cohorts. *Clin. Exp. Nephrol.* **2013**, *17*, 659–662. [CrossRef]
59. Göçeroğlu, A.; Berden, A.E.; Fiocco, M.; Floßmann, O.; Westman, K.W.; Ferrario, F.; Gaskin, G.; Pusey, C.D.; Hagen, E.C.; Noël, L.-H.; et al. ANCA-Associated Glomerulonephritis: Risk Factors for Renal Relapse. *PLoS ONE* **2016**, *11*, e0165402. [CrossRef]

60. Brix, S.R.; Stege, G.; Disteldorf, E.; Hoxha, E.; Krebs, C.; Krohn, S.; Otto, B.; Klätschke, K.; Herden, E.; Heymann, F.; et al. CC Chemokine Ligand 18 in ANCA-Associated Crescentic GN. *J. Am. Soc. Nephrol.* **2015**, *26*, 2105–2117. [CrossRef]
61. Pepper, R.J.; Draibe, J.B.; Caplin, B.; Fervenza, F.C.; Hoffman, G.S.; Kallenberg, C.G.; Langford, C.A.; Monach, P.A.; Seo, P.; Spiera, R.; et al. Association of Serum Calprotectin (S100A8/A9) Level with Disease Relapse in Proteinase 3-Antineutrophil Cytoplasmic Antibody-Associated Vasculitis. *Arthritis Rheumatol.* **2017**, *69*, 185–193. [CrossRef] [PubMed]
62. Závada, J.; Kideryová, L.; Pytlík, R.; Hrusková, Z.; Tesar, V. Reduced Number of Endothelial Progenitor Cells is Predictive of Early Relapse in Anti-Neutrophil Cytoplasmic Antibody-Associated Vasculitis. *Rheumatology* **2009**, *48*, 1197–1201. [CrossRef] [PubMed]
63. Monach, P.A.; Warner, R.L.; Lew, R.; Tómasson, G.; Specks, U.; Stone, J.H.; Fervenza, F.C.; Hoffman, G.S.; Kallenberg, C.G.M.; Langford, C.A. Serum Biomarkers of Disease Activity in Longitudinal Assessment of Patients with ANCA-Associated Vasculitis. *ACR Open Rheumatol.* **2022**, *4*, 168–176. [CrossRef] [PubMed]
64. Grayson, P.C.; Monach, P.A.; Pagnoux, C.; Cuthbertson, D.; Carette, S.; Hoffman, G.S.; Khalidi, N.A.; Koening, C.L.; Langford, C.A.; Maksimowicz-McKinnon, K.; et al. Value of Commonly Measured Laboratory Tests as Biomarkers of Disease Activity and Predictors of Relapse in Eosinophilic Granulomatosis with Polyangiitis. *Rheumatology* **2015**, *54*, 1351–1359. [CrossRef]
65. Yang, J.J.; Preston, G.A.; Pendergraft, W.F.; Segelmark, M.; Heeringa, P.; Hogan, S.L.; Jennette, J.C.; Falk, R.J. Internalization of Proteinase 3 is Concomitant with Endothelial Cell Apoptosis and Internalization of Myeloperoxidase with Generation of Intracellular Oxidants. *Am. J. Pathol.* **2001**, *158*, 581–592. [CrossRef]
66. Xiao, H.; Heeringa, P.; Hu, P.; Liu, Z.; Zhao, M.; Aratani, Y.; Maeda, N.; Falk, R.J.; Jennette, J.C. Antineutrophil Cytoplasmic Autoantibodies Specific for Myeloperoxidase Cause Glomerulonephritis and Vasculitis in Mice. *J. Clin. Investig.* **2002**, *110*, 955–963. [CrossRef]
67. Little, M.A.; Smyth, C.L.; Yadav, R.; Ambrose, L.; Cook, H.T.; Nourshargh, S.; Pusey, C.D. Antineutrophil Cytoplasm Antibodies Directed Against Myeloperoxidase Augment Leukocyte-Microvascular Interactions In Vivo. *Blood* **2005**, *106*, 2050–2058. [CrossRef] [PubMed]
68. Little, M.A.; Smyth, L.; Salama, A.D.; Mukherjee, S.; Smith, J.; Haskard, D.; Nourshargh, S.; Cook, H.T.; Pusey, C.D. Experimental Autoimmune Vasculitis: An Animal Model of Anti-Neutrophil Cytoplasmic Antibody-Associated Systemic Vasculitis. *Am. J. Pathol.* **2009**, *174*, 1212–1220. [CrossRef] [PubMed]
69. Pfister, H.; Ollert, M.; Fröhlich, L.F.; Quintanilla-Martinez, L.; Colby, T.V.; Specks, U.; Jenne, D.E. Antineutrophil Cytoplasmic Autoantibodies Against the Murine Homolog of Proteinase 3 (Wegener Autoantigen) Are Pathogenic In Vivo. *Blood* **2004**, *104*, 1411–1418. [CrossRef]
70. Little, M.A.; Al-Ani, B.; Ren, S.; Al-Nuaimi, H.; Leite, M., Jr.; Alpers, C.E.; Savage, C.O.; Duffield, J.S. Anti-Proteinase 3 Anti-Neutrophil Cytoplasm Autoantibodies Recapitulate Systemic Vasculitis in Mice with a Humanized Immune System. *PLoS ONE* **2012**, *7*, e28626. [CrossRef]
71. Koh, J.H.; Kemna, M.J.; Cohen Tervaert, J.W.; Kim, W.U. Editorial: Can an Increase in Antineutrophil Cytoplasmic Autoantibody Titer Predict Relapses in Antineutrophil Cytoplasmic Antibody-Associated Vasculitis? *Arthritis Rheumatol.* **2016**, *68*, 1571–1573. [CrossRef]
72. Tervaert, J.W.; van der Woude, F.J.; Fauci, A.S.; Ambrus, J.L.; Velosa, J.; Keane, W.F.; Meijer, S.; van der Giessen, M.; van der Hem, G.K.; The, T.H. Association Between Active Wegener's Granulomatosis and Anticytoplasmic Antibodies. *Arch. Intern. Med.* **1989**, *149*, 2461–2465. [CrossRef]
73. Kemna, M.J.; Damoiseaux, J.; Austen, J.; Winkens, B.; Peters, J.; van Paassen, P.; Cohen Tervaert, J.W. ANCA as a Predictor of Relapse: Useful in Patients with Renal Involvement but Not in Patients with Nonrenal Disease. *J. Am. Soc. Nephrol.* **2015**, *26*, 537–542. [CrossRef] [PubMed]
74. Fussner, L.A.; Hummel, A.M.; Schroeder, D.R.; Silva, F.; Cartin-Ceba, R.; Snyder, M.R.; Hoffman, G.S.; Kallenberg, C.G.; Langford, C.A.; Merkel, P.A.; et al. Factors Determining the Clinical Utility of Serial Measurements of Antineutrophil Cytoplasmic Antibodies Targeting Proteinase 3. *Arthritis Rheumatol.* **2016**, *68*, 1700–1710. [CrossRef]
75. Jones, R.B.; Tervaert, J.W.; Hauser, T.; Luqmani, R.; Morgan, M.D.; Peh, C.A.; Savage, C.O.; Segelmark, M.; Tesar, V.; van Paassen, P.; et al. Rituximab Versus Cyclophosphamide in ANCA-Associated Renal Vasculitis. *N. Engl. J. Med.* **2010**, *363*, 211–220. [CrossRef] [PubMed]
76. Stone, J.H.; Merkel, P.A.; Spiera, R.; Seo, P.; Langford, C.A.; Hoffman, G.S.; Kallenberg, C.G.; St Clair, E.W.; Turkiewicz, A.; Tchao, N.K.; et al. Rituximab Versus Cyclophosphamide for ANCA-Associated Vasculitis. *N. Engl. J. Med.* **2010**, *363*, 221–232. [CrossRef] [PubMed]
77. Specks, U.; Merkel, P.A.; Seo, P.; Spiera, R.; Langford, C.A.; Hoffman, G.S.; Kallenberg, C.G.; St Clair, E.W.; Fessler, B.J.; Ding, L.; et al. Efficacy of Remission-Induction Regimens for ANCA-Associated Vasculitis. *N. Engl. J. Med.* **2013**, *369*, 417–427. [CrossRef] [PubMed]
78. Guillevin, L.; Pagnoux, C.; Karras, A.; Khouatra, C.; Aumaître, O.; Cohen, P.; Maurier, F.; Decaux, O.; Ninet, J.; Gobert, P.; et al. Rituximab versus azathioprine for maintenance in ANCA-associated vasculitis. *N. Engl. J. Med.* **2014**, *371*, 1771–1780. [CrossRef]
79. Stone, J.H.; Merkel, P.A.; Seo, P.; Spiera, R.; Langford, C.A.; Hoffman, G.S. Extended Follow-Up of Treatment with Rituximab Versus Cyclophosphamide for Remission-Induction of ANCA-Associated Vasculitis: Which Subsets Are at Greatest Risk for Flare? *Arthritis Rheum.* **2011**, *63*, S946–S947.

80. Alberici, F.; Smith, R.M.; Jones, R.B.; Roberts, D.M.; Willcocks, L.C.; Chaudhry, A.; Smith, K.G.C.; Jayne, D.R.W. Long-Term Follow-Up of Patients Who Received Repeat-Dose Rituximab as Maintenance Therapy for ANCA-Associated Vasculitis. *Rheumatology* **2015**, *54*, 1153–1160. [CrossRef]
81. Charles, P.; Terrier, B.; Perrodeau, É.; Cohen, P.; Faguer, S.; Huart, A.; Hamidou, M.; Agard, C.; Bonnotte, B.; Samson, M.; et al. Comparison of Individually Tailored Versus Fixed-Schedule Rituximab Regimen to Maintain ANCA-Associated Vasculitis Remission: Results of a Multicentre, Randomised Controlled, Phase III Trial (MAINRITSAN2). *Ann. Rheum. Dis.* **2018**, *77*, 1143–1149. [CrossRef] [PubMed]
82. Bunch, D.O.; Mendoza, C.E.; Aybar, L.T.; Kotzen, E.S.; Colby, K.R.; Hu, Y.; Hogan, S.L.; Poulton, C.J.; Schmitz, J.L.; Falk, R.J.; et al. Relapse Risk from B Cell Phenotype: Decreased CD5+ B Cells Portend a Shorter Time to Relapse After B Cell Depletion in Patients with ANCA-Associated Vasculitis. *Ann. Rheum. Dis.* **2015**, *74*, 1784–1786. [CrossRef] [PubMed]
83. Md Yusof, M.Y.; Vital, E.M.; Das, S.; Dass, S.; Arumugakani, G.; Savic, S.; Rawstron, A.C.; Emery, P. Repeat Cycles of Rituximab on Clinical Relapse in ANCA-Associated Vasculitis: Identifying B Cell Biomarkers for Relapse to Guide Retreatment Decisions. *Ann. Rheum. Dis.* **2015**, *74*, 1734–1738. [CrossRef] [PubMed]
84. Kurz, T.; Weiner, M.; Skoglund, C.; Basnet, S.; Eriksson, P.; Segelmark, M. A Myelopoiesis Gene Signature During Remission in Anti-Neutrophil Cytoplasm Antibody-Associated Vasculitis Does Not Predict Relapses But Seems to Reflect Ongoing Prednisolone Therapy. *Clin. Exp. Immunol.* **2014**, *175*, 215–226. [CrossRef] [PubMed]
85. Bournazos, S.; Ravetch, J.V. Diversification of IgG Effector Functions. *Int. Immunol.* **2017**, *29*, 303–310. [CrossRef]
86. Kemna, M.J.; Plomp, R.; van Paassen, P.; Koeleman, C.A.M.; Jansen, B.C.; Damoiseaux, J.G.M.C.; Cohen Tervaert, J.W.; Wuhrer, M. Galactosylation and Sialylation Levels of IgG Predict Relapse in Patients with PR3-ANCA Associated Vasculitis. *eBioMedicine* **2017**, *17*, 108–118. [CrossRef]
87. Wojcik, I.; Wuhrer, M.; Heeringa, P.; Stegeman, C.A.; Rutgers, A.; Falck, D. Specific IgG Glycosylation Differences Precede Relapse in PR3-ANCA Associated Vasculitis Patients with and Without ANCA Rise. *Front. Immunol.* **2023**, *14*, 1214945. [CrossRef]
88. Prskalo, L.; Skopnik, C.M.; Goerlich, N.; Freund, P.; Wagner, L.; Grothgar, E.; Mirkheshti, P.; Klocke, J.; Sonnemann, J.; Metzke, D.; et al. Urinary CD4+ T Cells Predict Renal Relapse in ANCA-Associated Vasculitis. *J. Am. Soc. Nephrol.* **2024**, *35*, 483–494. [CrossRef]
89. Rhee, R.L.; Davis, J.C.; Ding, L.; Fervenza, F.C.; Hoffman, G.S.; Kallenberg, C.G.M.; Langford, C.A.; McCune, W.J.; Monach, P.A.; Seo, P.; et al. The Utility of Urinalysis in Determining the Risk of Renal Relapse in ANCA-Associated Vasculitis. *Clin. J. Am. Soc. Nephrol.* **2018**, *13*, 251–257. [CrossRef]
90. Lugli, G.; Buscemi, P.; Calatroni, M.; Alderotti, G.; Preciado, F.G.; Moroni, G.L.; Sinico, R.A.; Emmi, G.; Peyronel, F.; Little, M.; et al. Development of a relapse risk score in patients with ANCA-associated vasculitis treated with cyclophosphamide induction. *Nephrol. Dial. Transplant.* **2024**, *39*, gfae069.019. [CrossRef]
91. Samson, M.; Devilliers, H.; Thietart, S.; Charles, P.; Pagnoux, C.; Cohen, P.; Karras, A.; Mouthon, L.; Terrier, B.; Puéchal, X.; et al. Score to assess the probability of relapse in granulomatosis with polyangiitis and microscopic polyangiitis. *RMD Open* **2023**, *9*, e002953. [CrossRef] [PubMed]

diagnostics

MDPI

Review

Neutrophils and Platelets as Key Players in the Pathogenesis of ANCA-Associated Vasculitis and Potential Sources of Disease Activity Biomarkers

Anna Drynda [1], Marcin Surmiak [2], Stanisława Bazan-Socha [2], Katarzyna Wawrzycka-Adamczyk [2], Mariusz Korkosz [3], Jacek Musiał [2] and Krzysztof Wójcik [2,*]

[1] Doctoral School of Medical Sciences and Health Sciences, Jagiellonian University Medical College, 31-530 Cracow, Poland; anna.drynda@doctoral.uj.edu.pl

[2] 2nd Department of Internal Medicine, Faculty of Medicine, Jagiellonian University Medical College, 30-688 Cracow, Poland; marcin.surmiak@uj.edu.pl (M.S.); stanislawa.bazan-socha@uj.edu.pl (S.B.-S.); katarzyna.wawrzycka@uj.edu.pl (K.W.-A.); jacek.musial@uj.edu.pl (J.M.)

[3] Department of Rheumatology and Immunology, Jagiellonian University Medical College, 30-688 Cracow, Poland; mariusz.korkosz@uj.edu.pl

* Correspondence: krzysztof.wojcik@uj.edu.pl

Abstract

Anti-neutrophil cytoplasmic antibodies (ANCA)-associated vasculitis (AAV) is a heterogeneous group of small-vessel vasculitides, characterized by the presence of antibodies binding to myeloperoxidase (MPO) and proteinase-3 (PR3) found in neutrophil granules. Apart from being the target of ANCA, neutrophils actively contribute to the vicious cycle of inflammation and vascular damage in AAV. On the other hand, platelets have recently been recognized as essential for thrombosis and as inflammatory effectors that collaborate with neutrophils, reinforcing the generation of reactive oxygen species (ROS) and the formation of neutrophil extracellular traps (NETs) in those diseases. Neutrophils exhibit morphological and functional heterogeneity in AAV, reflecting the complexity of their contribution to disease pathogenesis. Since long-term immunosuppression may be related to serious infections and malignancies, there is an urgent need for reliable biomarkers of disease activity to optimize the management of AAV. This review summarizes the current understanding of the role of neutrophils and platelets in the pathogenesis of granulomatosis with polyangiitis (GPA) and microscopic polyangiitis (MPA), focusing on their crosstalk, and highlights the potential for identifying novel biomarkers relevant for predicting the disease course and its relapses.

Keywords: ANCA-associated vasculitis (AAV); neutrophils; platelets; myeloperoxidase (MPO); proteinase-3 (PR3); neutrophil extracellular traps (NETs); extracellular vesicles (EVs); biomarkers

1. Introduction

The anti-neutrophil cytoplasmic antibodies (ANCA)-associated vasculitis (AAV) comprises a group of autoimmune diseases characterized by inflammation of small and medium-sized blood vessels, often leading to multi-organ damage. According to the 2012 Revised International Chapel Hill Consensus Conference Nomenclature, AAV encompasses three main subtypes: granulomatosis with polyangiitis (GPA), microscopic polyangiitis (MPA), and eosinophilic granulomatosis with polyangiitis (EGPA) [1], with EGPA being the rarest and most distinct form due to its eosinophilic component. The presence of ANCA is a characteristic feature of AAV, with PR3-ANCA (proteinase-3 ANCA) associated with GPA and MPO-ANCA (myeloperoxidase ANCA) observed in MPA. Unlike GPA and MPA, where ANCA is detected in approximately 90% of cases, only 30–40% of EGPA cases are ANCA-positive, primarily with MPO-ANCA [2,3]. The heterogeneity of AAV presents significant challenges in diagnosis and management, as symptoms and disease severity vary.

Although any tissue can be involved, the respiratory tract and kidneys are most frequently affected, with complications such as pulmonary hemorrhage and rapidly progressive glomerulonephritis (RPGN) posing serious risks, including death [3–5]. Additionally, some patients exhibit overlapping features of different AAV subtypes, further complicating classification and prognosis [2,6,7]. Finally, the clinical presentation and disease trajectory may also change, making the long-term prognosis and treatment plans complex and challenging [8].

Given the typical relapse-remission pattern of AAV, remission induction and remission maintenance are fundamental paradigms in management. Remission induction in GPA and MPA depends on the severity of disease presentation. For patients with life- or organ-threatening manifestations, both the 2021 American College of Rheumatology/Vasculitis Foundation (ACR/VF) [9] and 2022 European Alliance of Associations for Rheumatology (EULAR) guidelines [10] recommend a combination of glucocorticoids (GC) and either rituximab (RTX) or cyclophosphamide (CYC). Maintenance of remission relies on intensive and long-term immunosuppression. In GPA and MPA, maintenance treatment with repeated doses of RTX is superior to azathioprine (AZA) and methotrexate (MTX) in reducing relapse rates, while AZA and MTX are recommended when RTX is contraindicated [11,12]. Mycophenolate mofetil (MMF) is considered a third-line treatment [9,10]. However, in some patients, discontinuing GC despite immunosuppressive therapy use may still be unfeasible [10].

Immunosuppressive treatment in AAV patients is associated with various complications, some of which can be severe and potentially fatal, particularly during long-term maintenance therapy. It has been shown that infections and malignancies rank among the top three long-term causes of death in AAV, being surpassed only by cardiovascular diseases, whose risk increases dose-dependently with GC use [13–15]. Therefore, it is crucial to balance therapy to reduce the risk of disease relapse and also minimize the side effects and toxicity of immunosuppression. Since no reliable clinical parameters are available, laboratory biomarkers are urgently needed to predict clinical trajectory and disease relapse.

Vasculitides are related to the inflammatory process that damages the walls of small and medium-sized blood vessels, resulting in impaired blood flow and ischemia [16,17]. The exact mechanisms underlying immunologic and cell responses, including preliminary triggers, have not been fully understood; however, the central role of neutrophils in the pathogenesis of AAV is unquestionable [18–21]. Platelets, on the other hand, have recently been considered as potential contributors to the inflammatory process underlying AAV. Moreover, there is growing evidence of crosstalk between neutrophils and platelets in various conditions [22–24], including AAV [25–28]. Given the relatively novel evidence on platelet involvement in AAV pathogenesis, we aim to review that issue. Furthermore, we recapitulate the known facts on the interplay between neutrophils and platelets in AAV and highlight the impact of this novel research on disease prognosis and optimal therapeutic approach in those patients.

2. Materials and Methods

A literature search was performed on PubMed and Embase for studies published in English up until April 2025, using MeSH and Emtree terms related to ANCA-associated vasculitis, neutrophils, and platelets. The titles and abstracts were screened for relevance to the review topic. Articles that did not provide new insights were excluded. Additional relevant articles were identified through citation searching. Due to substantially different pathogenesis and rarity, this review did not include data on EGPA.

3. Pathogenesis of ANCA-Associated Vasculitis—An Overview

The pathogenesis of AAV involves a complex interplay between innate and adaptive immunity. While ANCA and neutrophils are central to this process, their pathogenicity is modulated and amplified through interactions with monocytes, macrophages, B and T lymphocytes, the complement and coagulation systems, as well as platelets.

Monocytes and macrophages also contribute to vascular damage and immune activation. Circulating monocytes infiltrate inflamed tissues, differentiate into macrophages, and promote granulomatous inflammation. Monocytes are stimulated by ANCA to produce proinflammatory cytokines, such as TNF and IL-6 [29], and are a major source of tissue factor (TF) that links inflammation to thrombosis [30]. They also play a role in impaired clearance of apoptotic neutrophils, which may perpetuate inflammation and interfere with resolution [31]. Additionally, macrophages may respond to NET-derived molecules [32,33] and participate in antigen presentation and T-cell activation, thus bridging innate and adaptive immunity [34].

B cells are essential for the production of ANCA and also serve as antigen-presenting cells. Abnormal B-cell activation and survival, enhanced by elevated B-cell activating factor (BAFF), are observed in AAV and correlate with disease activity [35]. The clinical efficacy of rituximab confirms their crucial pathogenic role in AAV [36]. T cells, including Th1, Th17, CD8+, and regulatory T-cell subsets, are actively involved in both granulomatous inflammation and humoral activation. Dysregulated T-cell function contributes to ANCA production, tissue infiltration, and loss of tolerance. IL-17-producing Th17 cells are increased in active disease, and T cells specific for complementary PR3 peptides (cPR3) have been detected in patients with PR3-ANCA vasculitis [37,38].

The complement system is a crucial amplifier of inflammation. C5a promotes neutrophil priming and chemotaxis [39]. Crosstalk between complement and coagulation systems facilitates thrombin generation and propagates endothelial injury [40]. The coagulation cascade is closely intertwined with immune activation. AAV patients exhibit increased thrombotic risk, associated with neutrophil- and monocyte-derived tissue factors and thrombin-mediated platelet activation [30,41]. Thrombin not only promotes fibrin formation but also stimulates inflammation through PAR signaling, further connecting thrombosis and vasculitis pathophysiology [26,42].

4. Neutrophils

4.1. Cytokine-Dependent Regulation of Neutrophil Production Is Abnormally Upregulated in AAV

Neutrophils, or polymorphonuclear (PMN) leukocytes, are the most abundant type of leukocytes, constituting 50–70% of their total population. The average lifespan of neutrophils is relatively short, limited by programmed cell death, ranging from 7 to 9 h [43] to over 5 days [44]. Therefore, to maintain their count, about $1–2 \times 10^{11}$ neutrophils are produced daily in the bone marrow via neutropoiesis [45], a process dependent on granulocyte colony-stimulating factor (G-CSF) activity [46]. After maturation, neutrophils are retained in bone marrow for the next 4–6 days, forming a reserve pool, ready to be deployed in case of an infection, inflammation, or trauma [47]. Neutrophil retention and release are regulated by chemokine signaling, the expression of which is controlled also by G-CSF [48]. In MPA, high initial levels of circulating G-CSF were associated with the severity of central nervous system involvement and disease activity, according to the Birmingham Vasculitis Activity Scale (BVAS) [49]. After fulfilling a biological function, neutrophils undergo apoptosis in the bone marrow, spleen, or liver. Then, they are cleared by macrophages through efferocytosis [31], which modulates the neutropoiesis by a negative feedback loop. Macrophages release large amounts of interleukin (IL)-23, triggering IL-17 production by T, NK, and NKT cells, and further increasing G-CSF production. Interestingly, phagocytosis of neutrophils reduces IL-23 production by macrophages, leading to diminished neutropoiesis and cell release to the peripheral blood. On the other hand, when inflammation is amplified, the same cytokine axis intensifies neutrophil proliferation and maturation [50,51]. Patients with AAV exhibit a markedly elevated circulating neutrophil count [52]. In AAV, according to the study by Nogueira et al. [53], serum IL-17A levels were significantly higher in the acute phase of GPA than in healthy controls. Moreover, in the same study, patients with elevated IL-23 had more active disease and higher ANCA titers. Additionally, a study by Huang et al. documented a positive correlation between the neutrophil-to-lymphocyte ratio (NLR) and C-reactive protein (CRP) and an inverse with C3 level in those with MPO-ANCA [54]. Interestingly, a threshold NLR of at least 5.9 was related to increased disease severity and risk of relapse in follow-up [55]. Furthermore, an elevated delta neutrophil index (DNI) of at least 0.65, reflecting the proportion of immature granulocytes within the total neutrophil count, was associated with more severe disease at diagnosis; thus, it could likely serve as a predictor of relapse in GPA or MPA [56].

4.2. Neutrophil-Endothelium Interactions Mediate Adhesion, Migration and Inflammatory Amplification in AAV

As vascular wall damage in small vessels plays a key role in AAV, interactions between neutrophils and the endothelium are crucial to its pathogenesis. Under physiological conditions, neutrophils do not adhere to resting endothelium. Upon exposure to inflammatory stimuli, neutrophils migrate towards the inflammation site, where they undergo adhesion cascade and extravasation (Figure 1) [57–59].

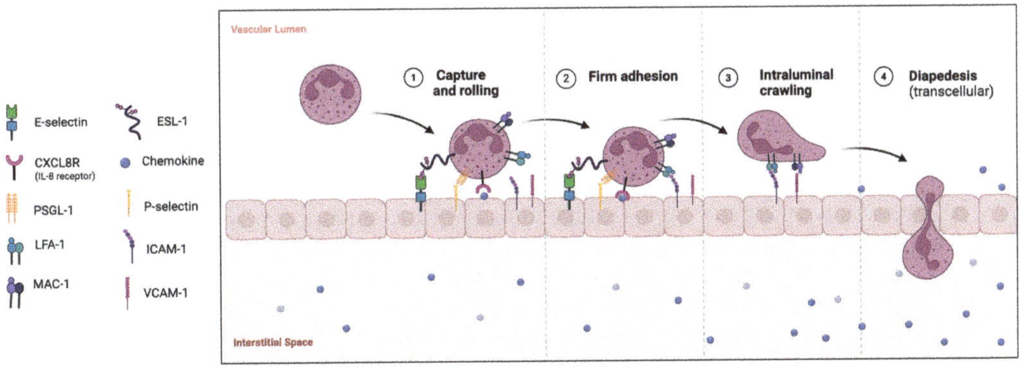

Figure 1. Neutrophil adhesion cascade preceding extravasation. This process involves capture, rolling, activation, firm adhesion, and intraluminal crawling. It depends on interactions of neutrophil glycoproteins with endothelial E- and P-selectins, whose expression is upregulated in inflammatory loci. Firstly, E- and P-selectin capture circulating neutrophils to the surface of endothelium by interacting with E-selectin ligand-1 (ESL-1) and P-selectin glycoprotein ligand 1 (PSGL1), respectively. The interaction of β_2 integrins, namely lymphocyte function-associated antigen-1 (LFA-1, $\alpha_L\beta_2$, CD11a/CD18) and macrophage-1 antigen (Mac-1, $\alpha_M\beta_2$, CD11b/CD18) with ligands such as vascular cell adhesion molecule (VCAM-1), intercellular adhesion molecule-1 (ICAM-1, CD54), and ICAM-2 on endothelial cells, ensures firm adhesion of neutrophils.

The expression of adhesion molecules, along with the deposition of plasma fibronectin on leukocytes, is enhanced by inflammation and endothelial damage. Both ANCA and tumor necrosis factor (TNF) increase β_2 integrin expression on neutrophils, further promoting their attachment and neutrophil aggregation, enhancing trapping of cell aggregates in capillaries [60]. Adhesion of neutrophils is followed by crawling along the surface of the endothelium, following the gradient of chemoattractants, adhesion receptors, and endothelial stiffness. Finally, neutrophils travel through the vascular wall via paracellular or, to a lesser extent, transcellular routes in the process of diapedesis, facilitated by the interaction of β_2 integrins, ICAM-1, platelet endothelial cell adhesion molecule 1 (PECAM-1), and junctional adhesion molecules [61]. In this context, the biological role of CD177, a novel IgG Fc receptor found on the neutrophil surface, should also be considered. It has been demonstrated that CD177 ligation causes the migratory arrest of neutrophils, likely triggered by β_2 integrins as signaling partners, including their higher expression and affinity, reduced internalization, and extracellular signal-regulated kinases (ERK)-driven suppression of chemoattractants stimuli, potentially leading to endothelial injury [62]. Next, studies on murine models and in vitro have shown that some adhesive molecules can increase neutrophil extracellular trap (NETs) formation, a process essential to AAV pathogenesis and tremendously enhancing local inflammatory response. For instance, Mac-1 augments lipopolysaccharides (LPSs)-related NET formation (NETosis), P-selectin after ligation to PSGL-1, while the β_2 integrin subfamily when triggered by β-glucan [60].

Semaphorin A4D (SEMA4D) is a glycoprotein engaged in neutrophil-endothelium interactions, considered a potential biomarker of disease activity. In typical physiological conditions, the membrane complex of CD100/SEMA4D serves as an inhibitory receptor on neutrophils, where it interacts with plexin-B2 (PLXNB2) expressed by endothelial cells. This interaction shields the endothelium from damage, mainly by suppressing neutrophil-driven immune responses by reducing the production of reactive oxygen species (ROS) and NETosis [63]. A disintegrin and metalloproteinase domain-containing protein 17 (ADAM17) is a protease responsible for cleavage membrane-bound proteins, including SEMA4D, converting it to a soluble form [63,64]. A study by Bertram et al. [64] has reported a higher circulating ADAM17 concentration in patients with active PR3-AAV with kidney involvement compared to those in remission or with nonvascular kidney diseases. Similarly, markedly elevated serum SEMA4D levels have been demonstrated in patients with AAV, depicting a positive association with the BVAS score, and they were higher than in other autoimmune diseases, such as rheumatoid arthritis or systemic lupus erythematosus (SLE) [63]. Furthermore, Wang et al. [65] demonstrated that neutrophils from AAV patients exhibited a notable reduction in cell-surface SEMA4D compared to healthy controls. These findings suggest increased proteolytic shedding of SEMA4D in AAV, likely mediated by ADAM17. Since membrane-bound SEMA4D contributes to endothelial protection by regulating neutrophil activation, its loss from the cell surface, resulting in elevated levels of soluble SEMA4D, may impair this regulatory mechanism and promote neutrophil-mediated vascular injury.

4.3. Neutrophil Granule Proteins, Reactive Oxygen Species Production and Extracellular Vesicles Shape the Inflammatory Environment in AAV

Neutrophils possess an armamentarium of mechanisms aimed at pathogen detection and destruction. Neutralization of ingested particles and pathogens relies on two main cytotoxic mechanisms—ROS generation in the oxidative burst, catalyzed by nicotinamide adenine dinucleotide phosphate (NADPH) oxidase [66], and activity of antibacterial proteins, originating from neutrophil granules [67].

Depending on the stage of neutrophil differentiation, the granules can be divided into four main types—azurophil, specific, gelatinase, and secretory [68]. Degranulation through exocytosis also serves as a targeted, defensive mechanism and further enhances inflammatory response, with secretory granules being the most available for exocytosis [69]. Azurophil granules, however, are particularly relevant in the context of autoimmune vasculitis. Among various potent antimicrobial proteins—such as defensins, cathelicidins, cathepsin B, and lysozyme—they also include MPO and PR3 [70–72]. This phenomenon is mainly related to epigenetic dysregulation [73]. Furthermore, expression of these proteins on the neutrophil surface is augmented upon stimulation by complement component 5a (C5a) and cytokines released after ANCA binding [74].

ROS damage cellular components by causing double-stranded DNA breaks [75], inducing lipid peroxidation that compromises membrane integrity [76], and oxidizing proteins, leading to their misfolding and loss of function [77]. Hydroperoxides of amino acids and their residues are generated during oxidative modification driven by ROS, propagating oxidative damage further within proteins [78]. In addition to direct endothelium damage, oxidative burst might play a role in the stimulation of NETosis [79] (Figure 2), as its inhibition decreases NET formation [80]. A study by Hilhorst et al. [81] suggested that kidney damage in AAV depends on an imbalance between ROS and antioxidant defenses. Oxidative burst and hypochlorous acid (HOCl) production in neutrophils due to MPO activation at diagnosis have been linked to the presence of active cellular crescents in MPA, whereas higher serum thiol concentrations correlated with fewer cellular crescents and reduced interstitial fibrosis. According to the same study, MPA patients display higher oxidative stress, characterized by increased serum HOCl and advanced oxidation protein products (AOPP) concentration compared to healthy individuals. Interestingly, Sun et al. [82] reported a decrease in AAV-associated organ damage and MPO deposition in the kidneys and lungs of rat models treated with astaxanthin, a potent antioxidant. Therefore, the level of systemic oxidative stress response could reflect disease activity in AAV, making it a promising direction for further research.

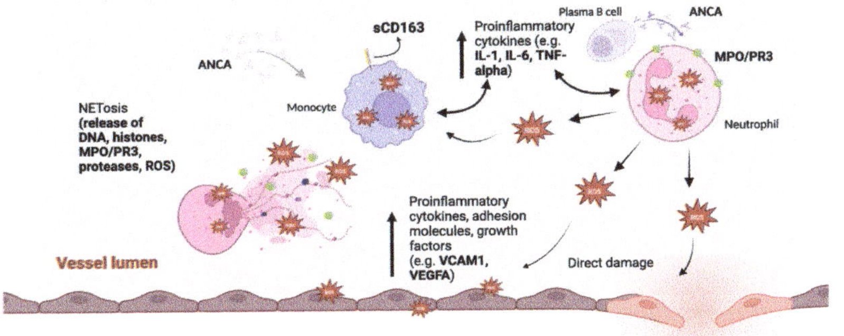

Figure 2. Reactive oxygen species (ROS) play a critical role in AAV. In addition to direct endothelial damage and perpetuating the inflammation via cytokine release, ROS generation is crucial for initiating NETosis. Monocytes and macrophages stimulated by ANCA, ROS, and inflammatory mediatiors release soluble CD163, which urine levels are a relatively novel biomarker of kidney vasculitis flare [83].

Beyond degranulation and ROS production, neutrophils also mediate inflammation via extracellular vesicles (EVs). EVs are an umbrella term for phospholipid bilayer-enclosed vesicles released by eukaryotic cells. Depending on their size, EVs can be divided into exosomes (50–150 nm) and microparticles (100–1000 nm) [84]. EVs regulate cell-to-cell communication, with different stimuli influencing the composition of their cargo, including proteins, nucleic acids, and lipids [85]. EVs cargo has been profiled in numerous studies investigating potential biomarkers in various conditions, such as cancer [86,87], neurological disorders [88], autoimmune diseases [89,90], and thrombosis [91]. Neutrophil-derived EVs were shown to carry ANCA-antigens, proinflammatory miRNA, and oxylipins. Interestingly, studies report a positive correlation between the BVAS and the levels of C3a, C5a, pentraxin 3 (PTX3) [92], and high mobility group box 1 (HMGB1) expressed on MPO-positive microparticles [93,94]. A recent study by our team [95] has reported that EVs from GPA patients, likely originating from neutrophils, encompass higher leukotriene B_4 (LTB_4) and 5-oxo-eicosatetraenoic acid (5-oxo-ETE) content compared to EVs from healthy controls. This study also shows that primed neutrophils stimulated with LTB_4 or 5-oxo-ETE exhibit a concentration-dependent increase in ROS production and dsDNA release. Another study of ours [96] shows that EVs released by IgG anti-PR3-activated neutrophils induce human umbilical vein endothelial cells (HUVECs) to produce proinflammatory cytokines via their miRNA content (most notably miR-223-3p and miR-142-3p). Furthermore, the expression of EVs-derived miR-223-3p and miR-664a-3p has been elevated in active GPA and correlated positively with BVAS, but also with circulating DNA-MPO complexes, suggesting a link to NETosis [97]. In a study by Glémain et al. [98], miR-142-3p and miR-451 from neutrophil-derived EVs have been implicated in promoting endothelial inflammation and damage. Furthermore, increased expression of miR-223, miR-142-3p, and miR-451 has been observed in peripheral blood of those with kidney involvement, suggesting their role in AAV progression.

4.4. *Phenotypic Diversity of Neutrophils, Including CD177$^+$ and Low-Density Subsets, Is Associated with Disease Activity in AAV*

In the past, neutrophils were thought to form a homogenous population of cells possessing uniform properties. However, this view has been challenged by findings enabled by the advent of high-resolution technologies [70]. Despite their short lifespan, neutrophils change in the process of aging. In addition to downregulating CXCR2 and L-selectin, it manifests by upregulating CXCR4, CD11b, and CD49 [99], accompanied by increased capacity to form NETs. These processes can be linked to the activation of pathogen-recognition receptors by pathogen associated molecular patterns (PAMPs) [100] and depend on changes in cortisol level and expression of circadian-clock genes, remaining in relation to circadian rhythm [101]. The abovementioned alterations promote neutrophils' homing and infiltrating tissues, where they act as sentinels. In the lungs, for instance, neutrophils adhere to the vascular lumen and reside in the interstitial spaces, retained by a mechanism that depends on CXCR4, making them a possible destination for aged neutrophils [102]. Evidence indicates that neutrophils might display differences in phenotype also across tissue [103,104]. Moreover, neutrophils display substantial diversity in morphology and function in pathological contexts of inflammation, infection, and cancer [105]. For instance, the proportion of circulating neutrophils expressing CD177 remains stable within an individual, regardless of age, gender, or activation state. However, their percentage can increase during pregnancy [106], GM-CSF therapy, or in patients with polycythemia vera [107]. Studies have revealed that variability in CD177 expression affects the surface display of PR3 [108]. Only CD177(+) neutrophils express PR3, and an increased proportion of these cells is linked to a higher risk of developing AAV [109] and a higher risk of relapse in GPA [110]. Stimulation of CD177 triggers degranulation and ROS production, especially in neutrophils expressing high levels of CD177 and PR3 [111]. Interestingly, that effect is attenuated by blocking the complement receptor integrin Mac-1 [112]. On the other hand, neutrophils of MPO-ANCA-positive individuals exhibit higher expression of LFA-1 compared to PR3-ANCA-positive ones, with this integrin expression associated with systemic and pulmonary components of the BVAS [113]. Furthermore, in AAV, neutrophils coexpressing CD177, LFA-1, Mac-1, CD80, CD86, CD100/SEMA4D, class II major histocompatibility complex (MHC II), TNF receptor (TNFR)1, and TNFR2 are detected in higher percentages, also in positive correlation with the BVAS [63,113–115].

Among neutrophil subsets described in a pathological context, particular attention is given to low-density neutrophils (LDNs), first identified in individuals with SLE [116]. LDNs can be separated from other granulocytes using a discontinuous density gradient and exhibit a density comparable to peripheral blood mononuclear cells (PBMCs). They have been observed in various conditions, including cancer [117], infections [118], and autoimmune disorders, such as rheumatoid arthritis [119] and psoriasis [120]. Studies based on autoimmune conditions suggest that LDGs are characterized by more pronounced proinflammatory properties [121,122], a higher tendency to undergo NETosis [123,124], and better promotion of Th17 cell differentiation compared to other subsets of neutrophils [125]. Interestingly, LDGs consisting of both mature CD10(+) and immature CD10() cells have been identified in AAV [126]. The CD10(−) subset displays downregulated CD16 and CD88/C5aR expression, an immature nuclear structure, and diminished responsiveness to stimulation by MPO-ANCA, which undermines their relevance in AAV pathogenesis [126]. On the other hand, LDGs co-expressing CD10, CD16, and CD88/C5aR can be induced by ANCA stimulation and likely play a role in activating the alternative complement pathway [127]. LDGs have been reported to correlate with disease activity in AAV [128]. However, it is important to note that LDNs encompass a broad spectrum of neutrophil phenotypes and have been observed in lower fraction also in healthy individuals [129]. The actual distinctiveness and relevance of neutrophil phenotypes have been questioned and attributed to the limitations of cell isolation methodology, making it one of the most controversial current aspects of neutrophil research [130,131].

4.5. Neutrophils Exhibit a Decreased Rate of Spontaneous Apoptosis and Enhanced NETosis in AAV

After completing their function, senescent neutrophils are removed from the inflamed tissue to avoid unnecessary perpetuation of the inflammation [70]. Besides homing to undergo apoptosis and efferocytosis, they can migrate in reverse or perish via different death processes, including pyroptosis, ferroptosis, necroptosis, necrosis, and NETosis [132]. In AAV, neutrophils show a decreased rate of spontaneous apoptosis in vitro, resulting in a prolonged lifespan, which suggests a tendency to accumulate at the inflammation site in vivo [133]. Delayed apoptosis observed in neutrophils of GPA patients involves both the intrinsic and extrinsic pathways and is likely driven by elevated levels of circulating factors such as GM-CSF, TNF, and soluble Fas cell surface death receptor (sFas) [134]. On the other hand, the opposite situation occurs in the case of NETosis in AAV. NETosis is a distinct form of cell death—as opposed to apoptosis, it involves the disintegration of neutrophil cell membrane paired with the release of NETs, which consist of granule contents combined with double-stranded DNA. This process is initiated by ROS generated through NADPH oxidase, which stimulates MPO to activate neutrophil elastase (NE) and promotes its translocation from azurophilic granules into the nucleus. There, NE cleaves histones and facilitates chromatin decondensation, aided by MPO, which acts synergistically. To reach the nucleus, NE must first degrade cytoplasmic F-actin. Notably, during NETosis, plasma membrane permeabilization occurs in a programmed manner, not due to physical disruption by expanding chromatin [135]. Upon release, chromatin immobilizes pathogens, and granule-derived proteins exert their antimicrobial effect, making this process a type of cell death and an effector neutrophil mechanism [136]. Moreover, it has been observed that, as in the case of unregulated necrosis, NETosis can drive a proinflammatory response instead of mitigating it, contributing to organ injury [137]. In AAV, neutrophils display enhanced NETosis compared to healthy individuals [138,139]. Although NET formation in AAV is often driven by ANCA, Kraaij et al. [139] suggest it can occur independently of them.

Even when IgG and IgA were depleted from AAV patient serum, NETosis still occurred in vitro, indicating the presence of additional humoral factors contributing to neutrophil activation and disease progression. MPO and PR3 are integral components of NETs, so their exposure may further drive ANCA production. In AAV, NETs enriched with PR3 and MPO have been detected in kidney tissues during active disease [140,141]. Interestingly, while both MPO and PR3 can form complexes with DNA, a study by our group [138] shows that MPO-DNA complexes are consistently present in all GPA patients, whereas PR3-DNA complexes can be detected only in some. Considering this, PR3-DNA complexes are of limited utility as NET formation markers in AAV, while MPO-DNA complexes appear to serve as a universal circulating marker of NET formation. In the same study, patients with active GPA exhibited elevated circulating levels of serine proteases, DNA-histone complexes, and MPO-DNA complexes. However, DNA-histone complexes were similarly elevated in GPA patients in remission and did not correlate with the BVAS score, further supporting the role of MPO-DNA complexes as a more reliable marker of NETosis. Additionally, increased levels of free circulating mitochondrial and genomic DNA have been identified as serum markers of GPA. Elevated circulating nucleosome levels, previously observed in AAV, further highlight the role of NETosis in disease pathology [142]. Moreover, fibrous DNA deposits containing PR3 and MPO can activate plasmacytoid dendritic cells (pDCs) and autoreactive B cells through a Toll-like receptor 9 (TLR-9)–dependent mechanism [143], potentially amplifying the autoimmune response. Interestingly, NET formation is not inextricably associated with cell death, as it can also occur via vital NETosis, contributing to the persistent, pathological immune response [144].

4.6. Neutrophil Effector Functions as an Emerging Therapeutic Target in AAV

In addition to their diagnostic and prognostic relevance, neutrophils and their proteases have gained attention as potential therapeutic targets in AAV. Rather than broadly suppressing immune responses, novel approaches aim to selectively inhibit neutrophil effector functions responsible for vascular injury. Preventing NETosis, for instance by PAD4 inhibitors, which prevent chromatin decondensation and NET release [145], seems particularly potential, but has not been evaluated in AAV yet. Similarly, inhibitors of neutrophil serine proteases [146,147] appear to be a compelling research direction in the search for agents to attenuate the inflammatory process in AAV. Although such inhibitors have not yet been evaluated in AAV, a study by Jerke et al. [148] on neutrophils derived from patients with Papillon-Lefèvre syndrome, who have a genetic deficiency in cathepsin C and consequently reduced protease activity, showed impaired neutrophil activation, lower surface expression of PR3, and significantly less endothelial damage. The same study further demonstrated that in human stem cell-derived neutrophils, where a specific cathepsin C inhibitor reduced levels of neutrophil serine proteases, membrane PR3 expression, PR3-ANCA-induced activation, and the transfer of active proteases to glomerular microvascular endothelial cells, which are the primary target in ANCA-induced necrotizing crescentic glomerulonephritis. Small-molecule inhibitors of spleen tyrosine kinase (Syk), central to ANCA-induced neutrophil activation via Fcγ receptors also bear a potential to become a new therapeutic target [149,150]. Notably, avacopan, an oral C5aR1 antagonist that has become a therapeutic option in AAV, prevents neutrophil priming and recruitment [151,152].

5. Platelets

Platelets are small, anucleate cells circulating for about 7–10 days in humans before being cleared in the spleen and liver. Platelet production, or thrombopoiesis, takes place primarily in the bone marrow. This process begins with hematopoietic stem cells (HSCs) differentiating into large, polyploid megakaryocytes, which then extend long, cytoplasmic protrusions known as proplatelets, ultimately demarcating their tips and releasing platelets into circulation [153]. Approximately 10^{11} platelets are produced daily [154]. While the roles of platelets in hemostasis and thrombosis have been extensively studied, their contributions to the immune response, particularly in autoimmune diseases, have only recently been recognized.

Although platelet counts are higher in patients with GPA compared to healthy individuals, no significant difference has been observed between those in remission and those with active disease [138,155]. Proposed mechanisms of count increase comprise interactions between platelet-derived sCD40L and matrix metalloproteinase-9 (MMP-9) [155] and between platelet-derived CCL5 and megakaryocytes [156]. A recent study by Lee et al. [157] has proposed a novel predictor based on platelet, neutrophil, monocyte, and lymphocyte counts—pan-immune-inflammation value (PIIV = neutrophil count ($\times 1000/\text{m}^3$) $\times$ monocyte count ($\times 1000/\text{m}^3$) $\times$ platelet count ($\times 1000/\text{mm}^3$)/lymphocyte count ($\times 1000/\text{m}^3$)). A high PIIV (cut-off point of at least 1011.3) at the onset of AAV has been postulated as an independent risk factor for all-cause mortality. Additionally, patients with GPA and MPA—especially those with kidney and pulmonary involvement—exhibit significantly elevated peripheral blood platelet count and platelet-to-lymphocyte ratio (PLR). PLR of 272.0 or greater has been linked to more severe disease activity [158,159]. On the other hand, in a study by Jin et al., lower platelet counts at presentation (cut-off point of 264.5 $\times$ 109/L) are suggested to be a predictor of worse kidney function, including end-stage kidney disease (ESKD), and death [160]. This observation is supported by a study by Sánchez Álamo et al., where lower platelet count was a predictor of mortality in AAV; however, the cut off value was within normal limits as well [161].

Platelets possess granules of three types: (1) alpha granules containing chemokines (CXCL7, CXCL4/PF4, CXL1/GROα, CXCL5, CCL5/RANTES, CCL3/MIP1α) [162], coagulation factors, PDGF receptors, TGF-β, P-selectin, fibrinogen, von Willebrand factor (vWF), and fibronectin; (2) dense granules storing calcium, magnesium, nucleotides (ADP, ATP), serotonin, and histamine; and (3) lysosomal granules, including glycohydrolases and proteases such as cathepsin, acid phosphatase, collagenase, and elastase. Dense bodies play a role in vasoconstriction and cytokine production primarily due to their high serotonin content [163,164]. In addition, platelets participate in immune responses by producing and releasing proinflammatory cytokines, most notably IL-1β [165]. They interact with specific receptors on leukocytes, such as monocytes, leading to cell activation. Platelets also express a diverse range of immune receptors, including chemokine receptors [166], Fc receptors [167], TLRs [24,168], and complement receptors [169–171]. The complement system plays a vital role in the pathogenesis of AAV [172]. Activation of the complement pathway leads to deposition of membrane attack complex (MAC) on the platelet surface and generation of C3a and C5a, further stimulating platelets [26].

In response to vascular damage, platelets undergo immediate changes in shape and function to participate in hemostasis or contribute to thrombosis in an unfavorable scenario. However, as platelets form heterogeneous subpopulations, chronic diseases involve shifts in their composition, altering platelet phenotypes [173]. Changes in platelet phenotypes can be driven by interactions between fully formed platelets and circulating inflammatory molecules or cells and by modulating platelet production by alterations in the megakaryocyte microenvironment. Such observations have been made in several disorders characterized by prolonged systemic inflammation, such as SLE [174], systemic sclerosis [175], and cancer [176]. For instance, chronic inflammatory states are characterized by increased platelet receptor expression and activity and the loss of surface receptors through cleavage and shedding [173]. However, as this is a relatively novel topic, it remains understudied and highlights a new direction for research in AAV monitoring.

6. Neutrophil-Platelet Crosstalk

Recent studies have shown that the progression of AAV involves interactions between activated platelets and neutrophils, as well as the interplay between the coagulation and complement systems

A study by Miao et al. [27] has investigated in AAV platelet-derived microparticles (PMP) containing proinflammatory cytokines, adhesion molecules, and growth factors, and has shown a positive correlation between PMP levels and erythrocyte sedimentation rate (ESR), CRP concentrations, and the BVAS score, particularly in relation to kidney involvement. The PMP level was also positively associated with both platelet and neutrophil counts and the percentage of neutrophils among leukocytes during the active phase of AAV. Upon exposure to cytokines such as TNF, but also C5a, and ANCA, neutrophils undergo an oxidative burst and degranulate, releasing microparticles containing tissue factors, which enhance NET formation. In turn, NETs not only enhance platelet adhesion [177] and aggregation [135], but also contribute to the activation of the coagulation cascade [178].

Both tissue factor and NETs components initiate the coagulation cascade, ultimately generating thrombin [22]. Thrombin then activates platelets through protease-activated receptors (PARs), leading to platelet degranulation and the release of P-selectin. Platelet receptors facilitate interactions with neutrophils, promoting ROS generation and further NET formation (Figure 3) [25,28]. These interactions damage the endothelium and trigger vWF release, which mediates platelet adhesion and aggregation, exacerbating vascular injury. Meanwhile, the activated neutrophils and platelets, through their membranes, microparticles, and NETs, stimulate the alternative complement pathway, increasing C5a levels. This positive feedback loop amplifies thrombin production and platelet/endothelial activation, perpetuating the inflammatory processes [179,180]. Activated platelets with bound fibrinogen can stimulate neutrophils, triggering an oxidative burst and facilitating neutrophil extravasation. Elevated plasma levels of platelet-derived soluble CD40L and CD62P/P-selectin complex correlate with disease activity in GPA [181]. The interaction between soluble CD40L and CD40 facilitates communication between platelets and endothelial cells, triggering the production of proinflammatory cytokines, such as IL-1β, IL-2, and TNF. This signaling also upregulates the expression of endothelial adhesion molecules, including ICAM-1, VCAM-1, and P-selectin, promoting the recruitment of leukocytes to the site of vascular damage. The sCD40L increases endothelial tissue factor expression and contributes to endothelial dysfunction by stimulating neutrophil ROS production. sCD40L can directly activate neutrophils, trigger ROS release, and upregulate Mac-1 [182]. It has been suggested that soluble P-selectin can serve as a biomarker of platelet activation [183]. The interaction of neutrophils and platelets mediated by P-selectin and PSGL enables their aggregation [184]. Patients with active GPA have more platelet-neutrophil aggregates and higher CD11b expression on neutrophils compared to healthy individuals. The percentage of platelet-neutrophil aggregates among neutrophils increases with BVAS [138]. The release of P-selectin from platelets stimulates NET formation; moreover, blocking its interaction with PSGL-1 substantially inhibits platelet-mediated NETosis [185]. In addition, according to a study by Matsumoto et al., platelets activated through TLR9 signaling release CXCL4, which in turn promotes the formation of NETs [28]. Interestingly, the TLR9–CXCL4 axis is upregulated in AAV. Platelets promote the formation of NETs also via activating neutrophils by TLR4 [168]. HMGB1 is a protein derived from platelets, capable of activating TLR4-dependant NETosis [186]. Higher serum levels of HMGB1 have also been linked to AAV with kidney involvement [187].

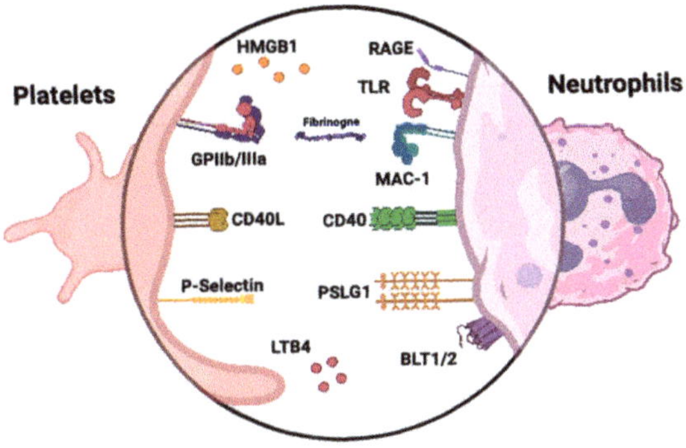

Figure 3. Platelet-neutrophil surface interactions in AAV. Upon activation, platelets express adhesion molecules and release inflammatory mediators that engage corresponding receptors on neutrophils. Notable interactions include P-selectin binding to PSGL-1 and platelet-derived HMGB1 engaging RAGE and TLRs on neutrophils, amplifying the inflammatory response through signaling pathways such as NF-κB and MAPK. Additionally, neutrophil MAC-1 interacts with platelet GPIIb/IIIa, facilitating firm adhesion. Leukotriene B4 (LTB4) and its receptors BLT1/2 contribute to neutrophil recruitment and activation.

Finally, the abovementioned CD177 has been shown not only to recognize β_2 integrins but also to bind to PR3 and PECAM-1, an immunoglobulin family protein found on endothelial cells, platelets, and neutrophils. However, evidence does not confirm its role in binding platelets to neutrophils or enhancing their interactions [62,188]. Further studies are needed to clarify that issue.

7. Biomarker Candidates in AAV Related to Neutrophils and Platelets

A summary of candidate biomarkers discussed in this study was presented in Table 1.

Table 1. An overview of neutrophil- and platelet-related biomarker candidates in AAV.

Biomarker	Source	Detection Method	Mechanism	Clinical Correlation and Relevance
ANCA	Autoantibodies	ELISA, IIF	Directly activate neutrophils via PR3/MPO binding	Established diagnostic and classification marker; titers may correlate with relapse [189].
MPO-DNA complexes	NETs	ELISA	Marker of NETosis, MPO bound to extracellular DNA	Correlate with disease activity and organ involvement [138].
Pentraxin-3 (PTX3)	NETs, activated neutrophils	ELISA	Acute-phase protein associated with NETs	Elevated in active disease; correlates with BVAS [92].
High Mobility Group Box 1 (HMGB1)	Neutrophils, platelets	ELISA	DAMP/alarmin promoting inflammation and NETosis	Increased in active AAV with kidney involvement [187].
Neutrophil-to-lymphocyte ratio (NLR)	Peripheral blood	Hematologic index	Indicator of systemic inflammation and neutrophil burden	Correlates with disease severity and relapse (cut-off ≥ 5.9) [55,190].
Delta Neutrophil Index (DNI)	Peripheral blood	Automated hematology analyzer	Reflects immature granulocyte population	Associated with relapse and severity (cut-off ≥ 0.65) [56].
CD177$^+$PR3$^+$ neutrophils	Neutrophils	Flow cytometry	Subset expressing surface PR3; more responsive to ANCA	Higher percentage in relapse-prone patients [110].
Low-density neutrophils (LDNs)	Neutrophils	Centrifugation in density gradient and flow cytometry	More pronounced proinflammatory properties and tendency to undergo NETosis	Correlates with BVAS [128], although it is unclear if LDNs form a truly distinct subset.
miR-223, miR-142-3p, miR-664a-3p	Neutrophil-derived EVs	RT-qPCR, miRNA sequencing	Proinflammatory miRNAs from neutrophile-derived vesicles	Correlate with BVAS and NETs [97].
P-selectin/sCD40L	Platelets	ELISA	Markers of platelet activation and endothelial crosstalk	Elevated in active GPA and correlate with NETs [180,184].

Table 1. *Cont.*

Biomarker	Source	Detection Method	Mechanism	Clinical Correlation and Relevance
Platelet-derived microparticles (PMPs)	Platelets	Flow cytometry, ELISA	Include TF, cytokines; promote NETs, coagulation	Correlate with ESR, CRP, BVAS, kidney involvement [27].
SEMA4D (soluble)	Neutrophils	ELISA	Cleaved from surface; loss facilitates NETosis	Elevated in active PR3-AAV [63].
Pan-Immune Inflammation Value (PIIV)	Peripheral blood	Hematologic index	Composite marker of neutrophil/monocyte/platelet burden	Predicts mortality risk (cut-off ≥ 1011.3) [158].

Although multiple studies have identified potential biomarker candidates in AAV, further research is necessary to confirm their clinical relevance and facilitate implementation, as most have not progressed beyond the discovery phase. Key challenges include standardizing assay methodologies, defining cut-offs, and verifying their added value in larger cohorts. International collaborative efforts, along with the development of integrative biomarker panels that combine multiple candidates, could accelerate the translational process.

8. Conclusions

Growing evidence shows that all essential neutrophil functions can be altered in AAV and are actively involved in disease pathogenesis. Furthermore, platelets play a crucial role in neutrophil activation and NET formation, ultimately leading to vascular damage. Potential predictors of AAV prognosis and biomarkers of disease activity related to neutrophils and platelets include indices calculated from blood counts (e.g., PLR), serum cytokine levels, surface antigen expression, and NET-associated components. However, further research is necessary to confirm their clinical relevance and facilitate implementation, especially as panels of multiple biomarkers. Neutrophil and platelet phenotypes represent a relatively novel and understudied area; therefore, changes in their composition and activation status may not only offer insights into AAV pathogenesis but also hold potential for disease monitoring.

Author Contributions: Conceptualization, A.D. and K.W.; methodology, A.D. and K.W.; software, M.S.; investigation, A.D. and S.B.-S.; writing—original draft preparation, A.D.; writing—review and editing, K.W., M.S., S.B.-S., K.W.-A., M.K. and J.M.; visualization, M.S.; supervision, K.W., M.S., K.W.-A., M.K. and J.M. All authors have read and agreed to the published version of the manuscript.

Funding: This research received no external funding.

Conflicts of Interest: The authors declare no conflicts of interest.

References

1. Jennette, J.C.; Falk, R.J.; Bacon, P.A.; Basu, N.; Cid, M.C.; Ferrario, F.; Flores-Suarez, L.F.; Gross, W.L.; Guillevin, L.; Hagen, E.C.; et al. 2012 revised International Chapel Hill Consensus Conference Nomenclature of Vasculitides. *Rheum. Arthritis Rheum.* **2013**, *65*, 180–186. [CrossRef]
2. Drynda, A.; Padjas, A.; Wójcik, K.; Dziedzic, R.; Biedroń, G.; Wawrzycka-Adamczyk, K.; Włudarczyk, A.; Wilańska, J.; Musiał, J.; Zdrojewski, Z.; et al. Clinical characteristics of EGPA patients in comparison to GPA subgroup with increased blood eosinophilia from Polvas Registry. *J. Immunol. Res.* **2024**, *2024*, 4283928. [CrossRef]
3. Wójcik, K.; Masiak, A.; Jeleniewicz, R.; Jakuszko, K.; Brzosko, I.; Storoniak, H.; Kur-Zalewska, J.; Wisłowska, M.; Madej, M.; Hawrot-Kawecka, A.; et al. Association of antineutrophil cytoplasmic antibody (ANCA) specificity with the demographic and clinical characteristics of patients with ANCA-associated vasculitides. *Pol. Arch. Intern. Med.* **2022**, *132*, 16187. [CrossRef] [PubMed]

4. Biedroń, G.; Włudarczyk, A.; Wawrzycka-Adamczyk, K.; Wójcik, K.; Musiał, J.; Bazan-Socha, S.; Zdrojewski, Z.; Masiak, A.; Czuszyńska, Z.; Majdan, M.; et al. Respiratory involvement in antineutrophil cytoplasmic antibody-associated vasculitides: A retrospective study based on POLVAS Registry. *Clin. Exp. Rheumatol.* **2021**, *40*, 720–726. [CrossRef] [PubMed]
5. Koirala, A.; Sharma, P.D.; Jhaveri, K.D.; Jain, K.; Geetha, D. Rapidly progressive glomerulonephritis. *Adv. Kidney Dis. Health* **2024**, *31*, 485–495. [CrossRef] [PubMed]
6. Iudici, M.; Puéchal, X.; Pagnoux, C.; Courvoisier, D.S.; Hamidou, M.; Blanchard-Delaunay, C.; Maurier, F.; Ruivard, M.; Quéméneur, T.; Aumaître, O.; et al. Significance of eosinophilia in granulomatosis with polyangiitis: Data from the French Vasculitis Study Group Registry. *Rheumatology* **2022**, *61*, 1211–1216. [CrossRef]
7. Quan, M.V.; Frankel, S.K.; Maleki-Fischbach, M.; Tan, L.D. A rare case report of polyangiitis overlap syndrome: Granulomatosis with polyangiitis and eosinophilic granulomatosis with polyangiitis. *BMC Pulm. Med.* **2018**, *18*, 181. [CrossRef]
8. Tomasson, G.; Grayson, P.C.; Mahr, A.D.; LaValley, M.; Merkel, P.A. Value of ANCA measurements during remission to predict a relapse of anca-associated vasculitis--a meta-analysis. *Rheumatology* **2011**, *51*, 100–109. [CrossRef]
9. Chung, S.A.; Langford, C.A.; Maz, M.; Abril, A.; Gorelik, M.; Guyatt, G.; Archer, A.M.; Conn, D.L.; Full, K.A.; Grayson, P.C.; et al. 2021 American College of Rheumatology/Vasculitis Foundation guideline for the management of Antineutrophil cytoplasmic antibody–associated vasculitis. *Arthritis Rheumatol.* **2021**, *73*, 1366–1383. [CrossRef]
10. Hellmich, B.; Sanchez-Alamo, B.; Schirmer, J.H.; Berti, A.; Blockmans, D.; Cid, M.C.; Holle, J.U.; Hollinger, N.; Karadag, O.; Kronbichler, A.; et al. Eular recommendations for the management of Anca-Associated Vasculitis: 2022 update. *Ann. Rheum. Dis.* **2024**, *83*, 30–47. [CrossRef]
11. Pagnoux, C.; Mahr, A.; Hamidou, M.A.; Boffa, J.-J.; Ruivard, M.; Ducroix, J.-P.; Kyndt, X.; Lifermann, F.; Papo, T.; Lambert, M.; et al. Azathioprine or methotrexate maintenance for ANCA-associated vasculitis. *N. Engl. J. Med.* **2008**, *359*, 2790–2803. [CrossRef] [PubMed]
12. Guillevin, L.; Pagnoux, C.; Karras, A.; Khouatra, C.; Aumaître, O.; Cohen, P.; Maurier, F.; Decaux, O.; Ninet, J.; Gobert, P.; et al. Rituximab versus azathioprine for maintenance in ANCA-associated vasculitis. *N. Engl. J. Med.* **2014**, *371*, 1771–1780. [CrossRef] [PubMed]
13. Flossmann, O.; Berden, A.; de Groot, K.; Hagen, C.; Harper, L.; Heijl, C.; Höglund, P.; Jayne, D.; Luqmani, R.; Mahr, A.; et al. Long-term patient survival in ANCA-associated vasculitis. *Ann. Rheum. Dis.* **2011**, *70*, 488–494. [CrossRef] [PubMed]
14. Smith, R. Complications of therapy for ANCA-associated vasculitis. *Rheumatol. Oxf. Engl.* **2020**, *59* (Suppl. S3), iii74–iii78. [CrossRef]
15. Sayer, M.; Chapman, G.B.; Thomas, M.; Dhaun, N. Cardiovascular disease in anti-neutrophil cytoplasm antibody-associated vasculitis. *Curr. Rheumatol. Rep.* **2023**, *26*, 12–23. [CrossRef]
16. Woywodt, A.; Streiber, F.; de Groot, K.; Regelsberger, H.; Haller, H.; Haubitz, M. Circulating endothelial cells as markers for ANCA-associated small-vessel vasculitis. *Lancet* **2003**, *361*, 206–210. [CrossRef]
17. Weidner, S.; Hafezi-Rachti, S.; Rupprecht, H.D. Thromboembolic events as a complication of antineutrophil cytoplasmic antibody-associated vasculitis. *Rheum. Arthritis Rheum.* **2006**, *55*, 146–149. [CrossRef]
18. Falk, R.J.; Jennette, J.C. Anti-Neutrophil cytoplasmic autoantibodies with specificity for myeloperoxidase in patients with systemic vasculitis and idiopathic necrotizing and crescentic glomerulonephritis. *N. Engl. J. Med.* **1988**, *318*, 1651–1657. [CrossRef]
19. Niles, J.L.; McCluskey, R.T.; Ahmad, M.F.; Arnaout, M.A. Wegener's granulomatosis autoantigen is a novel neutrophil serine proteinase. *Blood* **1989**, *74*, 1888–1893. [CrossRef]
20. Falk, R.J.; Terrell, R.S.; Charles, L.A.; Jennette, J.C. Anti-neutrophil cytoplasmic autoantibodies induce neutrophils to degranulate and produce oxygen radicals in vitro. *Proc. Natl. Acad. Sci. USA* **1990**, *87*, 4115–4119. [CrossRef]
21. Ewert, B.H.; Jennette, J.C.; Falk, R.J. Anti-myeloperoxidase antibodies stimulate neutrophils to damage human endothelial cells. *Kidney Int.* **1992**, *41*, 375–383. [CrossRef]
22. McDonald, B.; Davis, R.P.; Kim, S.J.; Tse, M.; Esmon, C.T.; Kolaczkowska, E.; Jenne, C.N. Platelets and neutrophil extracellular traps collaborate to promote intravascular coagulation during sepsis in mice. *Blood* **2017**, *129*, 1357–1367. [CrossRef]
23. Xu, X.R.; Yousef, G.M.; Ni, H. Cancer and platelet crosstalk: Opportunities and challenges for aspirin and other antiplatelet agents. *Blood* **2018**, *131*, 1777–1789. [CrossRef]
24. Tay, S.H.; Zharkova, O.; Lee, H.Y.; Toh, M.M.X.; Libau, E.A.; Celhar, T.; Narayanan, S.; Ahl, P.J.; Ong, W.Y.; Joseph, C.; et al. Platelet TLR7 is essential for the formation of platelet-neutrophil complexes and low-density neutrophils in lupus nephritis. *Rheumatology* **2024**, *63*, 551–562. [CrossRef]
25. Maugeri, N.; Baldini, M.; Ramirez, G.A.; Rovere-Querini, P.; Manfredi, A.A. Platelet-leukocyte deregulated interactions foster sterile inflammation and tissue damage in immune-mediated vessel diseases. *Thromb. Res.* **2012**, *129*, 267–273. [CrossRef]
26. Miao, D.; Li, D.Y.; Chen, M.; Zhao, M.H. Platelets are activated in ANCA-associated vasculitis via thrombin-PARs pathway and can activate the alternative complement pathway. *Arthritis Res. Ther.* **2017**, *19*, 252. [CrossRef] [PubMed]
27. Miao, D.; Ma, T.T.; Chen, M.; Zhao, M.H. Platelets release proinflammatory microparticles in anti-neutrophil cytoplasmic antibody-associated vasculitis. *Rheumatology* **2019**, *58*, 1432–1442. [CrossRef] [PubMed]

28. Matsumoto, K.; Yasuoka, H.; Yoshimoto, K.; Suzuki, K.; Takeuchi, T. Platelet CXCL4 mediates neutrophil extracellular traps formation in ANCA-associated vasculitis. *Sci. Rep.* **2021**, *11*, 222. [CrossRef] [PubMed]
29. Vegting, Y.; Vogt, L.; Anders, H.J.; de Winther, M.P.J.; Bemelman, F.J.; Hilhorst, M.L. Monocytes and macrophages in ANCA-associated vasculitis. *Autoimmun. Rev.* **2021**, *20*, 102911. [CrossRef]
30. Ivanov, I.I.; Apta, B.H.R.; Bonna, A.M.; Harper, M.T. Platelet P-selectin triggers rapid surface exposure of tissue factor in monocytes. *Sci. Rep.* **2019**, *9*, 13397. [CrossRef]
31. Greenlee-Wacker, M.C. Clearance of apoptotic neutrophils and resolution of inflammation. *Immunol. Rev.* **2016**, *273*, 357–370. [CrossRef]
32. Tan, H.; Zhang, S.; Zhang, Z.; Zhang, J.; Wang, Z.; Liao, J.; Qiu, X.; Jia, E. Neutrophil extracellular traps promote M1 macrophage polarization in gouty inflammation via targeting hexokinase-2. *Free Radic. Biol. Med.* **2024**, *224*, 540–553. [CrossRef]
33. Li, L.; Yu, X.; Liu, J.; Wang, Z.; Li, C.; Shi, J.; Sun, L.; Liu, Y.; Zhang, F.; Chen, H.; et al. Neutrophil Extracellular Traps Promote Aberrant Macrophages Activation in Behçet's Disease. *Front. Immunol.* **2021**, *11*, 590622. [CrossRef] [PubMed]
34. Hilhorst, M.; Shirai, T.; Berry, G.; Goronzy, J.J.; Weyand, C.M. T cell-macrophage interactions and granuloma formation in vasculitis. *Front. Immunol.* **2014**, *5*, 432. [CrossRef] [PubMed]
35. Tsuboi, K.; Noguchi, K.; Kitano, M.; Furukawa, T.; Hashimoto, T.; Azuma, N.; Matsui, K. Serum B cell activating factor (BAFF) as a biomarker for induction of remission with rituximab in ANCA-associated vasculitis. *Immunol. Med.* **2022**, *45*, 238–243. [CrossRef] [PubMed]
36. Stone, J.H.; Merkel, P.A.; Spiera, R.; Seo, P.; Langford, C.A.; Hoffman, G.S.; Kallenberg, C.G.; St Clair, E.W.; Turkiewicz, A.; Tchao, N.K.; et al. Rituximab versus cyclophosphamide for ANCA-associated vasculitis. *N. Engl. J. Med.* **2010**, *363*, 221–232. [CrossRef]
37. Alba, M.A.; Jennette, J.C.; Falk, R.J. Pathogenesis of ANCA-Associated Pulmonary Vasculitis. *Semin. Respir. Crit. Care Med.* **2018**, *39*, 413–424. [CrossRef]
38. Martinez Valenzuela, L.; Bordignon Draibe, J.; Fulladosa Oliveras, X.; Bestard Matamoros, O.; Cruzado Garrit, J.M.; Torras Ambrós, J. T-lymphocyte in ANCA-associated vasculitis: What do we know? A pathophysiological and therapeutic approach. *Clin. Kidney J.* **2019**, *12*, 503–511. [CrossRef]
39. Kimoto, Y.; Horiuchi, T. The Complement System and ANCA Associated Vasculitis in the Era of Anti-Complement Drugs. *Front. Immunol.* **2022**, *13*, 926044. [CrossRef]
40. Pryzdial, E.L.G.; Leatherdale, A.; Conway, E.M. Coagulation and complement: Key innate defense participants in a seamless web. *Front. Immunol.* **2022**, *13*, 918775. [CrossRef]
41. Vegting, Y.; Hanford, K.M.; Jongejan, A.; Gajadin, G.R.; Versloot, M.; van der Bom-Baylon, N.D.; Dekker, T.; Penne, E.L.; van der Heijden, J.W.; Houben, E.; et al. Cardiovascular risk in ANCA-associated vasculitis: Monocyte phenotyping reveals distinctive signatures between serological subsets. *Atherosclerosis* **2024**, *397*, 118559. [CrossRef]
42. Sun, X.J.; Chen, M.; Zhao, M.H. Thrombin Contributes to Anti-myeloperoxidase Antibody Positive IgG-Mediated Glomerular Endothelial Cells Activation Through SphK1-S1P-S1PR3 Signaling. *Front. Immunol.* **2019**, *10*, 237. [CrossRef]
43. Saverymuttu, S.H.; Peters, A.M.; Keshavarzian, A.; Reavy, H.J.; Lavender, J.P. The kinetics of 111indium distribution following injection of 111indium labelled autologous granulocytes in man. *Br. J. Haematol.* **1985**, *61*, 675–685. [CrossRef]
44. Pillay, J.; Braber, I.D.; Vrisekoop, N.; Kwast, L.M.; de Boer, R.J.; Borghans, J.A.M.; Tesselaar, K.; Koenderman, L. In vivo labeling with 2H2O reveals a human neutrophil lifespan of 5.4 days. *Blood* **2010**, *116*, 625–627. [CrossRef]
45. Dancey, J.T.; Deubelbeiss, K.A.; Harker, L.A.; Finch, C.A. Neutrophil kinetics in man. *J. Clin. Investig.* **1976**, *58*, 705–715. [CrossRef] [PubMed]
46. Richards, M.K.; Liu, F.; Iwasaki, H.; Akashi, K.; Link, D.C. Pivotal role of granulocyte colony-stimulating factor in the development of progenitors in the common myeloid pathway. *Blood* **2003**, *102*, 3562–3568. [CrossRef] [PubMed]
47. Rankin, S.M. The bone marrow: A site of neutrophil clearance. *J. Leukoc. Biol.* **2010**, *88*, 241–251. [CrossRef] [PubMed]
48. Summers, C.; Rankin, S.M.; Condliffe, A.M.; Singh, N.; Peters, A.M.; Chilvers, E.R. Neutrophil kinetics in health and disease. *Trends Immunol.* **2010**, *31*, 318–324. [CrossRef]
49. Ota, S.; Kotani, T.; Matsuda, S.; Nishioka, D.; Masuda, Y.; Unoda, K.; Hosokawa, T.; Ishida, S.; Takeuchi, T. Initial serum GM-CSF levels are associated with the severity of cerebral small vessel disease in microscopic polyangiitis patients. *J. Neuroimmunol.* **2021**, *359*, 577671. [CrossRef]
50. Stark, M.A.; Huo, Y.; Burcin, T.L.; Morris, M.A.; Olson, T.S.; Ley, K. Phagocytosis of apoptotic neutrophils regulates granulopoiesis via IL-23 and IL-17. *Immunity* **2005**, *22*, 285–294. [CrossRef]
51. Ley, K.; Smith, E.; Stark, M.A. IL-17A-producing neutrophil-regulatory Tn lymphocytes. *Immunol. Res.* **2006**, *34*, 229–242. [CrossRef] [PubMed]
52. Matsumoto, K.; Suzuki, K.; Yoshimoto, K.; Seki, N.; Tsujimoto, H.; Chiba, K.; Takeuchi, T. Significant association between clinical characteristics and immuno-phenotypes in patients with ANCA-associated vasculitis. *Rheumatology* **2020**, *59*, 545–553. [CrossRef] [PubMed]

53. Nogueira, E.; Hamour, S.; Sawant, D.; Henderson, S.; Mansfield, N.; Chavele, K.M.; Pusey, C.D.; Salama, A.D. Serum IL-17 and IL-23 levels and autoantigen-specific Th17 cells are elevated in patients with ANCA-associated vasculitis. *Nephrol. Dial. Transpl.* **2010**, *25*, 2209–2217. [CrossRef]
54. Huang, L.; Shen, C.; Zhong, Y.; Ooi, J.D.; Zhou, Y.O.; Chen, J.B.; Wu, T.; Meng, T.; Xiao, Z.; Lin, W.; et al. The association of neutrophil-to-lymphocyte ratio with all-cause mortality in Chinese patients with MPO-ANCA associated vasculitis. *Clin. Exp. Med.* **2020**, *20*, 401–408. [CrossRef]
55. Ahn, S.S.; Jung, S.M.; Song, J.J.; Park, Y.B.; Lee, S.W. Neutrophil to lymphocyte ratio at diagnosis can estimate vasculitis activity and poor prognosis in patients with ANCA-associated vasculitis: A retrospective study. *BMC Nephrol.* **2018**, *19*, 187. [CrossRef] [PubMed]
56. Yoo, J.; Ahn, S.S.; Jung, S.M.; Song, J.J.; Park, Y.B.; Lee, S.W. Delta Neutrophil Index Is Associated with Vasculitis Activity and Risk of Relapse in ANCA-Associated Vasculitis. *Yonsei Med. J.* **2018**, *59*, 397–405. [CrossRef]
57. Bazan-Socha, S.; Bukiej, A.; Marcinkiewicz, C.; Musial, J. Integrins in pulmonary inflammatory diseases. *Curr. Pharm. Des.* **2005**, *11*, 893–901. [CrossRef]
58. Ley, K.; Laudanna, C.; Cybulsky, M.I.; Nourshargh, S. Getting to the site of inflammation: The leukocyte adhesion cascade updated. *Nat. Rev. Immunol.* **2007**, *7*, 678–689. [CrossRef]
59. Halbwachs, L.; Lesavre, P. Endothelium-neutrophil interactions in ANCA-associated diseases. *J. Am. Soc. Nephrol.* **2012**, *23*, 1449–1461. [CrossRef]
60. Lelliott, P.M.; Nishide, M.; Pavillon, N.; Okita, Y.; Shibahara, T.; Mizuno, Y.; Yoshimura, H.; Obata, S.; Kumanogoh, A.; Smith, N.I. Cellular Adhesion Is a Controlling Factor in Neutrophil Extracellular Trap Formation Induced by Anti-Neutrophil Cytoplasmic Antibodies. *Immunohorizons* **2022**, *6*, 170–183. [CrossRef]
61. Halai, K.; Whiteford, J.; Ma, B.; Nourshargh, S.; Woodfin, A. ICAM-2 facilitates luminal interactions between neutrophils and endothelial cells in vivo. *J. Cell Sci.* **2014**, *127*, 620–629. [CrossRef] [PubMed]
62. Bai, M.; Grieshaber-Bouyer, R.; Wang, J.; Schmider, A.B.; Wilson, Z.S.; Zeng, L.; Halyabar, O.; Godin, M.D.; Nguyen, H.N.; Levescot, A.; et al. CD177 modulates human neutrophil migration through activation-mediated integrin and chemoreceptor regulation. *Blood* **2017**, *130*, 2092–2100. [CrossRef] [PubMed]
63. Nishide, M.; Nojima, S.; Ito, D.; Takamatsu, H.; Koyama, S.; Kang, S.; Kimura, T.; Morimoto, K.; Hosokawa, T.; Hayama, Y.; et al. Semaphorin 4D inhibits neutrophil activation and is involved in the pathogenesis of neutrophil-mediated autoimmune vasculitis. *Ann. Rheum. Dis.* **2017**, *76*, 1440–1448. [CrossRef] [PubMed]
64. Bertram, A.; Lovric, S.; Engel, A.; Beese, M.; Wyss, K.; Hertel, B.; Park, J.K.; Becker, J.U.; Kegel, J.; Haller, H.; et al. Circulating ADAM17 Level Reflects Disease Activity in Proteinase-3 ANCA-Associated Vasculitis. *J. Am. Soc. Nephrol.* **2015**, *26*, 2860–2870. [CrossRef]
65. Wang, L.; Li, X.; Song, Y.; Song, D.; Huang, D.M. The emerging roles of semaphorin4D/CD100 in immunological diseases. *Biochem. Soc. Trans.* **2020**, *48*, 2875–2890. [CrossRef]
66. Li, H.; Zhou, X.; Huang, Y.; Liao, B.; Cheng, L.; Ren, B. Reactive Oxygen Species in Pathogen Clearance: The Killing Mechanisms, the Adaption Response, and the Side Effects. *Front. Microbiol.* **2021**, *11*, 622534. [CrossRef]
67. Levy, O. Antimicrobial proteins and peptides of blood: Templates for novel antimicrobial agents. *Blood* **2000**, *96*, 2664–2672. [CrossRef]
68. Pham, C.T. Neutrophil serine proteases: Specific regulators of inflammation. *Nat. Rev. Immunol.* **2006**, *6*, 541–550. [CrossRef]
69. Faurschou, M.; Borregaard, N. Neutrophil granules and secretory vesicles in inflammation. *Microbes Infect.* **2003**, *5*, 1317–1327. [CrossRef]
70. Zhang, F.; Xia, Y.; Su, J.; Quan, F.; Zhou, H.; Li, Q.; Feng, Q.; Lin, C.; Wang, D.; Jiang, Z. Neutrophil diversity and function in health and disease. *Signal Transduct. Target Ther.* **2024**, *9*, 343. [CrossRef]
71. Cowland, J.B.; Borregaard, N. Granulopoiesis and granules of human neutrophils. *Immunol. Rev.* **2016**, *273*, 11–28. [CrossRef] [PubMed]
72. Nordenfelt, P.; Tapper, H. Phagosome dynamics during phagocytosis by neutrophils. *J. Leukoc. Biol.* **2011**, *90*, 271–284. [CrossRef] [PubMed]
73. Jennette, J.C.; Falk, R.J. Pathogenesis of antineutrophil cytoplasmic autoantibody-mediated disease. *Nat. Rev. Rheumatol.* **2014**, *10*, 463–473. [CrossRef] [PubMed]
74. Hong, Y.; Eleftheriou, D.; Hussain, A.A.; Price-Kuehne, F.E.; Savage, C.O.; Jayne, D.; Little, M.A.; Salama, A.D.; Klein, N.J.; Brogan, P.A. Anti-neutrophil cytoplasmic antibodies stimulate release of neutrophil microparticles. *J. Am. Soc. Nephrol.* **2012**, *23*, 49–62. [CrossRef]
75. Sharma, V.; Collins, L.B.; Chen, T.H.; Herr, N.; Takeda, S.; Sun, W.; Swenberg, J.A.; Nakamura, J. Oxidative stress at low levels can induce clustered DNA lesions leading to NHEJ mediated mutations. *Oncotarget* **2016**, *7*, 25377–25390. [CrossRef]
76. Mylonas, C.; Kouretas, D. Lipid peroxidation and tissue damage. *Vivo* **1999**, *13*, 295–309.
77. Sohal, R.S. Role of oxidative stress and protein oxidation in the aging process. *Free Radic. Biol. Med.* **2002**, *33*, 37–44. [CrossRef]

78. Michalski, R.; Zielonka, J.; Gapys, E.; Marcinek, A.; Joseph, J.; Kalyanaraman, B. Real-time measurements of amino acid and protein hydroperoxides using coumarin boronic acid. *J. Biol. Chem.* **2014**, *289*, 22536–22553. [CrossRef]

79. Azzouz, D.; Khan, M.A.; Palaniyar, N. ROS induces NETosis by oxidizing DNA and initiating DNA repair. *Cell Death Discov.* **2021**, *7*, 113. [CrossRef]

80. Leung, H.H.L.; Perdomo, J.; Ahmadi, Z.; Yan, F.; McKenzie, S.E.; Chong, B.H. Inhibition of NADPH oxidase blocks NETosis and reduces thrombosis in heparin-induced thrombocytopenia. *Blood Adv.* **2021**, *5*, 5439–5451. [CrossRef]

81. Hilhorst, M.; Maria, A.T.; Kavian, N.; Batteux, F.; Borderie, D.; Le Quellec, A.; van Paassen, P.; Guilpain, P. Impact of MPO-ANCA-mediated oxidative imbalance on renal vasculitis. *Am. J. Physiol. Renal. Physiol.* **2018**, *315*, F1769–F1776. [CrossRef] [PubMed]

82. Sun, R.L.; Shang, J.C.; Han, R.H.; Xing, G.Q. Protective effect of astaxanthin on ANCA-associated vasculitis. *Int. Immunopharmacol.* **2024**, *132*, 111928. [CrossRef] [PubMed]

83. Moran, S.M.; Monach, P.A.; Zgaga, L.; Cuthbertson, D.; Carette, S.; Khalidi, N.A.; Koening, C.L.; Langford, C.A.; McAlear, C.A.; Moreland, L.; et al. Urinary soluble CD163 and monocyte chemoattractant protein-1 in the identification of subtle renal flare in anti-neutrophil cytoplasmic antibody-associated vasculitis. *Nephrol. Dial. Transpl.* **2020**, *35*, 283–291. [CrossRef] [PubMed]

84. van der Pol, E.; Böing, A.N.; Harrison, P.; Sturk, A.; Nieuwland, R. Classification, functions, and clinical relevance of extracellular vesicles. *Pharmacol. Rev.* **2012**, *64*, 676–705. [CrossRef]

85. Dalli, J.; Montero-Melendez, T.; Norling, L.V.; Yin, X.; Hinds, C.; Haskard, D.; Mayr, M.; Perretti, M. Heterogeneity in neutrophil microparticles reveals distinct proteome and functional properties. *Mol. Cell Proteom.* **2013**, *12*, 2205–2219. [CrossRef]

86. Soung, Y.H.; Ford, S.; Zhang, V.; Chung, J. Exosomes in Cancer Diagnostics. *Cancers* **2017**, *9*, 8. [CrossRef]

87. Sun, J.; Sun, Z.; Gareev, I.; Yan, T.; Chen, X.; Ahmad, A.; Zhang, D.; Zhao, B.; Beylerli, O.; Yang, G.; et al. Exosomal miR-2276-5p in Plasma Is a Potential Diagnostic and Prognostic Biomarker in Glioma. *Front. Cell Dev. Biol.* **2021**, *9*, 671202. [CrossRef]

88. Pulliam, L.; Sun, B.; Mustapic, M.; Chawla, S.; Kapogiannis, D. Plasma neuronal exosomes serve as biomarkers of cognitive impairment in HIV infection and Alzheimer's disease. *J. Neurovirol.* **2019**, *25*, 702–709. [CrossRef]

89. Zheng, C.; Xie, L.; Qin, H.; Liu, X.; Chen, X.; Lv, F.; Wang, L.; Zhu, X.; Xu, J. The Role of Extracellular Vesicles in Systemic Lupus Erythematosus. *Front. Cell Dev. Biol.* **2022**, *10*, 835566. [CrossRef]

90. Ricco, C.; Eldaboush, A.; Liu, M.L.; Werth, V.P. Extracellular Vesicles in the Pathogenesis, Clinical Characterization, and Management of Dermatomyositis: A Narrative Review. *Int. J. Mol. Sci.* **2024**, *25*, 1967. [CrossRef]

91. Gasecka, A.; Böing, A.N.; Filipiak, K.J.; Nieuwland, R. Platelet extracellular vesicles as biomarkers for arterial thrombosis. *Platelets* **2017**, *28*, 228–234. [CrossRef] [PubMed]

92. Jonasdottir, A.D.; Antovic, A.; Qureshi, A.R.; Nordin, A.; Malmström, V.; Gunnarsson, I.; Bruchfeld, A. Pentraxin-3—A potential biomarker in ANCA-associated vasculitis. *Scand. J. Rheumatol.* **2023**, *52*, 293–301. [CrossRef] [PubMed]

93. Manojlovic, M.; Juto, A.; Jonasdottir, A.; Colic, J.; Vojinovic, J.; Nordin, A.; Bruchfeld, A.; Gunnarsson, I.; Mobarrez, F.; Antovic, A. Microparticles expressing myeloperoxidase as potential biomarkers in anti-neutrophil cytoplasmic antibody (ANCA)-associated vasculitides (AAV). *J. Mol. Med.* **2020**, *98*, 1279–1286. [CrossRef] [PubMed]

94. Antovic, A.; Mobarrez, F.; Manojlovic, M.; Soutari, N.; De Porta Baggemar, V.; Nordin, A.; Bruchfeld, A.; Vojinovic, J.; Gunnarsson, I. Microparticles Expressing Myeloperoxidase and Complement C3a and C5a as Markers of Renal Involvement in Antineutrophil Cytoplasmic Antibody-associated Vasculitis. *J. Rheumatol.* **2020**, *47*, 714–721. [CrossRef]

95. Surmiak, M.; Gielicz, A.; Stojkov, D.; Szatanek, R.; Wawrzycka-Adamczyk, K.; Yousefi, S.; Simon, H.U.; Sanak, M. LTB_4 and 5-oxo-ETE from extracellular vesicles stimulate neutrophils in granulomatosis with polyangiitis. *J. Lipid Res.* **2020**, *61*, 1–9. [CrossRef]

96. Surmiak, M.; Kosałka-Węgiel, J.; Polański, S.; Sanak, M. Endothelial cells response to neutrophil-derived extracellular vesicles miRNAs in anti-PR3 positive vasculitis. *Clin. Exp. Immunol.* **2021**, *204*, 267–282. [CrossRef]

97. Surmiak, M.; Wawrzycka-Adamczyk, K.; Kosałka-Węgiel, J.; Polański, S.; Sanak, M. Profile of circulating extracellular vesicles microRNA correlates with the disease activity in granulomatosis with polyangiitis. *Clin. Exp. Immunol.* **2022**, *208*, 103–113. [CrossRef]

98. Glémain, A.; Néel, M.; Néel, A.; André-Grégoire, G.; Gavard, J.; Martinet, B.; Le Bloas, R.; Riquin, K.; Hamidou, M.; Fakhouri, F.; et al. Neutrophil-derived extracellular vesicles induce endothelial inflammation and damage through the transfer of miRNAs. *J. Autoimmun.* **2022**, *129*, 102826. [CrossRef]

99. Casanova-Acebes, M.; Pitaval, C.; Weiss, L.A.; Nombela-Arrieta, C.; Chèvre, R.; A-González, N.; Kunisaki, Y.; Zhang, D.; van Rooijen, N.; Silberstein, L.E.; et al. Rhythmic modulation of the hematopoietic niche through neutrophil clearance. *Cell* **2013**, *153*, 1025–1035. [CrossRef]

100. Zhang, D.; Chen, G.; Manwani, D.; Mortha, A.; Xu, C.; Faith, J.J.; Burk, R.D.; Kunisaki, Y.; Jang, J.E.; Scheiermann, C.; et al. Neutrophil ageing is regulated by the microbiome. *Nature* **2015**, *525*, 528–532. [CrossRef]

101. Aroca-Crevillén, A.; Adrover, J.M.; Hidalgo, A. Circadian Features of Neutrophil Biology. *Front. Immunol.* **2020**, *11*, 576. [CrossRef] [PubMed]

102. Devi, S.; Wang, Y.; Chew, W.K.; Lima, R.; A-González, N.; Mattar, C.N.; Chong, S.Z.; Schlitzer, A.; Bakocevic, N.; Chew, S.; et al. Neutrophil mobilization via plerixafor-mediated CXCR4 inhibition arises from lung demargination and blockade of neutrophil homing to the bone marrow. *J. Exp. Med.* **2013**, *210*, 2321–2336. [CrossRef] [PubMed]
103. Watson, F.; Robinson, J.J.; Phelan, M.; Bucknall, R.C.; Edwards, S.W. Receptor expression in synovial fluid neutrophils from patients with rheumatoid arthritis. *Ann. Rheum. Dis.* **1993**, *52*, 354–359. [CrossRef]
104. Fortunati, E.; Kazemier, K.M.; Grutters, J.C.; Koenderman, L.; Van den Bosch, V.J. Human neutrophils switch to an activated phenotype after homing to the lung irrespective of inflammatory disease. *Clin. Exp. Immunol.* **2009**, *155*, 559–566. [CrossRef] [PubMed]
105. Sumagin, R. Phenotypic and Functional Diversity of Neutrophils in Gut Inflammation and Cancer. *Am. J. Pathol.* **2024**, *194*, 2–12. [CrossRef]
106. Dahlstrand Rudin, A.; Torell, A.; Popovic, J.; Stockfelt, M.; Jacobsson, B.; Rudin, A.; Christenson, K.; Lundell, A.C.; Bylund, J. Pregnancy is associated with a simultaneous but independent increase in circulating CD177pos and immature low-density granulocytes. *J. Leukoc. Biol.* **2025**, *117*, qiae255. [CrossRef]
107. Göhring, K.; Wolff, J.; Doppl, W.; Schmidt, K.L.; Fenchel, K.; Pralle, H.; Sibelius, U.; Bux, J. Neutrophil CD177 (NB1 gp, HNA-2a) expression is increased in severe bacterial infections and polycythaemia vera. *Br. J. Haematol.* **2004**, *126*, 252–254. [CrossRef]
108. Abdgawad, M.; Gunnarsson, L.; Bengtsson, A.A.; Geborek, P.; Nilsson, L.; Segelmark, M.; Hellmark, T. Elevated neutrophil membrane expression of proteinase 3 is dependent upon CD177 expression. *Clin. Exp. Immunol.* **2010**, *161*, 89–97. [CrossRef]
109. Witko-Sarsat, V.; Lesavre, P.; Lopez, S.; Bessou, G.; Hieblot, C.; Prum, B.; Noël, L.H.; Guillevin, L.; Ravaud, P.; Sermet-Gaudelus, I.; et al. A large subset of neutrophils expressing membrane proteinase 3 is a risk factor for vasculitis and rheumatoid arthritis. *J. Am. Soc. Nephrol.* **1999**, *10*, 1224–1233. [CrossRef]
110. Smargianaki, S.; Elmér, E.; Lilliebladh, S.; Ohlsson, S.; Pettersson, Å.; Hellmark, T.; Johansson, Å.C. Disease Activity and Tendency to Relapse in ANCA-Associated Vasculitis Are Reflected in Neutrophil and Intermediate Monocyte Frequencies. *J. Immunol. Res.* **2024**, *2024*, 6648265. [CrossRef]
111. Marino, S.F.; Jerke, U.; Rolle, S.; Daumke, O.; Kettritz, R. Competitively disrupting the neutrophil-specific receptor-autoantigen CD177, proteinase 3 membrane complex reduces anti-PR3 antibody-induced neutrophil activation. *J. Biol. Chem.* **2022**, *298*, 101598. [CrossRef]
112. Jerke, U.; Rolle, S.; Dittmar, G.; Bayat, B.; Santoso, S.; Sporbert, A.; Luft, F.; Kettritz, R. Complement receptor Mac-1 is an adaptor for NB1 (CD177)-mediated PR3-ANCA neutrophil activation. *J. Biol. Chem.* **2011**, *286*, 7070–7081. [CrossRef]
113. Matsumoto, K.; Kurasawa, T.; Yoshimoto, K.; Suzuki, K.; Takeuchi, T. Identification of neutrophil β2-integrin LFA-1 as a potential mechanistic biomarker in ANCA-associated vasculitis via microarray and validation analyses. *Arthritis Res. Ther.* **2021**, *23*, 136. [CrossRef]
114. Haller, H.; Eichhorn, J.; Pieper, K.; Göbel, U.; Luft, F.C. Circulating leukocyte integrin expression in Wegener's granulomatosis. *J. Am. Soc. Nephrol.* **1996**, *7*, 40–48. [CrossRef]
115. Hasegawa, M.; Nishii, C.; Ohashi, A.; Tomita, M.; Nakai, S.; Murakami, K.; Nabeshima, K.; Fujita, Y.; Ishii, J.; Hiki, Y.; et al. Expression of tumor necrosis factor receptors on granulocytes in patients with myeloperoxidase anti-neutrophil cytoplasmic autoantibody-associated vasculitis. *Nephron. Clin. Pract.* **2009**, *113*, c222–c233. [CrossRef] [PubMed]
116. Hacbarth, E.; Kajdacsy-Balla, A. Low density neutrophils in patients with systemic lupus erythematosus, rheumatoid arthritis, and acute rheumatic fever. *Rheum. Arthritis Rheum.* **1986**, *29*, 1334–1342. [CrossRef] [PubMed]
117. Vanhaver, C.; Aboubakar Nana, F.; Delhez, N.; Luyckx, M.; Hirsch, T.; Bayard, A.; Houbion, C.; Dauguet, N.; Brochier, A.; van der Bruggen, P.; et al. Immunosuppressive low-density neutrophils in the blood of cancer patients display a mature phenotype. *Life Sci. Alliance* **2023**, *7*, e202302332. [CrossRef] [PubMed]
118. Sun, R.; Huang, J.; Yang, Y.; Liu, L.; Shao, Y.; Li, L.; Sun, B. Dysfunction of low-density neutrophils in peripheral circulation in patients with sepsis. *Sci. Rep.* **2022**, *12*, 685. [CrossRef]
119. Wright, H.L.; Makki, F.A.; Moots, R.J.; Edwards, S.W. Low-density granulocytes: Functionally distinct, immature neutrophils in rheumatoid arthritis with altered properties and defective TNF signalling. *J. Leukoc. Biol.* **2017**, *101*, 599–611. [CrossRef]
120. Yu, N.; Qin, H.; Yu, Y.; Li, Y.; Lu, J.; Shi, Y. A Distinct Immature Low-Density Neutrophil Population Characterizes Acute Generalized Pustular Psoriasis. *J. Investig. Dermatol.* **2022**, *142*, 2831–2835.e5. [CrossRef]
121. Liu, Y.; Xia, C.; Chen, J.; Fan, C.; He, J. Elevated circulating pro-inflammatory low-density granulocytes in adult-onset Still's disease. *Rheumatology* **2021**, *60*, 297–303. [CrossRef] [PubMed]
122. Denny, M.F.; Yalavarthi, S.; Zhao, W.; Thacker, S.G.; Anderson, M.; Sandy, A.R.; McCune, W.J.; Kaplan, M.J. A distinct subset of proinflammatory neutrophils isolated from patients with systemic lupus erythematosus induces vascular damage and synthesizes type I IFNs. *J. Immunol.* **2010**, *184*, 3284–3297. [CrossRef] [PubMed]
123. Villanueva, E.; Yalavarthi, S.; Berthier, C.C.; Hodgin, J.B.; Khandpur, R.; Lin, A.M.; Rubin, C.J.; Zhao, W.; Olsen, S.H.; Klinker, M.; et al. Netting neutrophils induce endothelial damage, infiltrate tissues, and expose immunostimulatory molecules in systemic lupus erythematosus. *J. Immunol.* **2011**, *187*, 538–552. [CrossRef] [PubMed]

124. Torres-Ruiz, J.; Carrillo-Vázquez, D.A.; Leal-Alanis, A.; Zentella-Dehesa, A.; Tapia-Rodríguez, M.; Maravillas-Montero, J.L.; Nuñez-Álvarez, C.A.; Carazo-Vargas, E.R.; Romero-Hernández, I.; Juárez-Vega, G.; et al. Low-Density Granulocytes and Neutrophil Extracellular Traps as Biomarkers of Disease Activity in Adult Inflammatory Myopathies. *J. Clin. Rheumatol.* **2022**, *28*, e480–e487. [CrossRef]
125. Wu, H.; Zhen, Y.; Ma, Z.; Li, H.; Yu, J.; Xu, Z.G.; Wang, X.Y.; Yi, H.; Yang, Y.G. Arginase-1-dependent promotion of TH17 differentiation and disease progression by MDSCs in systemic lupus erythematosus. *Sci. Transl. Med.* **2016**, *8*, 331ra40. [CrossRef]
126. Ui Mhaonaigh, A.; Coughlan, A.M.; Dwivedi, A.; Hartnett, J.; Cabral, J.; Moran, B.; Brennan, K.; Doyle, S.L.; Hughes, K.; Lucey, R.; et al. Low Density Granulocytes in ANCA Vasculitis Are Heterogenous and Hypo-Responsive to Anti-Myeloperoxidase Antibodies. *Front. Immunol.* **2019**, *10*, 2603. [CrossRef]
127. Yuan, J.; Gou, S.J.; Huang, J.; Hao, J.; Chen, M.; Zhao, M.H. C5a and its receptors in human anti-neutrophil cytoplasmic antibody (ANCA)-associated vasculitis. *Arthritis Res. Ther.* **2012**, *14*, R140. [CrossRef]
128. Grayson, P.C.; Carmona-Rivera, C.; Xu, L.; Lim, N.; Gao, Z.; Asare, A.L.; Specks, U.; Stone, J.H.; Seo, P.; Spiera, R.F.; et al. Neutrophil-Related Gene Expression and Low-Density Granulocytes Associated with Disease Activity and Response to Treatment in Antineutrophil Cytoplasmic Antibody-Associated Vasculitis. *Arthritis Rheumatol.* **2015**, *67*, 1922–1932. [CrossRef]
129. Blanco-Camarillo, C.; Alemán, O.R.; Rosales, C. Low-Density Neutrophils in Healthy Individuals Display a Mature Primed Phenotype. *Front. Immunol.* **2021**, *12*, 672520. [CrossRef]
130. Silvestre-Roig, C.; Fridlender, Z.G.; Glogauer, M.; Scapini, P. Neutrophil Diversity in Health and Disease. *Trends Immunol.* **2019**, *40*, 565–583. [CrossRef]
131. Hardisty, G.R.; Llanwarne, F.; Minns, D.; Gillan, J.L.; Davidson, D.J.; Gwyer Findlay, E.; Gray, R.D. High Purity Isolation of Low Density Neutrophils Casts Doubt on Their Exceptionality in Health and Disease. *Front. Immunol.* **2021**, *12*, 625922. [CrossRef]
132. Pérez-Figueroa, E.; Álvarez-Carrasco, P.; Ortega, E.; Maldonado-Bernal, C. Neutrophils: Many Ways to Die. *Front. Immunol.* **2021**, *12*, 631821. [CrossRef]
133. Abdgawad, M.; Pettersson, Å.; Gunnarsson, L.; Bengtsson, A.A.; Geborek, P.; Nilsson, L.; Segelmark, M.; Hellmark, T. Decreased neutrophil apoptosis in quiescent ANCA-associated systemic vasculitis. *PLoS ONE* **2012**, *7*, e32439. [CrossRef] [PubMed]
134. Surmiak, M.; Hubalewska-Mazgaj, M.; Wawrzycka-Adamczyk, K.; Musiał, J.; Sanak, M. Delayed neutrophil apoptosis in granulomatosis with polyangiitis: Dysregulation of neutrophil gene signature and circulating apoptosis-related proteins. *Scand. J. Rheumatol.* **2020**, *49*, 57–67. [CrossRef] [PubMed]
135. Papayannopoulos, V. Neutrophil extracellular traps in immunity and disease. *Nat. Rev. Immunol.* **2018**, *18*, 134–147. [CrossRef] [PubMed]
136. Brinkmann, V.; Reichard, U.; Goosmann, C.; Fauler, B.; Uhlemann, Y.; Weiss, D.S.; Weinrauch, Y.; Zychlinsky, A. Neutrophil extracellular traps kill bacteria. *Science* **2004**, *303*, 1532–1535. [CrossRef]
137. Cahilog, Z.; Zhao, H.; Wu, L.; Alam, A.; Eguchi, S.; Weng, H.; Ma, D. The Role of Neutrophil NETosis in Organ Injury: Novel Inflammatory Cell Death Mechanisms. *Inflammation* **2020**, *43*, 2021–2032. [CrossRef]
138. Surmiak, M.; Hubalewska-Mazgaj, M.; Wawrzycka-Adamczyk, K.; Szczeklik, W.; Musiał, J.; Brzozowski, T.; Sanak, M. Neutrophil-related and serum biomarkers in granulomatosis with polyangiitis support extracellular traps mechanism of the disease. *Clin. Exp. Rheumatol.* **2016**, *34* (Suppl. S97), S98–S104.
139. Kraaij, T.; Kamerling, S.W.A.; van Dam, L.S.; Bakker, J.A.; Bajema, I.M.; Page, T.; Brunini, F.; Pusey, C.D.; Toes, R.E.M.; Scherer, H.U.; et al. Excessive neutrophil extracellular trap formation in ANCA-associated vasculitis is independent of ANCA. *Kidney Int.* **2018**, *94*, 139–149. [CrossRef]
140. Kessenbrock, K.; Krumbholz, M.; Schönermarck, U.; Back, W.; Gross, W.L.; Werb, Z.; Gröne, H.J.; Brinkmann, V.; Jenne, D.E. Netting neutrophils in autoimmune small-vessel vasculitis. *Nat. Med.* **2009**, *15*, 623–625. [CrossRef]
141. Aendekerk, J.P.; Ysermans, R.; Busch, M.H.; Theunissen, R.O.M.F.I.H.; Bijnens, N.; Potjewijd, J.; Damoiseaux, J.G.M.C.; Reutelingsperger, C.P.; van Paassen, P. Assessment of longitudinal serum neutrophil extracellular trap-inducing activity in anti-neutrophil cytoplasmic antibody-associated vasculitis and glomerulonephritis in a prospective cohort using a novel bio-impedance technique. *Kidney Int.* **2023**, *104*, 151–162. [CrossRef] [PubMed]
142. Surmiak, M.P.; Hubalewska-Mazgaj, M.; Wawrzycka-Adamczyk, K.; Szczeklik, W.; Musiał, J.; Sanak, M. Circulating mitochondrial DNA in serum of patients with granulomatosis with polyangiitis. *Clin. Exp. Immunol.* **2015**, *181*, 150–155. [CrossRef] [PubMed]
143. Ford, S.L.; O'Sullivan, K.M.; Kitching, A.R.; Holdsworth, S.R.; Gan, P.Y.; Summers, S.A. Toll-like Receptor 9 Induced Dendritic Cell Activation Promotes Anti-Myeloperoxidase Autoimmunity and Glomerulonephritis. *Int. J. Mol. Sci.* **2023**, *24*, 1339. [CrossRef] [PubMed]
144. Yousefi, S.; Mihalache, C.; Kozlowski, E.; Schmid, I.; Simon, H.U. Viable neutrophils release mitochondrial DNA to form neutrophil extracellular traps. *Cell Death Differ.* **2009**, *16*, 1438–1444. [CrossRef]
145. Gajendran, C.; Fukui, S.; Sadhu, N.M.; Zainuddin, M.; Rajagopal, S.; Gosu, R.; Gutch, S.; Fukui, S.; Sheehy, C.E.; Chu, L.; et al. Alleviation of arthritis through prevention of neutrophil extracellular traps by an orally available inhibitor of protein arginine deiminase 4. *Sci. Rep.* **2023**, *13*, 3189. [CrossRef]

146. Pan, T.; Tuoerxun, T.; Chen, X.; Yang, C.J.; Jiang, C.Y.; Zhu, Y.F.; Li, Z.S.; Jiang, X.Y.; Zhang, H.T.; Zhang, H.; et al. The neutrophil elastase inhibitor, sivelestat, attenuates acute lung injury in patients with cardiopulmonary bypass. *Front. Immunol.* **2023**, *14*, 1082830; Erratum in *Front. Immunol.* **2023**, *14*, 1165081. [CrossRef]
147. He, M.; Yang, Y.; Li, Y.; Zhou, X.; Xu, L.; Zhang, Z.; Zhang, H.; Li, Q. Therapeutic potential of elafin in airway inflammatory disease. *Eur. J. Inflamm.* **2024**, *22*, 1721727X241237437. [CrossRef]
148. Jerke, U.; Eulenberg-Gustavus, C.; Rousselle, A.; Nicklin, P.; Kreideweiss, S.; Grundl, M.A.; Eickholz, P.; Nickles, K.; Schreiber, A.; Korkmaz, B.; et al. Targeting Cathepsin C in PR3-ANCA Vasculitis. *J. Am. Soc. Nephrol.* **2022**, *33*, 936–947. [CrossRef]
149. Prendecki, M.; Gulati, K.; Pisacano, N.; Pinheiro, D.; Bhatt, T.; Mawhin, M.A.; Toulza, F.; Masuda, E.S.; Cowburn, A.; Lodge, K.M.; et al. Syk Activation in Circulating and Tissue Innate Immune Cells in Antineutrophil Cytoplasmic Antibody-Associated Vasculitis. *Arthritis Rheumatol.* **2023**, *75*, 84–97. [CrossRef]
150. McAdoo, S.P.; Prendecki, M.; Tanna, A.; Bhatt, T.; Bhangal, G.; McDaid, J.; Masuda, E.S.; Cook, H.T.; Tam, F.W.K.; Pusey, C.D. Spleen tyrosine kinase inhibition is an effective treatment for established vasculitis in a pre-clinical model. *Kidney Int.* **2020**, *97*, 1196–1207. [CrossRef]
151. Schreiber, A.; Xiao, H.; Jennette, J.C.; Schneider, W.; Luft, F.C.; Kettritz, R. C5a receptor mediates neutrophil activation and ANCA-induced glomerulonephritis. *J. Am. Soc. Nephrol.* **2009**, *20*, 289–298. [CrossRef]
152. Zimmermann, J.; Sonnemann, J.; Jabs, W.J.; Schönermarck, U.; Vielhauer, V.; Bieringer, M.; Schneider, U.; Kettritz, R.; Schreiber, A. Avacopan in Anti-Neutrophil Cytoplasmic Autoantibodies-Associated Vasculitis in a Real-World Setting. *Kidney Int. Rep.* **2024**, *9*, 2803–2808. [CrossRef]
153. Carminita, E.; Becker, I.C.; Italiano, J.E. What It Takes to Be a Platelet: Evolving Concepts in Platelet Production. *Circ. Res.* **2024**, *135*, 540–549. [CrossRef]
154. Ghalloussi, D.; Dhenge, A.; Bergmeier, W. New insights into cytoskeletal remodeling during platelet production. *J. Thromb. Haemost.* **2019**, *17*, 1430–1439. [CrossRef] [PubMed]
155. Willeke, P.; Kümpers, P.; Schlüter, B.; Limani, A.; Becker, H.; Schotte, H. Platelet counts as a biomarker in ANCA-associated vasculitis. *Scand. J. Rheumatol.* **2015**, *44*, 302–308. [CrossRef] [PubMed]
156. Machlus, K.R.; Johnson, K.E.; Kulenthirarajan, R.; Forward, J.A.; Tippy, M.D.; Soussou, T.S.; El-Husayni, S.H.; Wu, S.K.; Wang, S.; Watnick, R.S.; et al. CCL5 derived from platelets increases megakaryocyte proplatelet formation. *Blood* **2016**, *127*, 921–926. [CrossRef] [PubMed]
157. Lee, L.E.; Ahn, S.S.; Pyo, J.Y.; Song, J.J.; Park, Y.-B.; Lee, S.-W. Pan-immune-inflammation value at diagnosis independently predicts all-cause mortality in patients with antineutrophil cytoplasmic antibody-associated vasculitis. *Clin. Exp. Rheumatol.* **2021**, *39*, 88–93. [CrossRef]
158. Kucuk, H.; Tecer, D.; Goker, B.; Varan, O.; Babaoglu, H.; Guven, S.C.; Ozturk, M.A.; Haznedaroglu, S.; Tufan, A. Platelet/lymphocyte ratio and mean platelet volume in patients with granulomatosis with polyangiitis. *Adv. Rheumatol.* **2019**, *60*, 4. [CrossRef]
159. Park, H.J.; Jung, S.M.; Song, J.J.; Park, Y.B.; Lee, S.W. Platelet to lymphocyte ratio is associated with the current activity of ANCA-associated vasculitis at diagnosis: A retrospective monocentric study. *Rheumatol. Int.* **2018**, *38*, 1865–1871. [CrossRef]
160. Jin, Y.; Wang, F.; Tang, J.; Luo, L.; Huang, L.; Zhou, F.; Qi, E.; Hu, X.; Deng, S.; Ge, H.; et al. Low platelet count at diagnosis of anti-neutrophil cytoplasmic antibody-associated vasculitis is correlated with the severity of disease and renal prognosis. *Clin. Exp. Med.* **2024**, *24*, 70. [CrossRef]
161. Sánchez-Álamo, B.; Moi, L.; Bajema, I.; Faurschou, M.; Flossmann, O.; Hauser, T.; Hruskova, Z.; Jayne, D.; Luqmani, R.; Mahr, A.; et al. Long-term outcomes and prognostic factors for survival of patients with ANCA-associated vasculitis. *Nephrol. Dial. Transplant.* **2023**, *38*, 1655–1665. [CrossRef]
162. Flad, H.D.; Brandt, E. Platelet-derived chemokines: Pathophysiology and therapeutic aspects. *Cell Mol. Life Sci.* **2010**, *67*, 2363–2386. [CrossRef] [PubMed]
163. Sonmez, O.; Sonmez, M. Role of platelets in immune system and inflammation. *Porto Biomed. J.* **2017**, *2*, 311–314. [CrossRef] [PubMed]
164. Heijnen, H.; van der Sluijs, P. Platelet secretory behaviour: As diverse as the granules … or not? *J. Thromb. Haemost.* **2015**, *13*, 2141–2151. [CrossRef] [PubMed]
165. Berger, M.; Maqua, H.; Lysaja, K.; Mause, S.F.; Hindle, M.S.; Naseem, K.; Dahl, E.; Speer, T.; Marx, N.; Schütt, K. Platelets from patients with chronic inflammation have a phenotype of chronic IL-1β release. *Res. Pract. Thromb. Haemost.* **2023**, *8*, 102261. [CrossRef]
166. Clemetson, K.J.; Clemetson, J.M.; Proudfoot, A.E.; Power, C.A.; Baggiolini, M.; Wells, T.N. Functional expression of CCR1, CCR3, CCR4, and CXCR4 chemokine receptors on human platelets. *Blood* **2000**, *96*, 4046–4055. [CrossRef]

167. Worth, R.G.; Chien, C.D.; Chien, P.; Reilly, M.P.; McKenzie, S.E.; Schreiber, A.D. Platelet FcgammaRIIA binds and internalizes IgG-containing complexes. *Exp. Hematol.* **2006**, *34*, 1490–1495. [CrossRef]
168. Clark, S.R.; Ma, A.C.; Tavener, S.A.; McDonald, B.; Goodarzi, Z.; Kelly, M.M.; Patel, K.D.; Chakrabarti, S.; McAvoy, E.; Sinclair, G.D.; et al. Platelet TLR4 activates neutrophil extracellular traps to ensnare bacteria in septic blood. *Nat. Med.* **2007**, *13*, 463–469. [CrossRef]
169. Vik, D.P.; Fearon, D.T. Cellular distribution of complement receptor type 4 (CR4): Expression on human platelets. *J. Immunol.* **1987**, *138*, 254–258. [CrossRef]
170. Peerschke, E.I.; Ghebrehiwet, B. Platelet receptors for the complement component C1q: Implications for hemostasis and thrombosis. *Immunobiology* **1998**, *199*, 239–249. [CrossRef]
171. Del Conde, I.; Crúz, M.A.; Zhang, H.; López, J.A.; Afshar-Kharghan, V. Platelet activation leads to activation and propagation of the complement system. *J. Exp. Med.* **2005**, *201*, 871–879. [CrossRef]
172. Heras Benito, M. Complement in vasculitis associated with anti-neutrophil cytoplasm antibodies with renal involvement: Pathogenic, prognostic and therapeutic implications. *Med. Clin.* **2023**, *161*, 160–165. [CrossRef]
173. Aslan, J.E. Platelet Proteomes, Pathways, and Phenotypes as Informants of Vascular Wellness and Disease. *Arterioscler. Thromb. Vasc. Biol.* **2021**, *41*, 999–1011. [CrossRef] [PubMed]
174. Cornwell, M.G.; Bannoudi, H.E.; Luttrell-Williams, E.; Engel, A.; Barrett, T.J.; Myndzar, K.; Izmirly, P.; Belmont, H.M.; Clancy, R.; Ruggles, K.V.; et al. Modeling of clinical phenotypes in systemic lupus erythematosus based on the platelet transcriptome and FCGR2a genotype. *J. Transl. Med.* **2023**, *21*, 247. [CrossRef] [PubMed]
175. Yasuoka, H.; Sakata, K.; Yoshimoto, K.; Takeuchi, T. Phenotype of platelets are altered and activated in circulation of patients with systemic sclerosis. *Blood* **2018**, *132* (Suppl. S1), 3732. [CrossRef]
176. Holmes, C.E.; Levis, J.E.; Schneider, D.J.; Bambace, N.M.; Sharma, D.; Lal, I.; Wood, M.E.; Muss, H.B. Platelet phenotype changes associated with breast cancer and its treatment. *Platelets* **2016**, *27*, 703–711. [CrossRef]
177. Massberg, S.; Grahl, L.; von Bruehl, M.L.; Manukyan, D.; Pfeiler, S.; Goosmann, C.; Brinkmann, V.; Lorenz, M.; Bidzhekov, K.; Khandagale, A.B.; et al. Reciprocal coupling of coagulation and innate immunity via neutrophil serine proteases. *Nat. Med.* **2010**, *16*, 887–896. [CrossRef]
178. Brill, A.; Fuchs, T.A.; Savchenko, A.S.; Thomas, G.M.; Martinod, K.; De Meyer, S.F.; Bhandari, A.A.; Wagner, D.D. Neutrophil extracellular traps promote deep vein thrombosis in mice. *J. Thromb. Haemost.* **2012**, *10*, 136–144. [CrossRef]
179. Huang, Y.M.; Wang, H.; Wang, C.; Chen, M.; Zhao, M.H. Promotion of hypercoagulability in antineutrophil cytoplasmic antibody-associated vasculitis by C5a-induced tissue factor-expressing microparticles and neutrophil extracellular traps. *Arthritis Rheumatol.* **2015**, *67*, 2780–2790. [CrossRef]
180. de Bont, C.M.; Boelens, W.C.; Pruijn, G.J.M. NETosis, complement, and coagulation: A triangular relationship. *Cell Mol. Immunol.* **2019**, *16*, 19–27. [CrossRef]
181. Tomasson, G.; Lavalley, M.; Tanriverdi, K.; Finkielman, J.D.; Davis, J.C., Jr.; Hoffman, G.S.; McCune, W.J.; St Clair, E.W.; Specks, U.; Spiera, R.; et al. Relationship between markers of platelet activation and inflammation with disease activity in Wegener's granulomatosis. *J. Rheumatol.* **2011**, *38*, 1048–1054. [CrossRef]
182. Liu, X.; Gorzelanny, C.; Schneider, S.W. Platelets in Skin Autoimmune Diseases. *Front. Immunol.* **2019**, *10*, 1453. [CrossRef] [PubMed]
183. Ferroni, P.; Martini, F.; Riondino, S.; La Farina, F.; Magnapera, A.; Ciatti, F.; Guadagni, F. Soluble P-selectin as a marker of in vivo platelet activation. *Clin. Chim. Acta* **2009**, *399*, 88–91. [CrossRef] [PubMed]
184. Polanowska-Grabowska, R.; Wallace, K.; Field, J.J.; Chen, L.; Marshall, M.A.; Figler, R.; Gear, A.R.; Linden, J. P-selectin-mediated platelet-neutrophil aggregate formation activates neutrophils in mouse and human sickle cell disease. *Arterioscler. Thromb. Vasc. Biol.* **2010**, *30*, 2392–2399. [CrossRef]
185. Etulain, J.; Martinod, K.; Wong, S.L.; Cifuni, S.M.; Schattner, M.; Wagner, D.D. P-selectin promotes neutrophil extracellular trap formation in mice. *Blood* **2015**, *126*, 242–246. [CrossRef] [PubMed]
186. Tadie, J.M.; Bae, H.B.; Jiang, S.; Park, D.W.; Bell, C.P.; Yang, H.; Pittet, J.F.; Tracey, K.; Thannickal, V.J.; Abraham, E.; et al. HMGB1 promotes neutrophil extracellular trap formation through interactions with Toll-like receptor 4. *Am. J. Physiol. Lung Cell Mol. Physiol.* **2013**, *304*, L342–L349. [CrossRef] [PubMed]
187. Bruchfeld, A.; Wendt, M.; Bratt, J.; Qureshi, A.R.; Chavan, S.; Tracey, K.J.; Palmblad, K.; Gunnarsson, I. High-mobility group box-1 protein (HMGB1) is increased in antineutrophilic cytoplasmatic antibody (ANCA)-associated vasculitis with renal manifestations. *Mol. Med.* **2011**, *17*, 29–35. [CrossRef]
188. Pliyev, B.K.; Menshikov, M. Comparative evaluation of the role of the adhesion molecule CD177 in neutrophil interactions with platelets and endothelium. *Eur. J. Haematol.* **2012**, *89*, 236–244. [CrossRef]

189. Al-Soudi, A.; Vegting, Y.; Klarenbeek, P.L.; Hilhorst, M.L. Do Relapses Follow ANCA Rises? A Systematic Review and Meta-Analysis on the Value of Serial ANCA Level Evaluation. *Front. Med.* **2022**, *9*, 844112. [CrossRef]
190. Fonseca, J.A.; Gameiro, J.; Duarte, I.; Jorge, S.; Lopes, J.A. The neutrophil-to-lymphocyte ratio as a marker of vasculitis activity, severe infection and mortality in anca-associated vasculitis: A retrospective study. *Nefrol. (Engl. Ed.)* **2021**, *41*, 321–328. [CrossRef]

diagnostics

MDPI

Article

Distribution of Airway Findings in ANCA-Associated Vasculitis: A 20-Year Observational Analysis

Megan M. Sullivan [1,*], Maximiliano Diaz Menindez [2], Hassan Baig [3], Anushka Irani [4], Ronald Butendieck [4], Benjamin Wang [4], Florentina Berianu [4], Carolyn Mead-Harvey [5], Andy Abril [4] and Vikas Majithia [4]

1 Department of Internal Medicine, Division of Rheumatology, Mayo Clinic, Scottsdale, AZ 85259, USA
2 Department of Internal Medicine, Scottsdale, AZ 85259, USA; diazmenindez.maximiliano@mayo.edu
3 Department of Internal Medicine, Division of Pulmonology, Mayo Clinic, Jacksonville, FL 32224, USA; baig.hassan@mayo.edu
4 Department of Internal Medicine, Division of Rheumatology, Mayo Clinic, Jacksonville, FL 32224, USA; irani.anushka@mayo.edu (A.I.); butendieck.ronald@mayo.edu (R.B.); wang.benjamin@mayo.edu (B.W.); berianu.florentina@mayo.edu (F.B.); abril.andy@mayo.edu (A.A.); majithia.vikas@mayo.edu (V.M.)
5 Department of Quantitative Health Sciences, Mayo Clinic, Scottsdale, AZ 85259, USA; mead-harvey.carolyn@mayo.edu
* Correspondence: sullivan.megan2@mayo.edu; Tel.: +1-480-301-8368; Fax: +1-480-301-9066

Abstract: Objective: Pulmonary involvement is commonly observed in anti-neutrophil cytoplasmic antibody (ANCA)-associated vasculitis (AAV), presenting with manifestations such as diffuse alveolar hemorrhage, inflammatory infiltrates, pulmonary nodules, and tracheobronchial disease. We aimed to identify distinct subgroups of tracheobronchial disease patterns in patients with anti-neutrophil cytoplasmic antibody (ANCA)-associated vasculitis (AAV) using latent class analysis (LCA), and to evaluate their clinical characteristics and outcomes. **Methods:** We conducted a retrospective cohort study using electronic medical records of patients aged >18 years diagnosed with AAV and tracheobronchial disease between 1 January 2002 and 6 September 2022. Patients with follow-up <6 months were excluded. LCA was employed to identify disease subtypes based on 10 pre-defined indicators. Maximum likelihood estimation with 10 repetitions per model ensured robustness in model selection, guided by the Akaike information criterion (AIC). Patient and disease characteristics were summarized and compared across predicted classes. Statistical analyses included Kruskal–Wallis and Fisher's exact tests for continuous and categorical variables, respectively. The primary outcome was time to relapse of the tracheobronchial inflammation after starting immunosuppressive medication, analyzed using the Kaplan–Meier method and log-rank tests. Secondary outcomes included severity of pulmonary disease on pulmonary function tests, endoscopic interventions, tracheostomy, or mortality during follow-up. **Results:** Among 136 identified AAV patients assessed for tracheobronchial involvement, 111 (81.6%) were included after excluding 25 without tracheal or bronchial disease. Predominant findings included subglottic stenosis (91.0%), lower tracheal stenosis (16.2%), and bronchial stenosis (17.1%). LCA identified a three-class model as optimal: tracheal predominant (n = 94), tracheobronchial (n = 12), and bronchial predominant (n = 5). Tracheal predominant patients showed reduced risk of ear, eye, and lower respiratory manifestations, with milder obstruction on pulmonary function testing (PFT). Tracheobronchial-class patients were prone to saddle nose deformity (50%), extensive lower respiratory involvement (91.7%), and renal disease (66.7%). Bronchial predominant patients exhibited severe obstructive disease (median forced expiratory volume in 1 s (FEV1)% predicted: 58, IQR 34–66; FEV1/forced vital capacity (FVC) ratio: 56.9, interquartile range (IQR) 43–63.3) but lacked systemic AAV manifestations. LCA classes did not predict outcomes such as endoscopic intervention, tracheostomy, recurrent tracheobronchial narrowing, or mortality. **Conclusion:** LCA shows promise in subtype stratification of AAV patients, yet its utility in predicting outcomes and guiding treatment remains limited based on our analysis. Future studies with enhanced phenotypic data and larger cohorts are warranted to improve predictive accuracy.

Keywords: ANCA vasculitis; granulomatosis with polyangiitis; prognostication; tracheobronchial; subglottic stenosis; latent class analysis

1. Introduction

Anti-neutrophil cytoplasmic antibody (ANCA)-associated vasculitis (AAV) is a group of disorders including granulomatosis with polyangiitis (GPA), microscopic polyangiitis (MPA), and eosinophilic granulomatosis with polyangiitis (EGPA) [1,2]. These illnesses are complicated by small-vessel vascular inflammation that is associated with ANCA antibodies specific for proteinase-3 and myeloperoxidase.

GPA and MPA, and to a lesser degree EGPA, are well known to cause upper and lower respiratory manifestations [3] These can include pulmonary nodules, tracheobronchial involvement, diffuse alveolar hemorrhage, and less commonly, interstitial lung disease or bronchiectasis [4]. These manifestations can cause a variety of symptoms including hoarseness, cough, dyspnea, stridor, hemoptysis, and wheezing with upper airway involvement. Hemoptysis, pleuritic chest pain, and shortness of breath are common with lower airway involvement. Specifically, tracheobronchial disease has been reported in 19.3–23% of patients with AAV. In particular, subglottic stenosis, defined as narrowing of the airway between the vocal cords and the lower cricoid cartilage, is the most common manifestation of tracheobronchial AAV [5–10]. These are devastating complications which can lead to upper airway obstruction and potentially life-threatening disease [5–9]. Bronchial involvement occurs in approximately half of those with tracheal disease [7,11]. Despite the frequent upper airway involvement in AAV, there is a dearth of data about its epidemiology, outcomes, and prognosis, with only a few studies providing information about this manifestation.

Identification of patient subsets at particular risk for airway disease is a significant unmet need in AAV. The prevalence of tracheobronchial disease in patients with GPA has been the focus of a recent cohort where subglottic stenosis and endobronchial disease were reported in 10% and 6% of patients with GPA, respectively [7]. Interestingly, the tracheobronchial disease was reported to occur without disease activity in other organs and did not necessarily correlate to disease activity overall. This study suggested that certain epidemiologic characteristics of the patient, such as female sex and younger age of onset, may be associated with the phenotype of tracheobronchial disease and outcomes.

In contrast, a much higher prevalence of upper airway involvement of 70% was reported from a cohort in Iran but the involvement was not well defined [8,12]. In this cohort, upper airway involvement was associated with a higher disease-associated damage and worse outcomes. In a separate cohort from Turkey, ear–nose–throat (ENT) involvement that included bloody nasal discharge, sinusitis, subglottic stenosis, otomastoiditis, or hearing loss was 37%, but the individual prevalence was not defined [13]. ENT involvement was felt to be associated with better outcomes, but no differentiation was made regarding specific manifestations.

Lastly, in a separate cohort from Australia, the prevalence of tracheobronchial disease manifesting as subglottic and main bronchial airway stenosis was described in 17.1% of patients with GPA [14]. Many patients required multiple therapeutic endobronchial interventions to alleviate symptomatic airway obstruction. This report also highlighted the clinical dilemma that the stenotic lesion may result from ongoing active inflammatory disease or be related to exaggerated post-inflammatory cartilaginous fibrosis and structuring. It is unclear if these are amenable to immunosuppressive treatment with recent reports showing benefit with immunosuppressive therapy, particularly rituximab, as maintenance therapy [15,16].

The existence of specific subgroups within ANCA-positive patients experiencing tracheobronchial involvement that could guide prognostication and therapy remains unknown. Determining these phenotypic groups can prognosticate the outcomes and improve management decisions. LCA is a method used to differentiate potential groups and has been applied in similar instances [5,10]. LCA is considered superior to standard statistical methods for utilizing complex data to evaluate for "latent", or hidden subgroups that can be clinically relevant. Gu et al. utilized LCA to differentiate radiographic manifestations of microscopic polyangiitis, proposing a four-class model ("infiltrative", "fibrotic", "bronchiectatic", and "nonspecific") that correlated with disease manifestations, relapse rates, and cumulative survival [5]. Survival rates at one year were lowest for the infiltrative (51.9%) and fibrotic (62.5%) classes compared with the nonspecific (74.0%) and bronchiectatic (85.7%) classes. However, their analysis did not include tracheobronchial disease as a variable.

LCA has also been utilized in relapsing polychondritis, another disease process that can affect the tracheal and bronchial airways and is akin to ANCA vasculitis [17]. In this evaluation of 73 patients, LCA identified three subgroups which correlated with involved airway distribution, time to diagnosis, and disease severity.

We aimed to identify distinct subgroups of tracheobronchial disease patterns in patients with AAV using LCA, and to evaluate identified subgroups in regards to clinical characteristics and outcomes.

2. Patients and Methods

We conducted a retrospective cohort study using electronic medical records from three institutional Mayo Clinic sites (Minnesota, Florida, and Arizona). Patients aged >18 years diagnosed with AAV, based on the revised 2012 International Chapel Hill Consensus Nomenclature, and diagnosed with tracheobronchial disease between 1 January 2002 and 6 September 2022, were included. The diagnosis was based on a combination of histopathology findings and the type of ANCA involvement. Patients who were difficult to classify based on the Chapel Hill Consensus Nomenclature were labeled as "unspecified ANCA disease".

Evaluation for tracheobronchial disease could have been performed with laryngoscopy by otolaryngology or bronchoscopy with a pulmonologist. Patients with <6 months of follow-up were excluded. Clinical characteristics, pertinent serologic markers, and chest computed tomography (CT) findings were documented. Immunosuppressive regimens were documented along with the start date, end date, and reason for discontinuation. Immunosuppressive regimens included cyclophosphamide, rituximab, and methotrexate and these could be documented as induction agents or maintenance. Induction agents included rituximab or cyclophosphamide and were required to have been used within 6 months of the maintenance agent. Maintenance agents could include rituximab, methotrexate, mycophenolate, or azathioprine. Pulmonary function testing results included forced expiratory volume in the first second (FEV1) percent predicted and forced vital capacity (FVC), when available. Various demographic and clinical variables were collected and summarized as mean, standard deviation, median, interquartile range, and range for continuous variables, while categorical variables are summarized as count and percentage.

LCA was employed to identify disease subtypes using 10 pre-defined indicator variables: tracheal involvement, bronchial involvement, ANCA subtype (negative ANCA, PR3/C-ANCA, MPO/P-ANCA, or "other ANCA"), saddle nose deformity, presence of lung nodules and/or ground-glass opacities, symptoms in the eye, ear, or cardiovascular/gastrointestinal/nervous systems, renal involvement, and cutaneous involvement. Other ANCA was defined as any alternative combination of positive ANCA testing. Maximum likelihood estimation was performed with 10 repetitions per model. Models ranging from one to eight classes were estimated; models with more than eight classes were unstable and not considered further. Model selection was based on the AIC, with lower values indicating better fit. Additional fit and diagnostic criteria were assessed but did not influence the final model selection.

Patient and disease characteristics were summarized and compared across predicted classes using Kruskal–Wallis tests for continuous variables and Fisher's exact tests for categorical variables. Time to recurrence was defined as the duration from the initiation of first-line medication (including methotrexate, azathioprine, rituximab, or cyclophosphamide) to the first confirmed recurrence of airway inflammation observed during laryngoscopy or bronchoscopy. Patients without recurrence were censored at their last follow-up. Survival curves were estimated using the Kaplan–Meier method, and differences in survival among latent classes were assessed using log-rank tests. Analysis was performed in R version 4.2.2. and SAS version 9.4. LCA analysis was performed using the poLCA package [18].

3. Results

A total of 136 patients with AAV who had undergone assessment for tracheobronchial involvement (Figure 1) with laryngoscopy or bronchoscopy were identified. After excluding 25 who did not have identified tracheal or bronchial disease, 111 were included.

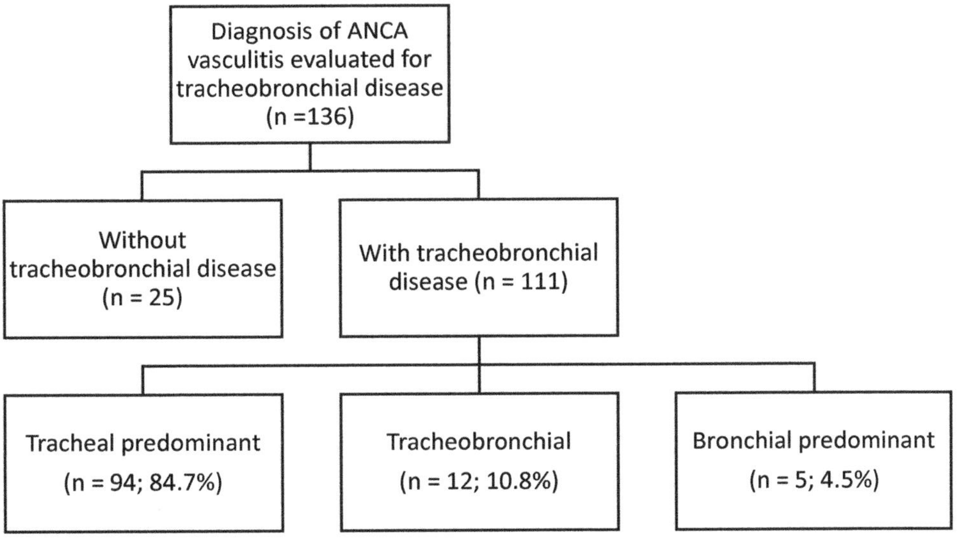

Figure 1. Flow chart of the study population.

3.1. Latent Classes Identified

A three-class model was deemed to be the best fit (Table 1). Table 2 identifies the baseline characteristics in each sub phenotype. The predicted probabilities of observing 10 variables per LCA classification are shown in Table 3. The first class identified, referred to as "tracheal predominant", was a group of 94 patients with mostly subglottic involvement without bronchial inflammation and with less lower respiratory disease (Table 3). The second group "tracheobronchial" consisted of 12 patients with a higher percentage (50%) exhibiting concomitant tracheal disease with bronchial inflammation and lower respiratory disease. The third group "bronchial predominant" held five patients. These patients lacked subglottic involvement.

Table 1. Model fit statistics for latent-class models from one to eight classes.

# of Classes	DF	AIC	BIC	Likelihood Ratio	Entropy
1	99	1173.376	1206	268.141	-
2	86	1160.303	1228	229.0679	1
3	73	1154.798	1258	197.5627	0.874
4	60	1166.587	1305	183.3519	0.81
5	47	1179.841	1353	170.606	0.779
6	34	1194.037	1403	158.802	0.816
7	21	1207.58	1451	146.3447	0.853
8	8	1221.306	1500	134.0711	0.879

Akaike Information Criterion (AIC) had the lowest value with the 3-class model indicating best fit. The entropy level for the 3-class model was also the highest at 0.874, suggesting that there was strong distinction between classes. This was coupled with a Bayesian information criterion (BIC) lower than that of models with higher number of classes, which suggests that further classification did not improve distinction between models. Additional abbreviations: DF, degrees of freedom.

Table 2. Baseline characteristics by predicted class assignment.

	Predicted Class				
Demographics	**Tracheal Predominant (N = 94)**	**Tracheo-Bronchial (N = 12)**	**Bronchial Predominant (N = 5)**	**Total (N = 111)**	***p*-Value**
Age at vasculitis diagnosis					0.171 [1]
Mean (SD)	42.3 (17.58)	32.8 (17.38)	35.8 (17.68)	41.0 (17.69)	
Median (IQR)	44.6 (26.5, 55.8)	27.0 (18.7, 46.9)	33.7 (25.1, 52.4)	43.6 (25.4, 55.1)	
Sex, n (%)					0.888 [2]
Female	72 (76.6%)	10 (83.3%)	4 (80.0%)	86 (77.5%)	
Male	22 (23.4%)	2 (16.7%)	1 (20.0%)	25 (22.5%)	
Ethnicity, n (%)					1.000 [2]
Caucasian	82 (87.2%)	11 (91.7%)	5 (100.0%)	98 (88.3%)	
Hispanic	7 (7.4%)	1 (8.3%)	0 (0.0%)	8 (7.2%)	
African American	2 (2.1%)	0 (0.0%)	0 (0.0%)	2 (1.8%)	
Native American	1 (1.1%)	0 (0.0%)	0 (0.0%)	1 (0.9%)	
Other	2 (2.1%)	0 (0.0%)	0 (0.0%)	2 (1.8%)	
Length of follow-up (weeks)					0.817 [1]
mean (SD)	480.1 (314.22)	504.9 (473.81)	409.4 (341.21)	479.6 (332.34)	
Median (IQR)	437.1 (209.0, 680.0)	299.9 (171.0, 977.8)	310.6 (111.4, 687.0)	420.9 (186.4, 697.1)	
Disease Characteristics					
Tracheal stenosis, n (%)	94 (100.0%)	12 (100.0%)	0 (0.0%)	106 (95.5%)	<0.001 [2]
Bronchial stenosis, n (%)	8 (8.5%)	6 (50.0%)	5 (100.0%)	19 (17.1%)	<0.001 [2]
Diagnosis, n (%)					>0.999 [2]
GPA	88 (93.6%)	12 (100.0%)	5 (100.0%)	105 (94.6%)	
MPA	4 (4.3%)	0 (0.0%)	0 (0.0%)	4 (3.6%)	
Unspecified ANCA-associated vasculitis	2 (2.1%)	0 (0.0%)	0 (0.0%)	2 (1.8%)	
ANCA, n (%)					0.098 [2]
negative ANCA	13 (13.8%)	0 (0.0%)	2 (40.0%)	15 (13.5%)	
PR3/C-ANCA	37 (39.4%)	8 (66.7%)	3 (60.0%)	48 (43.2%)	
MPO/P-ANCA	34 (36.2%)	2 (16.7%)	0 (0.0%)	36 (32.4%)	
Atypical ANCA	10 (10.6%)	2 (16.7%)	0 (0.0%)	12 (10.8%)	
Specific Organ Involvement					

Table 2. *Cont.*

Demographics	Tracheal Predominant (N = 94)	Tracheo-Bronchial (N = 12)	Bronchial Predominant (N = 5)	Total (N = 111)	*p*-Value
	Predicted Class				
Cutaneous, n (%)	9 (9.6%)	5 (41.7%)	0 (0.0%)	14 (12.6%)	0.019 [2]
Ear, n (%)	15 (16.0%)	12 (100.0%)	2 (40.0%)	29 (26.1%)	<0.001 [2]
Eye, n (%)	7 (7.4%)	2 (16.7%)	2 (40.0%)	11 (9.9%)	0.042 [2]
Saddle nose deformity, n (%)	13 (13.8%)	6 (50.0%)	0 (0.0%)	19 (17.1%)	0.011 [2]
* Lower respiratory, n (%)	34 (36.2%)	11 (91.7%)	4 (80.0%)	49 (44.1%)	<0.001 [2]
Renal, n (%)	14 (14.9%)	8 (66.7%)	0 (0.0%)	22 (19.8%)	<0.001 [2]
** Systemic, n (%)	12 (12.8%)	2 (16.7%)	0 (0.0%)	14 (12.6%)	0.828 [2]

[1] Kruskal–Wallis *p*-value; [2] Fisher's exact *p*-value; comparison of baseline characteristics by predicted class assignment. Abbreviations: SD, standard deviation; IQR, interquartile range; GPA, granulomatosis with polyangiitis; MPA, microscopic polyangiitis; ANCA, anti-neutrophil cytoplasmic antibody; PR3, proteinase-3; c-ANCA, cytoplasmic ANCA; MPO, myeloperoxidase; p-ANCA, perinuclear ANCA. *—indicates nodules, interstitial lung disease, or alveolar hemorrhage. **—indicates cardiac, nervous system, or renal involvement secondary to vasculitis.

Table 3. Probabilities of disease characteristics by predicted sub-phenotype classes.

Disease Characteristics	Bronchial Predominant	Tracheobronchial	Tracheal Predominant
Atypical ANCA	0.000	0.184	0.104
PR3	0.600	0.636	0.397
MPO	0.000	0.180	0.360
Negative ANCA	0.400	0.000	0.138
Subglottic involvement	0.000	1.000	1.000
Bronchial involvement	1.000	0.476	0.088
Saddle nose	0.000	0.458	0.143
Cutaneous	0.000	0.369	0.102
Ear	0.400	1.000	0.159
Eye	0.400	0.158	0.075
Lower respiratory involvement	0.800	0.911	0.362
Renal	0.000	0.618	0.155
Systemic	0.000	0.188	0.125

Class-conditional outcome probabilities were estimated from LCA modeling. Value in each cell is the probability of observing the disease characteristic for an individual in the predicted sub-phenotype. Cell color is determined by the value of the probability, with high probabilities given a darker shade and low probabilities given a lighter shade. Abbreviations: ANCA, anti-neutrophil cytoplasmic antibody; PR3, proteinase-3; MPO, myeloperoxidase.

3.2. Baseline Characteristics by Predicted Class Assignment

Table 2 summarizes the demographic and clinical characteristics of the cohort. Average age was 41.0 years, 86 (77.5%) patients were female, 98 (88.3%) were White. The majority, 105 (94.6%) patients, held a diagnosis of GPA as opposed to MPA or unspecified ANCA vasculitis. A total of 96 (86.5%) patients were positive for any ANCA type, 106 (95.5%) of patients had tracheal stenosis, and 19 (17.1%) had bronchial stenosis. Age, sex, and ethnicity were similar between predicted classes (Table 4). The median time of follow-up was 8.1 years (IQR 3.6–13.4).

Table 4. Outcomes by predicted class assignment.

	Predicted Class				
	Tracheal Predominant (N = 94)	Tracheo-Bronchial (N = 12)	Bronchial Predominant (N = 5)	Total (N = 111)	p-Value
Pulmonary Function Tests					
Available data, n (%) ****	72 (76.6%)	7 (58.3%)	5 (100.0%)	84 (75.7%)	0.201 [2]
FEV1% predicted					0.024 [1]
mean (SD)	86.8 (23.01)	77.1 (20.80)	55.4 (23.64)	84.0 (23.92)	
Median (IQR)	89.0 (73.0, 103.0)	75.0 (70.0, 95.0)	58.0 (34.0, 66.0)	88.0 (69.0, 102.0)	
FVC % predicted					0.505 [1]
mean (SD)	97.4 (18.87)	96.9 (6.07)	85.2 (24.14)	96.6 (18.52)	
Median (IQR)	100.5 (84.5, 109.5)	98.0 (90.0, 101.0)	92.0 (76.0, 96.0)	99.0 (85.5, 108.5)	
FEV1/FVC ratio					0.031 [1]
Mean (SD)	69.4 (13.48)	64.6 (15.86)	52.4 (17.12)	67.9 (14.37)	
Median (IQR)	73.0 (63.4, 78.3)	67.0 (58.7, 69.4)	56.9 (43.0, 63.3)	71.0 (60.4, 78.0)	
	Tracheobronchial Interventions				
Endoscopic dilation, n (%)	54 (57.4%)	9 (75.0%)	3 (60.0%)	66 (59.5%)	0.497 [2]
Number of dilations, n (%)					0.765 [2]
1	21 (38.9%)	3 (33.3%)	2 (66.7%)	26 (39.4%)	
2	9 (16.7%)	2 (22.2%)	0 (0.0%)	11 (16.7%)	
3	9 (16.7%)	3 (33.3%)	0 (0.0%)	12 (18.2%)	
4	15 (27.8%)	1 (11.1%)	1 (33.3%)	17 (25.8%)	
Number of dilations					0.863 [1]
Mean (SD)	2.3 (1.26)	2.2 (1.09)	2.0 (1.73)	2.3 (1.24)	
Median (IQR)	2.0 (1.0, 4.0)	2.0 (1.0, 3.0)	1.0 (1.0, 4.0)	2.0 (1.0, 4.0)	
Tracheostomy, n (%)	6 (6.4%)	1 (8.3%)	0 (0.0%)	7 (6.3%)	0.699 [2]
	Mortality				
Death during follow-up period, n (%)	2 (2.2%)	0 (0.0%)	0 (0.0%)	2 (1.9%)	1.000 [2]
Missing	2	1	0	3	

[1] Kruskal–Wallis p-value; [2] Fisher's exact p-value; **** Among patients in the tracheal predominant group who had PFTs, 3 were missing FEV1% predicted, 4 were missing FVC% predicted, and 5 were missing FEV1/FVC ratio. Abbreviations: FEV1, forced expiration volume over one minute; SD, standard deviation; IQR, interquartile range; FVC, forced vital capacity.

3.3. Immunosuppressive Management Within Cohort

Of the 111 patients, 44 (39.6%) utilized rituximab induction and maintenance in combination with another agent such as mycophenolate or methotrexate. Twenty-six (23.4%) patients utilized rituximab monotherapy as both induction and maintenance. Fifteen (13.5%) patients were treated with methotrexate without induction. Eight (7.2%) patients received induction therapy without maintenance. Of these 8 patients, 6 utilized rituximab, 1 utilized cyclophosphamide, and 1 was on a combination of rituximab and cyclophosphamide. Six (5.4%) patients were managed with azathioprine or mycophenolate without induction. Three (2.7%) patients utilized cyclophosphamide induction within 6 months of starting a maintenance agent (azathioprine, mycophenolate, or a combination). Four (3.6%) patients were not initiated on systemic immunosuppression. Three (2.7%)

patients were maintained on an immunosuppressive agent not previously listed. Two (1.8%) patients did not have medication history available.

3.4. Probabilities of Disease Characteristics by Predicted Sub-Phenotype Classes

Class 1, tracheal predominant, was noted to have the highest prevalence of anti-MPO positivity (36.2%), though this was not statistically significant. Ear and eye involvement were less frequent than in other classes (16.0% and 7.4% prevalence, respectively). Lower respiratory involvement was less common (36.2%).

Class 2, tracheobronchial, had the highest prevalence of saddle nose deformity (50%) and lower respiratory (91.7%), renal (66.7%), cutaneous (41.7%), and other systemic manifestations (16.7%) out of all three classes. This severity with widespread disease was not linked to specific ANCA status.

Class 3, bronchial predominant, had frequent lower respiratory involvement (80%) and lacked saddle nose deformity, cutaneous disease, renal involvement, or other systemic ANCA manifestations.

3.5. Outcomes by Predicted Class

Time to recurrence of tracheobronchial inflammation after initiating immunosuppressive therapy, defined as the time from first medication start date to first recurrence (or loss of follow-up), was compared between classes (Figure 2) without significant difference. Secondary outcomes are shown in Table 4. Endoscopic intervention was common (59.5%) though rates did not differ significantly between classes. The infrequent occurrences of tracheostomy and death were not different between classes (6.3% and 1.8%, respectively).

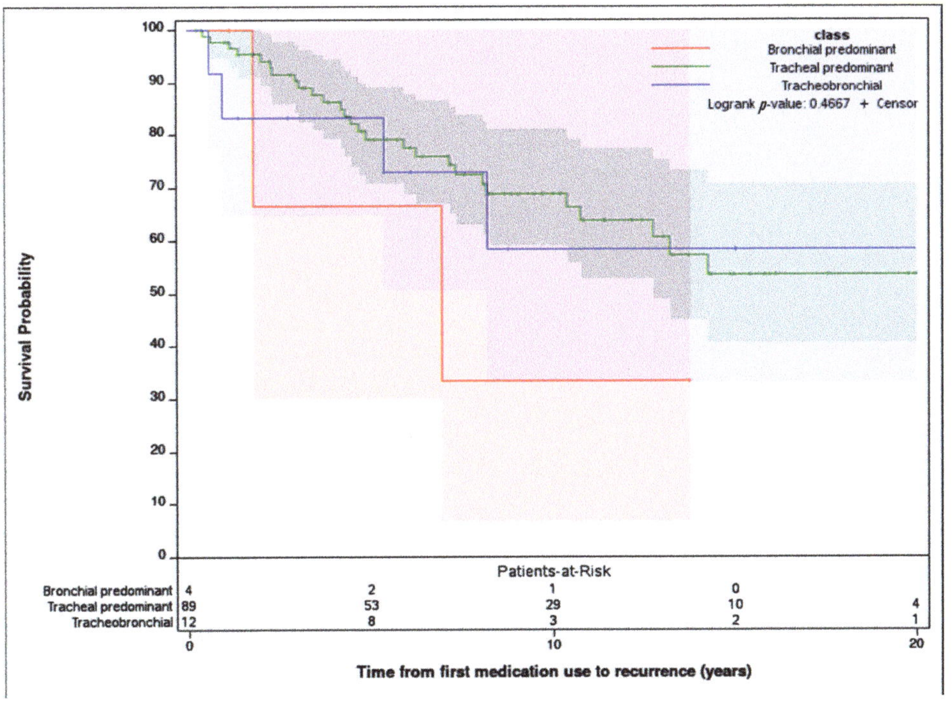

Figure 2. Relapse-free survival of tracheobronchial disease by predicted class. Shading represents the 95% confidence interval.

In the 84 (75.7%) patients who had pulmonary function testing available it was noted that median FEV1 percent predicted decreased with class allocation (89.0, 75.0, and 58.0, respectively, with a p value of 0.24). The FEV1/FVC ratio was also statistically significant across classes 1, 2, and 3 (73.0, 67.0, and 56.9, respectively, with a p value of 0.31).

4. Discussion

Tracheobronchial disease is a recognized consequence of ANCA-associated vasculitis, particularly GPA, and in this report, we have described a cohort of patients with AAV-associated tracheobronchial disease. Our findings align with previous reports, indicating that upper tracheal (subglottic) inflammation and stenosis are common [3,5–12,19,20].

As highlighted previously, there is a paucity of data regarding the epidemiology and outcomes of tracheobronchial disease in AAV with a limited number of studies available, and those that are available provide conflicting information [7,11–14]. The prevalence of tracheobronchial disease is felt to be around 20% but has been reported to be as high has 70% [8,12]. Previously, it has been reported that in patients with GPA, the subglottic stenosis variant of tracheobronchial disease may be more prevalent in younger and female patients with GPA and those with severe, destructive, sinonasal disease but a lack of renal disease [7]. Endobronchial disease was more prevalent in younger patients with positive PR3-ANCA, and those who has a history of ENT involvement. It remains unclear if the upper airway involvement is associated with a severe disease [7,8,10].

This analysis further builds on existing data and highlights the presence of sub-phenotypes within these cohorts. Patients with tracheal predominant disease were noted to have the highest prevalence of anti-MPO positivity and less common involvement of ear, eye, or lower respiratory tract. Tracheobronchial disease was associated with saddle nose deformity and lower respiratory, renal, cutaneous, and other systemic manifestations but not with specific ANCA status. The bronchial predominant subset had frequent lower respiratory involvement with obstructive lung disease, and lacked cutaneous, renal, or other systemic ANCA manifestations.

Most notably, systemic disease was seen in patients with more diffuse airway involvement, i.e., tracheobronchial disease, and less with isolated bronchial disease. These findings suggest that severe systemic presentation may herald a more severe upper airway involvement and vice-versa. The more frequent occurrence of renal disease in patients presenting with tracheobronchial disease suggests that this subset of patients should also be monitored closely for renal disease. Additionally, the degree of obstruction observed in pulmonary function tests was linked to both the tracheobronchial and bronchial predominant subgroups. Though the bronchial predominant group was small, there was an indication that those with isolated bronchial disease may have had less systemic manifestations.

It is important to note that this study observed less frequent involvement of the lower airways compared to earlier literature, with lower tracheal and bronchial disease each affecting less than 20% of the population. This discrepancy may be attributed to our study including patients who had undergone either laryngoscopy or bronchoscopy. Without bronchoscopy or chest computed tomography read by a skilled radiologist, the prevalence of lower airway involvement might have been underestimated.

Despite this limitation, LCA revealed three distinct subgroups with different phenotypic characteristics a useful construct that can be used during evaluation of these patients as well as for future research.

These innovative findings provide significant insight into the heterogeneity of the airway involvement in AAV and highlight the presence of three different phenotypic subgroups with prognostic and therapeutic implications. Clinicians can use these results to stratify the patients during evaluation to aggressively assess and closely follow for systemic disease and saddle nose deformities in patients with tracheobronchial disease, and potentially intervene early to improve the outcome. Furthermore, the findings provide a direction for additional studies in the future.

However, it is important to note that the phenotypic subgroups identified in this study did not show a correlation with outcomes outside of the degree of obstructive disease on pulmonary function testing, which seemed to be associated with bronchial airway involvement. Other outcomes, such as relapse rates of tracheobronchial disease following the initiation of immunosuppressive therapy or the necessity for endoscopic interventions like dilation and injection, did not correlate strongly. This lack of correlation is likely due to the small sample size, particularly in the bronchial predominant subgroup. Alternatively, this may also be due to a less aggressive use or the limited effectiveness of standard immunosuppressive therapies for tracheobronchial disease. The benefits of systemic immunosuppressive therapy for airway involvement are questionable based on current literature but there are instances of improved outcome with aggressive immunosuppressive therapy in addition to endoscopic or surgical interventions. Two recent studies show that immunosuppressive treatment, and in particular rituximab, may reduce the need for endoscopic interventions, supporting their use in AAV [15,16].

5. Conclusions

This LCA of patients with tracheobronchial disease and ANCA vasculitis identified distinct phenotypic subgroups, each characterized by unique disease features and association with distinct non-airway clinical manifestations. Despite these differences, our analysis did not reveal a significant association between these subgroups and clinical outcomes such as disease relapse or the need for endoscopic interventions. These findings suggest that while phenotypic heterogeneity exists, it may not directly translate into differences in clinical outcomes with the current treatment approaches. Future research should focus on further exploring the underlying mechanisms driving these subgroups and investigating whether more tailored or novel therapeutic strategies might improve outcomes for specific phenotypes. This could provide valuable insights for optimizing patient management and advancing personalized treatment in ANCA-associated tracheobronchial disease.

Author Contributions: Conceptualization, M.M.S. and V.M.; Methodology, M.M.S., A.A., and V.M.; Formal analysis, C.M.-H.; Data curation, M.M.S. and M.D.M.; Writing—original draft, M.M.S., R.B., B.W., C.M.-H., A.A. and V.M.; Writing—review & editing, M.M.S., H.B., A.I., R.B., B.W., F.B., A.A. and V.M.; Supervision, H.B., B.W. and F.B. All authors have read and agreed to the published version of the manuscript.

Funding: This research received no external funding.

Institutional Review Board Statement: The study was conducted in accordance with the Declaration of Helsinki, and approved under an exempt status by the Institutional Review Board of Mayo Clinic (protocol code 22-009660 on 10/13/2022).

Informed Consent Statement: Patient consent was waived due to the minimal risk status of the study and was performed as a retrospective chart review.

Data Availability Statement: Data can be provided by the authors upon request, with removal of identifiable information and anonymization of dates.

Conflicts of Interest: The authors declare no conflicts of interest.

References

1. Jennette, J.C.; Falk, R.J.; Bacon, P.A.; Basu, N.; Cid, M.C.; Ferrario, F.; Flores-Suarez, L.F.; Gross, W.L.; Guillevin, L.; Hagen, E.C.; et al. 2012 revised International Chapel Hill Consensus Conference Nomenclature of Vasculitides. *Arthritis Rheum.* **2012**, *65*, 1–11. [CrossRef]
2. Jennette, J.C.; Falk, R.J.; Andrassy, K.; Bacon, P.A.; Churg, J.; Gross, W.L.; Hagen, E.C.; Hoffman, G.S.; Hunder, G.G.; Kallenberg, C.G.; et al. Nomenclature of systemic vasculitides. Proposal of an international consensus conference. *Arthritis Rheum.* **1994**, *37*, 187–192. [CrossRef] [PubMed]
3. Gómez-Puerta, J.A.; Hernández-Rodríguez, J.; López-Soto, A.; Bosch, X. Antineutrophil cytoplasmic antibody-associated vasculitides and respiratory disease. *Chest* **2009**, *136*, 1101–1111. [CrossRef] [PubMed]
4. Sebastiani, M.; Manfredi, A.; Vacchi, C.; Cassone, G.; Faverio, P.; Cavazza, A.; Sverzellati, N.; Salvarani, C.; Luppi, F. Epidemiology and management of interstitial lung disease in ANCA-associated vasculitis. *Clin Exp Rheumatol* **2020**, *38*, 221–231. [PubMed]
5. Gu, Y.; Zhang, T.; Peng, M.; Han, Y.; Zhang, W.; Shi, J. Latent class analysis of chest CT abnormalities to define subphenotypes in patients with MPO-ANCA-positive microscopic polyangiitis. *Respir. Med.* **2024**, *226*, 107613. [CrossRef]
6. Horta-Baas, G.; Hernández-Cabrera, M.F.; Catana, R.; Pérez-Cristóbal, M.; Barile-Fabris, L.A. Subglottic stenosis in granulomatosis with polyangiitis (Wegener's granulomatosis): Report of 4 cases. *Reumatol. Clin.* **2016**, *12*, 267–273. [CrossRef] [PubMed]
7. A Quinn, K.; Gelbard, A.; Sibley, C.; Sirajuddin, A.; A Ferrada, M.; Chen, M.; Cuthbertson, D.; Carette, S.; A Khalidi, N.; Koening, C.L.; et al. Subglottic stenosis and endobronchial disease in granulomatosis with polyangiitis. *Rheumatology* **2019**, *58*, 2203–2211. [CrossRef] [PubMed]
8. Solans-Laqué, R.; Bosch-Gil, J.; Canela, M.; Lorente, J.; Pallisa, E.; Vilardell-Tarrés, M. Clinical features and therapeutic management of subglottic stenosis in patients with Wegener's granulomatosis. *Lupus* **2008**, *17*, 832–836. [CrossRef] [PubMed]
9. Taylor, S.C.; Clayburgh, D.R.; Rosenbaum, J.T.; Schindler, J.S. Progression and management of Wegener's granulomatosis in the head and neck. *Laryngoscope* **2012**, *122*, 1695–1700. [CrossRef]
10. Yamagata, M.; Ikeda, K.; Tsushima, K.; Iesato, K.; Abe, M.; Ito, T.; Kashiwakuma, D.; Kagami, S.; Iwamoto, I.; Nakagomi, D.; et al. Prevalence and Responsiveness to Treatment of Lung Abnormalities on Chest Computed Tomography in Patients With Microscopic Polyangiitis: A Multicenter, Longitudinal, Retrospective Study of One Hundred Fifty Consecutive Hospital-Based Japanese Patients. *Arthritis Rheumatol.* **2016**, *68*, 713–723. [CrossRef] [PubMed]
11. Marroquín-Fabián, E.; Ruiz, N.; Mena-Zúñiga, J.; Flores-Suárez, L.F. Frequency, treatment, evolution, and factors associated with the presence of tracheobronchial stenoses in granulomatosis with polyangiitis. Retrospective analysis of a case series from a single respiratory referral center. *Semin. Arthritis Rheum.* **2019**, *48*, 714–719. [CrossRef]
12. Babapoor, P.; Hajialilo, M.; Rahimi, M.; Esalatmanesh, K.; Rahmanpour, D.; Barahimi, A.; Khabbazi, A. Predictors of medications-free and long-term remission in anti-neutrophil cytoplasmic antibody-associated vasculitis: Real-world evidence. *Sarcoidosis Vasc. Diffuse Lung Dis.* **2024**, *41*, e2024011. [PubMed]
13. Toraman, A.; Gündüz, S. Predictors of renal and patient outcomes in anti-neutrophil cytoplasmic antibody-associated vasculitis: Our single-center, tertiary care experience. *Arch. Rheumatol.* **2021**, *36*, 445–457. [CrossRef] [PubMed]
14. Bell, P.T.; Sheehy, R.; Droney, L.; Prain, K.; Wong, R.; Keir, G.J. Pulmonary involvement in Anti-Neutrophil Cytoplasmic Antibody Associated Vasculitis: A single centre case series. *Respirol. Case Rep.* **2022**, *10*, e01058. [CrossRef] [PubMed]
15. Aden, A.A.; Awadallah, A.S.; Xie, K.Z.; Wallerius, K.P.; O'Byrne, T.J.; Bowen, A.J.; Edell, E.S.; Bayan, S.L.; Ekbom, D.C.; Koster, M.J. Medical Maintenance Therapy Following Laser Excision in Patients With Granulomatosis With Polyangiitis (GPA)-Associated Subglottic Stenosis. *Otolaryngol. Neck Surg.* **2024**, *171*, 180–187. [CrossRef]
16. Moroni, L.; Giudice, L.; Lanzillotta, M.; Cariddi, A.; Ramirez, G.A.; Bozzolo, E.P.; Germinario, B.; Gallina, G.; Viscardi, S.; Carretta, A.; et al. Role of systemic immunosuppression on subglottic stenosis in granulomatosis with polyangiitis: Analysis of a single-centre cohort. *Eur. J. Intern. Med.* **2023**, *114*, 108–112. [CrossRef]
17. Ferrada, M.; Rimland, C.A.; Quinn, K.; Sikora, K.; Kim, J.; Allen, C.; Sirajuddin, A.; Goodspeed, W.; Chen, M.; Grayson, P.C. Defining Clinical Subgroups in Relapsing Polychondritis: A Prospective Observational Cohort Study. *Arthritis Rheumatol.* **2020**, *72*, 1396–1402. [CrossRef] [PubMed]
18. Linzer, D.A.; Lewis, J.B. poLCA: An R Package for Polytomous Variable Latent Class Analysis. *J. Stat. Softw.* **2011**, *42*, 1–29. [CrossRef]
19. Langford, C.A.; Sneller, M.C.; Hallahan, C.W.; Hoffman, G.S.; Kammerer, W.A.; Talar-Williams, C.; Fauci, A.S.; Lebovics, R.S. Clinical features and therapeutic management of subglottic stenosis in patients with Wegener's granulomatosis. *Arthritis Rheum.* **1996**, *39*, 1754–1760. [CrossRef] [PubMed]
20. Sacoto, G.; Boukhlal, S.; Specks, U.; Flores-Suárez, L.F.; Cornec, D. Lung involvement in ANCA-associated vasculitis. *Presse Med.* **2020**, *49*, 104039. [CrossRef] [PubMed]

diagnostics

MDPI

Article

Comparative Analysis of Classification Criteria in IgG4-Related Disease and Evaluating Diagnostic Accuracy from a Retrospective Cohort in Clinical Practice

Marta Lopez-Gomez [1,2,3,*,†], Patricia Moya-Alvarado [3,4,5,*,†], Hye Sang Park [4,5], Mar Concepción Martín [6], Sara Calleja [7], Helena Codes-Mendez [3,4,5], Berta Magallares [3,5], Iván Castellví [3,4,5], Antonio J. Barros-Membrilla [8], Ana Laiz [4,5], César Diaz-Torné [4,5], Luis Sainz [4,5], Julia Bernárdez [5], Laura Martínez-Martinez [7] and Hèctor Corominas [3,4,5]

1 Rheumatology Department, Hospital Universitario Araba, 01009 Vitoria, Spain
2 Instituto de Investigación Biomédica BIORABA, Hospital Universitario Araba, 01009 Vitoria, Spain
3 Department of Medicine, Universitat Autònoma de Barcelona (UAB), 08193 Barcelona, Spain; hcodes@santpau.cat (H.C.-M.); berpauma@hotmail.com (B.M.); icastellvi@santpau.cat (I.C.); hcorominas@santpau.cat (H.C.)
4 Institut de Recerca Sant Pau (IR SANT PAU), 08041 Barcelona, Spain; hsang@santpau.cat (H.S.P.); alaiz@santpau.cat (A.L.); cdiazt@santpau.cat (C.D.-T.); lsainz@santpau.cat (L.S.)
5 Rheumatology Department, Hospital de la Santa Creu i Sant Pau, 08025 Barcelona, Spain; juliabernardez8@gmail.com
6 Gastroenterology Department, Hospital de la Santa Creu i Sant Pau, 08025 Barcelona, Spain; mconcepcion@santpau.cat
7 Immunology Department, Hospital de la Santa Creu i Sant Pau, IIB Sant Pau, UAB, 08025 Barcelona, Spain; scallejavara@gmail.com (S.C.); lmartinezma@santpau.cat (L.M.-M.)
8 Cardiology Department, Hospital de la Santa Creu i Sant Pau, 08025 Barcelona, Spain; abarros@santpau.cat
* Correspondence: marta.lopezigomez@osakidetza.eus (M.L.-G.); pmoyaa@santpau.cat (P.M.-A.)
† These authors contributed equally to this work.

Abstract: Introduction: We conducted a comprehensive comparative analysis of the Okazaki, Umehara, and American College of Rheumatology/European League Against Rheumatism (ACR/EULAR) classification criteria for diagnosing immunoglobulin G4-related disease (IgG4-RD). Materials and Methods: A retrospective study was conducted in a single tertiary hospital, using expert clinical judgment as the gold standard. We compared the diagnostic accuracy of the Okazaki, Umehara, and ACR/EULAR criteria in a cohort of 41 patients with suspected IgG4-RD. We assessed sensitivity, specificity, and positive and negative predictive values for each criterion, and conducted a separate analysis based on four IgG4-RD subtypes. Results: A total of 30 patients were confirmed to have IgG4-RD and 11 were identified as mimickers. The Umehara criteria demonstrated the highest sensitivity (83.33%), followed by the ACR/EULAR 2019 (66.67%) and Okazaki (60.0%) criteria. All three criteria exhibited 100% specificity, with overall diagnostic accuracy ranging from 70% to 88%. The areas under the curve (AUC) were 0.917 (Umehara), 0.800 (Okazaki), and 0.833 (ACR/EULAR 2019), indicating significant diagnostic effectiveness ($p < 0.000$). Subtype analysis revealed that the Umehara and ACR/EULAR 2019 criteria were more effective in diagnosing pancreato-hepato-biliary involvement (subtype 1), while the Okazaki and ACR/EULAR 2019 criteria were more effective in diagnosing retroperitoneal fibrosis and/or aortitis (subtype 2). Conclusions: Our study provides valuable insights into the diagnostic performance of the Okazaki, Umehara, and ACR/EULAR criteria for a cohort of patients with suspected IgG4-RD. The Umehara criterion demonstrated the highest sensitivity, suggesting its potential utility for screening purposes, while all three criteria showed consistent specificity.

Keywords: IgG4; diagnostic criteria; ACR/EULAR

1. Introduction

Immunoglobulin G4-related disease (IgG4-RD) is an immune-mediated chronic disorder characterized by intense inflammation, fibrosis, infiltration, and elevated IgG4 levels in peripheral blood affecting multiple organs [1–3]. This fibroinflammatory condition is characterized by an initial inflammatory phase driven by antigen-experienced lymphocytes secreting pro-fibrotic molecules, followed by a fibrotic phase marked by dense stromal reactions and leading to tissue distortion and organ damage.

While IgG4 antibodies normally resolve inflammation, in IgG4-RD, they may synergize with cytotoxic T cells to induce tissue injury. The antigens triggering the disease and the reasons for organ specificity remain unclear but suggest a breach of immunological tolerance as the potential initiating event [4]. IgG4-RD poses diagnostic challenges as it is often confused with neoplasms, infections, or other immunological conditions due to shared clinical, serological, and pathological features [5].

Although the prevalence of IgG4-RD in Europe has not specifically been described to date, it is estimated to be around 4.6 per 100,000 individuals, with a higher incidence among persons aged over 60 [6]. A multicenter observational study by Fernandez et al. [7] identified 55 Spanish patients with IgG4-RD, making this the largest series reported in Spain and contributing to an understanding of the disease. Singly [1] published estimates suggesting that the average time from symptom onset to disease diagnosis is two years.

Despite growing interest and scientific advances, diagnosing IgG4-RD remains a significant challenge for clinicians due to its complexity and heterogeneity. Moreover, IgG4-RD requires an integrated approach, involving comprehensive evaluation and proper coordination among different medical specialties.

The organs most frequently affected are the pancreas, retroperitoneum, salivary glands, and lymph nodes [7]. The average number of affected organs is 2.9 and isolated involvement of a single organ is very uncommon [4].

The IgG4-RD predilection for certain organs has been known since early on, although comprehensive assessments of consistent patterns in clinical manifestations were lacking until 2019, when, applying latent class analysis to an international cohort, the American College of Rheumatology (ACR)/European League against Rheumatism (EULAR) developed classification criteria for four homogeneous phenotypes of IgG4-RD, as follows: pancreato-hepato-biliary disease (31%), retroperitoneal fibrosis and/or aortitis (24%), head/neck-limited disease (22%), and Mikulicz syndrome with systemic involvement (22%) [1]. Notably, patients within each phenotype shared distinctive clinical, epidemiological, and serological features. Patients with head/neck limited disease were more likely to be female, Asian, and younger, and more frequently required histological confirmation for diagnosis. Patients with pancreato-hepatobiliary disease were more often referred to the emergency department due to symptom flare-ups. In the retroperitoneal fibrosis and Mikulicz syndrome patients, inflammatory markers were significantly higher and lower, respectively. Finally, patients with Mikulicz syndrome and systemic involvement had the highest median serum IgG4 concentrations [1]. This classification provides a framework for recognizing IgG4-RD phenotypes, enabling the description of biological differences, the assessment of biomarker performance in homogeneous cohorts, and the search for personalized follow-up and therapeutic strategies.

While no genetic risk factors have been definitively linked to gender differences in IgG4-RD, environmental factors like smoking and occupational exposures are more frequently observed in male patients, potentially contributing to the higher prevalence of the disease in men [8–11].

Definitive diagnosis requires rigorous clinical–pathological correlation, as clinical, laboratory, and imaging findings are often non-specific [12]. Serum IgG4 elevation (55–97% of cases) correlates with organ involvement but is of poor diagnostic utility [4,12]. The absence of disease-specific autoantibodies (e.g., ANCA, SSA/Ro, SSB/La, double-stranded DNA, RNP, and Sm), helps differentiate IgG4-RD from other autoimmune conditions [3]. Histological examination remains the diagnostic mainstay but can be challenging for certain organs (such as the retroperitoneum and ocular cavity). Whole-body computed tomography (CT) or fludeoxyglucose F18 (18FDG)-positron emission tomography (PET) scans are recommended at diagnosis for staging and to identify accessible biopsy sites [13].

For the above reasons, classification criteria have been established based on joint evaluation of clinical, serological, and histological findings. The Okazaki criteria [14] (Appendix A), introduced in 2009, were the first to establish a standardized approach to IgG4-RD diagnosis. These criteria rely on a combination of clinical features, serological findings, and histological evidence. While their simplicity and high specificity make them suitable for initial screening, their low sensitivity requires further evaluation. The Umehara criteria [15] (Appendix B), proposed in 2012, expanded on the Okazaki criteria by incorporating additional clinical and serological parameters. They categorize cases into possible, probable, or definitive IgG4-RD. While this classification system has enhanced sensitivity compared to the Okazaki criteria, its complexity and lower specificity warrant cautious interpretation. Globally, despite clear clinical suspicion indicating the presence of the condition, neither of those diagnostic criteria are optimal, making accurate diagnosis and timely intervention not only challenging, but also underscores their inadequacy in terms of capturing the full spectrum of conditions and manifestations.

To adequately enhance the ability to identify and manage patients with IgG4-RD, the development of new criteria became imperative. In 2019, ACR/EULAR experts introduced novel classification criteria for IgG4-RD [16] (Appendix C), based on a three-stage approach that integrates clinical findings, serological data, and radiological findings. While the sensitivity (82–85%) of the ACR/EULAR 2019 criteria is the highest of the three sets of criteria, its complexity requires careful consideration. One notable advantage of the ACR/EULAR 2019 criteria is the ability to classify patients as having IgG4-RD even when obtaining a biopsy is challenging and/or serum IgG4 levels fall within the normal range despite clinical suspicion of IgG4-RD. Additionally, the ACR/EULAR 2019 criteria streamline the identification of homogeneous IgG4-RD cases in clinical trials, improving the availability and implementation of criteria in research settings.

While existing classification systems have individually advanced IgG4-RD diagnosis, a comprehensive comparative analysis of their clinical performance remains unexplored. As a rare, relatively novel, and often underdiagnosed condition due to low clinical suspicion and complex and unfamiliar classification criteria, IgG4-RD necessitates a thorough evaluation of existing diagnostic frameworks.

This study aims to address this critical knowledge gap by conducting a comparative analysis of the diagnostic performance (sensitivity, specificity, and accuracy) of the Okazaki, Umehara, and ACR/EULAR 2019 criteria for a cohort of confirmed IgG4-RD patients. The rationale for this research is multifaceted: (1) to optimize the diagnostic approach and facilitate timely and accurate diagnoses, crucial for appropriate management and prevention of organ damage; (2) to provide evidence-based guidance to clinicians on the most appropriate criteria for various clinical contexts, thereby potentially improving diagnostic accuracy and patient outcomes; and (3) to advance IgG4-RD research by identifying the most robust classification criteria, thereby enhancing the homogeneity of patient cohorts in clinical trials and observational studies, leading to more reliable and generalizable research findings. By offering a clearer understanding of the strengths and limitations of each set of criteria, we seek to contribute to more accurate diagnoses, more effective treatments, and better outcomes for patients with this challenging condition. Our comparative analysis is anticipated to offer valuable insights into the relative strengths and limitations of each set of criteria and provide a nuanced understanding of their applicability across diverse clinical scenarios. Ultimately, our study strives to fill a crucial knowledge gap, inform clinical practice, guide future research, and accelerate scientific progress regarding IgG4-RD, with the overarching goal of improving care for patients affected by this complex disorder.

2. Materials and Methods

2.1. Study Design and Setting

A retrospective cross-sectional study was conducted at the rheumatology outpatient clinic of a tertiary hospital designated as a Spanish national reference center for systemic autoimmune diseases (XUEC CSUR, Hospital Sant Pau i de la Santa Creu, Barcelona, Spain). The study was approved by the Hospital Sant Pau i de la Santa Creu ethics committee following the good clinical practices protocol (IIBSP-EIG-2022-92) and was performed in accordance with the tenets of the 1964 Helsinki Declaration and its subsequent amendments.

2.2. Patients

All patients aged 18 years and older with suspected IgG4-RD based on clinical grounds and elevated IgG4 levels (>135 mg/dL) were included from January 2000 to January 2024. The patients were evaluated by experienced rheumatologists and categorized into two groups based on expert clinical judgment: those diagnosed as having and not having IgG4-RD (IgG4-RD group and non-IgG4-RD group, respectively).

2.3. Procedures

Obtained retrospectively from the hospital's electronic healthcare records were patient demographic data (sex, age, race) and disease-related variables, including clinical and laboratory parameters, histological findings, previous neoplasia, cause of death (any cause), and prescribed treatments.

The following specific clinical manifestations were also recorded: glandular involvement, pulmonary involvement, retroperitoneal fibrosis, autoimmune pancreatitis, renal involvement, aortitis, inflammatory aortic aneurysm, lower back pain, constitutional symptoms, fever, hypophysitis, pachymeningitis, orbital pseudotumor, and ocular involvement. Visceral involvement was assessed through imaging techniques including CT, PET, and/or nuclear magnetic resonance imaging (nMRI).

Recorded laboratory data included hemogram; total IgG and IgG4, C-reactive protein (CRP), erythrocyte sedimentation rate (ESR), and tests results for the presence or absence of anti-extractable nuclear antigens (ENA), rheumatoid factor, antinuclear antibodies (ANA), and various disease-specific autoantibodies (including anti-Ro/SSA, anti-La/SSB, anti-neutrophil cytoplasmic, anti-double stranded DNA, anti-RNP, anti-Sm, and plasmablasts). IgG4 quantification was performed from peripheral blood samples by turbidimetry using the Optilite kit. Reference values at our hospital were 3.9–86 mg/dL, though the upper limit of normal serum IgG4 concentration was set to 135 mg/dL, a threshold commonly used in Japanese diagnostic criteria for IgG4-RD [13,14]. Plasmablasts were identified through flow cytometry based on the expression of surface proteins (CD19 + IgM − IgD − CD27 + $CD38^{high}$).

The three classification sets of criteria (Okazaki: present or absent; Umehara: possible, probable, definitive; ACR/EULAR 2019: present or absent and quantitative according to a weighted numeric score) were evaluated across the entire patient cohort and compared for the four IgG4-RD subtypes (pancreatic-hepato-biliary disease; retroperitoneal fibrosis and/or aortitis; head/neck-limited disease, and Mikulicz syndrome with systemic involvement) [1].

Finally, histopathological confirmation, where available, was obtained for patients in both the IgG4-RD and non-IgG4-RD groups. However, in some cases, particularly those with deep-seated fibrotic disease such as retroperitoneal fibrosis, histological confirmation was not possible due to the invasive nature of biopsy procedures and the associated clinical risks, including bleeding and vascular complications. The presence of the following histopathological features was also recorded: lymphoplasmacytic infiltration, obliterative phlebitis, and/or glandular fibrosis.

2.4. Statistical Analysis

Patient demographic, clinical, and biochemical data were summarized using percentages, means, and standard deviations (SD), or medians and interquartile ranges (IQR), depending on the characteristics of the variable. Differences in values of continuous variables between IgG4-RD and non-IgG4-RD groups were analyzed by Student's *t*-test or the Mann–Whitney U test. Categorical variables were compared between groups using chi-square or Fisher's exact tests. IgG4 subtypes in terms of either demographic or laboratory values were compared by analysis of variance (ANOVA) for continuous variables and the chi-square test for categorical variables.

Sensitivity, specificity, positive predictive value (PPV), and negative predictive value (PPV) were calculated for the Okazaki, Umehara, and ACR/EULAR 2019 criteria (note that, for the sensitivity analysis of the Umehara criteria, the possible, probable, and definitive categories were either analyzed separately or collapsed into a single disease-positive category). Values were summarized using contingency tables for true positive (T+), false positive (F+), true negative (T−), and false negative (F−) values to obtain full information on sensitivity, specificity, and diagnostic odds ratios. A receiver operator characteristics (ROC) curve was plotted, and the area under the ROC curve (AUC) was calculated to evaluate the IgG4-RD diagnostic performance of each set of criteria.

All analyses were conducted for a significance level of 0.05. Analyses were performed using R v. 4.3.1 (R Core Team (2022). R: A language and environment for statistical computing. R Foundation for Statistical Computing, Vienna, Austria).

3. Results

3.1. General IgG4-RD Characteristics

Of the 41 patients with suspected IgG4-RD included in the study, 30 cases were confirmed as IgG4-RD based on expert clinical judgment and the remaining 11 cases were classified as non-IgG4-RD. The mean (SD) age at the time of IgG4-RD diagnosis was 61.79 (16.27).

Baseline characteristics for the IgG4-RD group and non-IgG4-RD group are described in Table 1. The definitive diagnoses of the 11 non-IgG4-RD patients were retroperitoneal fibrosis (n = 5), inflammatory aortic aneurysm (n = 3), autoimmune pancreatitis (n = 2), and hypophysitis (n = 1).

Table 1. Patient clinical characteristics (n = 41).

	IgG4-RD (n = 30)	**Non-IgG4-RD (n = 11)**	***p* Value**
Sex (male)	25 (83.3%)	4 (36.3%)	0.007
Race			
- Caucasian	28 (96.6%)	10 (90.9%)	0.47
- Asian	1 (3.4%)	1 (9.1%)	
Weight (kg), median (IQR)	83 (70.5–100.8)	84 (73.7–89.5)	0.665
Arterial hypertension	14 (46.7%)	4 (36.4%)	0.726
Dyslipidemia	14 (46.7%)	4 (36.4%)	0.726
Ischemic heart disease	6 (20%)	2 (18.2%)	1
Non-hematological neoplasia	1 (3.3%)	0 (0%)	1

Table 1. *Cont.*

	IgG4-RD (*n* = 30)	**Non-IgG4-RD (*n* = 11)**	***p* Value**
Glandular involvement	4 (13.3%)	0 (0%)	1
- 1 set	2 (6.7%)		
- >2 sets	2 (6.7%)		
Pulmonary involvement			1
- Peri-bronchovascular and septal thickening	5 (16.7%)	1 (9.1%)	
- Paravertebral-like thorax soft tissue	0 (0%)	0 (0%)	
- Wall thickening of thoracic aorta	0 (0%)	0 (0%)	
Pancreatic involvement	10 (33.3%)	3 (27.27%)	0.557
- Lobulation loss	1 (3.3%)	0 (0%)	
- Low density capsule edging	2 (6.7%)	2 (18.2%)	
- Pancreatic and biliary injury	7 (23.3%)	1 (9.1%)	
Renal involvement	14 (46.7%)	1 (9.1%)	0.267
- Hypocomplementemia	3 (10%)	0 (0%)	
- Thickening of renal pelvis	3 (10%)	1 (9.1%)	
- Bilateral low-density renal cortex	8 (%)	0 (0%)	
Retroperitoneal involvement	17 (56.7%)	4 (36.4%)	0.593
- Wall thickening of abdominal aorta	7 (23.3%)	2 (18.2%)	
- Iliac or infrarenal aortic soft peripheral tissue	10 (33.3%)	2 (18.2%)	
Fever	3 (10%)	0 (0%)	0.551
Constitutional syndrome	3 (10%)	0 (0%)	0.551
Lower back pain	6 (20%)	0 (0%)	0.167
Hydronephrosis	3 (10%)	0 (0%)	0.551
Aneurysm	10 (33.3%)	3 (27.3%)	1
Hypophysitis	1 (3.3%)	1 (9.1%)	0.47
Pachymeningitis	1 (3.3%)	0 (0%)	0.268

Table 1. *Cont.*

	IgG4-RD (n = 30)	Non-IgG4-RD (n = 11)	p Value
Orbital pseudotumor	0 (0%)	0 (0%)	1
Uveal involvement	0 (0%)	0 (0%)	1
Sclera involvement	1 (9.1%)	0 (0%)	0.268
IgG, median (IQR)	1196 (979.2–1536.2)	1137 (1006.5–1250)	0.233
IgG4, median (IQR)	90.5 (40.8–154.5)	47.0 (33.5–86)	0.05
Plasmablasts, median (IQR)	993.0 (255.5–1628.2)	24 (0–101)	0.004

Comparative analysis of the IgG4-RD (n = 30) and non-IgG4-RD (n = 11) groups revealed several significant differences. In the IgG4-RD group, males were more prevalent (83.3% vs. 36.3%; p = 0.007), median serum IgG4 levels were higher (90.5 vs. 47.0; p = 0.05), and the median plasmablast count in peripheral blood was significantly more elevated (993.0 vs. 24; p = 0.004). These findings highlight the utility of elevated IgG4 as a biomarker for diagnosing IgG4-RD and underscore the importance of integrating both clinical characteristics with serological biomarkers for accurate diagnosis.

All 30 patients in the IgG4-RD group had negative results for rheumatoid factor, ANA, and ENA.

Histological data are summarized in Table 2. Samples were obtained from nine patients in the IgG4-RD group, compared to just one patient in the non-IgG4-RD group (34.6% vs. 9.09%; p = 1.000). A notable limitation of this study is the lack of histological confirmation for most of the non-IgG4-RD patients. This was primarily due to the clinical presentation of these subjects, who exhibited retroperitoneal fibrosis associated with aortic aneurysm and mildly elevated serum IgG4 levels. The potential risks of retroperitoneal biopsies in such cases, including bleeding and vascular complications, were deemed to outweigh the diagnostic benefits.

Table 2. Histological characteristics.

	IgG4-RD (n = 30)	Non-IgG4-RD (n = 11)	p-Value
Histology	9 (34.6%)	1 (9.09%)	1.000
Histological location - Liver - Adenopathy - Salivary gland - Abdominal mass - Pleura - Renal	 1 (11.1%) 1 (11.1%) 2 (22.2%) 2 (22.2%) 1 (11.1%) 2 (22.2%)	1 (100.0%)	
Plasma cells	8 (88.9%)	1 (100.0%)	0.200
Phlebitis	2 (22.2%)	0 (0.0%)	1.000
Fibrosis	2 (22.2%)	0 (0.0%)	1.000

While no patients in the non-IgG4-RD group received intravenous methylprednisolone (IV-MTPD) boluses or steroid therapy, all patients in the IgG4-RD group underwent treatment with these interventions. This stark contrast in treatment approaches highlights a key difference in the management of the two patient cohorts. Two patients (6.7%) in the IgG4-RD group who received IV-MTPD boluses followed by oral prednisone (median dose (IQR) 55 (30–60) mg) as initial treatment showed a statistically significant difference ($p < 0.001$) compared to the non-IgG4-RD group. Additionally, four patients (13.3%) required treatment with rituximab (500 mg), administered in two infusions separated by 15 days and a maintenance dose over two weeks every six months.

3.2. Okazaki, Umehara, and ACR/EULAR 2019 Criteria

We evaluated these criteria in a cohort of 41 patients, including 30 with confirmed IgG4-RD and 11 without IgG4-RD.

Of the 30 patients diagnosed with IgG4-RD, 18 (60%) met the Okazaki criteria; 25 (83.33%) met the Umehara criteria, including 6 (20%) definitive, 2 (6.7%) probable, and 17 (56.7%) possible cases; and 20 (66.7%) met the ACR/EULAR 2019 criteria, with a median (IQR) value of 20.0 (20–44).

Table 3 summarizes the diagnostic performance of the Okazaki, Umehara, and ACR/EULAR 2019 criteria.

Table 3. Okazaki, Umehara, and ACR/EULAR 2019 diagnostic performance.

METRIC	OKAZAKI	UMEHARA	ACR/EULAR 2019
Confirmed IgG4-RD patients ($n = 30$)	18 (60%)	25 (83.33%)	20 (66.67%)
Sensitivity [95% CI]	60% [40.6–77.34%]	83.33% [65.28–94.36%]	66.67% [47.19–82.71%]
Specificity [95% CI]	100% [71.51–100%]	100% [71.51–100%]	100% [71.51–100%]
Accuracy [95% CI]	70.73% [54.46–83.87%]	87.8% [73.8–95.92%]	75.61% [59.7–87.64%]
Positive predictive value [95% CI]	100% [81.47–100%]	100% [86.28–100%]	100% [83.16–100%]
Negative predictive value [95% CI]	47.83% [26.82–69.41%]	68.75% [41.34–88.98%]	52.38% [29.78–74.29%]
Negative likelihood ratio [95% CI]	40% [25.81–62%]	16.67% [7.49–37.1%]	33.33% [20.1–55.29%]

Note: CI = confidence interval.

For the 30 IgG4-RD patients, sensitivity was highest for the Umehara criteria (83.33%; 95% CI: 65.28–94.36%), which correctly identified 25 patients, followed by the ACR/EULAR 2019 criteria (66.67%; 95% CI: 47.19–82.71%), identifying 20 patients, and the Okazaki criteria (60%; 95% CI: 40.6–77.34%), identifying 18 patients. Further stratification of patients according to the Umehara criteria into possible, probable, or definitive IgG4-RD, the sensitivity values were 56.67% (95% CI: 37.43–74.54%), 6.67% (95% CI: 0.82–22.07%), and 20% (95% CI: 7.71–38.57%), respectively.

Specificity for all three criteria was 100% (95% CI: 71.51–100%), with all 11 non-IgG4-RD patients correctly identified, and resulting in a PPV of 100% for each set of criteria.

Accuracy was highest for the Umehara criteria, which correctly classified 87.8% (95% CI: 73.8–95.92%) of the patients, followed by the ACR/EULAR 2019 criteria (75.61%; 95% CI: 59.7–87.64%) and the Okazaki criteria (70.73%; 95% CI: 54.46–83.87%).

The NPV was highest for the Umehara criteria at 68.75% (95% CI: 41.34–88.98%), followed by the ACR/EULAR 2019 criteria, at 52.38% (95% CI: 29.78–74.29%), and the Okazaki criteria, at 47.83% (95% CI: 26.82–69.41%).

The AUC values (Figure 1) were 0.917 for the Umehara criteria, 0.800 for the Okazaki criteria, and 0.833 and 0.864 for the ACR/EULAR 2019 criteria and numeric score, respectively, with all values showing significant diagnostic performance ($p < 0.000$).

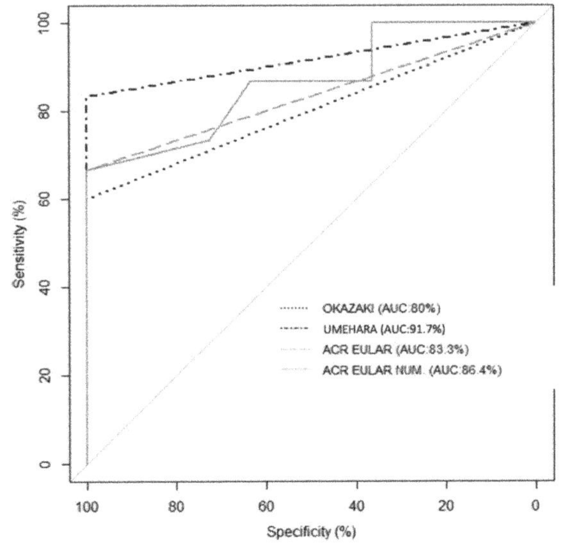

Figure 1. Area under the curve for the Okazaki, Umehara, and ACR/EULAR criteria.

3.3. Description of IgG4-RD Subtypes

The analysis of IgG4-RD subtypes revealed distinct patterns across four identified groups (Table 4). Subtype 1, comprising 26.7% of cases, was characterized by a strong male predominance (87.5%) and the most pronounced pancreatic involvement, with 75% of cases showing pancreatic–biliary injury. Subtype 2 was the most prevalent subtype, comprising 19 patients (63.3%). Was especially associated with hypertension (p = 0.066), aneurysms (47.4%) and retroperitoneal involvement. Pulmonary manifestations, specifically peribronchovascular and septal thickening, were exclusive to this subtype (26.3% of cases). Subtype 3 (head/neck-limited) was represented by a single case, limiting comparative analysis. Subtype 4 (Mikulicz-systemic involvement), with only two cases, showed a tendency for systemic manifestations, including aneurysm in one case.

Table 4. IgG4 subtypes.

	SUBTYPE 1 Pancreato-Hepato-Biliary ***n*** **= 8 (26.7%)**	**SUBTYPE 2 Retroperitoneal +/− Aortitis** ***n*** **= 19 (63.3%)**	**SUBTYPE 3 Head/Neck-Limited** ***n*** **= 1 (3.3%)**	**SUBTYPE 4 Mikulicz-Systemic Involvement** ***n*** **= 2 (6.7%)**	***p*** **Value**
Gender (male)	7 (87.5%)	16 (84.2%)	1 (100%)	1 (50%)	0.592
Race					
- Caucasian	8 (100%)	18 (94.7%)	1 (100%)	2 (100%)	1
- Asian	0 (0%)	1 (5.3%)	0 (0%)	0 (0%)	
Arterial hypertension	2 (25%)	12 (63.2%)	0 (0%)	0 (0%)	0.066
Dyslipidemia	3 (37.5%)	10 (52.6%)	0 (0%)	1 (50%)	0.83
Ischemic heart disease	0 (0%)	6 (31.6%)	0 (0%)	0 (0%)	0.321

Table 4. *Cont.*

	SUBTYPE 1 Pancreato-Hepato-Biliary n = 8 (26.7%)	SUBTYPE 2 Retroperitoneal +/− Aortitis n = 19 (63.3%)	SUBTYPE 3 Head/Neck-Limited n = 1 (3.3%)	SUBTYPE 4 Mikulicz-Systemic Involvement n = 2 (6.7%)	p Value
Non-hematological neoplasia	0 (0%)	1 (5.3%)	0 (0%)	0 (0%)	1
Glandular involvement					
- 1 set	0 (0%)	2 (10.5%)	0 (0%)	0 (0%)	1
- >2 sets	1 (12.5%)	1 (5.3%)	0 (0%)	0 (0%)	
Pulmonary involvement					
- Peri-bronchovascular and septal thickening	0 (0%)	5 (26.3%)	0 (0%)	0 (0%)	0.483
- Paravertebral-like thorax soft tissue	0 (0%)	0 (0%)	0 (0%)	0 (0%)	
Pancreatic involvement					
- Lobulation loss	0 (0%)	1 (5.3%)	0 (0%)	0 (0%)	
- Low-density capsule edging	2 (25%)	0 (0%)	0 (0%)	0 (0%)	<0.001
- Pancreatic-biliary injury	6 (75%)	1 (5.3%)	0 (0%)	0 (0%)	
Renal involvement					
- Hypocomplementemia	1 (12.5%)	2 (10.5%)	0 (0%)	0 (0%)	
- Thickening of renal pelvis	0 (0%)	3 (15.8%)	0 (0%)	0 (0%)	0.914
- Bilateral low-density renal cortex	1 (12.5%)	6 (31.57%)	0 (0%)	1 (50%)	
Retroperitoneal involvement					
- Wall thickening of abdominal aorta	0 (0%)	7 (36.8%)	0 (0%)	0 (0%)	0.001
- Iliac and infrarenal aortic soft peripheral tissue	0 (0%)	10 (52.6%)	0 (0%)	0 (0%)	

Table 4. *Cont.*

	SUBTYPE 1 Pancreato-Hepato-Biliary n = 8 (26.7%)	SUBTYPE 2 Retroperitoneal +/− Aortitis n = 19 (63.3%)	SUBTYPE 3 Head/Neck-Limited n = 1 (3.3%)	SUBTYPE 4 Mikulicz-Systemic Involvement n = 2 (6.7%)	p Value
Fever	0 (0%)	2 (10.5%)	0 (0%)	1 (50%)	0.293
Constitutional syndrome	0 (0%)	2 (10.5%)	0 (0%)	1 (50%)	0.293
Lower back pain	0 (0%)	6 (31.6%)	0 (0%)	0 (0%)	0.321
Hydronephrosis	0 (0%)	3 (15.8%)	0 (0%)	0 (0%)	0.663
Aneurysm	0 (0%)	9 (47.4%)	0 (0%)	1 (50%)	0.037
Hypophysitis	1 (12.5%)	0 (0%)	0 (0%)	0 (0%)	0.367
Okazaki 2009 criteria					
- Not met	4 (50%)	7 (36.8%)	0 (0%)	1 (50%)	0.902
- Met	4 (50%)	12 (63.2%)	1 (100%)	1 (50%)	
Umehara 2012 criteria					
- Not met	0 (0%)	5 (26.3%)	0 (0%)	0 (0%)	0.652
- Possible	4 (50%)	10 (52.6%)	1 (100%)	2 (100%)	
- Probable	1 (12.5%)	1 (5.3%)	0 (0%)	0 (0%)	
- Definitive	3 (37.5%)	3 (15.8%)	0 (0%)	0 (0%)	
ACR/EULAR 2019 criteria					
- Not met	2 (25%)	6 (31.6%)	1 (100%)	1 (50%)	0.653
- Met	6 (75%)	13 (68.4%)	0 (0%)	1 (50%)	
ACR/EULAR numeric value, median (IQR)	24.0 (19.8–34.0)	20.0 (12.0–23.5)	4.0 (4.0–4.0)	12.5 (8.2–16.8)	0.523
IgG, median (IQR)	1166.5 (853.2–1306.0)	1180.0 (985.5–1542.0)	1624.0 (1624.0–1624.0)	1355.5 (1261.8–1449.2)	0.390
IgG4, median (IQR)	72.0 (39.8–132.8)	84.0 (43.5–180.0)	153.0 (153.0–153.0)	297.0 (207.0–387.0)	0.45
Plasmablasts, median (IQR)	518.0 (0.0–862.2)	1005.0 (288.0–1657.5)	9680.0 (9680.0–9680.0)	1176.5 (1145.8–1207.2)	0.179

On comparing diagnostic criteria across groups, distinctive trends emerged. The diagnostic accuracies of Umehara's criteria and the ACR/EULAR 2019 criteria for subtype 1 were 50% and 75%, respectively. For subtype 2, ACR/EULAR 2019 demonstrated an accuracy of 68.4%, while the Okazaki's criteria exhibited an accuracy of 63.2%. These findings suggest that specific criteria may be more useful for the diagnosis of these particular subtypes. Finally, only the subtype 3 case met both Okazaki's and Umehara's criteria, while the two subtype 4 cases met Umehara's criteria.

4. Discussion

We evaluated the diagnostic performance of the Okazaki, Umehara, and ACR/EULAR 2019 IgG4-RD classification criteria for a cohort of 41 Spanish patients with suspected IgG4-RD, in 30 of whom the diagnosis was confirmed by expert clinical judgment. Sensitivity was highest for the Umehara criteria (83.3%), followed by the ACR/EULAR 2019 criteria (66.66%) and the Okazaki criteria (60.0%).

Regarding the Okazaki (2009) and Umehara (2011) criteria, sensitivity was suboptimal for our cohort, which would question their utility for IgG4-RD screening in clinical practice. For the ACR/EULAR 2019 criteria, our sensitivity value of 66.66% was lower than reported (85.5% and 82.0%) in the original validation studies [15]. This discrepancy can be attributed to several factors. Firstly, the inherent design of the ACR/EULAR 2019 criteria gives them a built-in advantage, as the pre-defined threshold values for sensitivity and specificity during the criteria development process effectively established a high pre-test probability. This approach inherently increased the likelihood of achieving superior diagnostic performance in the initial validation cohort. Secondly, our relatively small sample may have influenced our results, while potential differences between our cohort and the original validation cohorts (disease phenotypes, patient characteristics, geographic variations) may contribute to the observed differences. Consequently, the ACR/EULAR 2019 criteria may not achieve the same level of sensitivity when applied to different patient populations or in real-world clinical settings, as in our study. This underscores the importance of external validation studies in diverse populations to assess the true performance of diagnostic criteria outside their development cohort and to account for variations in patient demographics and clinical presentations across different settings.

Notably, in our cohort all three criteria demonstrated excellent specificity (100%) and PPV (100%). These findings align with previous studies highlighting the high specificity of these diagnostic criteria for IgG4-RD [13–15].

The Umehara criteria, when stratified into possible, probable, or definitive IgG4-RD categories, showed lower sensitivity than when stratified dichotomously (with/without IgG4-RD). This observation aligns with Carruthers et al. [11], who reported significantly reduced sensitivity (36%) when considering only the definitive category. These findings underscore the heterogeneous nature of IgG4-RD and the challenges associated with strict compliance with more stringent classification criteria in specific cases. To optimize diagnostic sensitivity and prevent the omission of true cases, our study highlights the importance of considering all classification criteria categories, rather than focusing solely on the category with the highest specificity.

Subgroup analysis revealed differing compliance patterns for the four IgG4-RD phenotypes (classified according to the Wallace et al. 2019 [1] categorization), suggesting the potential utility of applying specific criteria to identify certain disease subtypes.

In our cohort, retroperitoneal fibrosis and/or aortitis (subtype 2) was the most prevalent subtype, comprising 63.3% of our patients. This differs from the literature, which reports pancreato-hepato-biliary involvement (subtype 1) to be the most prevalent subtype, accounting for 31% of cases [1]. The greater prevalence of subtype 2 in our cohort can be attributed to the presence of a multidisciplinary specialized aorta monthly committee in our institution, which likely led to increased detection and referral of cases with retroperitoneal fibrosis and aortitis. The varying prevalence of subtypes in our cohort, along with differences in how well each subtype meets different diagnostic criteria, underscores the known heterogeneity of IgG4-related disease and highlights the challenges faced in creating universally applicable diagnostic criteria.

Aligning with previous reports advocating for customized diagnostic approaches based on phenotype-specific consideration [1,14,15], our findings underscore the importance of considering disease phenotypes when selecting appropriate diagnostic criteria. We found that the Umehara and ACR/EULAR 2019 criteria performed better for the pancreato-hepato-biliary subtype, whereas the Okazaki and ACR/EULAR 2019 criteria performed better for the retroperitoneal fibrosis and/or aortitis subtype [17]. Adams et al. [5] also found that the ACR/EULAR 2019 criteria were more effective for both pancreato-hepato-biliary and retroperitoneal fibrosis and/or aortitis subtypes, corroborating Martinez-Calabuig et al. [18], who found that the ACR/EULAR 2019 criteria were superior to the Umehara and Okazaki criteria in diagnosing these subtypes. Those findings overall suggest that the ACR/EULAR 2019 criteria can play a crucial role in enhancing diagnostic accuracy for the IgG4-RD pancreato-hepato-biliary and retroperitoneal fibrosis and/or aortitis subtypes, thereby potentially improving patient care and outcomes.

The mean age of IgG4-RD diagnosis in our cohort was 61.79 years, which aligns with Brito-Zerón et al.'s [19] observation that the disease predominantly affects older adults.

Likewise, men predominated among our patients with an IgG4-RD diagnosis, highlighting potential sex-specific differences in disease presentation and susceptibility. Although no definitive disparity hypothesis is supported, men with IgG4-RD typically exhibit more a frequent involvement of organs such as the pancreas and kidneys, accompanied by a more active B-cell response [6].

The main strength of our study is the novelty of simultaneously comparing all three sets of criteria (Okazaki, Umehara, and ACR/EULAR 2019) in a cohort of IgG4-RD patients which, to our knowledge, is the first such comparison to date. While previous studies have compared the ACR/EULAR 2019 and the Umehara criteria separately, no single study has comprehensively evaluated the diagnostic performance of all three criteria sets concurrently. Additionally, our cohort includes patients representing all four IgG4-RD phenotypes, although, importantly, there was a significant imbalance in their distribution, in contrast with the leading ACR/EULAR groups [1]. In our cohort, subtypes 2 and 1 were predominant, while subtypes 3 and 4 were only anecdotally represented. This disproportionate distribution makes it challenging to draw robust conclusions regarding the latter two groups. Consequently, while our study provides some insights into the potential utility of specific criteria for different subtypes, the reliability of these insights varies considerably across subtypes.

The strict selection of patients with a high pretest probability of IgG4-RD (based on stringent inclusion criteria and comprehensive evaluation) likely contributed to the observed 100% PPV across all three criteria and minimized the inclusion of false negatives, while meeting the classification criteria significantly increased the likelihood of true positives. These findings highlight the clinical utility and reliability of the diagnostic criteria in accurately identifying IgG4-RD cases within our study cohort.

The main limitations are the small sample size, reflecting the low prevalence of the disease, and the single-center nature of our study. Further studies with larger sample sizes are necessary to achieve greater robustness. We plan to include all potential cases of IgG4-RD evaluated in our hospital for a future multicenter study to validate our results. Another key limitation was that enrolled patients were selected based on high clinical suspicion of IgG4-related disease and elevated IgG4 levels. This selection process may not have captured the full clinical spectrum of the condition, as patients presenting with subtle or atypical manifestations, or those with normal IgG4 levels despite active disease, could have been inadvertently excluded. To help mitigate this potential selection bias, the final diagnosis was determined through comprehensive evaluation by physicians with specialized expertise in IgG4-RD. However, this approach does not entirely eliminate the possibility that the study population may not be fully representative of the broader IgG4-RD patient population.

Additionally, since histopathological confirmation is crucial to diagnosing IgG4-RD in a non-negligible proportion of cases, a significant limitation was the small number of biopsies performed. Consequently, we may have inadvertently excluded a subset of patients with the disease. The paucity of biopsies in our cohort was due to the predominance of IgG4-RD subtype 2 (retroperitoneal fibrosis and aortitis). As reported in the literature, retroperitoneal fibrosis often presents with a fibrotic phenotype, meaning that tissue sampling is not only technically difficult (due to the deep-seated nature and proximity to vital structures) but may also yield limited diagnostic information (prominent fibrosis but minimal inflammation) [20]. This makes diagnosis particularly challenging, especially in the absence of distinctive histopathological features. Therefore, despite the recognized importance of biopsy for definitive diagnosis, the anatomical and pathological characteristics of subtype 2 often render biopsies unfeasible or potentially hazardous, further complicating the diagnostic process. Consequently, while our study provides some insights into the potential utility of specific criteria for different subtypes, the reliability of these insights varies considerably across the subgroups due to their uneven representation.

5. Conclusions

This retrospective study provides a detailed comparative evaluation of the Okazaki, Umehara, and ACR/EULAR 2019 classification criteria for diagnosing IgG4-related disease (IgG4-RD) in a Spanish cohort. Although the overall sample size is small, our findings demonstrate that the Umehara criteria exhibit the highest sensitivity (83.33%), making them the most suitable for screening purposes. Meanwhile, all three sets of criteria showed perfect specificity and positive predictive value (PPV), effectively confirming the diagnosis of IgG4-RD.

The predominance of subtype 2 in our cohort, attributed to a specialized multidisciplinary approach at our center, further supports the importance of clinical context in the diagnosis of IgG4-RD. However, the uneven distribution of subtypes, particularly the underrepresentation of subtypes 3 and 4, limits the generalizability of our conclusions for these less prevalent subtypes.

The lack of histopathological confirmation in some cases, particularly in patients with deep-seated fibrotic disease, remains a limitation, emphasizing the need for alternative diagnostic strategies when biopsy is not feasible. Future multicenter studies with larger, more balanced cohorts and broader histopathological validation are needed to refine these diagnostic criteria and improve their applicability across different IgG4-RD phenotypes.

In summary, our results suggest that while no single set of criteria is universally optimal, the Umehara and ACR/EULAR 2019 criteria offer the highest diagnostic value, especially when applied to specific subtypes. The development of tailored diagnostic strategies based on disease phenotype, along with further validation in diverse populations, will be essential to improve the accuracy and utility of these criteria in clinical practice.

Author Contributions: Formal analysis, H.S.P.; Investigation, P.M.-A., M.C.M., S.C., H.C.-M., B.M., I.C., A.J.B.-M., A.L., C.D.-T., L.S., J.B., L.M.-M. and H.C.; Writing—original draft, M.L.-G. All authors have read and agreed to the published version of the manuscript.

Funding: This research was funded by Sociedad Española de Reumatología.

Institutional Review Board Statement: The study was conducted in accordance with the Declaration of Helsinki and approved by the Ethics Committee (IIBSP-EIG-2022-92) in 2021 in Hospital Sant Pau i de la Santa Creu, Barcelona, Spain.

Informed Consent Statement: Informed consent was obtained from all subjects involved in the study.

Data Availability Statement: The original contributions presented in the study are included in the article, further inquiries can be directed to the corresponding authors.

Conflicts of Interest: The authors declare no conflicts of interest.

Appendix A

Okazaki Criteria (Proposed by the Japanese Research Committee for IgG4-Related Systemic Sclerosing Disease) 2009

1. Focal or diffuse enlargement or lesions in one or more organs.
2. Serum IgG4 concentrations > 135 mg/dL
3. Histopathology
    (a) Lymphocytic and plasmocytic infiltrate with fibrosis, without neutrophilic infiltrate.

(b) IgG4 positive plasmocytic infiltrate greater than 10/cap or IgG4/IgG > 40% ratio of IgG4/IgG cells.
(c) Storiform fibrosis
(d) Obliterative phlebitis

The patient will be classified by meeting one of the following combinations of criteria:

- 1 + 2
- 1 + 3 (a + b)
- 2 + 3 (a + b)
- 3 (a + b + c + d)

Appendix B

Umehara Criteria 2011

1. Clinical examination showing characteristic diffuse/localized swelling or masses in one or more organs.
2. Hematologic examination showing elevated serum IgG4 concentrations (≥135 mg/dL).
3. Histopathologic examination showing:
   - Marked lymphocyte and plasmacyte infiltration and fibrosis.
   - IgG4-positive plasma cell infiltration: IgG4/IgG-positive cell ratio > 40% and >10 IgG4-positive plasma cells/high potency field (HPF).

The patient will be classified by meeting one of the following combinations of criteria: Definitive: (1) + (2) + (3); Probable: (1) + (3); Possible: (1) + (2)

Appendix C

ACR/EULAR 2019 Criteria

Exclusion Criteria

Clinical

- fever: recurrent temperature > 38 °C without clinical signs of infection
- lack of response to glucocorticoids at doses of at least 40 mg/day of prednisone (approx. 0.6 mg/kg/day) for 4 weeks

Serologic

- leukopenia or thrombocytopenia without alternative explanation
- peripheral eosinophilia > 3000 mm^3
- presence of ANCA antibodies
- presence of antinuclear antibodies anti-Ro, anti-La, anti-double-stranded DNA, anti-RNP, anti-Sm, anti-synthetase (e.g., anti-Jo1), antitopoisomerase III (Scl-70). This does not include antibodies of low specificity, such as rheumatoid factor, antinuclear antibodies (in screening), antimitochondrial antibodies, antimuscle smooth muscle antibodies, and antiphospholipid antibodies
- cryoglobulinemia.

Radiological

- radiological changes characteristic of neoplastic diseases or infections not sufficiently screened for
- rapid radiological progression
- anomalies in long bones compatible with Erdheim-Chester disease: multifocal osteosclerotic lesions in long bones
- splenomegaly: >14 cm without other explanations

Histopathologic

- cellular infiltrates that raise suspicion of a malignant neoplasm and have not been sufficiently analyzed

- markers related to an inflammatory myofibroblastic tumor
- evident neutrophilic inflammation
- necrotizing vasculitis
- evident necrosis (especially zonal necrosis)
- primary granulomatous inflammation
- characteristic signs of diseases related to macrophage/histiocyte disorders.

Histopathological

- cellular infiltrates that raise suspicion of a malignant neoplasm and have not been sufficiently analyzed
- markers related to an inflammatory myofibroblastic tumor
- evident neutrophilic inflammation
- necrotizing vasculitis
- evident necrosis (especially zonal necrosis)
- primary granulomatous inflammation
- characteristic signs of diseases related to macrophage/histiocyte disorders.

Exclusion of specific diseases

- multicentric Castleman's disease
- Crohn's disease
- ulcerative colitis
- Hashimoto's thyroiditis

Inclusion criteria: a point count should be performed.

Histopathology	
-biopsy that does not provide relevant information	0
-dense lymphocytic infiltrate	4
-dense lymphocytic infiltrate and obliterative phlebitis	6
-dense lymphocytic infiltrate and glandular fibrosis with or without obliterating phlebitis	13
Immunostaining	0–16
Serum IgG4 concentration	
-normal or undetermined	0
-above normal, but <2× upper limit of normal (ULN)	4
-from 2× to 5× LSN	6
≥5× LSN	11
Bilateral involvement of lacrimal glands, parotid, sublingual and submaxillary salivary glands	
-unaffected	0
-affectation of 1 pair	6
-involvement of ≥2 pairs	14
Chest	
-undetermined or none of the aforementioned elements are present	0
-peri-bronchovascular and septal thickening	4
-paravertebral band-like soft tissue in the thorax	10

Pancreas and biliary tract	
-undetermined or none of the aforementioned elements are present	0
-diffuse enlargement of the pancreas (loss of lobulation)	8
-diffuse enlargement of the pancreas and low-density capsule rim	11
-involvement of the pancreas (one of the above) and bile ducts	19
Kidney	
-undetermined or none of the aforementioned elements are present	0
-hypocomplemententemia	6
-thickening of the renal pelvis/soft tissue	8
– bilateral areas of low density in the renal cortex	10
Retroperitoneum	
-undetermined or none of the aforementioned elements are present	0
-diffuse thickening of the wall of the abdominal aorta	4
-peripheral or anterolateral soft tissue around the infrarenal aorta or iliac arteries	8

IgG4-related disease classification criteria are met if the entry criterion is met, there are no exclusion criteria, and the total score is $\geq$20.

References

1. Wallace, Z.S.; Zhang, Y.; Perugino, C.A.; Naden, R.; Choi, H.K.; Stone, J.H.; ACR/EULAR IgG4-RD Classification Criteria Committee. Clinical phenotypes of IgG4-related disease: An analysis of two international cross-sectional cohorts. *Ann. Rheum. Dis.* **2019**, *78*, 406–412. [CrossRef] [PubMed]
2. Tsoboi, H.; Honda, F.; Takahashi, H.; Ono, Y.; Abe, S.; Kondo, Y.; Matsumoto, I.; Sumida, T. Pathogenesis of IgG4-related disease. Comparison with Sjögren's syndrome. *Mod. Rheumatol.* **2020**, *30*, 7–16. [CrossRef] [PubMed]
3. Liu, Z.; Nie, Y.; Yu, P.; Lu, H.; Zhang, P.; Li, J.; Sun, R.; Li, J.; Sun, B.; He, X.; et al. The external validation of the 2019 ACR/EULAR classification criteria for IgG4-related disease in a large cohort from China. *Semin. Arthritis Rheum.* **2023**, *61*, 152202. [CrossRef] [PubMed]
4. Lanzillotta, M.; Mancuso, G.; Della-Torre, E. Advances in the diagnosis and management of IgG4 related disease. *BMJ* **2020**, *16*, 369. [CrossRef] [PubMed]
5. Adam, Z.; Zeman, D.; Cermak, A.; Dastych, M.; Doubková, M.; Horváth, T.; Skorkovská, Š.; Adamová, Z.; Řehák, Z.; Koukalová, R.; et al. IgG4-related disease. Clinical manifestation, differential diagnosis and recent International Diagnostic Criteria for IgG4-related disease. *Vnitr. Lek.* **2022**, *68*, 4–19. [CrossRef] [PubMed]
6. Akiyama, M.; Takeuchi, T. IgG4-Related Disease: Beyond Glucocorticoids. *Drugs Aging* **2018**, *35*, 275–287. [CrossRef] [PubMed]
7. Fernandez-Codina, A.; Martínez-Valle, F.; Pinilla, B.; López, C.; DeTorres, I.; Solans-Laqué, R.; Fraile-Rodríguez, G.; Casanovas-Martínez, A.; López-Dupla, M.; Robles-Marhuenda, Á.; et al. IgG4-Related Disease: Results From a Multicenter Spanish Registry. *Medicine* **2015**, *94*, e1275. [CrossRef] [PubMed]
8. Terao, C.; Ota, M.; Iwasaki, T.; Shiokawa, M.; Kawaguchi, S.; Kuriyama, K.; Kawaguchi, T.; Kodama, Y.; Yamaguchi, I.; Uchida, K.; et al. IgG4-related disease in the Japanese population: A genome-wide association study. *Lancet Rheumatol.* **2019**, *1*, e14–e22. [CrossRef] [PubMed]
9. Yamamoto, M.; Tanaka, T.; Aochi, S.; Uehara, M. HLA-DRB1 is associated with therapeutic responsiveness in IgG4-related disease. *Intern. Med.* **2024**, *63*, 207–211. [CrossRef] [PubMed]
10. Floreani, A.; Okazaki, K.; Uchida, K.; Gershwin, M.E. IgG4-related disease: Changing epidemiology and new thoughts on a multisystem disease. *J. Transl. Autoimmun.* **2020**, *4*, 100074. [CrossRef] [PubMed]
11. Pinheiro, F.A.G.; Pereira, I.A.; Souza, A.W.S.; Giardini, H.A.M.; Cordeiro, R.A. IgG4-related disease—Rare but you should not forget it. *Adv. Rheumatol.* **2024**, *64*, 35. [CrossRef] [PubMed]
12. Carruthers, M.; Khosroshahi, A.; Augustin, T.; Deshpande, V.; Stone, J.H. The diagnostic utility of serum IgG4 concentrations in IgG4-related disease. *Ann. Rheum. Dis.* **2015**, *74*, 14–18. [CrossRef] [PubMed]
13. Zhang, J.; Chen, H.; Ma, Y.; Xiao, Y.; Niu, N.; Lin, W.; Wang, X.; Liang, Z.; Zhang, F.; Li, F.; et al. Characterizing IgG4-related disease with 18F-FDG PET/CT: A prospective cohort study. *Eur. J. Nucl. Med. Mol. Imaging* **2014**, *41*, 1624–1634. [CrossRef] [PubMed]
14. Okazaki, K.; Uchida, K.; Koyabu, M.; Miyoshi, H.; Takaoka, M. Recent advances in the concept and diagnosis of autoimmune pancreatitis and IgG4-related disease. *J. Gastroenterol.* **2011**, *46*, 277–288. [CrossRef] [PubMed]

15. Umehara, H.; Okazaki, K.; Masaki, Y.; Kowano, M.; Yamamoto, M.; Saeki, T.; Matsui, S.; Yoshino, T.; Nakamura, S.; Kawa, S.; et al. Comprehensive diagnostic criteria for IgG4-related disease (IgG4-RD). *Mod. Rheumatol.* **2012**, *22*, 21–30. [CrossRef] [PubMed]
16. Wallace, Z.; Naden, R.; Chari, S.; Choi, H.; Della-Torre, E.; Dicaire, J.-F.; A Hart, P.; Inoue, D.; Kawano, M.; Khosroshahi, A.; et al. The 2019 American College of Rheumatology/European League Against Rheumatism Classification Criteria for IgG4-Related Disease. *Arthritis Rheumatol.* **2020**, *72*, 7–19. [CrossRef] [PubMed]
17. Okazaki, K.; Umehara, H. Are Classification Criteria for IgG4-RD Now Possible? The Concept of IgG4-Related Disease and Proposal of Comprehensive Diagnostic Criteria in Japan. *Int. J. Rheumatol.* **2012**, *2012*, 357071. [CrossRef] [PubMed]
18. Martinez Calabuig, P.; Gil, J.J.F.; Rueda, A.; Maicas, L.S.; Mazarío, R.G.; Barbera, L.A.; Abad, M.C.S.; Rivera, A.S.; Miralles, I.C.; Lerma, J.J.; et al. IgG4-related disease: 2010-2022 case revision and performance of diagnostic criteria. *Ann. Rheum. Dis.* **2023**, *82* (Suppl. S1), 1957.
19. Brito-Zerón, P.; Ramos-Casals, M.; Bosch, X.; Stone, J. The clinical spectrum of IgG4-related disease. *Autoimmun. Rev.* **2014**, *13*, 1203–1210. [CrossRef] [PubMed]
20. Wallace, Z.S.; Katz, G.; Hernandez-Barco, Y.G.; Baker, M.C. Current and future advances in practice: IgG4-related disease. *Rheumatol. Adv. Pract.* **2024**, *8*, rkae020. [CrossRef] [PubMed]

diagnostics

MDPI

Article

Disease Course and Long-Term Outcomes in Adult IgA Vasculitis Nephritis: A Prospective Observational Study

Fatih Yıldırım [1,*], Muhammet Emin Kutu [2], Yalkın Çalık [2], Kübra Kalkan [1], Gamze Akkuzu [1], Duygu Sevinç Özgür [1], Bilgin Karaalioğlu [1], Rabia Deniz [1], Gül Güzelant Özköse [1], Burak İnce [1] and Cemal Bes [1]

1 Department of Rheumatology, Başakşehir Çam and Sakura City Hospital, University of Health Sciences, 34480 İstanbul, Turkey; kalkankubra86@gmail.com (K.K.); gamzeakkuzu89@hotmail.com (G.A.); duygu_se_a@hotmail.com (D.S.Ö.); bilginkaraalioglu@gmail.com (B.K.); dr.rabiadeniz@gmail.com (R.D.); guzelant_gul@hotmail.com (G.G.Ö.); drburakince@gmail.com (B.İ.); cemalbes@hotmail.com (C.B.)

2 Department of Rheumatology, Bakırköy Dr Sadi Konuk Training and Research Hospital, University of Health Sciences, 34140 İstanbul, Turkey; mekutu@hotmail.com (M.E.K.); yclk04@hotmail.com (Y.Ç.)

* Correspondence: f08fatih@gmail.com; Tel.: +90-5374411328

Abstract: Background/Objectives: A limited number of previous studies have reported high rates of end-stage renal disease (ESRD) in adults with IgA vasculitis nephritis (IgAVN). Despite the high prevalence of the disease and the high rates of ESRD reported in the literature, no specific guidelines for adult patients have been established and there is no consensus on the management of the disease. This study aimed to prospectively investigate adults with IgAVN from a broad perspective. **Methods**: This investigation was designed as a prospective observational study and was conducted between 01.02.2022 and 01.10.2024. A total of 49 newly diagnosed adult (>18 years) patients with IgAVN were regularly followed up. At the end of the study, the renal remission rates, factors influencing remission, treatment data, treatment-related adverse events, and disease outcomes were determined. **Results**: The median follow-up time was 22 (IQR: 11–24) months. A total of 42 patients (87%) received immunosuppressive treatment in addition to the initial glucocorticoid treatment. Azathioprine (AZA) was the preferred (41%) first steroid-sparing agent. ESRD occurred in only one patient (2%), while a total of ten patients (20%) had an unfavorable outcome. The rate of nephrotic-range proteinuria (NRP) was significantly higher in the patients who did not achieve renal remission at the end of the 12-month follow-up period (9,7% vs. 60%; $p = 0.02$) and NRP was an independent risk factor for unfavorable outcomes [OR: 17.18; 95% CI: 1.31–224.95; $p = 0.03$]. A total of 16% of the patients developed an infection that required hospitalization during follow-up; these patients had a higher rate of IgAVN-associated acute kidney injury (62.5% vs. 22%; $p = 0.02$) and were significantly older (mean: 46 ± 15.3 vs. 65 ± 13.3; $p = 0.002$). One patient died of sepsis at 4 months and another died of a myocardial infarction at 32 months. **Conclusions**: These results suggest that adults with IgVAN do not have a high rate of ESRD if they receive effective immunosuppressive therapy. However, immunosuppressive therapy is associated with an increased risk of infection, particularly in the elderly. The presence of NRP is associated with lower long-term remission rates and has a predictive value for unfavorable outcomes.

Keywords: IgA vasculitis; nephritis; prognosis; mortality; ESRD

1. Introduction

Immunoglobulin A vasculitis (IgAV), also known as Henoch–Schönlein purpura (HSP), is a type of primary vasculitis characterized by the deposition of IgA1-immune complexes in

https://doi.org/10.3390/diagnostics15080957

small vessels [1]. Its annual incidence in adults has been reported to vary from 0.3/100,000 to 5.1/100,000 [2–4]. The disease classically involves the skin, joints, gastrointestinal tract, and kidneys. Renal involvement is the most common cause of morbidity and mortality and is the main determinant of the prognosis in patients with IgAV [5,6]. The renal involvement of the disease is essentially an immune complex glomerulonephritis and is termed IgA vasculitis nephritis (IgAVN) [7]. The rate of IgAVN in adult patients with IgAV has been reported to vary between 45% and 85% [8]. Hematuria is the most common and first manifestation of IgAVN, but proteinuria, nephrotic syndrome, nephritic syndrome, and acute kidney injury may also occur due to the disease [9]. Most of the data in the literature on IgAVN are derived from studies conducted in children. Studies comparing pediatric and adult patients with IgAVN have shown that the disease has a worse prognosis in adults [10,11]. The aim of this study was to prospectively investigate the disease course, outcomes, and treatment options in adults with IgAVN.

2. Materials and Methods

2.1. Study Design and Population

This investigation was designed as a prospective observational study and was conducted between February 2022 and October 2024 at the University of Health Sciences Başakşehir Çam and Sakura City Hospital Department of Rheumatology. A total of 49 patients aged ≥18 years with histopathological or clinically diagnosed IgAVN were included in the study. Patients with isolated IgA nephropathy and patients whose renal findings could be explained by another concurrent disease were excluded. All the patients were re-examined at 3-month intervals. Their renal functions, urine analysis results, proteinuria level, medications and doses, adverse events, and vasculitis damage scores were recorded at each visit. At the end of the study, the long-term (12-month) renal outcomes of the patients and the factors influencing these outcomes were determined. This study was approved by the hospital ethics committee (approval number: KAEK/2022.11.361) and was conducted according to the guidelines of the Declaration of Helsinki. Informed consent was obtained from all the patients.

2.2. Clinical Definitions

The EULAR/PRINTO/PRES classification criteria were used for the diagnosis of IgAV [12]. Renal involvement was defined as the presence of proteinuria (≥150 mg/24 h or ≥150 mg/g spot urine protein/creatinine ratio) and/or hematuria (≥5 red cells per high-power field). Acute kidney injury (AKI) was defined as an increase in serum creatinine of 0.3 mg/dL within 48 h or an increase in baseline serum creatinine of ≥50% within 7 days. The definitions of renal conditions (proteinuria, hematuria, AKI, CKD, and ESRD) were made in accordance with the Kidney Disease: Improving Global Outcomes (KDIGO) guidelines [13–15]. Renal remission was defined as proteinuria <300 mg/g supcr with a GFR≥ 60 mL/min/1.73 m^2 and using a glucocorticoid dose of ≤5 mg/day of prednisolone or equivalent. A relapse was defined as a >50% increase in proteinuria with hematuria or the reappearance of hematuria that was not explained by another medical condition other than vasculitis during a period after remission in patients with at least 3 months of follow-up. The definition of renal remission was determined by the investigators specifically for this study. Unfavorable outcomes were defined as established CKD (G3a-G5), renal replacement therapy, persistent proteinuria >500 mg/g supcr at the end of the follow-up, relapse disease, IgAVN-associated death, or a vasculitis damage index (VDI) score ≥1 at the end of the follow-up period.

2.3. Statistical Analysis

Statistical analyses were performed with the Statistical Package for the Social Sciences (SPSS) 26.0 (IBM, Chicago, IL, USA). The Kolmogorov–Smirnov test and the Shapiro–Wilk test were used to assess the normality of the data. Continuous variables were summarized as the mean ± standard deviation or median [interquartile range (IQR)] and categorical variables were summarized as percentages. Comparisons of continuous variables between groups were performed using a *t*-test or the Mann–Whitney U test after the distribution was evaluated, and the chi-square (χ^2) test or Fisher's exact test were used to compare categorical variables. The binary logistic regression analysis and multivariate Cox regression analysis methods were used to determine the predictors. A Kaplan–Meier estimation was performed to calculate the rate of the endpoint.

3. Results

3.1. Patient Characteristics and Presentation Signs

This study enrolled 49 adult patients (30 male; mean age: 49 ± 2.3 years) with newly diagnosed IgAVN. The median follow-up time was 22 (11–24) months. Of a total of 49 patients, 46 (94%) had skin involvement, 16 (32.6%) had joint involvement, and 11 (22.4%) had gastrointestinal involvement. Palpable purpura (94%) was the most common clinical sign at initial presentation, followed by hematuria (73.4%) and proteinuria (69.3%). Eleven patients (22.4%) had no renal pathology at initial presentation but developed renal involvement during follow-up. In patients who subsequently developed renal findings, the median time between the first visit and the renal findings was 30 (8–49) days. Regarding the renal findings, the patients most commonly had non-nephrotic proteinuria (73.4%) with active urinary sediment, 16.3% had nephrotic-range proteinuria, and 28.5% had acute kidney injury. Renal biopsy was performed in 55% of patients and a skin biopsy was performed in 94%. In all the patients with renal biopsies, pathological examination revealed increased mesangial cells and IgA deposits; all patients had evidence of mesangioproliferative glomerulonephritis. Glomerular crescent formation was present in 41% of the patients, but none of them had a crescent rate of more than 50%. The details of the histopathological findings can be found in the Supplementary Materials. The baseline demographic and clinical characteristics of the patients are shown in Table 1.

Table 1. Demographics and clinical characteristics of the patients.

	N = 49
Age, year; mean ± SD	49 ± 2.3
Male; *n*/*N* (%)	30 (6.2)
Follow-up time, month; median (IQR)	22 (11–24)
Organ system involvement; *n*/*N* (%)	
Skin	46 (94)
Joint	16 (32.6)
Gastrointestinal	11 (22.4)
Renal	49 (100)
Overall renal involvement; *n*/*N* (%)	
Nephrotic-range proteinuria	8 (16.3)
Non-nephrotic proteinuria	36 (73.4)
Isolated hematuria	5 (10.2)
Acute kidney injury	14 (28.5)

Table 1. *Cont.*

	N = 49
Overall renal outcomes; n/N (%)	
Persistent proteinuria (>500 mg/24 h)	6 (12)
Relapse	3 (6)
Chronic kidney disease (G3a–G5)	4 (8)
G3a	1 (2)
G3b	1 (2)
G4	1 (2)
G5	1 (2)
Established renal replacement therapy	1 (2)
VDI score (≥1); n/N (%)	10 (20)
Mortality; n/N (%)	
Sepsis	1 (2)
Myocardial infarction	1 (2)

SD: standard deviation; VDI: vasculitis damage index; G3a-G5: Kidney Disease: Improving Global Outcomes (KDIGO) chronic kidney disease stages—G3a: GFR 45–59; G3b: GFR 30–44; G4: GFR15–29; G5: GFR < 15—IQR: interquartile range.

3.2. Immunosuppressive Management Within the Cohort

The drugs and drug doses used in the treatment were decided by the clinicians without any guidelines. All the patients received a glucocorticoid treatment (53.1% pulse methylprednisolone), and the median glucocorticoid dose was 500 mg/day of methylprednisolone. Azathioprine (AZA) was the most commonly preferred first glucocorticoid-tapering agent (41%), followed by cyclophosphamide (CYC) (31%) and mycophenolate mofetil (MMF) (6%). In seven patients (14%), the glucocorticoid-tapering agent was changed to another for various reasons. The drugs used in the treatment and their effects on the renal outcomes are shown in Table 2.

Table 2. Treatment data of the patients.

	All of the Patients N = 49	Remission at 12 Months (+) vs. (−)/p-Value	VDI Score (≤1) vs. (>1)/p-Value	Unfavorable Renal Outcomes (+) vs. (−)/p-Value
All of the steroid-sparing agents; n/N (%)				
CYC	16 (33)			
AZA	25 (51)			
MMF	16 (33)			
MFA	1 (2)			
COLCH	5 (10)			
LEF	1 (2)			
TOCI	1 (2)			
First steroid-sparing agent; n/N (%)				
CYC	15 (31)	22.6 vs. 20/0.691	23.1 vs. 30/0.693	40 vs. 28.2/0.478
AZA	20 (41)	41.9 vs. 60/0.632	41 vs. 50/0.61	40 vs. 41/0.993
MMF	3 (6)			
COLC	3 (7)			
LEF	1 (2)			
None	7 (14)			
Steroid-sparing agent after cyclophosphamide; n/N (%)				
AZA	5/13 (38)	40 vs. 0/0.633	27.3 vs. 50/0.569	50 vs. 27.3/0.409
MMF	8/13 (62)	60 vs. 100/0.634	54.5 vs. 50/0.66	50 vs. 54.5/1.000
Steroid-sparing agent switch; n/N (%)				
AZA > MMF (adverse event)	4/42 (10)			
AZA > MMF (inadequate response)	1 (2)			
CYC > MMF (adverse event)	1 (2)			
CYC > AZA > TOCI (inadequate response for arthritis)	1 (2)			

Table 2. *Cont.*

	All of the Patients N = 49	Remission at 12 Months (+) vs. (−)/p-Value	VDI Score (≤1) vs. (>1)/p-Value	Unfavorable Renal Outcomes (+) vs. (−)/p-Value
Initial glucocorticoid dosage (prednisolone or equivalent MP); n/N (%)				
Pulse (≥250 mg/day)	26 (53.1)	48.4 vs. 80/0.342	48.7 vs. 70/0.296	70 vs. 48.7/0.22
1 mg/kg/day	8 (16.3)	19.4 vs. 0/0.64	17.9 vs. 10/0.477	10 vs. 17.9/0.541
0.5–1 mg/kg/day	7 (14.3)	9.7 vs. 0/0.633	12.8 vs. 20/0.624	20 vs. 12.8/0.565
≤0.5 mg/kg/day	8 (16.3)	19.4 vs. 0/0.561	15.4 vs. 0/0.32	0 vs. 15.4/0.187
Total glucocorticoid (prednisolone) exposure (gr); mean ± SD	3.1 ± 0.2	2.2 ± 1.3 vs. 3.5 ± 1.2 ***/0.01***	3.0 ± 1.6 vs. 4.6 ± 1.6 /0.06	4.3 ± 1.8 vs. 2.8 ± 1.3 ***/0.006***

CYC: cyclophosphamide; AZA: azathioprine; MMF: mycophenolate mofetil; MFA: mycophenolic acid; COLC: colchicine; LEF: leflunomide; TOCI: tocilizumab; MP: methylprednisolone; VDI: vasculitis damage index; SD: standard deviation.

3.3. One-Year Renal Remission Rates and Factors Influencing Remission

A total of 36 patients reached the one-year follow-up point, and 86% of the patients were in remission at 12 months. The rate of NRP was significantly higher in patients who did not achieve renal remission at the end of the 12-month follow-up period (9.7% vs. 60%; $p = 0.02$). The one-year remission rates and the factors influencing remission are shown in Table 3.

Table 3. Factors associated with long-term renal remission.

	Renal Remission (+) at 12 Months N − 31	Renal Remission (−) at 12 Months N = 5	p-Value
Age; mean ± SD	48.6 ± 16	56.6 ± 19.8	0.322
Male; n/N (%)	17 (54.8)	2 (40)	0.651
Renal involvement; n/N (%)			
Nephrotic-range proteinuria	3 (9.7)	3(60)	***<0.02***
Non-nephrotic proteinuria	22 (71)	2 (40)	0.333
Isolated hematuria	4 (12.9)	0 (0)	0.398
Isolated proteinuria	2 (6.5)	0 (0)	0.559
Acute kidney injury	10 (32.3)	2 (40)	0.733
Other system involvement; n/N (%)			
Skin involvement	31 (100)	4 (80)	0.135
Joint involvement	10 (32.3)	1 (20)	0.515
Gastrointestinal involvement	7 (22.6)	0 (0)	0.554
Baseline laboratory findings; n/N (%)			
CRP (mg/L); median (IQR)	40.8 (7–116)	13.5 (2.1–22.8)	0.112
GFR; median (IQR)	102 (80–119)	93 (45–119)	0.742
Serum albumin, <3.5 gr/dL; n/N (%)	7 (22.6)	0 (0)	0.556
Serum IgA level; mean ± SD	3.6 ± 1.3	2.9 ± 1	0.513
SII; median (IQR)	975 (516–1585)	807 (473–1199)	0.478
BVAS; median (IQR)	12 (7–13)	12 (7–13.5)	0.732
Five-factor score, >1; n/N (%)	14 (45.2)	3 (60)	0.651
Initial glucocorticoid dosage (prednisolone), mg/day; median (IQR)	80 (60–1000)	1000 (500–1000)	0.09
Comorbid systemic disease; n/N (%)			
Hypertension	10 (32.1)	2 (40)	0.541
Type 2 diabetes mellitus	10 (32.2)	1 (20)	0.512
Comorbid rheumatic disease; n/N (%)			
FMF	3 (9.7)	0 (0)	0.631
AS	2 (6.5)	0 (0)	0.739
Predisposing factor; n/N (%)			
None	17 (54.8)	3 (40)	0.615
Infection	11 (35.5)	3 (60)	0.351
Drug	7 (22.6	0 (0)	0.312

CRP: C-reactive protein; IQR: interquartile range; GFR: glomerular filtration rate; SII: systemic immune–inflammation index; BVAS: Birmingham vasculitis activity score; FMF: familial Mediterranean fever; AS: ankylosing spondylitis; SD: standard deviation.

3.4. Overall Unfavorable Outcomes and Associated Factors

A total of 10 patients had unfavorable outcomes at the end of the follow-up period. The presence of NRP was an independent risk factor for unfavorable outcomes [OR: 17.18; 95% CI: 1.31–224.95; $p = 0.03$]. The unfavorable outcomes and the factors associated with them are shown in Table 4. The vasculitis damage index (VDI) was used to assess disease- and medication-related damage. A total of 20% of the patients had a high VDI score (>1) at the end of the follow-up period. Patients with high VDI scores had a significantly higher total glucocorticoid exposure than those without (2.8 ± 1.3 gr vs. 4.4 ± 1.8 gr; $p = 0.005$) (Table 2). A total of 16% of the patients developed an infection that required hospitalization during the follow-up period. There was no difference in glucocorticoid exposure or the glucocorticoid-tapering agents used between patients with and without an infection that required hospitalization. However, the patients who developed an infection requiring hospitalization had a higher rate of IgAVN-associated AKI (62.5% vs. 22%; $p = 0.02$), and these patients were significantly older (mean 46 ± 15,3 vs. 65 ± 13,3; $p = 0.002$) (Table 5). The mortality rate was 4%. End-stage renal disease (ESRD) and renal replacement therapy occurred in only one patient, and this patient died due to sepsis in the 4th month. Another patient died of a heart attack at 32 months; he was in remission with no unfavorable outcomes. During the entire follow-up period, relapsed disease occurred in three (6%) patients (Table 1).

Table 4. Factors associated with unfavorable outcomes and multivariate regression analysis.

	Unfavorable Outcomes (+) N = 10	Unfavorable Outcomes (−) N = 39	*p*-Value	Regression Analysis	
				OR (95% CI)	*p*-Value
Age, >60 years; *n/N* (%)	6 (60)	8 (20.5)	***0.01***	1.32 (0.02–73.32)	0.891
Male; *n/N* (%)	5 (50)	25 (64.1)	0.418		
Baseline laboratory					
CRP (mg/L); median (IQR)	22.8 (9.7–46.8)	40.8 (6.5–121)	0.444		
ESR (mm/h); mean ± SD	41.1 ± 30.7	43.3 ± 27.7	0.846		
GFR; median (IQR)	95 (70–115)	93 (80–110)	0.92		
Serum albumin (gr/dL); mean ± SD	3.9 ± 0.5	3.8 ± 0.6	0.591		
BVAS; median (IQR)	10 (6–13.2)	12 (9–15)	0.215		
Five-factor score, >2; *n/N* (%)	4 (40)	3 (7.7)	***0.02***	0.60 (0.23–15.97)	0.764
SII; median (IQR)	689 (335–1110)	978 (516–2135)	0.483		
Baseline renal condition; *n/N* (%)					
Crescent on biopsy (+)	4/4 (100)	10/16 (62.5)	0.266		
Proteinuria (>500 mg/day)	9 (90)	19 (48.7)	***0.03***	3.52 (0.33–37.14)	0.291
Acute kidney injury	2 (20)	4 (10.3)	0.581		
Nephrotic-range proteinuria (>3.5 gr/day)	6 (60)	2 (5.1)	***0.001***	***17.18 (1.31–224.95)***	***0.03***
Other system involvement; *n/N* (%)					
Skin	9 (90)	37 (94.9)	0.56		
Joint	3 (30)	13 (33)	0.84		
Gastrointestinal	2 (20)	9 (23.1)	0.83		
Renal remission; *n/N* (%)					
at 12 months	4/8 (50)	27/28 (96.4)	***0.005***	0.06 (0.02–2.53)	0.14

Table 4. *Cont.*

	Unfavorable Outcomes (+) N = 10	Unfavorable Outcomes (−) N = 39	p-Value	Regression Analysis	
				OR (95% CI)	p-Value
Glucocorticoid dosage,					
Pulse steroid (>250 mg/day/MP); n/N (%)	7 (70)	19 (48.7)	0.22		
Total steroid exposure (gr/PR); mean ± SD	4.3 ± 1.8	2.8 ± 1.3	***0.006***	2.49 (0.93–6.60)	0.06
First steroid-tapering agent; n/N (%)					
AZA	4 (40)	16 (41)	0.95		
CYC	4 (40)	11 (28.2)	0.47		
Comorbid systemic disease; n/N (%)					
Hypertension	4 (40)	11 (28.2)	0.47		
Type 2 diabetes mellitus	4 (40)	11 (28.2)	0.47		
Comorbid rheumatic disease; n/N (%)					
FMF	0 (0)	5 (12.8)	0.23		
AS	0 (0)	2 (5.1)	0.46		
Predisposing factor; n/N (%)					
None	2 (2)	18 (46.2)	0.16		
Infection	6 (60)	13 (33.3)	0.12		
Drug	1 (10)	11 (28.2)	0.23		

CRP: C-reactive protein; IQR: interquartile range; ESR: erythrocyte sedimentation rate; GFR: glomerular filtration rate; SII: systemic immune–inflammation index; BVAS: Birmingham vasculitis activity score; FMF: familial Mediterranean fever; AS: ankylosing spondylitis; AZA: azathioprine; CYC: cyclophosphamide; MP: methylprednisolone; PR: prednisolone; SD: standard deviation.

Table 5. Factors associated with infections that required hospitalization.

	Serious Infection (+) N = 8	Serious Infection (−) N = 41	p-Value
Age; mean ± SD	46 ± 15.3	65 ± 13.3	***0.002***
Gender; n/N (%)			
Male	5 (62)	25 (61)	0.931
Female	3 (38)	16 (39)	0.942
Comorbidities; n/N (%)			
Type 2 DM	4 (50)	11 (23)	0.072
FMF	1 (12.5)	4 (9.8)	0.601
AS	0 (0)	2 (4.9)	0.694
Total steroid exposure (gr); mean ± SD	3.6 ± 1.2	3.1 ± 1.7	0.382
First steroid-tapering agent used; n/N (%)			
CYC	3 (37)	12 (29)	0.68
AZA	2 (25)	18 (43.9)	0.444
MMF	2 (25)	1 (2.4)	0.062
Renal conditions during the follow-up period; n/N (%)			
NRP	3 (37.5)	5 (12.2)	0.113
AKI	5 (62.5)	9 (22)	***0.02***
CKD	2 (25)	2 (4.9)	0.125

SD: standard deviation; FMF: familial Mediterranean fever; AS: ankylosing spondylitis; CYC: cyclophosphamide; MMF: mycophenolate mofetil; NRP: nephrotic-range proteinuria; AKI: acute kidney injury; DM: diabetes mellitus; AZA: azathioprine; CKD: chronic kidney disease.

4. Discussion

It is generally accepted that renal involvement is more common and severe in adults with IgAV compared to children and is a major determinant of long-term morbidity and mortality [10]. The main management strategies of IgAVN are aimed at preventing the development of ESRD. In previous studies, the rate of ESRD in adult patients with IgAVN has been reported to be between 11% and 27% [16–19]. These ESRD rates seem to be comparable to those of ANCA-associated vasculitides (granulomatous polyangiitis and microscopic polyangiitis) and lupus nephritis [20,21]. In our study, only one (2%) patient developed ESRD. There may be several reasons for the lower rate of ESRD in this study. In previous studies, a significant proportion of patients (<40%) did not receive immunosuppressives other than glucocorticoids, whereas in this study, 87% of the patients received immunosuppressives in addition to the initial glucocorticoid treatment; the majority of previous studies had a retrospective design, whereas this study was prospective; patients were followed up closely at 3-month intervals and treatment changes were implemented promptly; and this study had a relatively shorter follow-up period (median of 22 months).

In cases of vasculitic renal involvement, it is crucial to define renal remission in clinical practice. However, there is not yet an internationally accepted definition of renal remission for IgAVN. Some previous studies have defined remission as the absence of proteinuria and hematuria with a stable GFR, while others have defined remission based on proteinuria alone. We believe that the dose of glucocorticoids used should be considered when defining renal remission, and we included the glucocorticoid dose in the definition of remission in this study. The remission rates were 86% at 12 months and 87% overall in this cohort. Previous studies have reported short-term remission rates of 10%-76.9% and long-term rates of 20%-80.8% [14,19,22,23]. Differences in the definition of remission, the lack of standardized treatment regimens, and genetic and geographical factors may be responsible for these different remission rates. It is clear that there is a need for internationally accepted, standardized remission definitions. Knowledge of the factors associated with remission rates and unfavorable renal outcomes may have implications for treatment and follow-up planning. In this study, NRP was a negative risk factor for achieving remission at 12 months. There is a paucity of studies that have examined the factors that influence long-term remission in IgAVN patients. However, a study published in 2019 by J Tan et al. revealed that IgAVN patients with nephrotic syndrome had lower remission and higher ESRD rates than others, which is similar to the findings of our study [24].

At the end of this study, 20% of the patients had unfavorable outcomes. In previous studies, an advanced age, the presence of hypertension, some histopathological findings (endocapillary proliferation, glomerular sclerosis and necrosis, and tubular atrophy and fibrosis), decreased GFR and proteinuria >1 g/day at presentation, and the presence of nephrotic syndrome were associated with unfavorable outcomes [18,24–27]. In our cohort, the rate of proteinuria >1 gr/day at presentation, the rate of NRP, and the five-factor score were significantly higher in the group of patients with unfavorable outcomes; in addition, the remission rates at 12 months were lower and the total glucocorticoid exposure was higher in this group. However, the multivariate regression analysis revealed only the presence of NRP as an independent risk factor for unfavorable outcomes. An elevated creatinine level and a low GFR at presentation have been highlighted as being associated with unfavorable outcomes in several previous studies [16,17,25]. In this study, there was no difference in unfavorable outcomes between patients with and without a low GFR at presentation; we believe this is related to the early and effective immunosuppressive treatment, given our high remission rates.

Looking at the treatment data in this study, all the patients received glucocorticoid therapy at different doses and for different durations, and 87% of the patients also received immunosuppressive therapy. In fact, it is still unclear how to treat adult patients with IgAVN. There are no high-level evidence-based studies on the efficacy of oral or intravenous pulse glucocorticoid therapy in adult patients with IgAVN. Data on the benefit of glucocorticoid therapy in IgAVN come from studies in children or patients with IgA nephropathy [28–30]. In 1998, Niaudet P and Habib R reported the clinical and histopathological benefits of pulse methylprednisolone in a study conducted with 38 pediatric patients with crescentic glomerulonephritis and nephrotic syndrome, although there was no control group in the study [30]. In our study, 53% of the patients received intravenous pulse methylprednisolone (methylprednisolone, >250 mg/day). There was no significant difference between the pulse methylprednisolone and non-pulse groups in terms of the 12-month remission rates and the overall unfavorable outcomes. In this study, AZA was the most frequently preferred drug as the first-line glucocorticoid-sparing agent, followed by CYC and MMF. There are no studies revealing that AZA is effective in adult patients with IgAVN, although it is a frequently preferred drug for these patients. Limited data on the efficacy of AZA come from studies with a low level of evidence in pediatric patients [31,32]. Similarly, although the literature data on MMF are limited, two retrospective studies conducted in China have previously reported that MMF may be beneficial in adult patients with IgAVN [23,33]. In our cohort, 33% of the patients received MMF as the glucocorticoid-sparing agent. Although CYC is now a relatively less preferred drug in rheumatic diseases than in the past due to the risk of toxicity, it is recommended as a first-line drug because of its potency and rapid effect in severe life- or organ-threatening diseases (e.g., ANCA-associated vasculitis and lupus nephritis) [34,35]. The efficacy of CYC in adult patients with IGAVN has not been demonstrated in the limited number of previous studies [22,36]. However, the current KDIGO guidelines recommend the use of CYC in combination with steroids in the presence of rapidly progressive glomerulonephritis *(RPGN)* in patients with IgAVN [14]. In our cohort, 44% of the patients receiving CYC presented with AKI, 73% had crescent formation (<50%) on renal biopsies, the mean proteinuria level was 2.3 g/day, 25% had an unfavorable outcome, and 13% developed stage G3a CKD. These data suggest that clinicians may prefer CYC in cases with severe disease at presentation. There was no significant difference in the remission rates or unfavorable outcomes between the selected first-line glucocorticoid-sparing agent groups. Frankly, there are no specific guidelines for the treatment of adult IgAVN. In the current KDIGO guideline, IgAVN is included with IgAN to a limited extent. It is emphasized that these recommendations apply only to renal involvement and are largely based on data from studies of IgAN. However, the guideline recommends strict blood pressure control and lifestyle modification for at least 3 months with ACEis/ARBs (angiotensin-converting enzyme inhibitors/angiotensin receptor blockers) prior to steroid treatment for IgAN without RPGN, and the same recommendation is made for IgAVN. Despite the similarity in the histopathological findings, the clinical courses of these two diseases are very different. Even in the absence of RPGN, this recommendation worries rheumatologists. It is clear that more disease-specific studies are needed to formulate recommendations with high-level evidence for the treatment of IgAVN [14].

In systemic vasculitis, it is very important for clinicians to objectively determine disease- and treatment-related damage. There are no studies in the literature that have investigated disease/treatment-related damage in adult patients with IgAVN. However, Gazel U et al. published a study on the assessment of damage in patients with IgAV in 2020. In that study, the VDI score was used to perform a damage assessment; in total, 24.7% of the patients had at least one damage item, and the damage was related to the disease itself rather than the treatment [37]. In this study, the VDI was also used to perform a disease/treatment-related damage assessment. A total of 22% of the patients had at least one damage item. The total glucocorticoid exposure was significantly higher in the high-damage score group than in the no-damage group. However, high damage scores were more related to the disease than to the treatment (64% vs. 36%).

In previous reports of adult IgAVN cohorts, serious infection rates have been reported to be between 2% and 4% [16,22,23]. In this study, during the follow-up period, 16% of our patients developed infections that required hospitalization. There was no difference between patients with and without serious infections in terms of the total glucocorticoid exposure and the glucocorticoid-tapering agents used. However, patients who developed serious infections were significantly older than those who did not, and the rate of AKI at presentation was significantly higher in this group. It is known that AKI creates an immunosuppressive status, and infections are important causes of mortality during the recovery period in patients with an AKI [38,39]. In a study published in 2016, Hong S et al. showed that the mortality was higher in patients with late-onset IgAV compared with early-onset patients and that infections were an important cause of mortality [40]. The higher rate of serious infections in this study compared to previous studies may be explained by the more frequent use of immunosuppressives and the more effective doses. Literature data on this issue are very limited and more detailed studies are needed. In previous studies, the relapse rate in patients with IgAVN has been reported to vary between 13% and 22.6% [23,33,40]. In this study, the relapse rate was 6%. Similarly to remission, a standardized definition for relapse has not been established to date. Differences in the definition of relapse and the treatments administered may explain the variable relapse rates. In our cohort, one patient died from sepsis and another patient died from a heart attack. The patient who died from sepsis was not in remission and was receiving renal replacement therapy. In the cohort analysis published by Pillebout E et al. in 2002, the mortality rate was 26% after 14.8 years of follow-up. This was a high rate, and the most common cause of mortality was cancer [17]. Subsequently, Coppo R et al. reported a mortality rate of 5.1% in a cohort with a follow-up of 5.5 years in 2006; Oh HJ et al. reported a rate of 2.2% in a cohort with a follow-up of 5.2 years in 2012; and Guan Y et al. reported a rate of 7.4% in a cohort with a follow-up of 8.5 years in 2023 [19,41,42]. The most common causes of death were cancer/cerebrovascular attack, unknown causes, and infections, respectively. It was striking that cancer was the leading cause of mortality and that disease-related complications were in the background. It is clear that more comprehensive studies are needed to determine the factors associated with mortality in patients with IgAVN.

Our study has some limitations. Only 55% of the patients included in the study had a renal biopsy, which may have influenced the clinicians' treatment preferences or the histopathological findings that affected the prognosis. The cohort consisted of a relatively small number of patients, resulting in wide confidence intervals for the parameters found to be significant in the regression analyses. Finally, there was no control group for the treatment groups.

5. Conclusions

These results suggest that contrary to popular belief, the renal prognosis of adults with IgVAN is not poor if they receive effective immunosuppressive therapy. The presence of NRP is associated with low remission rates, and it has predictive value for unfavorable outcomes. Patients with NRP should be followed-up more closely and treated more stringently. Effective immunosuppressive treatment and close follow-up can achieve high remission rates and significantly reduce the risk of ESRD in adults with IgAVN, but immunosuppressive therapy may also carry a high risk of infection, particularly in the elderly. It is clear that further prospective controlled trials are needed for the rational management of adult patients with IgAVN. Future research should focus on the treatment of different subgroups (for the elderly, in cases of nephrotic disease, etc.).

Supplementary Materials: The following supporting information can be downloaded at: https://www.mdpi.com/article/10.3390/diagnostics15080957/s1, Table S1: Histopathological features of the patients. Dataset S1: Dataset form.

Author Contributions: Conceptualization: F.Y. and M.E.K.; methodology: F.Y. and B.İ.; formal analysis: Y.Ç.; investigation: F.Y.; resources: F.Y.; data curation: F.Y., Y.Ç., K.K., G.A., D.S.Ö., B.K., G.G.Ö. and R.D.; writing—original draft preparation: F.Y.; writing—review and editing: C.B.; supervision: C.B. All authors have read and agreed to the published version of the manuscript.

Funding: This research received no external funding.

Institutional Review Board Statement: This study was conducted in accordance with the Declaration of Helsinki and was approved in 9 January 2022 by the ethics committee (Decision number: KAEK/2022.11.361) of Başakşehir Çam and Sakura City Hospital, İstanbul, Turkey.

Informed Consent Statement: Informed consent was obtained from all the subjects involved in this study.

Data Availability Statement: The data can be provided by the authors upon request, with the removal of identifiable information and the anonymization of dates.

Conflicts of Interest: The authors declare no conflicts of interest.

References

1. Jennette, J.C.; Falk, R.J.; Bacon, P.A.; Basu, N.; Cid, M.C.; Ferrario, F.; Flores-Suarez, L.F.; Gross, W.L.; Guillevin, L.; Hagen, E.C.; et al. Revised international chapel hill consensus conference nomenclature of vasculitides. *Arthritis Rheum.* **2013**, *65*, 1 11. [CrossRef] [PubMed]
2. Hočevar, A.; Rotar, Z.; Ostrovršnik, J.; Jurčić, V.; Vizjak, A.; Dolenc Voljč, M.; Lindič, J.; Tomšič, M. Incidence of IgA vasculitis in the adult slovenian population. *Br. J. Dermatol.* **2014**, *171*, 524–527. [CrossRef] [PubMed]
3. Watts, R.A.; Jolliffe, V.A.; Grattan, C.E.; Elliott, J.; Lockwood, M.; Scott, D.G. Cutaneous vasculitis in a defined population—clinical and epidemiological associations. *J. Rheumatol.* **1998**, *25*, 920–924. [PubMed]
4. García-Porrúa, C.; González-Gay, M.A. Comparative clinical and epidemiological study of hypersensitivity vasculitis versus henoch-schönlein purpura in adults. *Semin. Arthritis Rheum.* **1999**, *28*, 404–412. [CrossRef]
5. Parums, D.V. A Review of IgA vasculitis (henoch-schönlein purpura) past, present, and future. *Med. Sci. Monit.* **2024**, *30*, e943912. [CrossRef]
6. Davin, J.C.; Coppo, R. Henoch-schönlein purpura nephritis in children. *Nat. Rev. Nephrol.* **2014**, *10*, 563–573. [CrossRef]
7. Hilhorst, M.; van Paassen, P.; van Breda Vriesman, P.; Cohen Tervaert, J.W. Immune complexes in acute adult-onset henoch-schonlein nephritis. *Nephrol. Dial. Transpl.* **2011**, *26*, 3960–3967. [CrossRef]
8. Rieu, P.; Noël, L.H. Henoch-schönlein nephritis in children and adults. morphological features and clinicopathological correlations. *Ann. Med. Interne.* **1999**, *150*, 151–159.
9. Calvo-Río, V.; Loricera, J.; Mata, C.; Martín, L.; Ortiz-Sanjuán, F.; Alvarez, L.; González-Vela, M.C.; González-Lamuño, D.; Rueda-Gotor, J.; Fernández-Llaca, H.; et al. Henoch-schönlein purpura in northern spain: Clinical spectrum of the disease in 417 patients from a single center. *Medicine* **2014**, *93*, 106–113. [CrossRef]
10. Rostoker, G. Schönlein-henoch purpura in children and adults: Diagnosis, pathophysiology and management. *BioDrugs* **2001**, *15*, 99–138. [CrossRef]
11. Lu, S.; Liu, D.; Xiao, J.; Yuan, W.; Wang, X.; Zhang, X.; Zhang, J.; Liu, Z.; Zhao, Z. Comparison between adults and children with henoch-schönlein purpura nephritis. *Pediatr. Nephrol.* **2015**, *30*, 791–796. [CrossRef] [PubMed]
12. Ruperto, N.; Ozen, S.; Pistorio, A.; Dolezalova, P.; Brogan, P.; Cabral, D.A.; Cuttica, R.; Khubchandani, R.; Lovell, D.J.; O'Neil, K.M.; et al. EULAR/PRINTO/PRES criteria for henoch-schönlein purpura, childhood polyarteritis nodosa, childhood wegener granulomatosis and childhood takayasu arteritis: Ankara 2008. part i: Overall methodology and clinical characterisation. *Ann. Rheum. Dis.* **2010**, *69*, 790–797. [CrossRef] [PubMed]
13. KDIGO 2024 Clinical practice guideline for the evaluation and management of chronic kidney disease. *Kidney Int.* **2024**, *105*, S117–S314. [CrossRef] [PubMed]
14. KDIGO 2021 Clinical practice guideline for the management of glomerular diseases. *Kidney Int.* **2021**, *100*, S1–S276. [CrossRef]

15. Khwaja, A. KDIGO Clinical practice guidelines for acute kidney injury. *Nephron. Clin. Pract.* **2012**, *120*, c179–c184. [CrossRef]
16. Coppo, R.; Mazzucco, G.; Cagnoli, L.; Lupo, A.; Schena, F.P. Long-term prognosis of henoch-schönlein nephritis in adults and children. Italian group of renal immunopathology collaborative study on henoch-schönlein purpura. *Nephrol. Dial. Transpl.* **1997**, *12*, 2277–2283. [CrossRef]
17. Pillebout, E.; Thervet, E.; Hill, G.; Alberti, C.; Vanhille, P.; Nochy, D. Henoch-schönlein purpura in adults: Outcome and prognostic factors. *J. Am. Soc. Nephrol.* **2002**, *13*, 1271–1278. [CrossRef]
18. Shrestha, S.; Sumingan, N.; Tan, J.; Alhous, H.; McWilliam, L.; Ballardie, F. Henoch schönlein purpura with nephritis in adults: Adverse prognostic indicators in a UK population. *QJM* **2006**, *99*, 253–265. [CrossRef]
19. Coppo, R.; Andrulli, S.; Amore, A.; Gianoglio, B.; Conti, G.; Peruzzi, L.; Locatelli, F.; Cagnoli, L. Predictors of outcome in henoch-schönlein nephritis in children and adults. *Am. J. Kidney Dis.* **2006**, *47*, 993–1003. [CrossRef]
20. Moiseev, S.; Novikov, P.; Jayne, D.; Mukhin, N. End-stage renal disease in ANCA-associated vasculitis. *Nephrol. Dial. Transpl.* **2017**, *32*, 248–253. [CrossRef]
21. Tektonidou, M.G.; Dasgupta, A.; Ward, M.M. Risk of end-stage renal disease in patients with lupus nephritis, 1971-2015: A systematic review and bayesian meta-analysis. *Arthritis Rheumatol.* **2016**, *68*, 1432–1441. [CrossRef] [PubMed]
22. Pillebout, E.; Alberti, C.; Guillevin, L.; Ouslimani, A.; Thervet, E. Addition of cyclophosphamide to steroids provides no benefit compared with steroids alone in treating adult patients with severe henoch schönlein purpura. *Kidney Int.* **2010**, *78*, 495–502. [CrossRef] [PubMed]
23. Ren, P.; Han, F.; Chen, L.; Xu, Y.; Wang, Y.; Chen, J. The combination of mycophenolate mofetil with corticosteroids induces remission of henoch-schönlein purpura nephritis. *Am. J. Nephrol.* **2012**, *36*, 271–277. [CrossRef] [PubMed]
24. Tan, J.; Tang, Y.; Xu, Y.; Yan, S.; Xu, Y.; Tan, L.; Zhong, Z.; Tarun, P.; Qin, W. The clinicopathological characteristics of henoch-schönlein purpura nephritis with presentation of nephrotic syndrome. *Kidney Blood Press. Res.* **2019**, *44*, 754–764. [CrossRef]
25. Huang, X.; Wu, X.; Le, W.; Hao, Y.; Wu, J.; Zeng, C.; Liu, Z.; Tang, Z. Renal prognosis and related risk factors for henoch-schönlein purpura nephritis: A chinese adult patient cohort. *Sci. Rep.* **2018**, *8*, 5585. [CrossRef]
26. Yun, D.; Kim, D.K.; Oh, K.-H.; Joo, K.W.; Moon, K.C.; Kim, Y.S.; Lee, K.; Han, S.S. MEST-C Pathological score and long-term outcomes of child and adult patients with henoch-schönlein purpura nephritis. *BMC Nephrol.* **2020**, *21*, 33. [CrossRef]
27. Hočevar, A.; Ostrovršnik, J.; Jurčić, V.; Tomšič, M.; Rotar, Ž. Short-term outcome of patients with adult iga vasculitis: A single-center experience. *Front. Med* **2023**, *10*, 1210307. [CrossRef]
28. Lv, J.; Wong, M.G.; Hladunewich, M.A.; Jha, V.; Hooi, L.S.; Monaghan, H.; Zhao, M.; Barbour, S.; Jardine, M.J.; Reich, H.N.; et al. Effect of oral methylprednisolone on decline in kidney function or kidney failure in patients with IgA nephropathy: The testing randomized clinical trial. *JAMA* **2022**, *327*, 1888–1898. [CrossRef]
29. Ronkainen, J.; Koskimies, O.; Ala-Houhala, M.; Antikainen, M.; Merenmies, J.; Rajantie, J.; Ormälä, T.; Turtinen, J.; Nuutinen, M. Early prednisone therapy in henoch-schönlein purpura: A randomized, double-blind, placebo-controlled trial. *J. Pediatr.* **2006**, *149*, 241–247. [CrossRef]
30. Niaudet, P.; Habib, R. Methylprednisolone pulse therapy in the treatment of severe forms of schönlein-henoch purpura nephritis. *Pediatr. Nephrol.* **1998**, *12*, 238–243. [CrossRef]
31. Bergstein, J.; Leiser, J.; Andreoli, S.P. Response of crescentic henoch-schoenlein purpura nephritis to corticosteroid and azathioprine therapy. *Clin. Nephrol.* **1998**, *49*, 9–14. [PubMed]
32. Foster, B.J.; Bernard, C.; Drummond, K.N.; Sharma, A.K. Effective therapy for severe henoch-schonlein purpura nephritis with prednisone and azathioprine: A clinical and histopathologic study. *J. Pediatr.* **2000**, *136*, 370–375. [CrossRef] [PubMed]
33. Han, F.; Chen, L.; Ren, P.; Le, J.; Choong, P.; Wang, H.; Xu, Y.; Chen, J. Mycophenolate mofetil plus prednisone for inducing remission of henoch-schönlein purpura nephritis: A retrospective study. *J. Zhejiang. Univ. Sci. B* **2015**, *16*, 772–779. [CrossRef] [PubMed]
34. Hellmich, B.; Sanchez-Alamo, B.; Schirmer, J.H.; Berti, A.; Blockmans, D.; Cid, M.C.; Holle, J.U.; Hollinger, N.; Karadag, O.; Kronbichler, A.; et al. EULAR recommendations for the management of ANCA-associated vasculitis: 2022 update. *Ann. Rheum. Dis.* **2024**, *83*, 30–47. [CrossRef]
35. Fanouriakis, A.; Kostopoulou, M.; Andersen, J.; Aringer, M.; Arnaud, L.; Bae, S.-C.; Boletis, J.; Bruce, I.N.; Cervera, R.; Doria, A.; et al. EULAR recommendations for the management of systemic lupus erythematosus: 2023 update. *Ann. Rheum. Dis.* **2024**, *83*, 15–29. [CrossRef]
36. Audemard-Verger, A.; Terrier, B.; Dechartres, A.; Chanal, J.; Amoura, Z.; Le Gouellec, N.; Cacoub, P.; Jourde-Chiche, N.; Urbanski, G.; Augusto, J.F.; et al. Characteristics and management of IgA vasculitis (henoch-schönlein) in adults: Data from 260 patients included in a french multicenter retrospective survey. *Arthritis Rheumatol.* **2017**, *69*, 1862–1870. [CrossRef]
37. Gazel, U.; Colak, S.; Sari, A.; Cansu, D.Ü.; Yazici, A.; Cefle, A.; Bes, C.; Karadag, O.; Omma, A.; Direskeneli, H.; et al. Damage assessment in adult IgA vasculitis. cross-sectional results of a multicentre cohort. *Clin. Exp. Rheumatol.* **2020**, *38* (Suppl. S124), 155–160.
38. Gist, K.M.; Faubel, S. Infection post-AKI: Should we worry? *Nephron* **2020**, *144*, 673–676. [CrossRef]

39. Griffin, B.R.; You, Z.; Holmen, J.; SooHoo, M.; Gist, K.M.; Colbert, J.F.; Chonchol, M.; Faubel, S.; Jovanovich, A. Incident infection following acute kidney injury with recovery to baseline creatinine: A propensity score matched analysis. *PLoS ONE* **2019**, *14*, e0217935. [CrossRef]
40. Hong, S.; Ahn, S.M.; Lim, D.H.; Ghang, B.; Yang, W.S.; Lee, S.K.; Kim, Y.G.; Lee, C.K.; Yoo, B. Late-onset IgA vasculitis in adult patients exhibits distinct clinical characteristics and outcomes. *Clin. Exp. Rheumatol.* **2016**, *34* (Suppl. S97), S77–S83.
41. Oh, H.J.; Ahn, S.V.; Yoo, D.E.; Kim, S.J.; Shin, D.H.; Lee, M.J.; Kim, H.R.; Park, J.T.; Yoo, T.H.; Kang, S.W.; et al. Clinical outcomes, when matched at presentation, do not vary between adult-onset henöch-schönlein purpura nephritis and IgA nephropathy. *Kidney Int.* **2012**, *82*, 1304–1312. [CrossRef] [PubMed]
42. Guan, Y.; Liu, S.; Hao, C.M.; Lai, L. Effect of nonimmune factors on renal prognosis in adult IgA vasculitis with nephritis: A long-term retrospective cohort study. *J. Rheumatol.* **2023**, *50*, 1032–1038. [CrossRef] [PubMed]

diagnostics

MDPI

Case Report

Hepatic Vascular Involvement in Adenosine Deaminase 2 Deficiency (DADA2): Case Reports and Literature Review †

Mihaela Sparchez [1,2,*], Laura Damian [3], Mihai Adrian Socaciu [4], Otilia Fufezan [2] and Zeno Sparchez [5]

1 Second Pediatric Discipline, "Iuliu Hatieganu" University of Medicine and Pharmacy, 400177 Cluj-Napoca, Romania
2 Emergency Clinical Hospital for Children Cluj-Napoca, 4000370 Cluj-Napoca, Romania
3 Department of Rheumatology, Emergency County Clinical Hospital Cluj, 400006 Cluj-Napoca, Romania
4 Department of Medical Imaging, "Iuliu Hatieganu" University of Medicine and Pharmacy, 400162 Cluj-Napoca, Romania
5 Department of Internal Medicine, "Iuliu Hatieganu" University of Medicine and Pharmacy, 400162 Cluj-Napoca, Romania
* Correspondence: mihaelaspirchez@gmail.com

† Meeting Abstract. Proceedings of the 23rd Paediatric Rheumatology European Society Congress: Part One, Genoa, Italy, 28 September–1 October 2016.

Abstract

Background and Clinical Significance: Deficiency of Adenosine Deaminase 2 (DADA2) is a rare monogenic vasculopathy characterised by systemic inflammatory and immunodeficiency features. Although neurological and haematological manifestations are well-documented, hepatic vascular involvement remains underappreciated. This report aims to describe the clinical and imaging characteristics of hepatic vascular involvement in a patient with DADA2 and to illustrate the evolution of hepatic lesions during long-term Etanercept therapy. In addition, we provide a synthesis of the available evidence on hepatic manifestations in DADA2, emphasising vascular pathology, clinical presentation, and therapeutic implications. **Case Presentation:** We describe a girl with early-onset DADA2 presenting with recurrent systemic inflammation, hypogammaglobulinaemia, vasculopathy, and two childhood strokes, followed by the development of multiple FNH-like hepatic nodules on CEUS and MRI with persistently elevated GGT. Genetic testing confirmed biallelic ADA2 mutations, and treatment with Etanercept led to sustained clinical stabilisation and marked regression of liver lesions over a nine-year follow-up period. Her older sister, carrying the same mutations, showed a milder phenotype without hepatic involvement but experienced a mesenteric vascular event. **Conclusions**: Large regenerative nodules with an FNH-like appearance on CEUS or MRI have not been previously reported in this setting. In our patient, Etanercept therapy produced a favourable hepatic response, reflected by a significant reduction in both the number and size of the lesions. Our case contributes to the understanding of liver disease in DADA2 and the influence of imaging and treatment on the hepatic manifestations of the condition.

Keywords: deficiency of adenosine deaminase 2; hepatic vascular involvement; nodular regenerative hyperplasia; FNH-like lesions; portal hypertension; vasculitis; immunodeficiency

1. Introduction

Deficiency of Adenosine Deaminase 2 (DADA2) is a monogenic autoinflammatory and immunodeficiency disorder first described in 2014 [1]. Caused by biallelic mutations in the

ADA2 gene (*CECR1*), DADA2 is characterised by systemic vasculopathy, recurrent fever, immunodeficiency, cytopenias, and variable organ involvement [1]. While neurological, haematological, and rheumatological manifestations have been extensively reported, hepatic involvement remains less well-characterised [2,3]. Nevertheless, emerging evidence suggests that hepatic vascular manifestations—including nodular regenerative hyperplasia, hepatoportal sclerosis, portal hypertension, and Budd–Chiari syndrome [4,5]—are an underrecognized but significant component of the DADA2 phenotype.

Meyts and Aksentijevich (2018) [2] and Lee et al. (2022) [3] provided comprehensive reviews of the clinical spectrum of DADA2, highlighting multi-organ vasculopathy but only briefly mentioning hepatic manifestations. More systematic phenotypic surveys, such as those by Barron et al. (2021) [4] and Maccora et al. (2023) [5], have explicitly documented hepatic involvement, reporting hepatomegaly, elevated liver enzymes, and biopsy findings of vascular pathology.

The vasculopathy associated with this rare monogenic disorder primarily affects small- and medium-sized arteries. Biallelic loss-of-function mutations in the ADA2 gene cause immune dysregulation, leading to a skewed macrophage polarisation towards a pro-inflammatory M1 phenotype, endothelial dysfunction, and increased TNF-α production. This results in inflammation of the vessel walls, necrosis, and subsequent vascular occlusion or aneurysm formation [2,3].

Histological data from cohorts and case series reveal a recurring pattern of vascular injury in the liver (compromised endothelial integrity, endothelial cellular activation and inflammation) [1]. Barron et al. (2021) [4] reported that 12% of patients developed portal hypertension, with biopsy findings including nodular regenerative hyperplasia (NRH), hepatoportal sclerosis, and portal vasculopathy. Springer et al. (2018) [6] similarly identified NRH as a key lesion, implicating small-vessel injury as a central pathogenic mechanism. Zhou et al. (2014) [1] included patients with liver biopsy evidence of vascular inflammation in their seminal description of DADA2, providing early evidence of hepatic involvement.

Nodular regenerative hyperplasia (NRH) denotes a diffuse transformation of the hepatic parenchyma into multiple small regenerative nodules, characterised by the absence of fibrosis. It involves the entire liver and can lead to non-cirrhotic portal hypertension. This condition probably stems from intrahepatic microvascular injury and hypoperfusion, which cause hepatocyte injury and the formation of regenerative nodules. Histologically, it is characterised by numerous small regenerative nodules separated by compressed hepatic plates, with no fibrous septa [7,8].

In NRH, regenerative nodules typically measure 1–3 mm in diameter, although larger lesions—up to 1–2 cm—may also occur. These have been referred to as large regenerative nodules or multiacinar regenerative nodules, defined histologically as regenerative nodules containing more than one portal tract [9,10]. Some of these larger nodules exhibit imaging characteristics similar to focal nodular hyperplasia (FNH) and are therefore described as FNH-like lesions [11]. According to current literature, there is no clear consensus on whether these lesions represent a variant of large regenerative nodules (LRN) or a distinct pathological entity [11]. FNH-like lesions have been described in children in association with a variety of liver conditions that alter hepatic perfusion and increase arterial inflow, including Budd–Chiari syndrome [11], congestive hepatopathy, Fontan-associated liver disease [12], sinusoidal obstruction syndrome after chemotherapy or hematopoietic stem cell transplantation [13], autoimmune hepatitis [11,14], cavernous transformation of the portal vein, hereditary hemorrhagic telangiectasia, and common variable immunodeficiency [11].

To date, no cases of focal nodular hyperplasia-like (FNH-like) hepatic lesions have been explicitly reported in patients with DADA2.

https://doi.org/10.3390/diagnostics16020189

Mechanistically, hepatic manifestations seem to reflect the systemic vasculopathy linked to DADA2. Endothelial dysfunction, TNF-driven vascular inflammation, and defective perivascular repair mechanisms have been described (Lee et al. 2022) [3]. The liver, with its dual blood supply and dense sinusoidal network, may be particularly vulnerable to microvascular injury, leading to reactive or regenerative lesions and non-cirrhotic portal hypertension.

Literature evidence is extremely sparse on Budd–Chiari syndrome (BCS) associated with DADA2, suggesting it is a rare or underreported condition.

Clinically, hepatic involvement in DADA2 ranges from asymptomatic enzyme abnormalities to overt complications of non-cirrhotic portal hypertension and end-stage liver disease. However, elevated liver enzymes and hepatosplenomegaly are the most common clinical signs of liver-related disease [1,15,16]. Barron et al. (2021) [4] observed that liver fibrosis was detectable by transient elastography in approximately 25% of cases, while 7 of 56 patients developed portal hypertension with clinical consequences such as splenomegaly and varices. Colangelo et al. (2023) [17] described a striking case of Budd–Chiari syndrome, demonstrating that hepatic venous outflow obstruction can also occur. Case series from Iran (Ashari et al. 2023) [18] and other international cohorts have reported hepatomegaly, elevated transaminases, and hepatosplenomegaly in subsets of patients.

The diagnosis of NRH is often difficult because its histopathologic features may be interpreted variably, and most patients lack specific symptoms or laboratory abnormalities [14]. It may, however, be accompanied by slightly elevated ALP and gamma-glutamyltransferase levels, with a gradual increase over the years leading to chronic cholestasis, non-cirrhotic portal hypertension, or cirrhosis [11].

This article aims to synthesise current evidence on hepatic vascular involvement in DADA2, delineate key patterns, and discuss clinical implications, while adding a novel observation to the hepatic phenotype of the disease: large regenerative nodules of focal nodular hyperplasia appearance (FNH-like) in one patient and a favourable evolution of these lesions under anti-TNF therapy.

2. Case Presentation

2.1. Case 1

The first case involved a girl born to non-consanguineous parents and with no significant pathology in the family.

At 1.66 years of age, she suddenly presented with a high fever, a nonspecific maculopapular rash, arthralgia, and myalgia, accompanied by elevated levels of acute phase reactants and a rapid response to steroids. One year later, these symptoms recurred. A skin biopsy revealed interstitial granulomatous dermatitis associated with vasculopathy.

At the age of 3, she began experiencing recurrent cranial nerve palsies and livedo reticularis, followed by two stroke events at age 4—one ischemic and the other hemorrhagic. Magnetic resonance angiography revealed no signs of cerebral vasculitis, and a brain biopsy performed during the surgical procedure for the hemorrhagic stroke showed only extravasation of erythrocytes and fibrin deposition around small vessels without significant inflammation. The antibody profile was negative, including antinuclear antibodies, antineutrophil cytoplasmic antibodies, autoantibodies associated with autoimmune hepatitis, and antiphospholipid antibodies. Additionally, clotting tests were within the normal range.

Hypogammaglobulinemia with global immunoglobulin deficiency was present from the onset of the disease and persisted over time. She could not be classified as having common variable immunodeficiency (CVID) because her total serum IgG levels were not

https://doi.org/10.3390/diagnostics16020189

consistently below 500 mg/dL. As part of a research study, she was also found to have a complete C4B deficiency.

At the age of 5, she developed moderate thrombocytopenia that persisted for the following 3 years.

At 5.5 years of age, ultrasound revealed multiple diffuse hyperechoic hepatic lesions measuring 1–2 cm and mild splenomegaly. On contrast-enhanced ultrasound (CEUS), the lesions exhibited arterial-phase hyperenhancement with centrifugal filling and became isoenhancing during the portal and late phases (Figure 1). These features were interpreted as consistent with large regenerative nodules of focal nodular hyperplasia-like appearance (FNH-like). At this stage, serum GGT levels were elevated and remained persistently high, peaking at 120 U/L. Serum transaminases (AST and ALT) were only slightly elevated, with ALT sometimes remaining within the normal range.

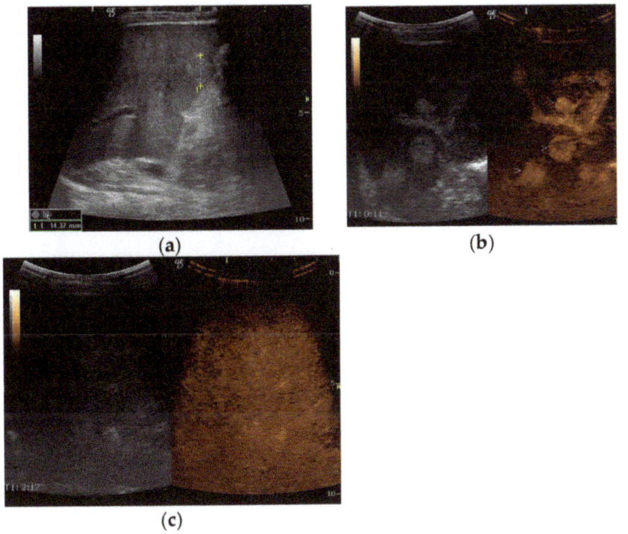

(a) (b) (c)

Figure 1. Initial ultrasound (US) of the liver before treatment. (**a**) Grey-scale US showing a hyperechoic nodule in the right lobe; (**b**) Contrast-enhanced ultrasound (CEUS). Arterial phase. Multiple round hyperenhancing nodules in the right lobe (marked with the symbol '>' on the image); (**c**) CEUS in parenchymal phase. The nodules are isoenhanced and no longer detectable.

MRI showed multiple hyperenhancing focal lesions visible in the arterial phase, disseminated throughout the entire hepatic parenchyma; most were isointense on T2w and native T1w images, iso- or hyperintense in the late phase, with no washout. The lesions were relatively similar in size (10–25 mm) and imaging features (Figure 2).

A liver biopsy was not performed at that time due to the increased risk of bleeding given our patient's thrombocytopenia, the absence of severe liver damage or other risk factors for primary liver malignancies and typical radiologic features of FNH-like nodules.

During the first two years of her condition, only high doses of corticosteroids were effective in controlling the disease manifestations. Treatments such as methotrexate, azathioprine, cyclosporine, and cyclophosphamide proved ineffective. In contrast, mycophenolate mofetil (MMF) combined with high monthly doses of intravenous immunoglobulin led to prompt and sustained improvements in clinical symptoms and acute-phase reactants, allowing for a gradual reduction in steroid dosage. With MMF treatment, no recurrences were observed; however, the FNH-like lesions showed slow progression.

https://doi.org/10.3390/diagnostics16020189

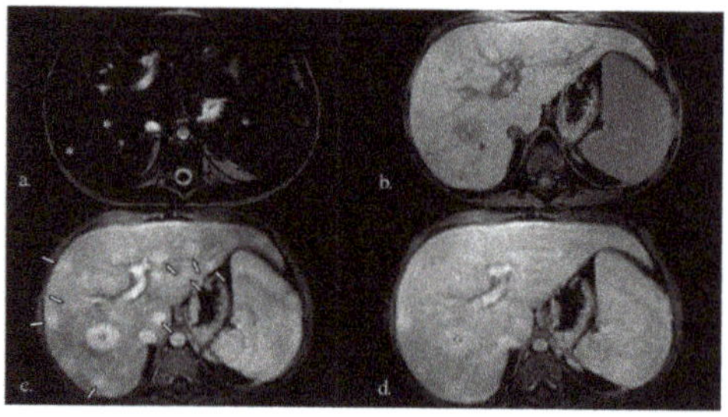

Figure 2. Initial MRI examination of the liver. (**a**) Native T2-weighted; (**b**) Native fat-saturated T1-weighted; Gd-enhanced fat-saturated T1-weighted in the arterial (**c**) and late (**d**) phases. Multiple hyperenhancing focal lesions are visible in the arterial phase (arrows, asterisks), most are isointense on T2w and native T1w images, iso- or hyperintense in the late phase, with no washout. The lesions are relatively similar in size (10 to 25 mm) and imaging features. Two of the lesions (asterisks) are slightly hyperintense on T2w and hypointense on native T1w, while still enhancing after Gd injection.

At the age of 8, genetic testing revealed two homozygous pathogenic mutations in the ADA2 gene (*p.G326R* and *p.V458D*). Plasma ADA2 enzyme activity was notably low, measured at 3 mU/mL/h. The patient was commenced on Etanercept, which effectively controlled systemic inflammation, thrombocytopenia, and vascular symptoms. Over the following 9 years, no neurological events occurred. She is hemiparetic due to the previous stroke, and some disease features persist, including hypogammaglobulinemia and livedo reticularis.

Remarkably, under anti-TNF treatment, there has been a significant improvement in liver lesions, as evidenced by reductions in both their size and number on repeated liver imaging (Figures 3 and 4), along with normalisation of GGT levels in subsequent years. Improvement was evident after just one year of treatment and continued to progress until the patient reached 17 years of age. Splenomegaly persisted without evidence of portal hypertension, and liver stiffness on elastography decreased slightly over time (6.1 kPa before Etanercept and 5.6 kPa after treatment).

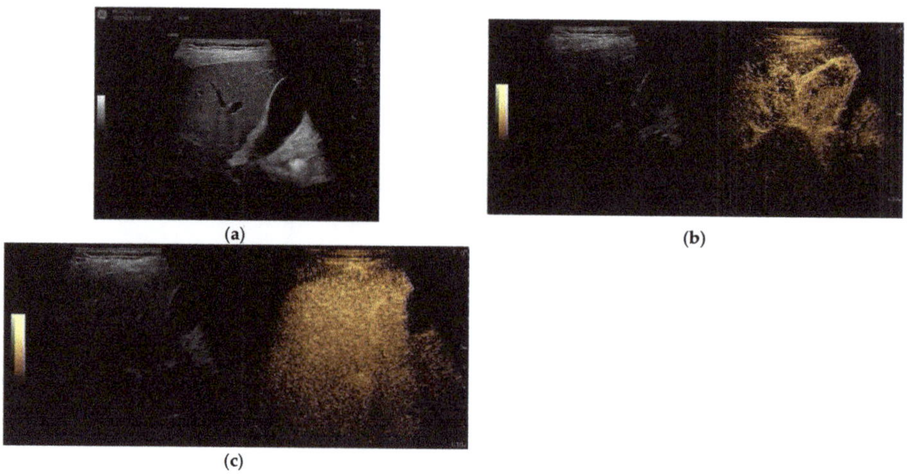

Figure 3. Ultrasound (US) evaluation after 9 years of Etanercept treatment. (**a**) B Mode US shows no evident liver nodules; (**b**) Contrast-enhanced ultrasound (CEUS) arterial phase shows an inhomogeneous pseudonodular enhancement of the right lobe; (**c**) CEUS in parenchymal phase—no hypoenhanced nodules are seen.

https://doi.org/10.3390/diagnostics16020189

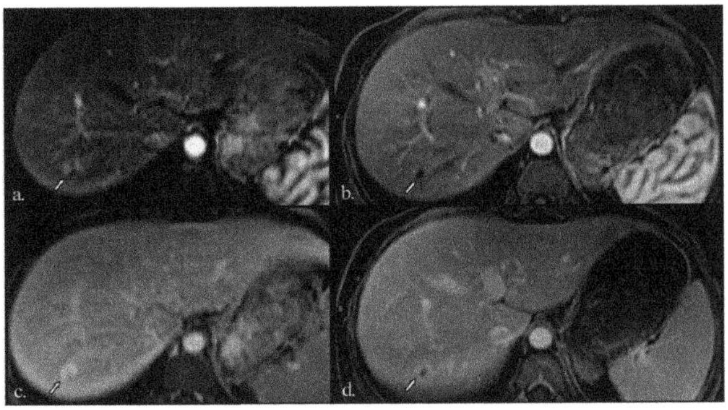

Figure 4. Subsequent MRI examinations after 5 years (**a**,**c**) and 9 years (**b**,**d**) of Etanercept treatment since the initial assessment. Gd-enhanced fat-saturated T1-weighted images in the arterial (**a**,**b**) and late (**c**,**d**) phases. Only one lesion (arrow) remains visible, showing hyperenhancement in the periphery and a central scar with progressive, incomplete filling in the late phases. The lesion has shrunk in the last examination.

The timeline (Figure 5) shows the progression of disease manifestations, liver involvement, and treatment response in patient 1.

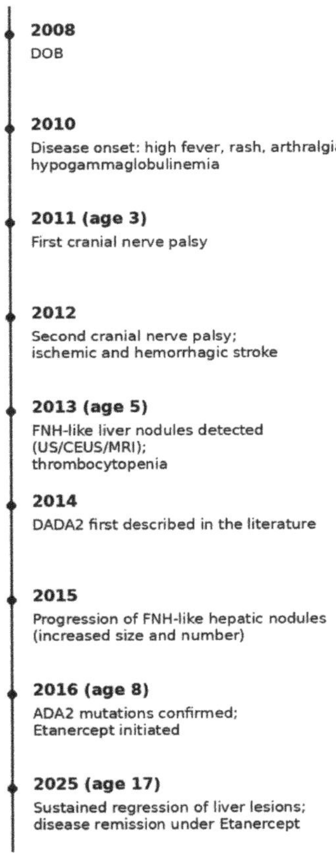

Figure 5. Concise timeline of disease progression, liver involvement, and treatment response in Patient 1 with DADA2.

https://doi.org/10.3390/diagnostics16020189

2.2. Case 2

The older sister of the patient described above, who shares the same homozygous pathogenic mutations in the ADA2 gene, exhibited a later onset of clinical symptoms (at 6.5 years old), including persistent fever, myalgia, livedo reticularis, vascular purpura, painful subcutaneous nodules, systemic arterial hypertension, recurrent abdominal pain, and a highly persistent inflammatory response. In her case, the immunodeficiency phenotype appeared milder, with slightly reduced IgM levels and normal IgG and IgA levels. She did not show any hepatic vascular involvement of the disease, nor did she develop neurological symptoms. However, at 7.5 years of age, she experienced a massive intestinal bleed, preceded by acute abdominal pain, considered a vascular complication affecting the mesenteric vessels. The source of the bleeding was not identified on endoscopic and imaging studies. At the last assessment, during ongoing Etanercept treatment, patient 2 was in persistent clinical remission with no new complications.

3. Discussion

The literature indicates that hepatic vascular involvement is a significant yet often overlooked aspect of DADA2. While neurological and haematological symptoms are predominant, up to one-third of patients may exhibit biochemical, radiological, or histopathological signs of liver disease. The most consistent observation across reports is nodular regenerative hyperplasia, indicating noncirrhotic portal hypertension due to small vessel vasculopathy. Cases of Budd–Chiari syndrome highlight that hepatic venous outflow obstruction can also occur, extending the spectrum of hepatic features.

No prior reports have documented focal nodular hyperplasia-like (FNH-like) lesions in DADA2, highlighting the novelty of this observation within the disease's hepatic spectrum.

The underestimation of liver involvement probably arises from two factors: firstly, subtle or subclinical hepatic disease can be missed without systematic screening; secondly, the multisystem impact of DADA2 may overshadow hepatic symptoms in clinical practice. Nevertheless, the clinical significance is considerable. Portal hypertension carries risks such as variceal bleeding, hypersplenism, and reduced quality of life. Moreover, progressive liver disease may persist despite TNF inhibition, raising questions about the timing of treatment and the possible role of hematopoietic stem cell transplantation in refractory cases.

Comparative analysis with other systemic vasculopathies shows that hepatic involvement in DADA2 is unique in its frequent presentation as non-cirrhotic portal hypertension, rather than typical inflammatory hepatitis. This emphasises the vascular, rather than parenchymal, nature of hepatic injury in DADA2.

Nodular regenerative hyperplasia of the liver occurs in patients with the immunodeficiency phenotype of DADA2, as well as in those with hypogammaglobulinaemia disorders, particularly common variable immunodeficiency (CVID). NRH is the characteristic hepatic lesion in CVID, and relevant parallels with DADA2 have been drawn regarding this liver complication [8,14]. This relationship is also observed in our siblings. Only the one with significant hypogammaglobulinemia developed large regenerative nodules of focal nodular hyperplasia-like appearance (FNH-like), even though they share the same homozygous pathogenic mutations in the ADA2 gene.

Structural changes related to NRH can be detected on imaging studies such as ultrasound, CT or MRI; however, the radiologic findings are often nonspecific, and a definitive diagnosis typically requires clinical correlation and histopathologic confirmation [7,19,20]. FNH-like lesions, in contrast, exhibit more distinctive and characteristic imaging features than smaller regenerative nodules, which sometimes allow a confident radiologic diagnosis when interpreted in the proper clinical context [11,13].

https://doi.org/10.3390/diagnostics16020189

Grey-scale ultrasound detection of NRH is challenging, particularly for an inexperienced sonographer, because nodules are usually small and commonly isoechoic, and they affect the entire hepatic parenchyma diffusely. Moreover, in our patient, many larger nodules were identified with CEUS, highlighting its additional value in evaluating such cases.

Contrast-enhanced ultrasound has been sporadically explored for evaluating NRH. Evidence is limited to isolated case reports [21]. Due to the diffuse and micronodular nature of NRH, the technique lacks sensitivity and specificity. CEUS may occasionally reveal non-specific or misleading enhancement patterns, so its findings should always be interpreted in conjunction with clinical data, cross-sectional imaging, and histopathological confirmation. Currently, no validated CEUS criteria are available for the identification of NRH.

Larger hepatic lesions, such as those resembling focal nodular hyperplasia (FNH), can be more accurately characterised using CEUS. These lesions typically exhibit intense centrifugal arterial-phase enhancement, followed by isoechoic enhancement during the portal venous and delayed phases [22]. The development of advanced CEUS techniques, together with higher-resolution contrast agents and emerging microbubble or molecular contrast media, is expected to improve the detection and characterisation of microvascular alterations seen in nodular regenerative hyperplasia (NRH).

In our patient, CEUS provided additional value in characterising the hepatic lesions. The presence of larger, hyperenhancing nodules with centrifugal arterial-phase filling and isoenhancement in the portal and late phases was consistent with FNH-like regenerative nodules. Depending on the clinical context, however, malignant lesions should be considered in the differential diagnosis.

Magnetic resonance imaging (MRI) supports the assessment of liver nodules. While more sensitive than ultrasound in detecting subtle parenchymal heterogeneity, MRI findings in NRH are often nonspecific, typically showing diffuse reticular or micronodular enhancement without a dominant mass or fibrous septa. These features help differentiate NRH from cirrhosis and focal nodular hyperplasia; however, histological confirmation remains crucial for an accurate diagnosis [7,20].

Conversely, larger or macro regenerative nodules (LRN) or FNH-like lesions show arterial hyperenhancement but no late-phase washout. They are typically similar in native and post-contrast features to FNH nodules, which are mostly found in adult women. Still, they are usually multiple, relatively homogeneous in size, and seem to have arterial flow overexpression as the leading cause. Usual MRI features of these nodules include: iso- to hypointensity on T2-weighted (T2w) images, iso- to hyperintensity natively on T1w images, no diffusion restriction, homogenous or "spoke-wheel" enhancement in the Gd-enhanced arterial phase, and no wash-out in the venous and late phase. A central scar with arterial hypoenhancement and late-phase enhancement can also be common [11,23]. The use of hepato-biliary contrast (i.e., Gadoxetic acid) will show either isoenhancement or hyperenhancement in the hepato-biliary phase, which can help distinguish from hepatocellular carcinoma or liver adenoma (where some wash-out is to be expected in the hepato-biliary phase) [11,13,24,25].

Considering current evidence, the most recent consensus recommends abdominal ultrasonography with Doppler as the primary imaging modality for evaluating the liver and spleen in DADA2. This approach reflects recognition that patients may develop noncirrhotic portal hypertension and vascular or inflammatory hepatic lesions, including focal nodular hyperplasia and nodular regenerative hyperplasia [26].

An MRI was also performed in our patient to provide a more detailed characterisation of the hepatic nodules. Multiple hyperenhancing focal lesions were identified during the arterial phase; most appeared isointense on T2-weighted and native T1-weighted images

https://doi.org/10.3390/diagnostics16020189

and iso- to hyperintense in the late phase, without evidence of washout. The nodules were relatively uniform in size and imaging appearance. Typical native and post-contrast features consistent with FNH were present in most lesions, except for two nodules that were T1 hypointense and T2 hyperintense. This finding suggests some heterogeneity among large regenerative nodules that do not always conform to classical imaging patterns. Given that these nodules also regressed during follow-up under therapy, they are unlikely to represent a different pathology. The native T1 hypointensity and T2 hyperintensity most likely reflect increased water content within the lesions, without a specific underlying cause.

Although suggested by magnetic resonance imaging or ultrasound scan, diagnosis must be histologically confirmed [14]. Being an invasive procedure with an increased risk of bleeding in the context of our patient's thrombocytopenia and in the absence of severe liver damage, the liver biopsy was withheld in the first year after the diagnosis. After TNF inhibitors demonstrated effectiveness in reducing the number of nodules and their size, the procedure was no longer considered beneficial for the patient.

In the absence of histologic confirmation, alternative diagnoses were considered. Malignant hepatic nodules may complicate conditions associated with liver fibrosis (such as Budd–Chiari syndrome), but they are rare in autoimmune-related liver disease. Other benign entities, including hepatic hemangiomatosis or biliary hamartomas, were unlikely, as they would typically exhibit markedly hyperintense T2-weighted signals. The longitudinal evolution under Etanercept therapy, however, provides more substantial support for DADA2-related regenerative nodules.

Available data suggest that anti-TNF agents (Etanercept, Adalimumab, or Infliximab) significantly improve survival and overall disease control in DADA2, although their effect on hepatic involvement remains inconsistent. Data from the National Human Genome Research Institute shows that TNF inhibition decreases systemic inflammation and improves endothelial integrity in blood vessels, and may even reverse endothelial damage at the clinical, molecular, and histological levels [27].

While anti-TNF therapy has transformed the prognosis of DADA2 patients, its impact on hepatic manifestations remains uncertain. Some reports suggest stabilisation of liver disease with anti-TNF therapy, while others document progression of portal hypertension despite systemic disease control (Table 1) [4,6,28]. This raises the possibility that hepatic injury, once established, may be irreversible or only partially responsive to treatment.

Table 1. Anti-TNF therapy and hepatic outcomes in DADA2.

Study/ Source	Year	No. of Patients	Hepatic Manifestation(s)	Effect of Anti-TNF Therapy	Comments/Notes
Barron et al. [4]	2021	60	Portal hypertension, nodular regenerative hyperplasia, increased liver stiffness	Mixed outcomes: some stabilisation, others progression despite systemic disease control	Liver stiffness improved in a few cases; portal hypertension persisted or worsened in others
Springer et al. [6]	2018	2 adult siblings	NRH, end-stage liver disease	One patient improved systemically; another developed irreversible hepatic failure	Suggests established liver damage may be refractory to TNF inhibition
Ombrello et al. [28]	2015	24 (NIH cohort)	Hepatomegaly, vascular involvement	Reported stabilisation in some hepatic findings; no detailed long-term data	Early report supporting TNF blockade as mainstay, without liver-specific endpoints

https://doi.org/10.3390/diagnostics16020189

Table 1. *Cont.*

Study/ Source	Year	No. of Patients	Hepatic Manifestation(s)	Effect of Anti-TNF Therapy	Comments/Notes
Lee et al. [26]	2023	Consensus/ review	Multisystem vasculopathy (hepatic manifestations included)	Effective for vasculitic and hematologic features; hepatic response uncertain	Highlights lack of controlled data on hepatic disease progression
Deuitch et al. [27]	2022	Mechanistic study	endothelial cell model	TNF inhibition restores endothelial function in vitro	Supports biological plausibility, but no clinical hepatic outcomes reported

One reported DADA2 patient exhibited clinical symptoms from early childhood, including primary vasculopathy, hypogammaglobulinaemia, a history of stroke, and liver disease [6]. He was diagnosed in his 40s and began Etanercept, which proved effective in controlling the disease activity. However, he died 18 months after his initial DADA2 diagnosis and one year after starting Etanercept, due to complications related to end-stage liver disease (nodular regenerative hyperplasia of the liver with portal hypertension and varices). In this case, the NHGRI group observed intact endothelial layers in postmortem brain and lung biopsies, suggesting that anti-TNF therapy was effective in those vascular territories. However, it does not demonstrate a definitive clinical effect on portal hypertension [27]. Overall, this case demonstrates the importance of early diagnosis and treatment to minimise organ damage and prevent life-threatening complications in patients with DADA2.

While a recent consensus on the evaluation and management of DADA2 patients emphasises the benefit of anti-TNF therapy for vascular/neurologic disease, the authors state that evidence for efficacy against non-vascular manifestations (including hepatic disease) is more limited [26].

In our patient, the FNH-like lesions showed an early positive response after starting Etanercept, with a noticeable decrease in both the size and number of nodules. This improvement was maintained, as imaging performed nine years into continuous anti-TNF therapy showed substantial regression of the hepatic nodules. To our knowledge, this is the first documented case of FNH-like liver lesions in DADA2 that show long-term improvement with anti-TNF treatment.

Available data—mostly from small cohorts and case reports—underscore the need for prospective, liver-focused monitoring of DADA2 patients receiving TNF inhibitors.

4. Conclusions

Hepatic vascular involvement represents a clinically significant yet frequently underrecognised component of the DADA2 phenotype. Diffuse nodular liver infiltration—consistently reported as regenerative nodular hyperplasia—has been described in some patients with the immunodeficiency phenotype of DADA2, underscoring the need for systematic liver evaluation. NRH-type involvement should be considered in individuals with abnormal liver function tests and features of portal hypertension, with biopsy required for confirmation.

Large regenerative nodules with an FNH-like appearance on CEUS or MRI have not previously been documented in this setting. In our patient, Etanercept therapy produced a favourable hepatic response, reflected by a significant reduction in both the number and size of the lesions. Our case contributes to the understanding of liver disease in DADA2 and the influence of imaging and treatment on the hepatic manifestations of the condition.

https://doi.org/10.3390/diagnostics16020189

Author Contributions: M.S. developed the manuscript and contributed to the clinical evaluation, diagnostic work-up, and treatment management of the patients. Z.S. provided US and CEUS monitoring of our patient and offered expertise with imaging considerations. L.D. contributed to long-term follow-up and took over patient care after the transition to adult services. M.A.S. and O.F. contributed to the acquisition and analysis of the magnetic resonance images. All authors have read and agreed to the published version of the manuscript.

Funding: This research received no external funding.

Institutional Review Board Statement: Not applicable, being a descriptive, not an interventional case report.

Informed Consent Statement: Written informed consent has been obtained from the patients for publication of this paper.

Data Availability Statement: The original contributions presented in this study are included in the article. Further inquiries can be directed to the corresponding author.

Acknowledgments: We thank all contributors involved in the diagnosis, imaging evaluation, and therapeutic management of these patients. This article is a revised and expanded version of a conference paper [29], which was presented as a poster at the 23rd Paediatric Rheumatology European Society Congress, Genoa, Italy, 28 September–1 October 2016.

Conflicts of Interest: The authors declare no conflicts of interest.

Abbreviations

The following abbreviations are used in this manuscript:

DADA2	Deficiency of adenosine deaminase 2
FNH	Focal nodular hyperplasia
CEUS	Contrast-enhanced ultrasound
US	Ultrasound
MRI	Magnetic resonance imaging
TNF	Tumour Necrosis Factor
GGT	Gamma-glutamyl transpeptidase
NRH	Nodular regenerative hyperplasia

References

1. Zhou, Q.; Yang, D.; Ombrello, A.K.; Zavialov, A.V.; Toro, C.; Stone, D.L.; Chae, J.J.; Rosenzweig, S.D.; Bishop, K.; Barron, K.S.; et al. Early-onset stroke and vasculopathy associated with mutations in ADA2. *NEIJM* **2014**, *370*, 911–920. [CrossRef]
2. Meyts, I.; Aksentijevich, I. Deficiency of Adenosine Deaminase 2 (DADA2): Updates on the phenotype, genetics, pathogenesis, and treatment. *J. Clin. Immunol.* **2018**, *38*, 569–578. [CrossRef]
3. Lee, P.Y.; Aksentijevich, I.; Zhou, Q. Mechanisms of vascular inflammation in deficiency of adenosine deaminase 2 (DADA2). *Semin. Immunopathol.* **2022**, *44*, 269–280. [CrossRef] [PubMed]
4. Barron, K.S.; Aksentijevich, I.; Deuitch, N.T.; Stone, D.L.; Hoffmann, P.; Videgar-Laird, R.; Soldatos, A.; Bergerson, J.; Toro, C.; Cudrici, C.; et al. The spectrum of the deficiency of adenosine deaminase 2, An observational analysis of a 60-patient cohort. *Front. Immunol.* **2021**, *12*, 811473. [CrossRef]
5. Maccora, I.; Maniscalco, V.; Campani, S.; Carrera, S.; Abbati, G.; Marrani, E.; Mastrolia, M.V.; Simonini, G. A wide spectrum of phenotypes of deficiency of adenosine deaminase 2. *Orphanet J. Rare Dis.* **2023**, *18*, 183. [CrossRef]
6. Springer, J.M.; Gierer, S.A.; Jiang, H.; Kleiner, D.; Deuitch, N.; Ombrello, A.K.; Grayson, P.C.; Aksentijevich, I. Deficiency of Adenosine Deaminase 2 in adult siblings: Many years of a misdiagnosed disease with severe consequences. *Front. Immunol.* **2018**, *9*, 1361. [CrossRef]
7. Hartleb, M.; Gutkowski, K.; Milkiewicz, P. Nodular regenerative hyperplasia: Evolving concepts on underdiagnosed cause of portal hypertension. *World J. Gastroenterol.* **2011**, *17*, 1400–1409. [CrossRef]
8. Barge, S.; Grando, V.; Nault, J.C.; Broudin, C.; Beaugrand, M.; Ganne-Carrié, N.; Roulot, D.; Ziol, M. Prevalence and clinical significance of nodular regenerative hyperplasia in liver biopsies. *Liver Int.* **2016**, *36*, 1059–1066. [CrossRef]

https://doi.org/10.3390/diagnostics16020189

9. Ames, J.T.; Federle, M.P.; Chopra, K. Distinguishing clinical and imaging features of nodular regenerative hyperplasia and large regenerative nodules of the liver. *Clin. Radiol.* **2009**, *64*, 1190–1195. [CrossRef] [PubMed]
10. Ueda, T.; Starkey, J.; Mori, K.; Fukunaga, K.; Shimofusa, R.; Motoori, K.; Minami, M.; Kondo, F. A pictorial review of benign hepatocellular nodular lesions: Comprehensive radiological assessment incorporating the concept of anomalous portal tract syndrome. *J. Hepatobiliary Pancreat. Sci.* **2011**, *18*, 386–396. [CrossRef] [PubMed]
11. Nolan, P.E.; Catania, R.; Vendrami, C.L.; Borhani, A.A.; Miller, F.H. Large Regenerative Nodules and Focal Nodular Hyperplasia-Like Lesions: Definition, Pathogenesis, and Imaging Findings. *Radiol. Clin. N. Am.* **2022**, *60*, 795–808. [CrossRef]
12. Hilscher, M.B.; Wells, M.L.; Venkatesh, S.K.; Cetta, F.; Kamath, P.S. Fontan-associated liver disease. *Hepatology* **2022**, *75*, 1300–1321. [CrossRef]
13. Alfares, B.A.; Sieben, L.; Li, W.; Cervio, G.; Minetto, J.; Sierre, S.; Kaliciński, P.; Markiewicz-Kijewska, M.; Kolesnik, A.; Franchi-Abella, S.; et al. Incidence and risk factors for portal vein complications after pediatric liver transplantation: A retrospective cohort analysis from the PORTAL registry. *Liver Transpl.* **2025**, *Epub ahead of print*. [CrossRef]
14. Pecoraro, A.; Crescenzi, L.; Varricchi, G.; Marone, G.; Spadaro, G. Heterogeneity of Liver Disease in Common Variable Immunodeficiency Disorders. *Front. Immunol.* **2020**, *11*, 338. [CrossRef]
15. Batu, E.D.; Karadag, O.; Taskiran, E.Z.; Kalyoncu, U.; Aksentijevich, I.; Alikasifoglu, M.; Özen, S. Case Series of adenosine deaminase 2-deficient patients emphasizing treatment and genotype-phenotype correlations. *J. Rheumatol.* **2015**, *42*, 1532–1534. [CrossRef] [PubMed]
16. Elkan, P.N.; Pierce, S.B.; Segel, R.; Walsh, T.; Barash, J.; Padeh, S.; Zlotogorski, A.; Berkun, Y.; Press, J.J.; Mukamel, M.; et al. Mutant adenosine deaminase 2 in a polyarteritis nodosa vasculopathy. *NEJM* **2014**, *370*, 921–931. [CrossRef]
17. Colangelo, A.; Tromby, F.; Cafaro, G.; Gerli, R.; Bartoloni, E.; Perricone, C. Vasculitis associated with adenosine deaminase 2 deficiency. *Reumatismo* **2023**, *75*, 144–151. [CrossRef] [PubMed]
18. Ashari, K.A.; Aslani, N.; Parvaneh, N.; Assari, R.; Heidari, M.; Fathi, M.; Sharabian, F.T.; Ronagh, A.; Shahrooei, M.; Moafi, A.; et al. A case series of ten + one deficiency of adenosine deaminase 2 (DADA2) patients in Iran. *Pediatr. Rheumatol.* **2023**, *21*, 55. [CrossRef] [PubMed]
19. Force, J.; Saxena, R.; Schneider, B.P.; Storniolo, A.M.; Sledge, G.W., Jr.; Chalasani, N.; Vuppalanchi, R. Nodular Regenerative Hyperplasia after Treatment with Trastuzumab Emtansine. *J. Clin. Oncol.* **2016**, *34*, e9-12. [CrossRef]
20. Ozaki, K.; Goshima, S. Hyperintense liver lesions on hepatobiliary phase of gadoxetic acid-enhanced magnetic resonance imaging: Clinical insights and significance. *Abdom. Radiol.* **2025**, *Epub ahead of print*. [CrossRef]
21. Caturelli, E.; Ghittoni, G.; Ranalli, T.V.; Gomes, V.V. Nodular regenerative hyperplasia of the liver: Coral atoll-like lesions on ultrasound are characteristic in predisposed patients. *Br. J. Radiol.* **2011**, *84*, e129–e134. [CrossRef] [PubMed] [PubMed Central]
22. Newerla, C.; Schaeffer, F.; Terracciano, L.; Hohmann, J. Multiple FNH-Like Lesions in a Patient with Chronic Budd-Chiari Syndrome: Gd-EOB-Enhanced MRI and BR1 CEUS Findings. *Case Rep. Radiol.* **2012**, *2012*, 685486. [CrossRef] [PubMed]
23. Rousseau, C.; Ronot, M.; Sibileau, E.; Boulay-Coletta, I.; Lewin, M.; Duchatelle, V.; Vilgrain, V.; Zins, M. Central element in liver masses, helpful, or pitfall? *Abdom. Imaging* **2015**, *40*, 1904–1925.
24. Dioguardi Burgio, M.; Ronot, M.; Salvaggio, G.; Vilgrain, V.; Brancatelli, G. Imaging of Hepatic Focal Nodular Hyperplasia: Pictorial Review and Diagnostic Strategy. *Semin. Ultrasound CT MR* **2016**, *37*, 511–524. [CrossRef] [PubMed]
25. Vernuccio, F.; Ronot, M.; Dioguardi Burgio, M.; Cauchy, F.; Choudhury, K.R.; Dokmak, S.; Soubrane, O.; Valla, D.; Zucman-Rossi, J.; Paradis, V.; et al. Long-term Evolution of Hepatocellular Adenomas at MRI Follow-up. *Radiology* **2020**, *295*, 361–372. [CrossRef]
26. Lee, P.Y.; Davidson, B.A.; Abraham, R.S.; Alter, B.; Arostegui, J.I.; Bell, K.; Belot, A.; Bergerson, J.R.E.; Bernard, T.J.; Brogan, P.A.; et al. Evaluation and management of deficiency of adenosine deaminase 2. *JAMA Netw. Open* **2023**, *6*, E2312357. [CrossRef]
27. Deuitch, N.T.; Yang, D.; Lee, P.Y.; Yu, X.; Moura, N.S.; Schnappauf, O.; Ombrello, A.K.; Stone, D.; Kuehn, H.S.; Rosenzweig, S.D.; et al. TNF inhibition in vasculitis management in adenosine deaminase 2 deficiency (DADA2). *J. Allergy Clin. Immunol.* **2022**, *149*, 1812–1816.e6. [CrossRef]
28. Ombrello, A.; Stone, D.; Hoffmann, P.; Jones, A.; Barham, B.; Barron, K.; Flegel, W.; Sheldon, S.; Zhou, Q.; Hershfield, M.; et al. The deficiency of adenosine deaminase type 2-results of therapeutic intervention. *Pediatr. Rheumatol.* **2015**, *13*, O40. [CrossRef]
29. Sparchez, M.; Damian, L.; Sparchez, Z. Severe systemic vasculitis associated with primary immunodeficiency in two siblings. *Pediatr. Rheumatol.* **2017**, *15: 37*, P150, Proceedings of the 23rd Paediatric Rheumatology European Society Congress: Part one. [CrossRef]

https://doi.org/10.3390/diagnostics16020189

MDPI AG
Grosspeteranlage 5
4052 Basel
Switzerland
Tel.: +41 61 683 77 34

Diagnostics Editorial Office
E-mail: diagnostics@mdpi.com
www.mdpi.com/journal/diagnostics

www.ingramcontent.com/pod-product-compliance
Lightning Source LLC
Chambersburg PA
CBHW061614210926
51850CB00009B/2324

Laser Assisted Manufacturing

Guest Editors

Swee Leong Sing
Wai Yee Yeong

MDPI

Basel • Beijing • Wuhan • Barcelona • Belgrade • Novi Sad • Cluj • Manchester

Guest Editors
Swee Leong Sing
Department of Mechanical Engineering
National University of Singapore
Singapore

Wai Yee Yeong
Singapore Centre for 3D Printing
School of Mechanical and Aerospace Engineering
Nanyang Technological University
Singapore

Editorial Office
MDPI AG
Grosspeteranlage 5
4052 Basel, Switzerland

This is a reprint of the Special Issue, published open access by the journal *Quantum Beam Science* (ISSN 2412-382X), freely accessible at: https://www.mdpi.com/journal/qubs/special_issues/laser_assisted.

For citation purposes, cite each article independently as indicated on the article page online and as indicated below:

Lastname, A.A.; Lastname, B.B. Article Title. *Journal Name* **Year**, *Volume Number*, Page Range.

ISBN 978-3-7258-4267-4 (Hbk)
ISBN 978-3-7258-4268-1 (PDF)
https://doi.org/10.3390/books978-3-7258-4268-1

Contents

About the Editors

Swee Leong Sing

Swee Leong Sing is an Assistant Professor at the Department of Mechanical Engineering, National University of Singapore (NUS). Prior to joining NUS in August 2021, he was a Presidential Postdoctoral Fellow at the Singapore Centre for 3D Printing (SC3DP) and School of Mechanical and Aerospace Engineering (MAE), Nanyang Technological University (NTU), Singapore, after being awarded the prestigious fellowship in 2020.

Swee Leong has been active in the 3D printing field. He obtained his BEng (Hons) in Aerospace Engineering and PhD in Mechanical Engineering with a topic in additive manufacturing (AM) in 2012 and 2016, respectively. Swee Leong's research focuses on using advanced manufacturing techniques as enablers for materials development and to create strategic values for the industries. He is also active in inter-disciplinary research and translational work. Swee Leong has worked on numerous 3D printing projects with government agencies, universities, research institutes, and industrial collaborators. Swee Leong has filed five patents pertaining to 3D printing processes and materials. He has published more than 90 peer reviewed journal and conference articles. Swee Leong currently has an h-index of 39 with more than 9000 citations (Web of Science, 30 April 2025).

Wai Yee Yeong

Professor Wai Yee Yeong is the winner of the TCT Women in 3D Printing Innovator Award 2019 and features on the Singapore 100 Women in Tech List 2021. Her work is well-recognized, with an H-index of 73 and more than 23,000 citations on Google Scholar. She has filed multiple patents and knowhows, with a keen interest in Bioprinting and the 3D printing of new materials. On academic fronts, she is the Associate Editor for two international journals and has authored three textbooks on 3D printing. Prof Yeong serves as Program Director in the Singapore Centre for 3D Printing and HP-NTU Digital Manufacturing Corp Lab. Prof Yeong was awarded the NRF Investigatorship (Class of 2022) in her pursuit for groundbreaking and high-risk research. She is also the Chair of the School of Mechanical and Aerospace Engineering at Nanyang Technological University, Singapore.

quantum beam science

MDPI

Article

Blue Diode Laser Welding of Commercially Pure Titanium Foils

Tim Pasang [1,*], Pai-Chen Lin [2], Wojciech Z. Misiolek [3], Jia-Yuan Wei [2], Shinichiro Masuno [4], Masahiro Tsukamoto [4], Eiji Hori [4], Yuji Sato [4], Yuan Tao [5], Danang Yudhistiro [6] and Salahuddin Yunus [6]

1 Department of Mechanical and Manufacturing Engineering and Technology, Oregon Institute of Technology, Klamath Falls, OR 97601, USA
2 AIM-HI, National Chung Cheng University, No. 168, Section 1, Daxue Rd, Minxiong Township Chiayi County 62102, Taiwan; imepcl@ccu.edu.tw (P.-C.L.); k6816512@gmail.com (J.-Y.W.)
3 Loewy Institute, Department of Materials Science and Engineering, Lehigh University, Bethlehem, PA 18015, USA; wzm2@lehigh.edu
4 Joining and Welding Research Institute (JWRI), Osaka University, Osaka 567-0047, Japan; masuno.snicr@gmail.com (S.M.); tukamoto@jwri.osaka-u.ac.jp (M.T.); hori@jwri.osaka-u.ac.jp (E.H.); sato@jwri.osaka-u.ac.jp (Y.S.)
5 Department of Mechanical Engineering, Auckland University of Technology, Auckland 1010, New Zealand; yuan.tao@aut.ac.nz
6 Department of Mechanical Engineering, Universitas Jember, Jember 68121, Jawa Timur, Indonesia; danang.ft@unej.ac.id (D.Y.); salahudin.teknik@unej.ac.id (S.Y.)
* Correspondence: tim.pasang@oit.edu; Tel.: +1-541-851-5262

Abstract: The need for thin foil welding is increasing significantly, particularly in the electronic industries. The technologies that are currently available limit the joining processes in terms of materials and their geometries. In this paper, a series of trials of fusion welding (bead-on- plate) of commercially pure titanium (CPTi) foils were conducted using a blue diode laser (BDL) welding method. The power used was 50 W and 100 W for 0.1 mm and 0.2 mm thick foils, respectively. Following welding, various samples were prepared to examine the weld profiles, microstructures, hardness, tensile strength, and fracture surface characteristics. The results showed that the base metal (BM) had an annealed microstructure with equiaxed grains, while the weld zones contained martensite (α') with large grains. The hardness increased in both regions, from around 123 HV to around 250 HV, in the heat-affected zone (HAZ) and fusion zone (FZ) areas. The tensile tests revealed that the strengths of the welded samples were slightly lower than the unwelded samples, i.e., UTS = 300–350 MPa compared with 325–390 MPa for the unwelded samples. Fracture took place within the BM area. All of the samples, welded and unwelded, showed identical fracture mechanisms, i.e., microvoid coalescence or ductile fracture. The weld zone experienced very small strains (elongation) at fracture, which indicates a good weld quality.

Keywords: blue diode laser (BDL) welding; digital image correlation (DIC); commercially pure titanium (CP Ti); bead-on-plate; mechanical properties; fracture surface

1. Introduction

The blue diode laser (BDL) is one of the laser technologies that is commonly used in applications such as lights for projectors and general lighting. However, many more potential applications are possible in the near future if the laser's power and brightness can be increased [1,2]. A new generation of blue diode laser (BDL) has recently been developed at the Joining and Welding Research Institute (JWRI), Osaka University, in collaboration with Shimadzu Corporation, Japan. The welding machine has a power of up to 100 W and an energy density of 1.3 × 106 W/cm^2 at the end of the output fiber. This new device uses a GaN-based diode [1] and is expected to be used as a light source for various applications, including welding of the so-called difficult-to-weld metals such as gold, copper, and other reflective metals as well as in 3D printing of such metals because blue light can be efficiently absorbed by these metals [1,2]. Given its very small spot beam size, BDL technology can also be applied extensively to thin foil manufacturing, such as in cutting and/or welding processes. Joining (welding) of thin foils has always been required, for example, in battery cell applications [3]. In addition, with a very small spot size, the heat distortion is also minimized, which means post-weld heat treatment to remove residual stresses may not be required [1]. Furthermore, it is also expected to contribute to reducing the processing time and electrical power consumption in these applications, which is not possible with conventional modules. More details about the BDL machine developed at the JWRI can be found in the paper by Tojo et al. [1].

The need for thin foil welding is increasing significantly, particularly in electronic industries. The technologies that are currently available are limiting the joining processes in terms of materials and their geometries. Several welding experiments on thin foils have been reported where the infra-red or direct laser was utilized, but none have reported on titanium foils. Ventrella and co-authors [4] used infra-red laser technology to weld 0.1 mm thick stainless steel 316 L foils. Following the experimental work and analyses, they concluded that the quality of the thin foil weld was good in terms of the mechanical properties. Abe et al. [5] utilized a direct diode laser to weld 0.05 mm SS304 stainless steel without any spatter and reported a nearly equal strength as the un-welded samples. Kim [6] reported their findings following welding of a 0.05 mm thick AM350 stainless steel foil onto SS304 stainless steel with a thickness of 1 mm. They concluded that the beam diameter played a significant role in thin foil welding, and further recommended that a smaller beam diameter would be preferred. Pakmanesh et al. [7] performed a lap joint of a 316 L stainless steel foil using a pulsed Nd:YAG laser to optimize the process parameters. It was concluded that the underfill and undercut increased with the increased power. On the one hand, the underfill increased with a reduced frequency; however, on the other hand, the undercut increased with an increased high frequency. The authors managed to overcome the presence of these defects by superimposing different responses. The above-mentioned welding methods are, however, not suitable for bright and reflective metals such as copper, and gold; therefore, the development of new technology is still needed.

Limited articles have been published on blue laser or blue diode lasers related to welding, cladding, and materials processing, and they are summarized in the following. Das et al. [3] performed welding of multi-layered stainless steel (SS316L) by stacking 20 layers of micro-foils with a thickness of 0.025 mm onto a 0.2 mm thick SS316L foil sandwich and welded them together. They suggested that this welding technique is suitable for industrial needs, especially for electrical micro joining, as it results in free cracks, low porosity, and low spatter. Zediker et al., conducted welding on copper using a blue laser with a power of 500 W and a spot size of 215 μm. They were able to perform welding at an angle of 90°. The authors reported that neither porosity nor spatter was found [8]. In addition, Zediker et al., performed a full penetration bead-on-plate welding on copper with a power of 600 W and a spot size diameter of 200 μm. They concluded that the shorter wavelength, such as that of the blue laser, is well absorbed by copper [9]. Wang et al., used a blue diode laser of 250 W for material processing for successful laser irradiation on a steel sample [10]. Suwa et al., developed a blue laser for processing copper foils and melting copper powder, with a power of 100 W and a core diameter of 100 μm. The blue laser is called BLUE IMPACT, and they stated this new laser technology can improve the manufacturing quality of copper for electronic and automotive applications [11]. Another blue laser that was recently developed was reported by Konning et al., at Coherent DILAS. The authors reported two types of modules, both with a wavelength of 450 nm—one module with 500 W power and a 200 μm core diameter, and the second with 550 W power with a 400 μm core fiber. The intention of this newly developed laser technology was for material processing [12]. The BDL technology at JWRI has been successfully used for cladding pure copper on a stainless steel (SS304) substrate [13,14]. Hummel et al. [15] conducted a feasibility study by conducting micro-welding of copper using a diode laser with a wavelength of 450 nm (no other detail was provided, but presumably a BDL) and 150 W of power. The thickness of the copper samples ranged from 150 μm to 1 mm. It was concluded that the butt and lap joints could be satisfactorily achieved up to a thickness of 500 μm with a speed of up to 10 mm/s. Xu et al. [16] compared the cladding characteristics of copper on martensitic stainless steels using TIG and diode laser methods. They found out the laser cladding had fine microstructures, a narrow heat-affected zone, and excellent wear resistance compared with the TIG method. Separately, Boese et al. [17] reviewed blue laser technology with added power and brightness, and suggested that this technology allowed for welding copper samples and that it also improved the ability to weld dissimilar metals, for example, copper to stainless steels or copper to aluminum alloys.

In this paper, the results from the recent investigation on the welding of CP Ti foils using the BDL welding method are presented. The purpose of this work was to establish if BDL could be applied to the welding of thinner metallic foils and higher welding speeds. At this stage, the focus of the work was on relatively less-bright metals such as titanium to identify the possible parameters for the subsequent welding of the thin copper or gold foils. The microstructure and the strength of the welds were examined. In addition to the hardness and tensile testing results, a digital image correlation (DIC)—a post-processing feature following the tensile testing—was also conducted to gain a better understanding of the weld response to tensile stresses. The fracture surfaces from the tensile testing were also examined with the scanning electron microscope (SEM) and are reported in this paper.

2. Experimental Procedures

2.1. Materials

The material used in this investigation was commercially pure titanium (CP Ti) Grade 2 foil with a thickness of 100 μm and 200 μm. The nominal composition of the material is given in Table 1.

Table 1. Chemical composition of commercially pure titanium (CP Ti) in wt.%.

Material	Ti	Fe	H	N	O	C
CP Ti	Balance	<0.3	<0.015	<0.03	<0.25	<0.1

2.2. Welding Procedures

Bead-on-plate using a blue diode laser welding technique was performed at the Joining and Welding Research Institute (JWRI), Osaka University, Japan. Prior to welding, the foils were cleaned thoroughly with ethanol to ensure they were free from dirt, grease, and other surface contaminations. The system employed up to six diode laser modules with a single module power of around 20 W. The focal spot of the laser light had a top-hat profile of 100 μm diameter. The welding was performed without any filler metal (autogenous) with the following parameters: 50 and 100 W of power and a welding speed of 20 and 30 mm/s for the 100 μm and 200 μm thick foils, respectively, and a wavelength of 450 nm. Note that the speed used in this investigation was 2–3 times higher than what was reported previously [9]. Pure argon gas (purity of up to 99.9%) was used as shielding with a flow of 25 L/min. The welding heat input was estimated to be between 1 and 5 J/mm.

The schematic diagram of the BDL welding used in this investigation is given in Figure 1. More details about the BDL system at JWRI have been provided by Sato et al. [13] and Asano et al. [14].

2.3. Metallography

For the microstructural and microhardness examinations, metallographic samples were prepared from the welded specimens. The samples were cut in the normal to the welding direction. They were mounted in a conductive bakelite resin. The mounted samples were ground using SiC paper up to 2400 grit size and were polished down to 0.05 μm using colloidal silica on polishing cloths. The polished samples were etched with

Kroll's reagent (100 mL H_2O + 2 mL HF + 5 mL HNO_3) and were examined using an Olympus BX51M optical microscope to characterize the microstructures.

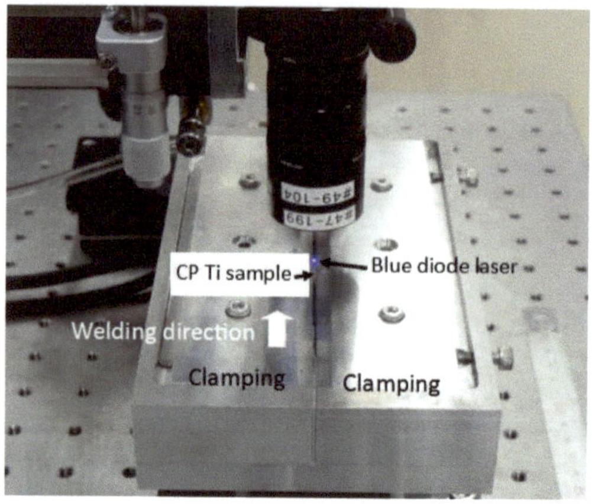

Figure 1. Blue diode laser (BDL) welding set up.

2.4. Mechanical Testing

2.4.1. Microhardness

To produce the hardness profiles, micro-hardness tests were conducted on the polished and etched samples using a Vickers machine (Leco AMH 55, St. Joseph, MI, USA) with a load of 50 g and a dwell time of 10 s. Indentations were made on the base metal (BM), heat-affected zone (HAZ), and the fusion zone (FZ). The results were then plotted to determine the hardness profiles.

2.4.2. Tensile Testing

Tensile testing was conducted on dog bone-shaped samples using the Shimadzu Universal Testing Machine model AG-IS (Shimadzu, Kyoto, Japan) with a crosshead speed of 0.07 mm/s. Three samples were tested for each welding condition. The dimensions of the samples are shown in Figure 2. The tensile testing machine used was equipped with a digital image correlation (DIC) system with a couple of 5.0 Megapixel CCD cameras. This non-contact technique was employed to measure the overall strain, its distribution, and the local strain gradients at the fracture locations. The post-processing of the DIC was performed and analyzed using the VIC-3D system (Correlated Solutions, Irmo, SC 29063, USA).

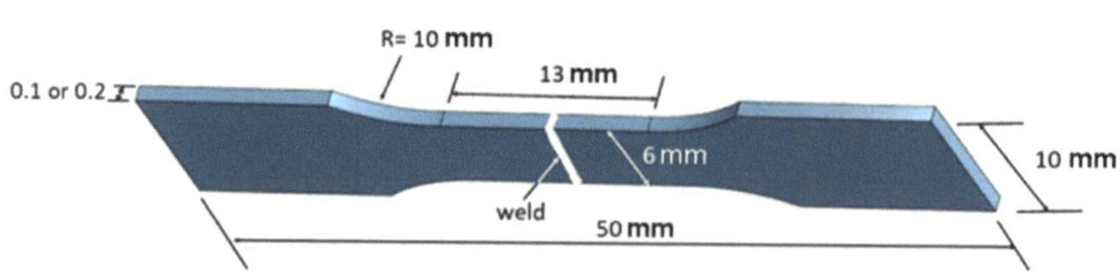

Figure 2. Schematic diagram of the dog-bone sample with dimensions (in mm).

2.4.3. Fracture Surface Examination

A scanning electron microscope (SEM), Hitachi SU70 (Hitachi High-Technologies Corporation, Minato-ku, Tokyo, Japan), was employed to study the fracture surfaces following tensile testing. The samples were prepared using ultrasonic cleaning for 10 min using ethanol prior to the SEM examinations.

3. Results and Discussions

The general appearance of the CP Ti foils with weldments are shown in Figure 3.

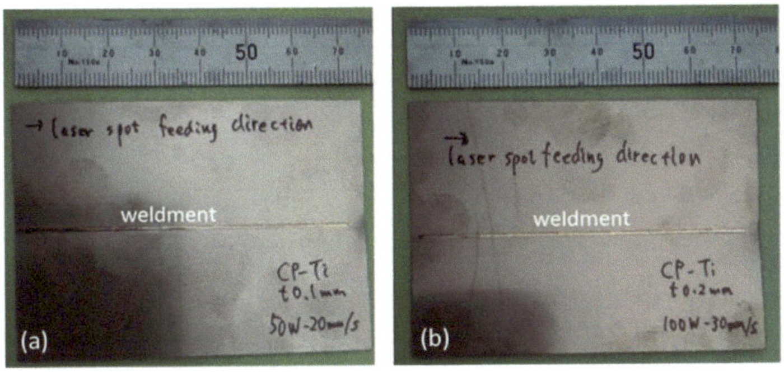

Figure 3. Welded CP Ti foils: (**a**) 100 μm thick and (**b**) 200 μm thick.

A full penetration bead-on-plate was achieved for both foils (Figures 3 and 4) with the parameters indicated in Section 2.2. The weldments showed a V-shaped configuration for the FZ and HAZ zones (Figure 4). The width of the weldments was up to 450 μm and 200 μm on the face and the root surfaces for the 100 μm thick foil, and up to 700 μm and 250 μm for the 200 μm thick foil for the face and root surfaces, respectively. It is also worth mentioning that there was very little distortion during metallography handling of the weldments. The slight bend of the 0.1 mm sample (Figure 4a) might be due to the handling of the sample after welding or during the metallography sample preparation.

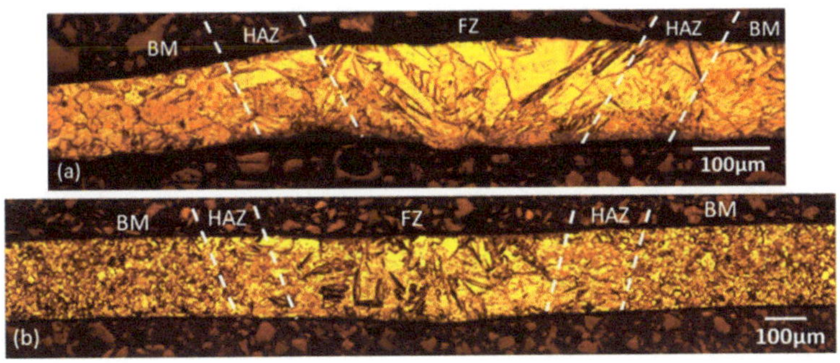

Figure 4. Optical micrographs showing weld profiles: (**a**) 100 μm thick welded with 50 W of power and at a speed of 20 mm/s, and (**b**) 200 μm thick welded with 100 W of power and at a speed of 30 mm/s.

The microstructure of the base metal showed an annealed structure with equiaxed grains (Figure 4). They were approximately between 5 and 10 μm in diameter. In the FZ area, the grains were fairly large, i.e., up to 20 μm in width and 100 μm in length. The grain size in the HAZ was smaller than for the grains in the FZ, but larger than in the BM area. A few cases of twin grains were also observed within the base metal and the weld zones. It was also noted that the weld zones, particularly in FZ (Figure 5), contained the α' structure (martensite), which is the main strengthening element in titanium alloys, including the high-grade CP Ti used in this investigation [18–25]. In addition, lamellar α phases were also present in the weld zone, especially in the FZ area [18,23,24]. More detailed information regarding the microstructures of CP Ti welds can be found in Danielson et al. [18] and Lathabai et al. [22].

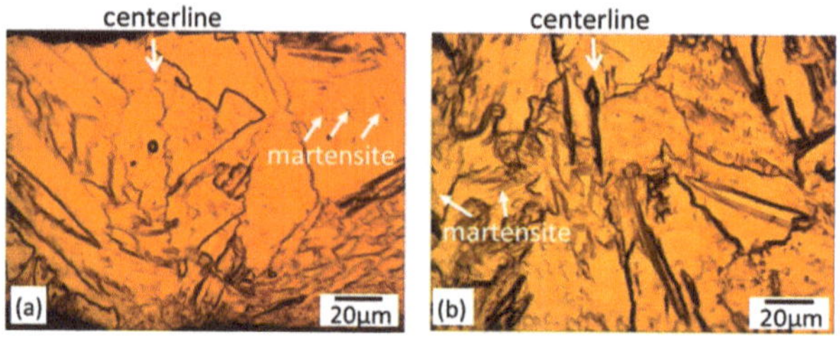

Figure 5. High magnification optical micrographs showing the weld centerlines and martensite (α′) phase on the (**a**) 100 μm thick foil welded with 50 W of power and at a speed 20 mm/s, and the (**b**) 200 μm thick foil welded with 100 W of power and at a speed of 30 mm/s.

The results from the microhardness testing showed that HAZ and FZ had higher hardness compared with the base metal (Figures 6 and 7). This probably is due to the presence of α′ (martensite) in WZ. The presence of α′ is associated with a fast cooling rate because both samples were fairly thin. Danielson et at. reported an increase in the weld zone area due to a high oxygen content [18]. In addition, the hardness of the 100 μm thick foil on the HAZ area increased earlier than that of the 200 μm thick foil due to its thinner size; hence, it had arguably faster cooling rates and more martensite (α′) compared with the later foil.

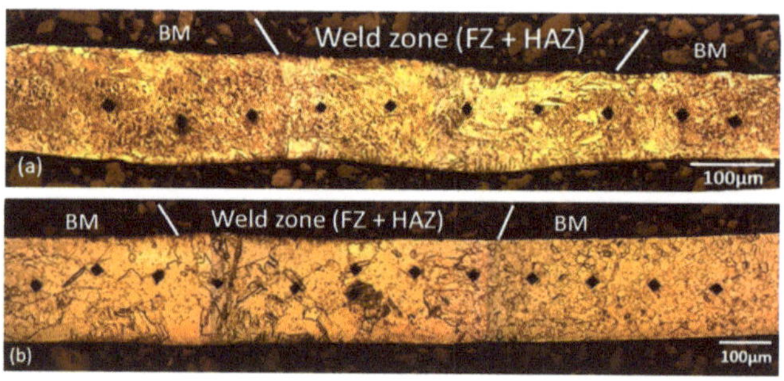

Figure 6. Hardness indentations on metallographically prepared samples: (**a**) 100 μm and (**b**) 200 μm thick foil samples.

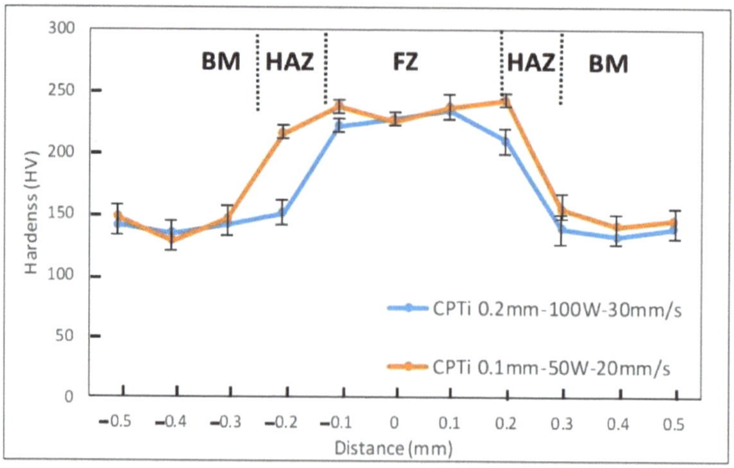

Figure 7. Hardness profiles of the welded samples for two different foils.

The tensile testing results are presented in Table 2. The results from the DIC analysis are presented in Figures 8–11.

Table 2. Tensile data of both the welded (BOP) and unwelded samples.

Material	Thickness (µm)	Power (Watt)	Welding Speed (mm/s)	Yield Strength (MPa)	Tensile Strength (MPa)	Elongation (%)	Fracture Location
CP Ti (BOP)	100	50	20	140	300	20	BM
				145	306	20	BM
				148	305	22	BM
CP Ti (BOP)	200	100	30	310	355	23	BM
				300	350	25	BM
				301	350	25	BM
CP Ti unwelded	100	N/A	N/A	170	325	24	N/A
	200	N/A	N/A	320	390	28	N/A

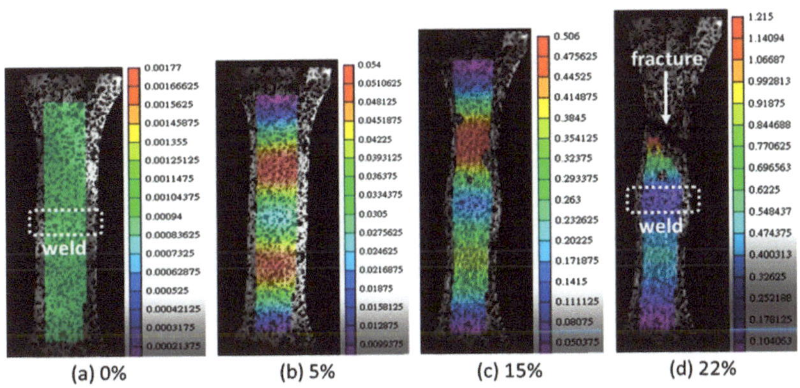

Figure 8. Pictures from digital image correlation (DIC) of CP Ti, 100 µm, 50 W, and 20 mm/s during tensile testing showing sample conditions at various percentages of strain (**a**) at 0%, (**b**) 5%, (**c**) 15%, and (**d**) 22%, which correspond to fracture. Note: the numbers associated with the images are local strains × 100%.

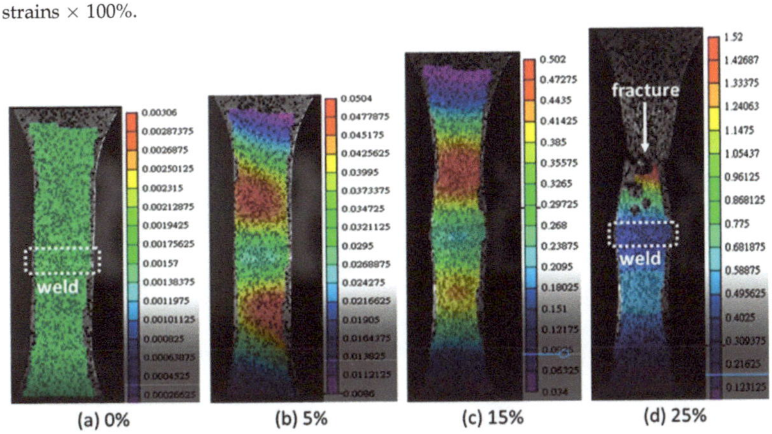

Figure 9. Images from the digital image correlation (DIC) of CP Ti, 200 µm, 100 W, and 30 mm/s during tensile testing showing sample conditions at various percentages of strain (**a**) at 0%, (**b**) 5%, (**c**) 15%, and (**d**) 25%, which correspond to fracture. Note: the numbers associated with the images are local strains × 100%.

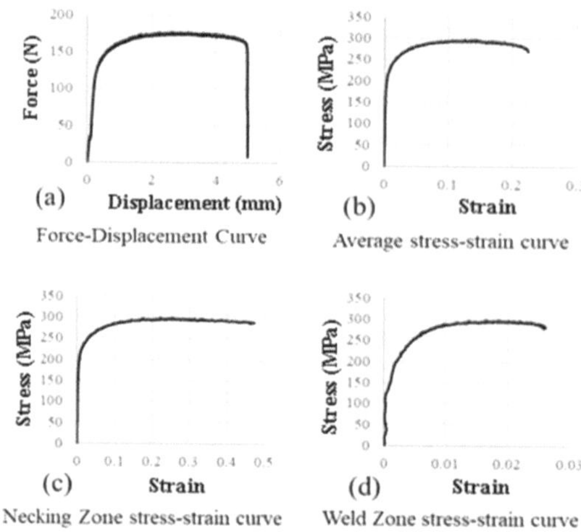

Figure 10. Diagrams showing (**a**) force−displacement curves and (**b**–**d**) stress−strain curves representing various stages/places during tensile testing on the 100 μm thick foil, with 50 W of power and at a speed of 20 mm/s.

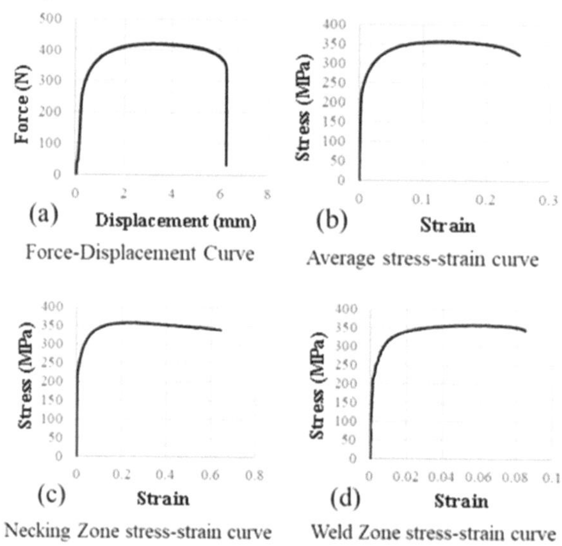

Figure 11. Diagrams showing (**a**) force−displacement curves and (**b**–**d**) stress−strain curves representing various stages/places during tensile testing on the 200 μm thick foil, with 100 W of power and at a speed of 30 mm/s.

Figures 8 and 9 show the strains within the samples at various location along the gauge length for the 100 μm and 200 μm thick foils, respectively. At an early stage, e.g., roughly less than 5% strain (Figures 8b and 9b), it is obvious that localized strains (necking) started to take place on each side (outside) of the weld zone, as indicated by the red color. Necking continued within these areas until the strains reached around 15 to 17% before a localized necking at a "single" location prior to fracture (Figures 8d and 9d). Figures 8d and 9d present the strain experienced by the samples upon fracture, i.e., around 22% and 25% for the 100 μm and 200 μm thick samples, respectively. The reason for the slightly higher percentage of strain (i.e., higher elongation) on the 200 μm thick samples could be due to their thicker sizes, which may delay the localized strain taking place. All of the tested samples fractured outside the weldments, which indicated a good weld quality and strong joints (also shown and confirmed by the high hardness in the weld zones).

Following the tensile testing, the DIC results were post-processed, and various relationships were derived including force vs. displacement, stress vs. strain, stress vs. strain at the necking zone, and stress vs. strain at the weld zone (Figures 10 and 11). These diagrams provide detailed information about the loads, displacements, stresses, and strains across the gauge lengths, weld zones, and fracture locations. The maximum forces recorded during the tensile testing were around 180 N for the 100 μm thick foil and around 420 N for the 200 μm thick foil. The displacements of the samples were found to be around 5 mm and 6.2 mm for the 100 μm and 200 μm thick foils, respectively. The unwelded foil samples had higher strengths (UTS) and elongations than the welded samples, which was, arguably, due to the uniform stress and strain distribution along the entire sample's gauge length. Additionally, the unwelded foil samples presented uniform strength distribution within the entire gauge, resulting in one localized deformation site (necking). For the welded samples, the presence of weldment (shown by the fine weld line) in the middle of the gauge length limited the stress and strain distribution to a much more limited volume in the test sample. In other words, the much smaller actual gauge size is found on each side of the weldment. Hence, relatively the early fracture resulted in slightly lower strengths and elongations compared with the unwelded samples. More detailed information about the strengths (both the yield and ultimate tensile strengths) can be seen in Table 2.

The strains deduced from the DIC system are presented in Figures 10b–d and 11b–d. The average strains (measured on the whole gauge length) showed 0.22 (22%) and 0.25 (25%) for the 100 μm and 200 μm thick samples, respectively. Within the necking zone, the 100 μm thick samples experienced a 0.46 (46%) strain compared with the 0.61 (61%) strain on the 200 μm thick samples. The DIC may also provide strains specifically in the weld zone area. The strain within the 100 μm thick samples was around 0.026 (2.6%), while the 200 μm thick sample had a strain of around 0.085 (8.5%). The weld zones area clearly did not experience significant strains compared with the other areas of the samples, which indicates a good weld quality (weld defects, if any, were not detected) and strong joints.

As indicated in Table 2, fractures for all of the welded samples occurred at the base metal (BM) locations. The examination of the fracture surfaces using scanning electron microscopy (SEM) showed a relatively highly ductile behavior with the presence of dimples throughout the surfaces (Figure 12). No indication of weld defects, such as porosity, gas bubbles, or lack of penetration, was observed. The presence of dimples on the fracture surface indicated a micro-void coalescence mechanism present for both specimen thicknesses.

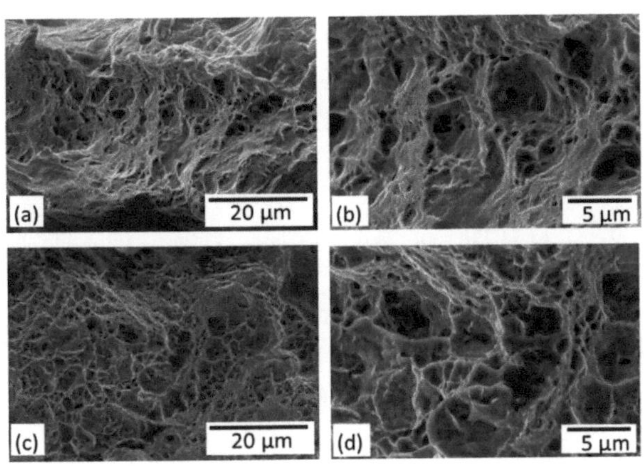

Figure 12. SEM micrographs showing fracture surfaces of (**a**,**b**) 100 μm, 50 W, and 20 mm/s, and (**c**,**d**) 200 μm, 100 W, and 30 mm/s.

4. Summary

Based on the performed investigation, the following can be concluded:

1. The blue diode laser (BDL) can be successfully used to perform welding on thin metallic foils such as CP Ti with thicknesses of 100 μm and 200 μm, and with a speed of up to 30 mm/s.
2. Although the samples were fairly thin, there was no distortion observed on the welded samples associated with the BDL process.
3. The weld zone (FZ and HAZ) displayed a high hardness (strengths) compared with the base metal (BM). This is due to the formation of α' (martensite) within the HAZ and FZ.
4. Based on the DIC results, the strains observed were concentrated within the BM where the fracture eventually took place. The samples fractured with a microvoid coalescence (ductile) mechanism where dimples can be observed throughout the fracture surfaces. This implies good weld quality and strong weld joints.

Author Contributions: Conceptualization, T.P.; methodology, experiments, writing—draft preparation, and editing, P.-C.L.; experiments and analysis, W.Z.M.; analysis and editing, J.-Y.W.; experiments and visualization, S.M.; experiments, M.T., supervision and funding acquisition, E.H.; experiments and investigation, Y.S.; investigation and supervision, Y.T.; experiments and analysis, D.Y., experiments and data curation, S.Y., experiments and data analysis. All authors have read and agreed to the published version of the manuscript.

Funding: This research was funded by JWRI, Osaka University, UNDER, JIJRec, 2019.

Acknowledgments: The work on the blue diode laser (BDL) has been promoted by the New Energy and Industrial Technology Development Organization (NEDO) project under "Development of advanced laser processing with intelligence based on high-brightness and high-efficiency laser technologies (2016–2020)" project. One of the authors (T.P.) would like to thank JWRI for its generous support under the JIJRec scheme in order to be able to carry out the experiments at JWRI, Osaka University. In addition, two co-authors (T.P. and W.Z.M.) would also like to thank the Lowey Institute at Lehigh for their continued support up until the completion of this manuscript.

Conflicts of Interest: The authors declare no conflict of interest.

References

1. Tojo, K.; Masuno, S.; Higashino, R.; Tsukamoto, M. Project Works towards Goal of Next-Generation Laser Processing System with High-Power Blue Diode Lasers. Available online: https://www.industrial-lasers.com/cutting/article/16485172/japan-develops-blue-laser-for-advanced-materials-processing (accessed on 1 September 2018).
2. Nakamura, S.; Pearton, S.; Fasol, G. *The Blue Laser Diode: The Complete Story*, 2nd ed.; Springer Science and Business Media: New York, NY, USA, 2000.
3. Das, A.; Fritz, R.; Finuf, M.; Masters, I. Blue laser welding of multi-layered AISI 316L stainless steel micro-foils. *Opt. Laser Technol.* **2020**, *132*, 106498. [CrossRef]
4. Ventrella, V.A.; Berretta, J.R.; de Rossi, W. Pulsed Nd: YAG laser seam welding of AISI 316L stainless steel thin foils. *J. Mater. Process. Technol.* **2010**, *210*, 1838–1843. [CrossRef]
5. Abe, N.; Funada, Y.; Imanaka, T.; Tsukamoto, M. Micro welding of thin stainless steel foil with a direct diode laser. *Trans. JWRI* **2005**, *34*, 19–23.
6. Kim, J.; Kim, S.; Kim, K.; Jung, W.; Youn, D.; Lee, J.; Ki, H. Effect of beam size in laser welding of ultra-thin stainless steel foils. *J. Mater. Process. Technol.* **2016**, *233*, 125–134. [CrossRef]
7. Pakmanesh, M.R.; Shamanian, M. Optimization of pulsed laser welding process parameters in order to attain minimum underfill and undercut defects in thin 316L stainless steel foils. *Opt. Laser Technol.* **2018**, *99*, 30–38. [CrossRef]
8. Zediker, M.; Fritz, R.; Finuf, M.; Pelaprat, J. Laser welding components for electric vehicles with a high-power blue laser system. *J. Laser Appl.* **2020**, *32*, 022038. [CrossRef]
9. Zediker, M.S.; Fritz, R.D.; Finuf, M.J.; Pelaprat, J.M. Stable keyhole welding of 1 mm thick copper with a 600 W blue laser system. *J. Laser Appl.* **2019**, *31*, 022404. [CrossRef]
10. Wang, H.; Kawahito, Y.; Yoshida, R.; Nakashima, Y.; Shiokawa, K. Development of a high-power blue laser (445 nm) for material processing. *Opt. Lett.* **2017**, *42*, 2251–2254. [CrossRef] [PubMed]

11. Suwa, M.; Wakabayashi, N.; Hiroki, T.; Tojo, K.; Masuno, S.-I.; Higashino, R.; Tsukamoto, M. Development of BLUE IMPACT, a 450nm-wavelength light source for laser processing. In Proceedings of the High-Power Diode Laser Technology XVII, Proc. SPIE 10900, San Francisco, CA, USA, 3–5 February 2019. [CrossRef]
12. Könning, T.; Drovs, S.; Stoiber, M.; König, P.; Kissel, H.; Harth, F.; Köhler, B.; Biesenbach, J.; König, H.; Lell, A.; et al. High brightness fiber coupled diode lasers at 450 nm. In Proceedings of the High-Power Diode Laser Technology XVII, Proc. SPIE 10900, San Francisco, CA, USA, 3–5 February 2019. [CrossRef]
13. Sato, Y.; Tsukamoto, M.; Shobu, T.; Funada, Y.; Yamashita, Y.; Hara, T.; Sengoku, M.; Sakon, Y.; Ohkubo, T.; Yoshida, M.; et al. In situ X-ray observations of pure-copper layer formation with blue direct diode lasers. *Appl. Surf. Sci.* **2019**, *480*, 861–867. [CrossRef]
14. Asano, K.; Tsukamoto, M.; Sechi, Y.; Sato, Y.; Masuno, S.-I.; Higashino, R.; Hara, T.; Sengoku, M.; Yoshida, M. Laser metal deposition of pure copper on stainless steel with blue and IR diode lasers. *Opt. Laser Technol.* **2018**, *107*, 291–296. [CrossRef]
15. Hummel, M.; Schöler, C.; Häusler, A.; Gillner, A.; Poprawe, R. New approaches on laser micro welding of copper by using a laser beam source with a wavelength of 450 nm. *J. Adv. Join. Process.* **2020**, *1*, 100012. [CrossRef]
16. Xu, G.; Kutsuna, M.; Liu, Z.; Yamada, K. Comparison between diode laser and TIG cladding of Co-based alloys on the SUS403 stainless steel. *Surf. Coat. Technol.* **2006**, *201*, 1138–1144. [CrossRef]
17. Boese, E.; Finuf, M.; Zediker, M.; Pelaprat, J.M. Blue Lasers Add Power and Brightness. Available online: https://www.industrial-lasers.com/welding/article/14173138/blue-lasers-add-power-and-brightness (accessed on 20 May 2020).
18. Danielson, P.; Wilson, R.; Alman, D. Microstructure of Titanium Welds. *Adv. Mater. Process.* **2003**, *161*, 39–42.
19. Karpagaraj, A.; Shanmugam, N.S.; Sankaranarayanasamy, K. Some studies on mechanical properties and microstructural characterization of automated TIG welding of thin commercially pure titanium sheets. *Mater. Sci. Eng. A* **2015**, *640*, 180–189. [CrossRef]
20. Choi, B.H.; Choi, B.K. The effect of welding conditions according to mechanical properties of pure titanium. *J. Mater. Process. Technol.* **2008**, *201*, 526–530. [CrossRef]
21. Li, C.; Muneharua, K.; Takao, S.; Kouji, H. Fiber laser-GMA hybrid welding of commercially pure titanium. *Mater. Des.* **2009**, *30*, 109–114. [CrossRef]
22. Lathabai, S.; Jarvis, B.L.; Barton, K.J. Comparison of keyhole and conventional gas tungsten arc welds in commercially pure titanium. *Mater. Sci. Eng. A* **2001**, *299*, 81–93. [CrossRef]
23. Liu, H.; Nakata, K.; Zhang, J.X.; Yamamoto, N.; Liao, J. Microstructural evolution of fusion zone in laser beam welds of pure titanium. *Mater. Charact.* **2012**, *65*, 1–7. [CrossRef]
24. Pasang, T.; Tao, Y.; Azizi, M.; Kamiya, O.; Mizutani, M.; Misiolek, W.Z. Welding of Titanium alloys. *MATEC Web Conf.* **2017**, *123*, 1–6. [CrossRef]
25. Lütjering, G.; Williams, J.C. *Titanium*; Springer: Berlin, Germany, 2007.

quantum beam science

MDPI

Article

Laser Cleaning as Novel Approach to Preservation of Historical Books and Documents on a Paper Basis

Vadim Parfenov [1,*], Alexander Galushkin [2], Tatiana Tkachenko [2] and Vladimir Aseev [3]

1 Department of Photonics, St. Petersburg Electrotechnical University, 197376 St. Petersburg, Russia
2 St. Petersburg Branch of the Archive of the Russian Academy of Sciences, 199034 St. Petersburg, Russia; lkrd@rambler.ru (A.G.); restlaser@gmail.com (T.T.)
3 Faculty of Photonics, National Research University ITMO, 197101 St. Petersburg, Russia; aseev@oi.ifmo.ru
* Correspondence: vaparfenov@etu.ru

Abstract: The purpose of this work is the study of laser cleaning of historical paper. The effect of laser exposure of the paper reflectance, fracture resistance and acidity was investigated. The paper surface roughness before and after laser treatment was analyzed by optical and scanning electron microscopy. It was shown that use of multi-pulse micromachining in combination with high-speed scanning of laser beams provides high safety for paper cleaning. The optimal parameters of laser radiation for effective and safe cleaning are a power density of about 2×105 W/cm^2 at a wavelength of 1.06 μm, pulse repetition rate is 20 kHz; and a beam scanning speed of 200 mm/s–500 mm/s. The selective laser cleaning method for books and documents was proposed. Selective cleaning is achieved by means of high-precision control of the trajectory of movement of laser beams.

Keywords: laser cleaning; paper; books; documents; contaminants; cultural heritage; restoration

1. Introduction

The use of laser technology in the field of preservation of cultural heritage (CH) is a new but rapidly developing scientific and technical direction. Most often, lasers are used to determine the chemical composition, structural diagnostics, and documentation of works of art. These applications are based on the use of laser spectroscopy, interferometry, holography, and 3D scanning [1–3]. The restoration exploits laser cleaning technology, which allows solving the problems of removing natural layers and anthropogenic pollution from the surface of CH objects. However, despite the fact that lasers were first used in restoration almost 50 years ago, to date, only the technology of cleaning the stone has been developed. Laser restoration of other, primarily organic materials is still in the process of conducting exploratory research [3–19]. This is due to the fact that in the process of laser treatment, damage to their surface may occur, which is unacceptable according to the canons of restoration.

This article is devoted to the development of technology of cleaning of books and documents in the paper base. Cleaning paper sheets of dirt is a necessary and very time-consuming operation in the restoration of books and documents. Wax stains, soot and dust pollution, biological lesions, the so-called "fly ash", etc., are subject to removal. However, traditional methods of restoration cleaning do not always give satisfactory results. Thus, mechanical cleaning (based on the use of an eraser, rubber crumb or abrasive sandpaper with fine grain) violates the integrity of the surface structure of the paper, and reduces the thickness of the sheets, which ultimately negatively affects their mechanical strength. In addition, some of the removed dirt remains in the upper layer of the damaged paper surface in the form of dust. It should also be noted that there are often cases when the physical condition of books, especially the dilapidation of the lower corners of the book block sheets, in principle does not allow the use of mechanical cleaning. As an alternative to mechanical cleaning, water washing and chemical treatment with organic solvents and enzymes are sometimes used. Although such methods may be effective, they cannot be used to clean handwritten documents, as well as books with unstable printing ink.

For these reasons, the search for alternative methods of restoration of books and documents is currently relevant. One possible approach to solving this problem may be the use of laser cleaning. The first experimental works on the use of lasers for this purpose was carried out in the late 1990s [4,5], but is still being carried out by a few scientific groups in Europe [6–18]. These works show the possibility of using a laser for cleaning, but the method is not yet widely used. For this, it is necessary to develop appropriate technologies and specialized laser systems suitable for a wide range of contaminants.

Therefore, the purpose of this work is to develop a method for laser cleaning of documents and books with different types of paper.

2. Experimental

Model samples of paper that differed by chemical composition as well as fragments of historical documents and books of XVI-XIX centuries were used in experiments (Table 1).

Table 1. List of samples.

Label	Paper Composition	Dating
	Model samples	
B-2	100% sulphate cellulose	XX century
B-5	100% sulphate cellulose, kaolin filler, ash content–5.2%	XX century
B-6	100% Linen half-mass	XX century
B-19	100% sulphate cellulose, kaolin filler, ash content–4.6%	XX century
B-25	100% cotton half-mass, kaolin filler, ash content–9.3%	XX century
Pag paper	100% flax fiber, sizing-starch	XX century
	Historical paper	
Russian typographic book		beginning of the XIX century
Russian handwritten book		XVII century
Arabic manuscript		Late of 19th century
Arabic manuscript		Medieval

A pulsed ytterbium fiber laser generating at the wavelength of 1.06 μm was used for paper cleaning.

For all paper samples, reflection spectra were measured, whiteness of the paper, its acidity (pH) and fracture resistance were determined. Measurements were taken before and after laser cleaning. Reflection spectra were measured on a LAMBDA 900 spectrophotometer (manufactured by PerkinElmer LLC, Santa Clara, CA, USA) in the wavelength range of 300–2500 nm with a scanning step of 1 nm. The whiteness of the paper was measured on an FMSh-56 M ball photometer. An electron scanning microscope JSM-35 (JEOL Ltd., Tokyo, Japan) was used for surface study.

3. Results and Discussion

3.1. Choosing a Laser for Paper Cleaning

Laser cleaning of paper is based on the use of physical effects, which is called photoablation. Photoablation is the contaminant particles' ejection by photons as a result of their absorption by dirt material to be removed in the process of cleaning. The concept of the use of laser radiation for selective removal from the surface of an optically absorbing different substance, for instance, a secondary encrustation, was first demonstrated in 1965 by Arthur Schawlow, one of the laser inventors, who evaporated selectively absorbing black pigments of printing ink from a strongly reflecting white sheet of paper [20]. Later, in 1972 John Asmus first demonstrated the laser cleaning of Cultural Heritage objects [21]. Nowadays, basic physical principles of laser cleaning are well known and described in the scientific literature (see, for instance [2,22,23]).

The first step towards the development of laser technology for paper restoration is the choice of such laser radiation parameters that allow for high efficiency in cleaning books and documents. However, laser output parameters must be so they do not cause any negative consequences (including carbonization as well as changes in color, acidity, porosity and other physical and chemical properties of the paper). When choosing the type of laser and its output characteristics, it is necessary to keep in mind that paper is a very fragile, easily damaged material. It is a porous-capillary body in the form of a "carcass" formed by cellulose fibers connected to each other by chemical hydrogen bonds. Under the influence of heat, mechanical stresses and chemical reagents, the paper fibers are easy to damage.

It is known from the scientific literature that various types of lasers were used for paper cleaning, including excimer lasers (in particular, the XeCl laser with a radiation wavelength of 308 nm and the KrF laser with wavelength of 248 nm), as well as a solid-state Nd: YAG laser operating either at the main wavelength or at the wavelengths of the second, third and fourth harmonics (with wavelength of 1064 nm, 532 nm, 355 nm and 266 nm, respectively) [2,4–13]. In all cases, pulsed laser radiation was used. In particular, when working with a solid-state Nd:YAG laser, a Q-switched generation regime with a pulse duration of 10 ns–30 ns is usually used. As for the pulse repetition rate, it is usually in the range 1 Hz–100 Hz (maximum—1 kHz).

In order to choose the optimal laser wavelength for efficient and safe cleaning of books and documents, the spectral characteristics of the paper measured at the initial stage of our work. Measurements of the reflectance spectra give information on the spectral bandwidth where paper has maximum absorption. Since paper is a scattering medium, we used an integrating sphere. Results of these measurements are shown in Figure 1.

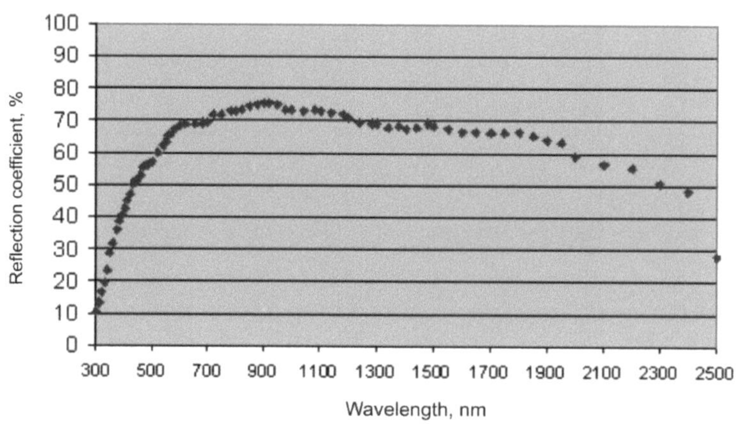

Figure 1. Reflection coefficient of paper versus laser radiation wavelength (for sheet of a Russian typographic book of the beginning of the XIX century made of wood pulp).

Then, we measured the reflectance of paper sheets of historical books and documents These measurements were conducted using a LAMBDA 900 spectrophotometer (manufacturer—PerkinElmer LLC, Santa Clara, CA, USA). A diaphragm with a diameter of 10 mm was used to select the measurement area. The area included typical paper contaminations: traces of silicate glue and rust, dust and dirt stains, grease stains, moisture traces, etc. Obtained spectra are presented in Figure 2.

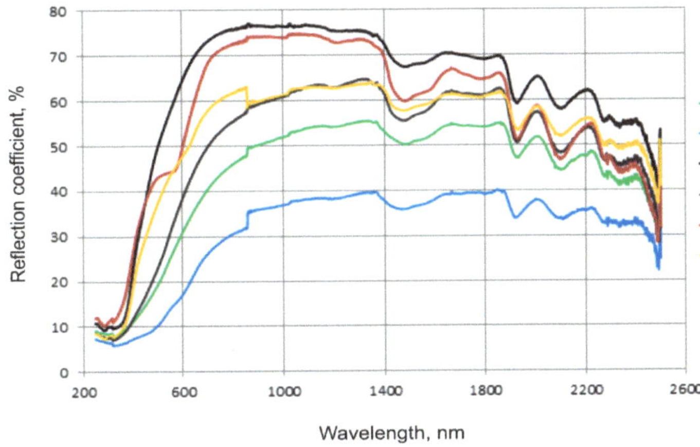

Figure 2. Reflection coefficient of paper with contaminants versus laser radiation wavelength.

From Figures 1 and 2, one can see that all the recorded spectra are identical to each other, and the differences are only in the absolute values of the reflection coefficient, which depend on the specific type of surface contamination. The most important finding is that the paper has the lowest reflectance values in the UV region of the spectrum. Consequently, the use of short-wave lasers for cleaning books and documents can be dangerous for their state of preservation due to the significant absorption of radiation energy by the paper. Indeed, the authors of some works (see, for example, [5]) reported damage to paper during its cleaning by an excimer laser with a radiation wavelength of 308 nm. From the graph in Figure 1 it is also clear that the maximum value of the reflection coefficient of the paper is in the range of 900 nm–1100 nm. Therefore, it is advisable to use lasers with a wavelength of radiation in this spectral region, and the best "candidates" for this role are solid-state neodymium lasers, as well as fiber ytterbium lasers with wavelength of about 1 micrometer. It is obvious that when using such lasers, the effect of their radiation on the surface of the paper cleaned of impurities will be insignificant, which ensures its safety during laser processing.

As for paper with contaminants on the surface from Figure 2, one can see that in the wavelength range of 900 nm–1100 nm, samples with dust contamination and under the lobes have lower reflection coefficients (about 35–60%) than samples with grease, silicate glue and stains of unknown origin (about 60–70%). In this case, the maximum value of the reflection coefficient (about 80%) has a sample with fat spots. It is clear that using lasers with a wavelength of about 1 micrometer with enough one can remove contaminants if the intensity of radiation will be enough high.

Another important parameter of laser radiation in the treatment of materials is the pulse repetition rate. Since at a fixed level of the average laser output power, an increase in the frequency leads to a decrease in the energy density of a single pulse, it is obvious that this allows for a higher "delicacy" of paper processing by reducing the thermal energy generated as a result of its absorption of laser radiation. It is for this reason that, unlike other scientific groups involved in study of laser paper cleaning, the authors of this work decided to check the possibility of using very high values of the repetition rate of laser pulses (at the level of tens of kilohertz). With all the above parameters, the effect of the laser on the paper becomes similar to the so-called multi-pulse laser micro-processing, which is widely used in industrial processing of materials. For the first time, the idea of using this approach in the restoration of paper was expressed by one of the authors of this article in 2007 [24].

However, it should be noted that to ensure maximum safety of paper processing, it is important not only to reduce the pulse energy density, but also to eliminate the cumulative effect of the thermal effect of laser radiation. Local temperature increase, which can occur during prolonged exposure to the same area of the surface, may cause negative effects—color change and even charring of the paper. To avoid this, it is necessary to ensure a very fast and uniform movement of the laser beam on the surface of the paper sheet. This problem can be solved by using high-speed laser beam scanning systems. For this purpose, you can use, for example, 2-coordinate scanners based on galvanometric mirrors, which are used in lasers for marking and engraving. In this case, each time the laser beam passes over the surface of the paper sheet, very thin layers of dirt will be removed. If the cleaning level is insufficient, the processing can be continued by re-scanning the entire sheet or its individual sections.

Based on the above considerations, in the experiments on paper cleaning, a pulsed solid–state fiber ytterbium laser was used. It has the following output characteristics: radiation wavelength—1.06 μm; maximum average power—10 W; pulse duration—10 ns; maximum pulse repetition rate—100 kHz.

3.2. Characterization of Paper before and after Laser Cleaning

The scheme of the experimental setup is shown in Figure 3a. The laser beam was focused onto the surface of paper and the sample was scanned (the spot diameter of focused laser beam was about 50 μm). The general view of the experimental setup in the process of laser cleaning of paper is shown in Figure 3b.

Laser processing parameters have been determined to ensure the safe and efficient removal of contaminants from the paper surface. Safe cleaning does mean the absence of such negative side effects as charring (carbonization), discoloration and roughness change of the paper surface. The maximum removal efficiency without paper damage was obtained at an average power of 4 W, while the pulse repetition rate was 20 kHz. Thus, the power density in the spot was about 2×105 W/cm^2. The beam scanning speed was varied in the range of 200 mm/s–500 mm/s, and the laser processing area was 4×6 cm^2.

At the first stage, there was a study of the effect of laser processing on the physical, mechanical and chemical properties of paper and its wear resistance. The following parameters of paper properties were determined: fracture strength, pH value of aqueous extraction and whiteness. In the field of book restoration, exactly these parameters characterize the safety of any restoration treatment. Accelerated thermal aging of the studied samples (105 °C, 72 h) was carried out to study the effect of laser processing on the durability of paper. To reduce the thermal effect of the laser on the paper, high-speed scanning in two mutually perpendicular directions was used. The paper samples were lasered on both sides of the sheet. The values of the index of resistance to destruction of paper samples of various compositions after laser processing of its surface (on both sides) are presented in Table 2.

The maximum effect of laser cleaning on the mechanical strength of paper was in samples B-2 (from 100% sulfate pulp) and B-6 (from 100% half-mass of flax). For these samples, the average value of the number of double kinks (ndk) decreased by 12–20%, and the decrease in fracture resistance occurs only in the longitudinal direction. For other types of paper (B-5, B-19, B-25 and Pag paper), the fracture resistance index does not decrease after laser processing.

A slight increase in the ndk in the transverse direction was also observed. The nature of fracture resistance in mutually perpendicular directions is different, in the longitudinal direction it is determined by the strength and elasticity of the fiber, and in the transverse direction it depends on the strength of the interfiber bonds. Heating to a temperature of 220 °C leads to dehydration, which reduces the elasticity of the paper and leads to a decrease in the tear resistance of the paper. This is proved by a small weight loss associated with the dehydration of cellulose fiber, which was observed during DSC analysis in [25]. At the same time, the removal of hygroscopic water should lead to strengthening of hydrogen bonds, which make the main contribution to the energy of interfiber bonds in paper. Laser exposure leads to heating of the paper and similar processes can be observed in this case.

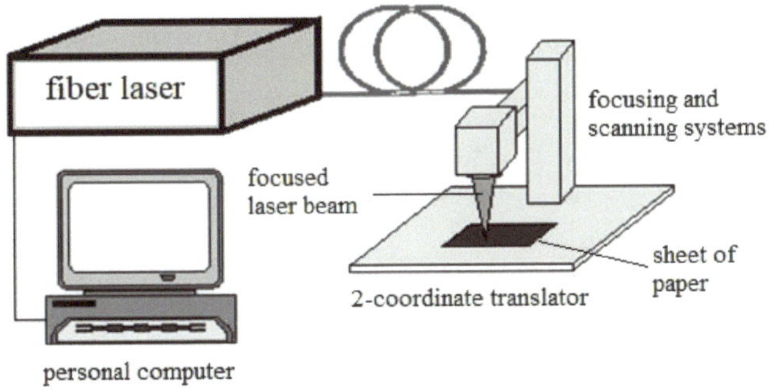

(a)

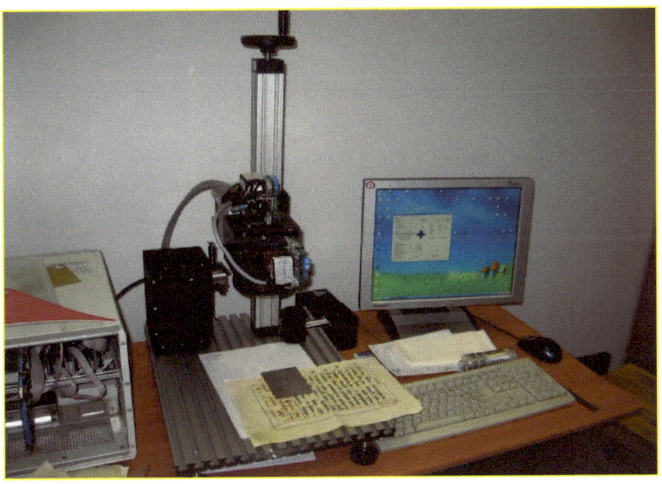

(b)

Figure 3. Experimental setup for laser treatment of paper: (**a**)—diagram of experimental setup; (**b**)—general view.

Table 2. The effect of laser processing on the physical and mechanical properties of paper (index-fracture resistance).

	Paper Composition	Fracture Resistance (Number of Permissible Double Kinks)					
		Control			After Laser Treatment		
		Longitudinal Direction	Transverse Direction	Average Value	Longitudinal Direction	Transverse Direction	Average Value
B-2	100% sulphate cellulose	208	160	184	150	174	162
B-5	100% sulphate cellulose, kaolin filler, ash content–5.2%	14	31	22	13	36	24

Table 2. *Cont.*

	Paper Composition	Fracture Resistance (Number of Permissible Double Kinks)					
		Control			After Laser Treatment		
		Longitudinal Direction	Transverse Direction	Average Value	Longitudinal Direction	Transverse Direction	Average Value
B-6	100% Linen half-mass	630	274	452	469	284	376
B-19	100% sulphate cellulose, kaolin filler, ash content-4.6%	134	92	113	170	97	134
B-25	100% cotton half-mass, kaolin filler, ash content-9.3%	10	7	8	10	8	9
Pag paper	100% flax fiber, sizing-starch	9	9	9	9	9	9

The whiteness and acidity index values of paper samples before and after laser treatment (Table 3) show that paper properties (related to whiteness and pH) do not change.

Table 3. The effect of laser treatment on the whiteness of the paper and the value of the acidity index (pH).

Cipher of Sample	Control		After laser Treatment	
	Whiteness,%	pH	Whiteness,%	pH
B-5	73.0	5.1	72.0	4.8
B-19	72.0	7.2	72.0	7.0
B-25	83.0	7.3	82.0	7.6
Rag paper	58.0	4.9	58.0	4.9

Analyzing the data of accelerated thermal aging of the samples, it can be concluded that laser processing did not affect the durability of the paper. Changes in fracture resistance, brightness, and pH values of the laser-treated and control samples were identical (see Table 4).

Table 4. Changes in the physical, mechanical, optical, and chemical properties of control paper samples and laser-treated paper samples after thermal aging (100 °C, 72 h).

Cipher of Sample	Thermal Aging									
	Control					After Laser Treatment				
	Fracture Resistance (n.p.k.)			White, %	pH	Fracture Resistance (n.p.k.)			White, %	pH
	Longitudinal Direction.	Transverse Direction	Average Value			Longitudinal Direction.	Transverse Direction	Average Value		
B-5	9	20	14	69.0	4.9	7	22	14	69.0	4.8
B-19	168	116	142	70.0	6.9	192	113	152	69.0	7.0
B-25	10	8	9	82.0	7.6	10	7	8	81.0	7.4
Rag paper	4	5	4	55.0	4.5	4	6	5	55.0	4.5

Visual inspection of the cleaning areas (using an optical stereomicroscope) showed that as a result of a single laser treatment, a significant part of the contamination is removed without disturbing the microrelief of the paper surface and its color characteristics. After completing a series of test tests on model images that demonstrated the safety of the selected laser and its output characteristics on the properties of paper, experiments were conducted on laser cleaning of original historical documents—a sheet of a handwritten book of the XVII century, as well as a page of a Russian typographic book of the early XIX century with typical types of contamination. As a result of laser treatment, the main surface contamination was removed in both cases. The condition of the paper before and after laser cleaning, as well as when working with model samples, was monitored using an optical microscope. Additionally, an scanning electronic microscope (SEM) JSM-35 was also used. Optical microscopic and SEM images shown in Figures 4–6 allow us to conclude that laser processing does not lead to a violation of the surface morphology and structure of the cellulose fibers of the paper. In addition, there are no changes in its color. It was confirmed by means of colorimetric measurements including the original measuring technique described in one of our recent publications [17].

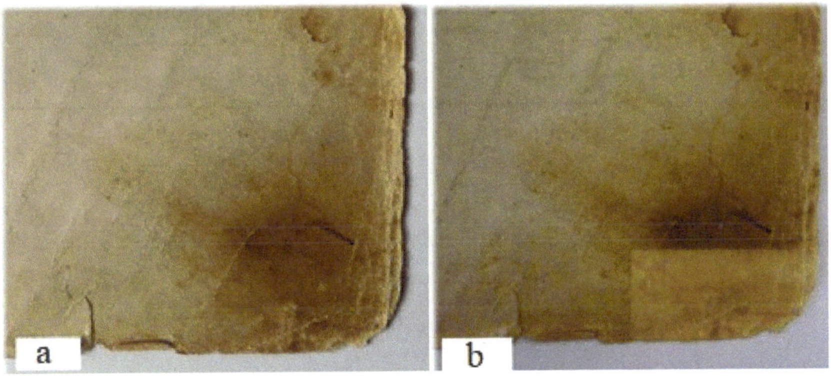

Figure 4. Flyleaf of a Russian typographic book (the beginning of the XIX century) with characteristic surface contamination: (**a**)—before laser cleaning; (**b**)—after laser treatment (light yellow rectangle in the lower right part of the sheet).

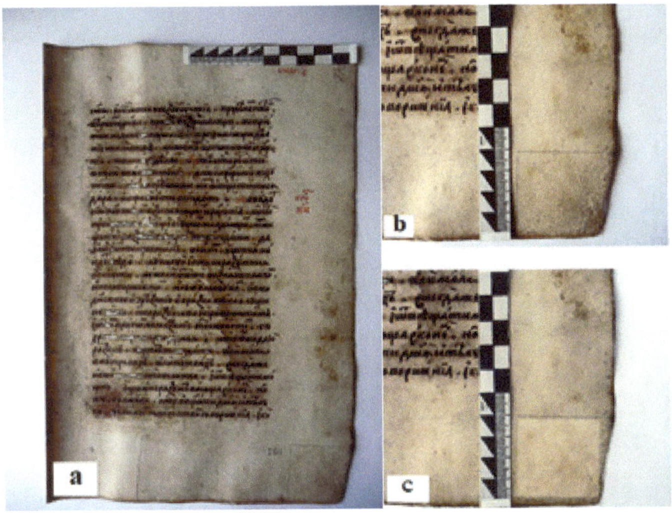

Figure 5. Page of a Russian handwritten book of the XVII century with characteristic surface contamination: (**a**)—the initial state; (**b**)—the lower right corner marked with a pencil—the experimental area for clearing with a laser; (**c**)—the same section of the page after laser processing.

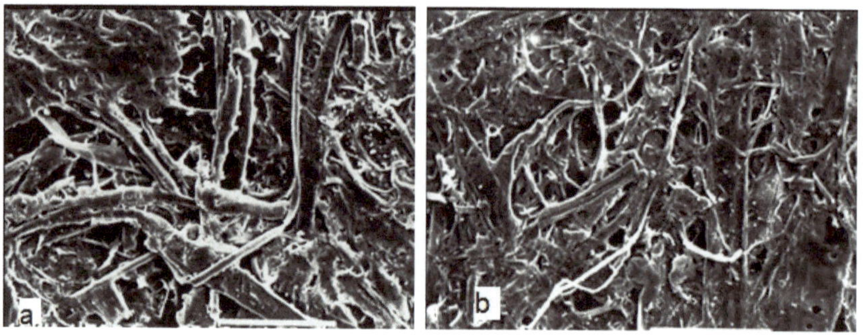

Figure 6. Images of the surface of a sheet of handwritten paper book obtained on an electronic scanning microscope: (**a**)—the initial state, (**b**)—after cleaning with a laser.

It should be noted that Fourier Transform Infrared spectroscopy makes it possible to control the chemical changes of paper after laser treatment at the molecular level, but in our work such measurements have not been conducted since from scientific literature it is known (see, for instance [11]) that with the right choice of laser exposure, such a negative side effect can be prevented.

Therefore, our experiments confirmed high efficiency and safety of laser cleaning of paper.

3.3. Selective Laser Cleaning

Consider the security of such processing for the entire page, which may include text and pictures. Since the absorption of carcasses and ink differs from the absorption of paper, it is necessary to study the effect of laser cleaning on such objects.

The preliminary experiments were carried out on a sheet of modern Russian strong paper "type 1000" on which typewritten text was printed in black ink. Laser cleaning removed the text from the paper, along with the dirt.

Then, a fragment of a sheet of a medieval Arabic handwritten book with text written in multi-colored ink (red and black) was cleaned. The text in red ink has not changed. Removal of surface dirt from the paper also led to partial removal of black ink (Figure 7).

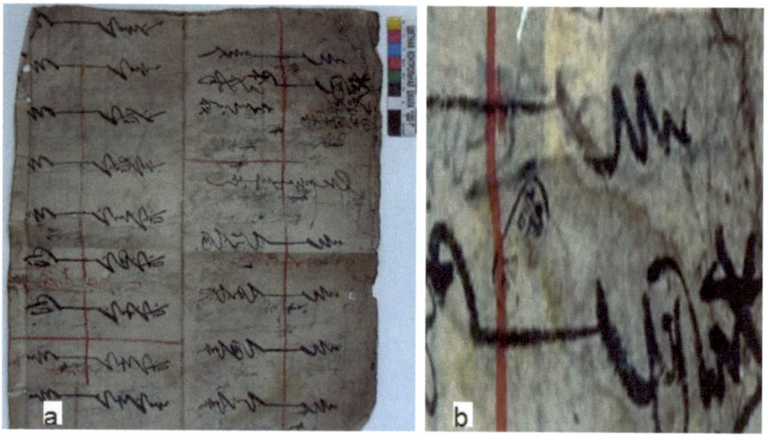

Figure 7. Images of a sheet of medieval Arabic manuscript: (**a**)—a general view, (**b**)—a fragment (a light rectangle in the middle at the top) cleaned by a laser.

From a later Arabic manuscript (19th century), both black and red ink were partially removed by laser treatment (see Figure 8). That is, if a pencil, iron gall and soot ink were used to write books, then special protection measures must be taken during their laser cleaning. Aniline ink does not require any special protection procedures.

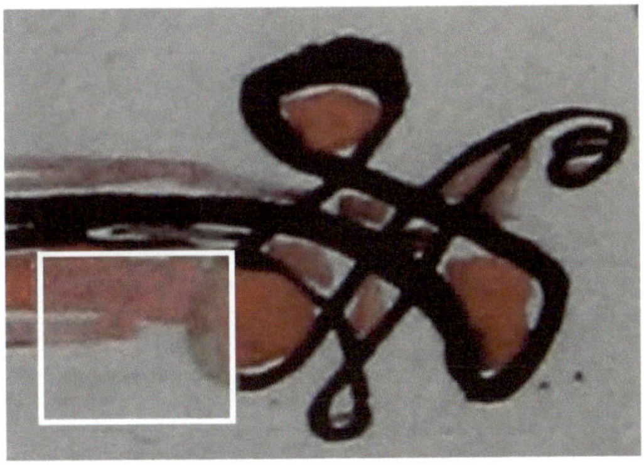

Figure 8. A fragment of an Arabic manuscript page after laser processing (the white square shows the area processed by the laser).

To ensure the safety of paper documents, it is necessary to exclude the effect of laser radiation on text and drawings applied by handwriting and printing. Thus, for the restoration of books and documents, it is necessary to use selective laser cleaning.

It should be noted that the idea of selective purification has already been described in [26]. Laser cleaning the BAM (Federal Institute for Materials Research and Testing, Berlin, Germany) prototype (designed by W. Kautek) was based on the use of a Nd:YAG laser (generating at 1064 nm or 532 nm) with a maximum repetition rate of up to 1 kHz and an energy density of ~10 J/cm^2. Increasing the repetition rate to 35 kHz while maintaining a power density of 10 J/cm^2 allowed us to reduce the energy of a single pulse, which is safer for paper heating.

The method of selective cleaning by zones was developed on model samples, which were sheets of modern office paper with laser-printed text. Coal dust was applied to the surface of the paper to simulate contamination. To remove from the processing area areas containing text, their inverted vector image (mask image) was sent to the scanning system operation control program. The mask image was created by cropping the original sheet image with text and converting it using CorelDRAW X7 (designed by Corel Inc., Ottawa, ON, Canada).

With laser cleaning, it is necessary to ensure a very precise alignment of the processed area of the paper sheet with the scanning field in order to avoid the risk of damaging text and graphic information. For this, a combination of special fiducial marks (previously applied to the processed area of paper) and the so-called overall frame was made. Reference marks are applied to the treated surface to align it with the working area of the laser.

During the experiments, an artificially polluted sheet of paper was treated with a focused laser beam. The results of laser processing of the model sample sheet are shown in Figure 9. As one can see from these photos (on the left—a sheet of paper in its original state, on the right—after laser cleaning), the contamination was successfully removed, but the typographic text remained unchanged. This confirms the effectiveness of the proposed technical solution.

At the final stage of the work, experiments were carried out on the selective cleaning of authentic historical documents. In particular, a page of an early 20th-century Arabic book was used for this purpose. A small area of the text sheet was selected for cleaning. After completing all the preparatory technological stages (it is described in details in [17]), it was necessary to accurately position the processing area selected on the book sheet relative to the laser working area. The processing area was a rectangle drawn in pencil (see Figure 10).

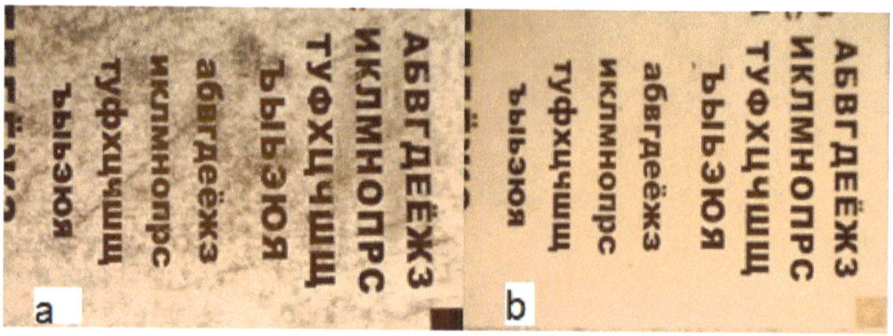

Figure 9. A model sample of paper with simulation of contaminants on the surface: (**a**)—before cleaning, (**b**)—after laser treatment.

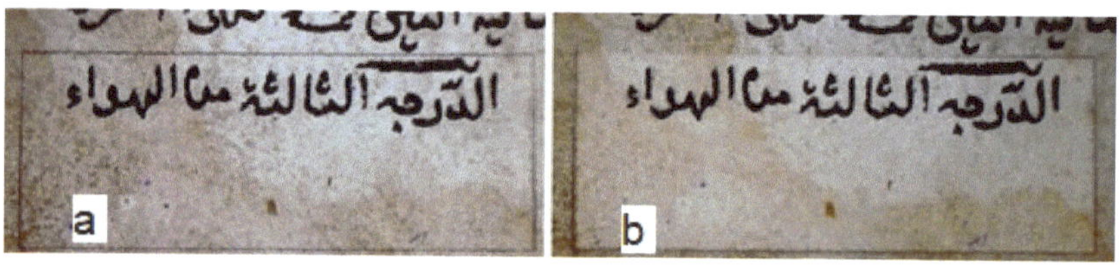

Figure 10. A fragment of antique Arabic manuscript: (**a**)—before cleaning, (**b**)—after laser treatment.

As can be seen from Figure 10, during the experiment it was possible to successfully perform selective cleaning—the book sheet was cleared of surface contamination, but the original text was saved in the laser processing zone.

The analysis of the cleaning was evaluated visually. Figure 11 shows a photo of a small fragment of a book sheet with typographic text before and after cleaning. It clearly shows that the integrity and readability of the letters of the typographic text is well preserved during the laser processing.

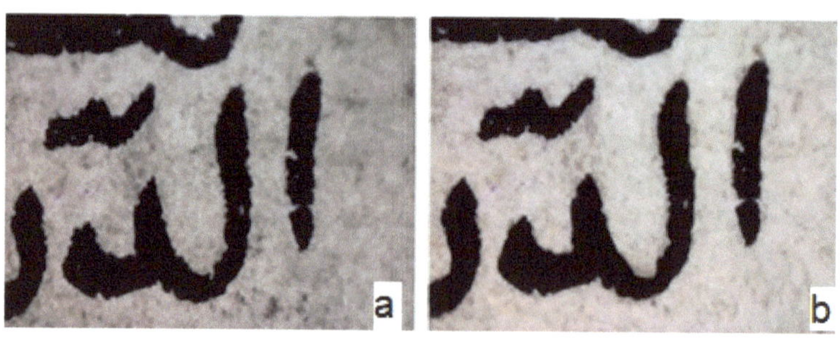

Figure 11. A small fragment of antique Arabic manuscript: (**a**)—before cleaning, (**b**)—after laser treatment.

4. Conclusions

Based on the experimental results obtained, the following main conclusions can be drawn:

1. Laser cleaning of paper using a pulsed IR laser with wavelength of about 1 μm provides high efficiency and safety of divestment of historical books and documents.
2. The use of multi-pulse micromachining in combination with high-speed scanning of laser beam provides high safety for paper cleaning. The optimal parameters of

laser cleaning of paper are: pulse duration—about 10 ns; average power—of about 4 W (power density of about 2 × 105 W/cm^2); pulse repetition rate—about 20 kHz; scanning speed—200 mm/s–500 mm/s.

3. To ensure the safety of books and documents during laser cleaning, it is necessary to exclude the impact of laser radiation on the text and drawings to avoid their damage. It can be achieved using a high-precision laser beam scanning system that allows you to display typographic text and graphic information from the laser processing area.

Author Contributions: Conceptualization, V.P.; methodology, V.P. and A.G.; validation, V.P., T.T., A.G., and V.A., investigation, V.P., T.T. and A.G.; resources, V.P. and V.A.; data curation, V.P. and A.G.; writing— V.P.; writing—review and editing, V.P., V.A. and A.G.; supervision, V.P.; project administration, V.P. All authors have read and agreed to the published version of the manuscript.

Funding: This research received no external funding.

Data Availability Statement: Not applicable.

Acknowledgments: The authors would like to acknowledge L.G. Levashova, S.V. Titov, A.N. Gerashchenko (present name—A.Adelberg) and A.A. Efimov, who took part in the experiments, for their contribution to the obtained results.

Conflicts of Interest: The authors declare no conflict of interest.

References

1. Fotakis, C.; Anglos, D.; Zafiropulos, V.; Georgiou, S.; Tornari, V. Lasers in the Preservation of Cultural Heritage. In *Principles and Applications*; CRC Press, Taylor & Francis Group: Boca Rayton, FL, USA, 2007.
2. Cooper, M. *Laser Cleaning in Conservation: An Introduction*; Butterworth-Heinemann: Oxford, UK, 1998.
3. Markov, V.B.; Mironyuk, G.I. Holography in museums of the Ukraine. In *Three-Dimensional Holography: Science, Culture, Education;* SPIE: Bellingham, WA, USA, 1991; Volume 123, pp. 340–347.
4. Friberg, T.R.; Zafiropulos, V.; Petrakis, Y.; Fotakis, C. Removal of fungi and stains from paper substrates using laser cleaning strategies. In *Lasers in the Conservation of Artworks (LACONA I)*; Restauratorenblatter (Special Isuue); Kautek, W., Konig, E., Eds.; Mayer & Comp: Vienna, Austria, 1997; pp. 79–82.
5. Kolar, J.; Strlic, M.; Pentzien, S.; Kautek, W. Near-UV, visible and IR pulsed laser light interaction with cellulose. *Appl. Phys. A* **2000**, *71*, 87–90. [CrossRef]
6. Kolar, J.; Strlic, M.; Müller-Hess, D.; Gruber, A.; Troschke, K.; Pentzien, S.; Kautek, W. Laser cleaning of paper using Nd:YAG laser running at 532 nm. *J. Cult. Herit.* **2003**, *4*, 185–187. [CrossRef]
7. Pilch, E.; Pentzien, S.; Madebach, H.; Kautek, W. Anti-Fungal Laser Treatment of Paper: A Model Study with a Laser Wavelength of 532 nm. Lasers in the Conservation of Artworks. *Springer Proc. Phys.* **2005**, *100*, 19–27. [CrossRef]
8. Kautek, W.; Pentzien, S. Laser Cleaning System for Automated Paper and Parchment Cleaning. *Springer Proc. Phys.* **2005**, *100*, 403–410.
9. Strlic, M.; Selih, V.; Kolar, J.; Kocar, D. Optimisation and on-line acoustic monitoring of laser cleaning of soiled paper. *Appl. Phys.* **2005**, *81*, 943–951. [CrossRef]
10. Bilmes, G.M.; Freisztav, C.M.; Cap, N. Laser cleaning of 19th century papers and manuscripts assisted by digital image processing. In *Lasers in the Conservation of Artworks*; Castillejo, M., Moreno, P., Oujja, M., Radvan, R., Ruiz, J., Eds.; Taylor & Francis Group: London, UK, 2008. [CrossRef]
11. Brandt, N.N.; Chikishev, A.Y.; Itoh, K.; Rebrikova, N.L. ATR-FTIR and FT Raman spectroscopy and laser cleaning of old paper samples with foxings. *Laser Phys.* **2009**, *19*, 483–492. [CrossRef]
12. Arif, S.; Kautek, W. Laser cleaning of paper: Cleaning efficiency and irradiation dose. *Stud. Conserv.* **2015**, *60*, S97–S105. [CrossRef]
13. Ciofini, D.; Osticioli, I.; Micheli, S.; Montalbano, L.; Siano, S. Laser Removal of Mold and Foxing Stains from Paper Artifacts: Preliminary Investigation. In *Fundamentals of Laser-Assisted Micro- and Nanotechnologies 2013*; SPIE Proceedings: Bellingham, WA, USA, 2013. [CrossRef]
14. Zekou, E.; Tsilikas, I.; Chatzitheodoridis, E.; Serafetinides, A. Laser paper cleaning: The method of cleaning historical books. In Proceedings of the 19th International Conference and School on Quantum Electronics: Laser Physics and Applications, Sozopol, Bulgaria, 5 January 2017; SPIE Proceedings: Bellingham, DC, USA, 2017; Volume 10226. [CrossRef]
15. Rosati, C.; Ciofini, D.; Osticioli, I.; Giorgi, R.; Tegli, S.; Siano, S. Laser removal of mold growth from paper. *Appl. Phys. A Mater. Sci. Process.* **2014**, *117*, 253–259. [CrossRef]
16. Balakhnina, I.A.; Brandt, N.N.; Chikishev, A.Y.; Shpachenko, I.G. Single-pulse two-threshold laser ablation of historical paper. *Laser Phys. Lett.* **2018**, *15*, 065605. [CrossRef]

17. Parfenov, V.A.; Titov, S.V. Technical and Technological Aspects of Laser Cleaning for Books and Documents. In Proceedings of the 2019 IEEE Conference of Russian Young Researchers in Electrical and Electronic Engineering (EIConRus), St. Petersburg, Russia, 28–30 January 2019; pp. 903–906. [CrossRef]
18. Atanassova, V.; Yankov, G.; Zahariev, P.; Grozeva, M. Laser treatment of contaminations on paper: A preliminary study. In Proceedings of the Conference "Applicazioni Laser nel Restauro (APLAR), Venezia, Italy, 7–8 November 2019; pp. 433–445.
19. Abdel-Maksouda, G.; Emamb, H.; Ragab, N.M. From Traditional to Laser Cleaning Techniques of Parchment Manuscripts: A ReviewAdvanced Research in Conservation Science. *Adv. Res. Conserv. Sci.* **2020**, *1*, 52–76.
20. Schawlow, A.L. Lasers. *Science* **1965**, *149*, 13–22. [CrossRef] [PubMed]
21. Lazzarini, L.; Asmus, J.; Marchesini, M.L. Laser for cleaning of statuary, initial results and potentialities. In Proceedings of the 1st Int. Symp. on the Deterioration of Building Stone, La Rochelle, France, 11–16 September 1972; pp. 89–94.
22. Luk'yanchuk, B.S. *Laser Cleaning*; World Scientific Publishing Company, Inc.: Singapore, 2002.
23. Kovalenko, V.S. Laser micro-and nanoprocessing. *Int. J. Nano.* **2006**, *1*, 173–180. [CrossRef]
24. Mokrushin Yu., M.; Parfenov, V.A. Use of copper-vapor laser for restoration of artworks. *J. Opt. Technol.* **2008**, *75*, 476–477. [CrossRef]
25. Vilesova, M.S.; Lazareva, C.Y.; Saprykina, N.P.; Tkachev, B.I.; Levashova, L.G.; Khalizova, E.M. Study of thermal transformations of paper. In Proceedings of the International Conference "Library of Academy of Sciences: Ten Years after Fire", St.Petersburg, Russia, 16–18 February 1997; pp. 135–139.
26. Kautek, W. Laser Cleaning of Paper and Other Organic Materials. Available online: http://www.science4heritage.org/COSTG7/booklet/chapters/org.htm (accessed on 27 June 2022).

quantum beam science

MDPI

Article

Effect of Process Parameters on Laser Powder Bed Fusion of Al-Sn Miscibility Gap Alloy

Chiara Confalonieri *, Riccardo Casati and Elisabetta Gariboldi *

Department of Mechanical Engineering, Politecnico di Milano, Via La Masa 1, 20156 Milan, Italy; riccardo.casati@polimi.it

* Correspondence: chiara.confalonieri@polimi.it (C.C.); elisabetta.gariboldi@polimi.it (E.G.)

Abstract: Al-Sn binary system is a miscibility gap alloy consisting of an Al-rich phase and a Sn-rich phase. This system is traditionally applied in bearings and more recently found application as form-stable phase change material (PCM) exploiting solid-liquid phase transition of Sn. A careful choice of production process is required to avoid macro-segregation of the two phases, which have different densities and melting temperatures. In the present study, the additive manufacturing process known as laser powder bed fusion (LPBF) was applied to an Al-Sn alloy with 20% volume of Sn, as a rapid solidification process. The effect of process parameters on microstructure and hardness was evaluated. Moreover, feasibility and stability with thermal cycles of a lattice structure of the same alloy were experimentally investigated. An Al-Sn lattice structure could be used as container for a lower melting organic PCM (e.g., a paraffin or a fatty acid), providing high thermal diffusivity thanks to the metallic network and a "safety system" reducing thermal diffusivity if the system temperature overcomes Sn melting temperature. Even if focused on Al-Sn to be applied in thermal management systems, the study offers a contribution in view of the optimization of manufacturing processes locally involving high solidification rates and reheat cycles in other miscibility gap alloys (e.g., Fe-Cu) with similar thermal or structural applications.

Keywords: phase change materials; Al-Sn; miscibility gap alloys; selective laser melting; powder bed laser fusion

1. Introduction

Al-Sn binary systems are miscibility gap alloys (MGAs), i.e., they consist of two phases which are immiscible in solid state. In more detail, the two phases are almost pure Al and pure Sn. Thanks to their anti-wear performance, these alloys have been widely used in bearings [1]. More recently, they were studied as form-stable phase change materials (PCMs), specifically composite materials in which the Sn-rich active phase undergoing a solid/liquid transition is mixed to a high-melting Al-rich phase [2,3]. The latter can provide structural properties as well as modify thermal and other characteristics of the material. PCMs can be used in thermal energy applications since they can store the latent heat associated to an endothermic transition (e.g., melting) and release it when the transition is reversed (e.g., solidification). Furthermore, the material can be used to limit the maximum temperature of the system, at least within certain heat input limits.

Simple casting of molten MGAs results in both micro-segregation of the lower melting phase at grain boundaries of the high-melting one, and in macro-segregation of the low-melting phase in the last solidifying regions [4]. Contrarily, powder metallurgy and rapid solidification processes can result in a more homogeneous and finer phase distribution. Powder metallurgy has been applied either for Al-Sn based bearing materials by Zhu et al. [1,5–7] and for metallic Al-Sn based PCMs by Confalonieri et al. [3,8,9] and Sugo et al. [2]. With these kind of techniques, the homogeneous and fine phase distribution is provided through compaction and sintering of homogeneous powder blends, which are not, or only partially, melted, thus preventing macro-segregation of low-melting phase. On the other hand, rapid solidification methods involve complete melting of base material in form of powders or homogeneous ingots. The following solidification with high cooling rate entraps low-melting phase in the network created by primary nucleation of high-melting one. Several techniques are reported in literature to obtain fast solidification of Al-Sn based alloys, like laser alloying (Zhai et al. [4], Makhatha et al. [10]), high-velocity oxyfuel (Marrocco et al. [11]), and melt spinning (Lucchetta et al. [12], Kim and Cantor [13], Zhang W. et al. [14], and Zhang Z. et al. [15]). Confalonieri and Gariboldi [16] studied the possibility of using laser powder bed fusion (LPBF) as rapid solidification process in which a blend of Al and Sn powders is locally melted through a pulse laser. In laser-based powder bed systems, a powder layer is first applied on a building platform, then a laser melts it locally according to the input 3D model, and finally the platform is lowered; the cycle is repeated until the part is fully built, embedded in the powder bed [17]. Confalonieri and Gariboldi [16] observed that the extremely fine microstructure obtained for Al-Sn alloy with LPBF was similar to the finest microstructures obtained from compressed ball-milled powders [8,9]. This microstructure can provide high hardness and wear resistance [1], as well as interesting thermal properties. In more detail, a fine distribution of Al-Sn phases results in a relatively fast thermal storage followed by a more gradual heat release in a wide range of temperatures, thus reducing thermal stresses during cooling [3,9]. The advantage of using LPBF is, therefore, the possibility to couple a suitable microstructure for conventional Al-Sn based MGA applications in bearings or as PCMs, with the design freedom typical of an additive manufacturing technique compared to the limitations of powder metallurgy involving compression and sintering.

The present paper aims to study the effect of LPBF process parameters on the properties of Al-Sn alloy with Al/Sn ratio equal to 80/20, in view of its application in thermal storage and thermal management devices. Differently from typical LPBF applications, the classical target of reducing discontinuities like pores and cracks is flanked by the need to control phase distribution and to have a microstructurally stable material over several thermal cycles. Once the relationship between parameters and microstructure is established, the material designer can select the proper parameters according to the features required by the specific application. The results of this study can also be helpful to produce other MGAs through LPBF. For example, Fe-Cu based MGAs are investigated for their higher thermal conductivity with respect to steels and high strength [18,19], as well as for the possibility of using them as PCMs [2].

In addition to simple parallelepiped samples, a 3D lattice structure was produced to prove the feasibility to print a complex structure. The microstructure of the materials was investigated by electron microscopy. Material hardness was measured by Vickers tests. The thermal stability was evaluated by experimenting possible operating conditions for PCMs.

Lattice structures could be used as a container for a low-melting PCM [20,21]. This kind of hybrid system contains two PCM systems: a low-melting one, such as paraffin (melting temperature range: 6–108 °C [22]) or fatty acids (with melting temperature in a slightly narrow melting range), which stores latent heat in the temperature range of interest; and a high-melting one (e.g., Al-Sn), which enhances thermal diffusivity to the overall system thanks to the metallic network [23] and also can act as "safety system" by reducing thermal diffusivity upon its phase transition if the system temperature increases too much. The presence of the low-melting PCM, with high wettability on Al alloys could also avoid the formation of Sn particles at the material surface.

2. Materials and Methods

Commercially pure Al (ECKA Granules Germany GmbH, Fürth, Germany) and pure Sn (STAGNO 106, Metalpolveri S.r.l., Gussago (BS), Italy) powders were mixed to obtain a blend with 20% volume of Sn, corresponding to about 40% in mass. Both powders had high purity (>99.7% mass). Al powder had grain size lower than 45 μm, while Sn powder contained also coarser particles (>106 μm: 0.1%, >45 μm: 15–45%, <45 μm: 55–85%). SEM micrographs of powders are shown in Figure 1. Before the mixing processes, powders were sieved separately with a −63 μm mesh, to remove coarse particles and agglomerates. Then, they were blended in a tumbler mixer (Adler T-0) with about 1/3 of empty space in the jar, for 1 h at 20 rpm at room temperature.

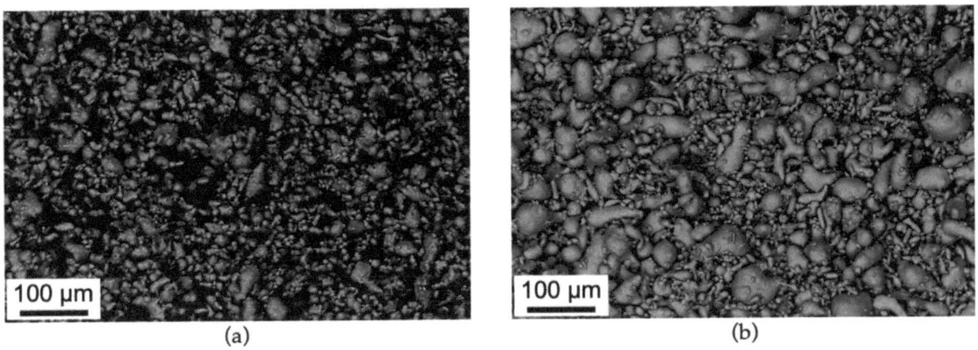

Figure 1. SEM micrographs of Al (**a**) and Sn (**b**) powders.

LPBF process was carried out using a pulsed laser Renishaw (Wotton-under-Edge, United Kingdom) AM 250 system equipped with a Reduced Build Volume apparatus (powder bed 90 mm × 90 mm). Using a pulsed laser, powders are melted by discrete and partially overlapped laser spots, which are exposed to the radiation for a given time (exposure time) [24]. The process was carried out in protective Ar atmosphere to reduce contamination from oxygen (oxygen content < 1000 ppm). A meander scanning strategy was applied and the scanning direction was rotated by 67° after each layer completion. The selected process parameters were in the range of typical values for Al alloys [24]. Layer thickness (25 μm), laser power (200 W), and exposure time (160 μs) were the same for all the samples. On the other hand, different values for hatch distances (d_h), i.e., the distance between the parallel adjacent scanned tracks, and point distance (d_p), i.e., distance between two neighbor points exposed to the pulsed laser, were selected, as reported in Table 1.

Table 1. Sample names and VED calculated accordingly to Equation (1).

		Point Distance, d_p [μm]			
		60	80	100	120
Hatch distance, d_h [μm]	60	A 356 J/mm^3	B 267 J/mm^3	C 213 J/mm^3	
	80	D 267 J/mm^3	E 200 J/mm^3	F 160 J/mm^3	
	100	G 213 J/mm^3	H 160 J/mm^3	I 128 J/mm^3	L 107 J/mm^3
	120			M 107 J/mm^3	N 89 J/mm^3

Volumetric energy density (also referred as specific energy, and expressed in J/mm^3) can be evaluated according to Equation (1), by approximating the scanning speed (v) as the ratio between point distance (d_p) and exposure time (t_{exp}):

$$\underline{E} = \frac{P}{d_h \cdot v \cdot l} \approx \frac{P \cdot t_{exp}}{d_h \cdot d_p \cdot l} \quad (1)$$

where P is the laser power, d_h is the hatch distance, and l is the layer thickness. Calculated values for each set of parameters are in Table 1. Two batches of samples were produced (A-I1, L-N); powders for the second batch were dried in a desiccator with silica for about 24 h before LPBF.

Specimens are parallelepipeds, with size 8 × 8 × 4 mm^3 for batch 1 (A-I1) and 10 × 8 × 4 mm^3 for batch 2 (L-N). Furthermore, a longer sample (40 × 9 × 5 mm^3), called I2, that was cut in smaller pieces for testing, and two lattice structures (with geometry shown in Figure 2 and produced with combination of parameters I) were added to the specimens of batch 2.

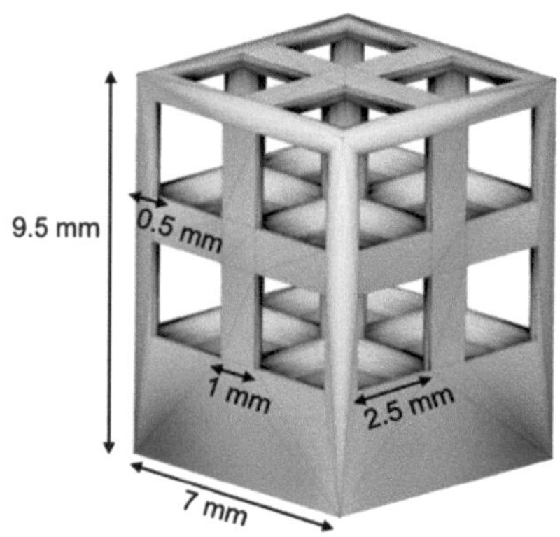

Figure 2. Three-dimensional model of lattice structure.

Characterization of parallelepiped samples consisted of the analysis of microstructure and hardness. Samples were sectioned, mounted, and ground with abrasive papers followed by polishing with diamond suspensions down to 1 μm. For microstructural characterization, both Optical Microscopy (OM, Eclipse LV150NL, Nikon, Tokyo, Japan) and Scanning Electron Microscopy (SEM, EVO 50, Zeiss, Jena, Germany) were used to evaluate materials features at different scale levels. Micrographs were analyzed using ImageJ software [25], measuring area fraction of pores, pore features, and crack density. In more detail, analyzed pore features are [26–28]:

- Equivalent diameter ($\varnothing_{eq}$), i.e., calculated diameter of a circle with the same area as the pore;
- Circularity, i.e., $4{\cdot}\pi{\cdot}$area/perimeter^2, which tends to 1 if the particle is round and smooth, and tends to 0 if it has irregular surface and/or elongated shape;
- Solidity, i.e., ratio between pore area and the minimum convex area that can cover the pore, which tends towards 1 if the pore has a convex shape, and tends towards zero if the boundary is irregular.

Crack density (d_{cracks}) is the average distance between cracks measured on a section parallel to building direction at low magnification.

Vickers microhardness tests were done on samples built on the diagonal of process parameter matrix shown in Table 1 (A, E, I, N). HV was measured along the sample direction parallel to the building direction, using a Future-tech FM-700 microhardness tester with a load of 4.91 N and a dwell time of 15 s. The test was repeated at least five times per sample choosing indentation points randomly on the sample surface to obtain an average value of hardness.

Analysis of lattice structures focused on evaluation of their behavior during thermal cycling reproducing operative conditions. Therefore, one of the lattice structures underwent 100 thermal cycles between 180 °C and 280 °C at a heating/cooling rate of ~27 °C/min, in protective Ar atmosphere to avoid oxidation of molten Sn. Photographs were taken before and after thermal cycles to observe possible changes.

3. Results

3.1. Low Magnification Analysis

Specimens printed with the two jobs are shown in Figure 3. The upper surface can have accumulated material at corners of the parallelepipeds, as pointed out by arrows for sample A in Figure 3. The accumulated material form peaks that are taller and wider as the VED increases, especially in samples from A to E. On the other hand, the samples with the lowest VED have an almost flat upper surface.

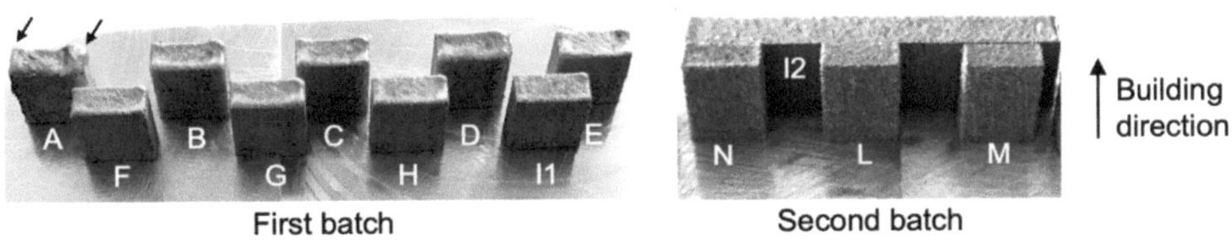

Figure 3. Photographs of parallelepiped samples before removal from support; arrows indicate accumulated material at corners of upper surface in sample A.

Optical micrographs of samples with the related process parameters are shown in Figure 4. At this relatively low magnification, Al and Sn phases are too fine to be distinguished; thus, specimens appear as consisting of a homogeneous grey metallic matrix with black areas corresponding to discontinuities, i.e., pores or cracks.

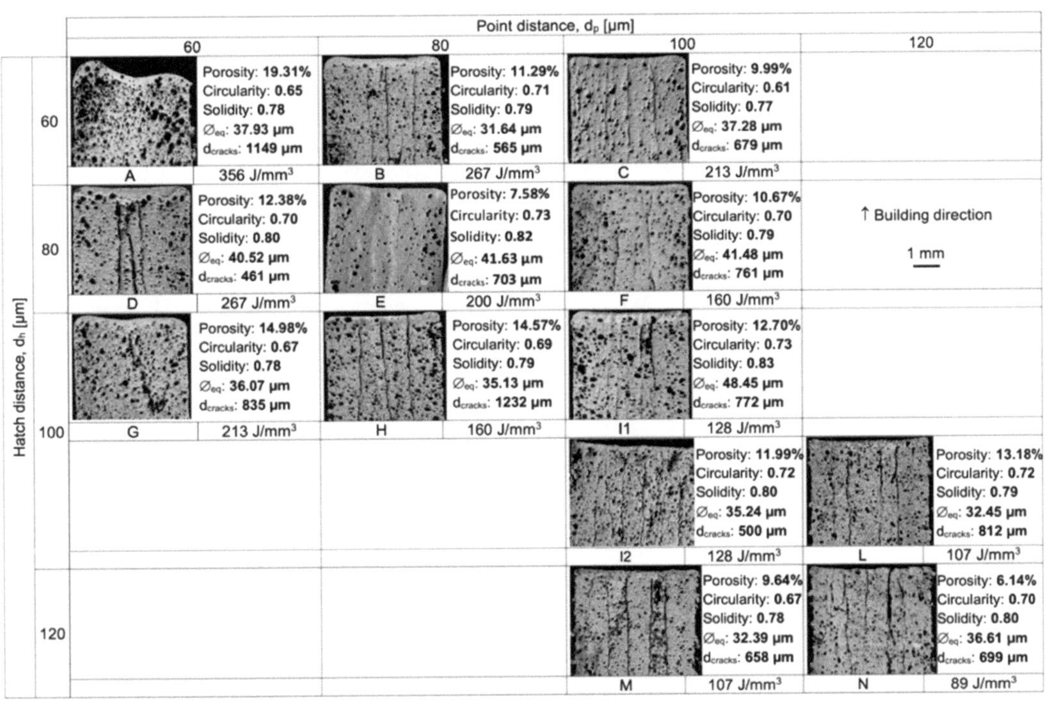

Figure 4. Optical micrographs, process parameters (hatch distance and point distance) and features of samples (porosity, circularity, solidity, equivalent diameter $\varnothing_{eq}$, and crack density d_{cracks}). Shown sections are parallel to building direction (vertical).

The average area fraction of pores (later on simply referred as porosity) as measured on OM micrographs ranges between 6% and 19%, with the highest value for the highest calculated VED (A) and the lowest ones for the lowest VED (N) and the central condition (E) (Figures 4 and 5). The other specimens have porosity between 9% and 15%, but, as shown in Figure 5, there is not a clear trend, neither considering the calculated VED variation nor single parameter (hatch or point distance) variation. Average values of circularity and solidity equal to about 0.7 and 0.8, respectively (Figure 4), show that pores tend to have a spherical shape with smooth surface. Considering pore size, the average equivalent diameter is between 30 μm and 50 μm for all samples (Figure 4).

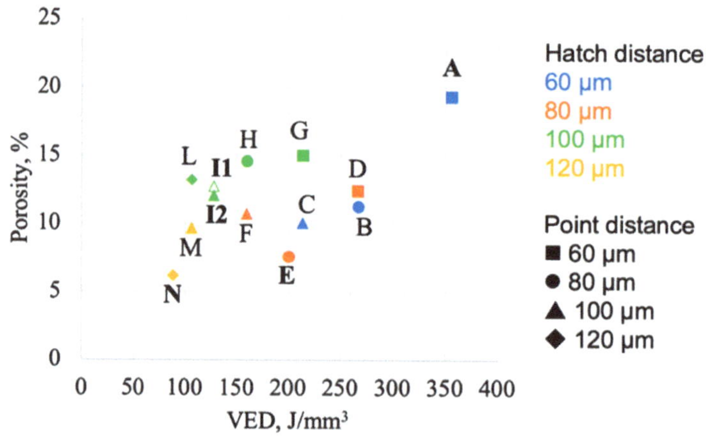

Figure 5. Porosity for each sample as function of VED.

The most significant differences between specimens can be found in pore size distribution (Figure 6) and pore location in the plane parallel to build direction (Figure 4). In all the samples, most of pores (40–50%) have equivalent diameter lower than 50 μm and the percentage of pores per size decreases as equivalent diameter reduces (Figure 6a). As shown in Figure 6b, the standard deviation of equivalent diameter generally reduces with VED. The high standard deviation of specimen I1, here represented with open symbol, is related to the presence of interconnected big pores, considered as a single one by ImageJ software during particles analysis. Figure 6b suggests that high energy samples have a wider pore size range, between ~10 μm and ~100 μm, with respect to low energy ones, generally with bigger pores concentrated near the external surface and in correspondence with the upper surface peaks mentioned above (Figure 4). By reducing the VED, the standard deviation of equivalent diameter reduces as well, i.e., pore size distribution becomes narrower, and the arrangement of pores in the sample tends to be more homogeneous. Such features, that were observed on longitudinal sections of the specimens, have also been confirmed by analyses of transversal sections of samples. For sake of comparison, see OM image of samples A, E, I1, and N in Figure 7.

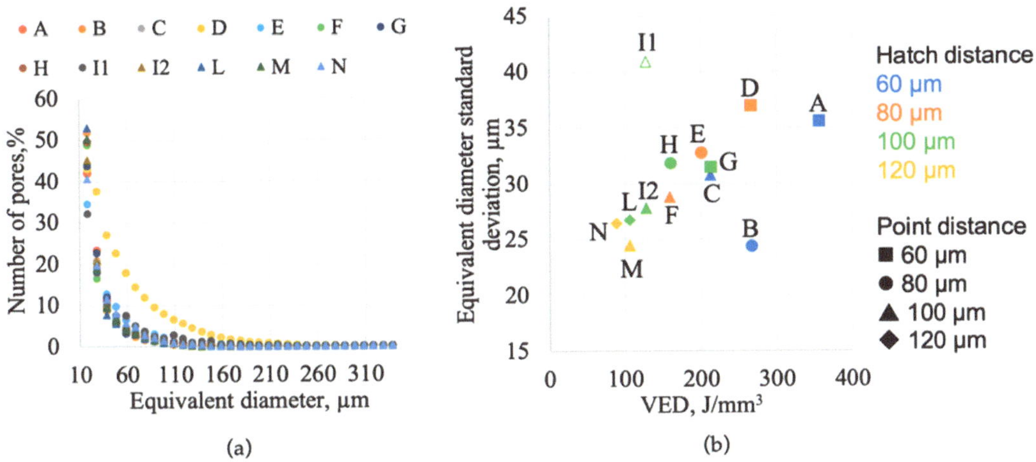

Figure 6. Pore size distribution described through: (**a**) percentage of pores per equivalent diameter (each point corresponds to an equivalent diameter range ± 5 µm), and (**b**) standard deviation of equivalent diameter as function of VED.

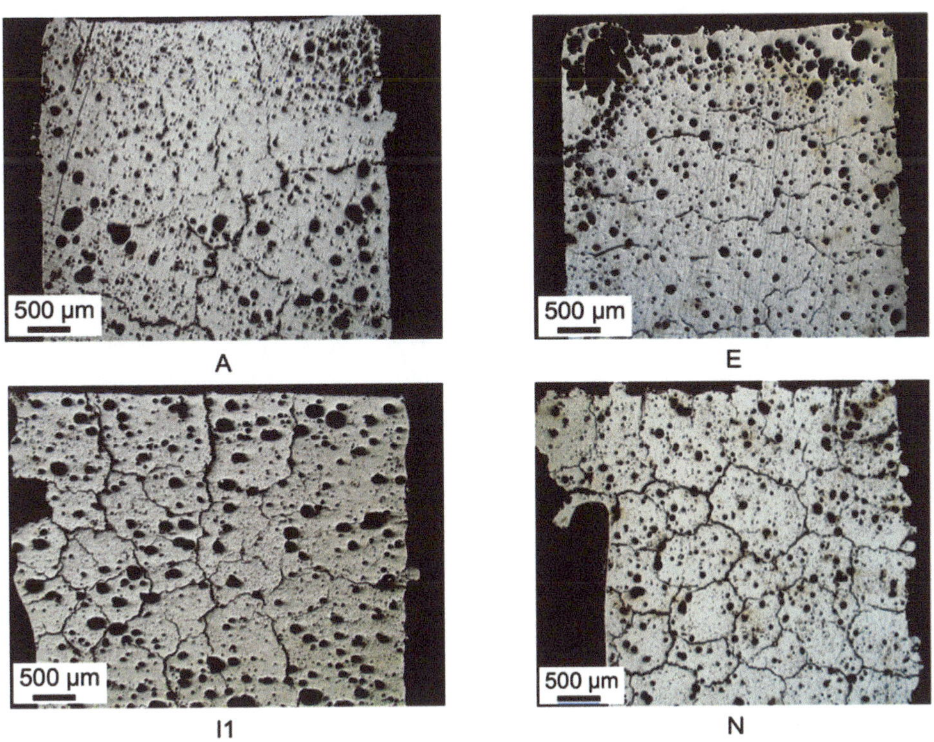

Figure 7. OM micrograph of samples A, E, I1, and N: section perpendicular to the building direction.

Vertical cracks (Figure 4) are generally parallel to the building direction, while cracks in sections perpendicular to building direction (Figure 7) tend to form a continuous network. In both sections, sample A (i.e., the one produced with the highest VED) displays few small cracks, concentrated especially in the region close to the building platform. On the other hand, the number of cracks increases as VED reduces. Considering crack position, they tend to concentrate in the middle of the sample at high energies, while they are more spread within the sample and interconnected in transverse direction at low energies. The minimum average distances between vertical cracks are 461 μm for sample D, while for the other samples this value ranges between 565 μm and 1232 μm or even higher. The range is compatible with the crack network distribution observed on transversal sections.

3.2. SEM Analysis

SEM micrographs of samples on diagonal of parameter matrix are shown in Figure 8, with increasing VED from A to N sample. Sn (bright contrast) and Al phases (dark contrast) can be distinguished in the SEM micrographs. The horizontal bands are formed by the grains grown between consequent layers in the production process; at low energies, Sn-rich zones are observed in these bands, highlighting the shape of molten pools. By decreasing energy, a finer structure is observed. The size of the Sn particles dispersed in Al phase is between ~2 μm and ~100 nm in sample A. In sample N, fine Sn films are formed along with Sn particles. The film is ~100 nm thick and the small particles are ~100 nm in size.

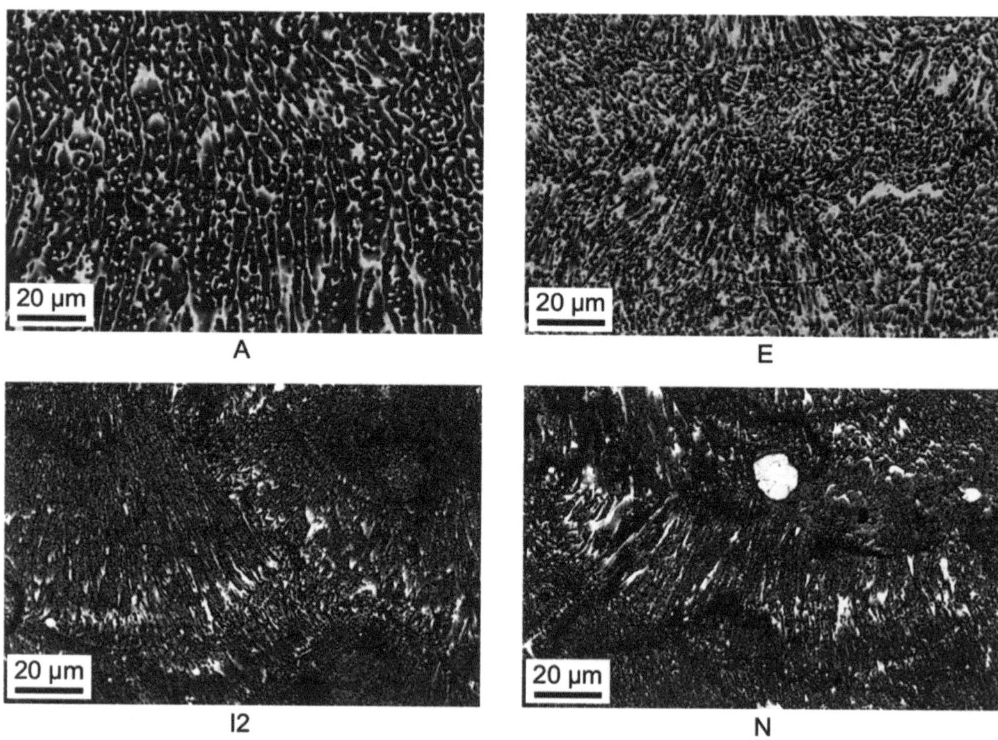

Figure 8. SEM micrographs (BSE) of samples A, E, I2, and N at 3000× magnification.

In all the samples, round-shape Sn particles with diameter of ~15 μm are observed (e.g., see sample N in Figure 8 and samples I and E in Figure 9). These particles seldomly show inner porosities (Figure 9b). Focusing on cracks (Figure 9), it is possible to notice that they can be partially or fully filled with Sn.

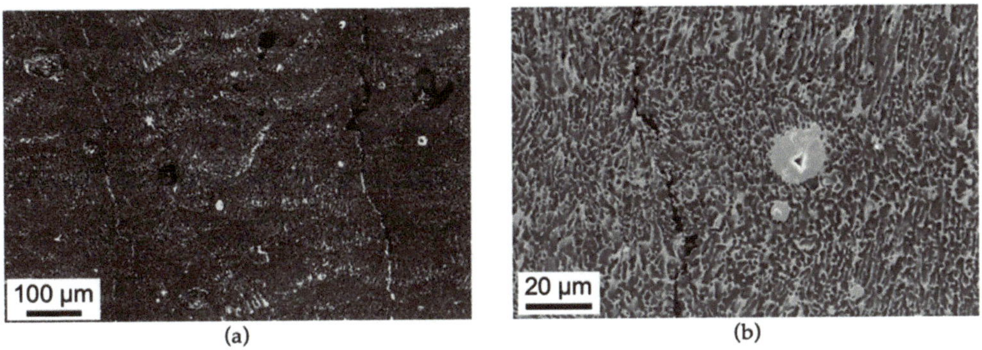

Figure 9. SEM micrographs (BSE) of sample I (**a**) and sample E (**b**) showing cracks at different orders of magnitude.

3.3. Vickers Microhardness

Results of Vickers microhardness measurements for samples on diagonal of parameters matrix are shown in Figure 10. Samples from the first batch (A, E, and I1) have hardness values of about 30 HV, while values for second-batch samples (I2 and N) are slightly above 40 HV.

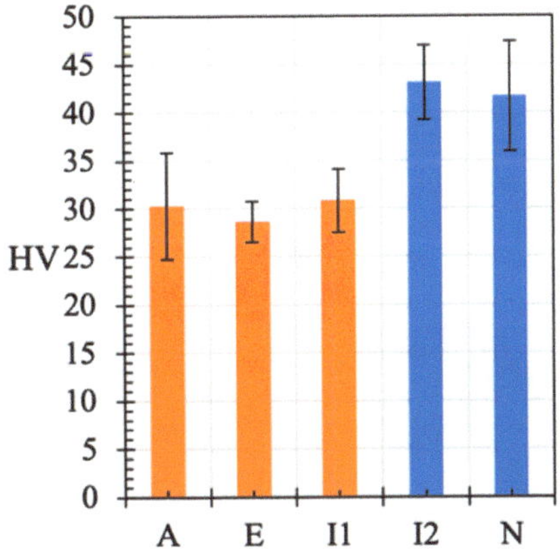

Figure 10. Vickers microhardness numbers for samples on the diagonal of parameter matrix (i.e., those with same hatch distance and point distance). Orange series and blue series indicate samples belonging to the first batch and to the second batch, respectively.

3.4. Lattice Structures

Lattice structures were produced using parameters I, i.e., hatch distance and point distance of 100 µm, correspondingly to those of sample I2. In as-built conditions (Figure 11a), the obtained structure does not show evident deformations or discrepancies with the CAD model. Poor surface quality is observed in the down-skin of horizontal trusses. After 100 thermal cycles between 180 °C and 280 °C, only a minimal deformation is observed in one of the upper corners (dashed ellipse in Figure 11b). Furthermore, Sn droplets (pointed out with arrows in Figure 11b) appear seldomly on surfaces.

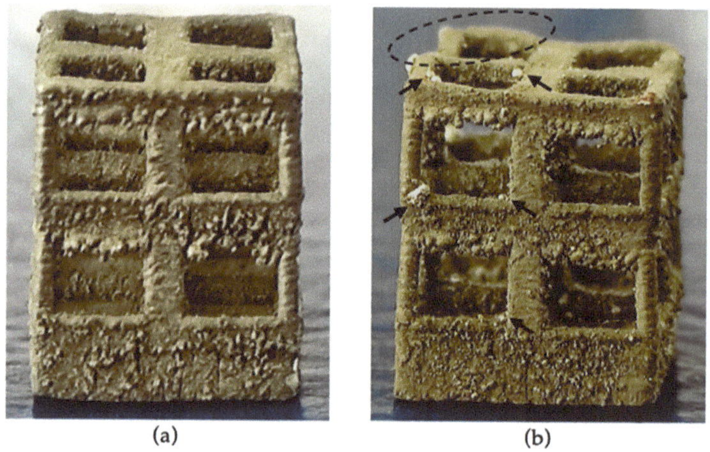

Figure 11. Photographs of lattice structures in as-produced conditions (**a**) and after 100 cycles across Sn melting temperature (**b**). In image (**b**), the dashed ellipse highlights a deformed region of the lattice, and the arrows point out Sn droplets.

SEM micrographs of the as-built lattice surface (Figure 12a) show the absence of surface cracks in vertical trusses, which are 0.5 mm or 1 mm wide. On the other hand, vertical cracks appear on horizontal trusses, which are 7 mm long. The distance between cracks ranges from 250 μm to 700 μm, with an average value of ~400 μm. The lowest average distances between longitudinal cracks can be found in the most highly constrained regions, i.e., at lattice nodes where 1 mm thick trusses converge, and at the bottom part of the lattice, in direct contact with the bulk Al substrate. After thermal cycling, lattice surface shows relatively coarse Sn droplets with diameter of hundreds of microns (Figure 12b), as well as small droplets with diameter below 50 μm and thread-like Sn whiskers (Figure 12c).

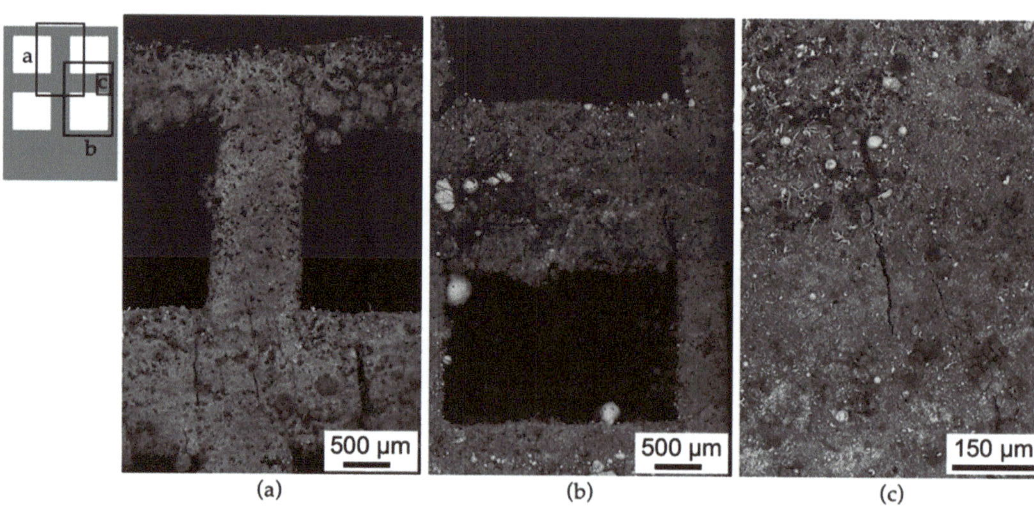

Figure 12. SEM micrographs (SE) of lattice structure surface before (**a**) and after (**b**,**c**) thermal cycling. The schema shows micrographs position.

4. Discussion

4.1. Effect of Process Parameters on Microstructure

Various process parameters affected microstructural features, as phase distribution, discontinuities (pores and cracks) and topology of the upper surface. The main physical principle that lies behind them is that the energy input (here considered in terms of VED) during LPBF affects the local thermal history of the material. The laser scanning induces fast melting and solidification of the material and the formation of steep thermal gradients affecting also the already printed material, with a complex set of consequences on the microstructure of MGA. As observed in a previous work by Confalonieri and Gariboldi [16], Al-20%vol Sn alloy produced through LPBF has an extremely fine microstructure thanks to the high cooling rate of the molten pool. This small size of microstructural features is comparable with those observed for the same alloy produced through ball milling, compression and sintering [3,8,9]. In addition, a similar microstructure was obtained with LPBF by Zafari and Xia [19] for MGA Fe-20%vol Cu. During cooling, due to the immiscibility of the two phases, Al grains solidify first, while Sn is segregated at grain boundaries reducing primary grain growth [19]. If, due to high energy input, the cooling rate is relatively slow and extensive remelting occurs during deposition of upper layers, Al cells are relatively coarse and the structure appears generally homogeneous, see samples A and E in Figure 8. As VED decreases, the microstructure becomes finer with Al cells elongated in vertical cooling direction with Sn at boundaries; at the same, Sn agglomerates form especially at the bottom of the melting pool, "trapped" during the fast solidification, as previously discussed by the authors in [16]. Thus, low VED results in less homogeneous microstructure. With this phase distribution, which was not significantly modified by the upper layer deposition, the former molten pools can be more easily appreciated. These various types of microstructures can affect thermal diffusivity of the system, leading to an isotropic or anisotropic behavior accordingly [16].

Porosity changes significantly in each sample in terms of quantity, size, and location. The investigated values of hatch distance and point distance do not have a clear effect on porosity, which, in any case, seems to be more affected by the overall VED. To further analyze the correlation between process parameters and porosity, an alternative description of energy density values suggested by Ferro et al. [29] was applied (Equation (2)).

$$\underline{\mathrm{E}} = \frac{\mathrm{C}(\mathrm{P}, \mathrm{t_{exp}}, \alpha, \beta, \phi)}{\mathrm{d_h}\sqrt{\mathrm{d_p}}} \Longrightarrow \underline{\mathrm{E}} \propto \frac{1}{\mathrm{d_h}\sqrt{\mathrm{d_p}}} \quad (2)$$

This expression includes thermal transport phenomena (α = powder thermal diffusivity, β = absorption coefficient, ϕ = spot size diameter). It relates the VED to the inverse of the product between hatch distance and the square root of point distance, while in Equation (1) the inverse proportionality of VED is with the product between hatch distance and the point distance. Accordingly, considering that C parameter is the same for all the samples, porosity and standard deviation of equivalent diameter are plot as function of $(d_h \times d_p{}^{0.5})^{-1}$ in Figure 13. Despite the change in VED dependency on hatch and point distance, the plots show the same trends observed in Figures 5 and 6b, i.e., the point series does not follow a clear law. The complexity in relating process parameters to microstructural features can be ascribed to the peculiar features that characterize an MGA. In more detail, it should be considered that heat transfer phenomena, especially at low temperature, are significantly affected by the phase transition of low-melting phase and thermal properties cannot be considered constant with temperature, thus heat transport cannot be easily modelled.

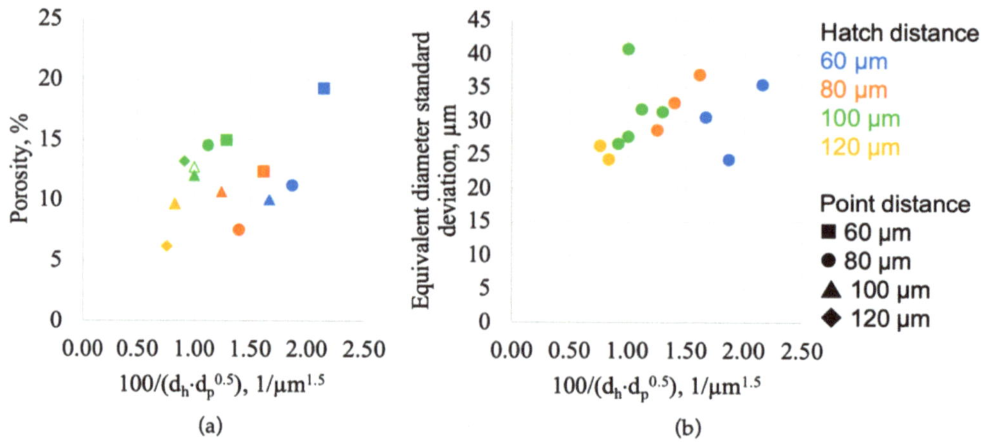

Figure 13. Porosity for each sample (**a**) and standard deviation of equivalent diameter (**b**) as function of $(d_h \times d_p^{0.5})^{-1}$, representing the alternative description of VED according to [29].

In the investigated MGAs the formation of pores can be ascribed to two main causes: presence of gases in the molten pool and Sn particles detachment during specimen preparation (artifact). The presence of gas in the molten pool, which gives rise to spherical-shape pores, can be related to several causes [30]. First, shielding gas (Ar in the present case) can be trapped in the molten pool due to turbulence, which is more likely to occur at high VED. At the same time, turbulence in the molten pool is known to concurrently lead to the formation of peaks on upper surface of specimens [30]. In addition, moisture initially adsorbed by the powders can also be responsible for porosity [31]. Comparing samples I1 and I2, produced with the same parameters in the two batches, it is possible to observe that the one produced with dried powders (I2) smaller average pore size has a slightly lower amount of porosity (almost 1% less). The last gas-related cause for porosity is the evaporation of Sn due to the higher absorptivity of Sn with respect to Al and the high energies involved to melt Al, since it is necessary to break the Al oxide layer and to compensate the high laser reflectivity [32,33]. Despite the specific cause for pore formation, pore size tends to reduce with VED, since gas expansion is lower as temperature decreases and turbulence of molten pool is lower as well.

Gas pores tend to form closer to the external regions of the sample and to be bigger as VED increases. In facts, the outer regions of the samples are the hottest, because (i) they are affected by slower cooling rates, due to the fact that the surrounding unmolten powder has lower thermal diffusivity than the compacted material, and (ii) the laser direction is inverted following the meander scanning strategy, resulting in close consecutive laser pulses. This phenomenon is clearly more emphasized as VED increases together with more turbulence in the molten pool. On the other hand, lower VED values result in lower temperatures and, consequently, lower porosity, that is spread more homogeneously throughout the analyzed sections.

Vertical cracks are mainly caused by thermal stresses related to solidification shrinkage [18]. Sn has a solidification temperature much lower than Al, which means that solid and liquid coexist in a wide temperature range, thus promoting hot cracking. High VED, causing slower cooling rates and less severe thermal gradients, reduces cracks, especially in the inner part of samples that is more constrained. Moreover, as previously mentioned, the outer areas of high-VED specimens are hotter than the core, so cracks tend to concentrate in the middle of the sample, whereas cracks are distributed throughout the section in low-VED samples.

Hardness of the alloy can be considered as constant for samples produced in the same job. The difference between the hardness of samples of the two batches (+25% in batch

2 samples), can be reasonably ascribed to the effect of moisture. Dried powder (batch 2) shows less and smaller pores and higher hardness. Within samples of the same batch, considering that coarse discontinuities (e.g., cracks and big pores) were avoided during HV measurements, microstructural differences are probably too small to affect significantly hardness. Comparing the obtained values with earlier studies, hardness values obtained for the first batch (~30 HV) are close to values for cast and press-and-sintered Al-Sn alloys with the same nominal composition [1,34]. Hardness of samples from the second batch (~40 HV) are close to those of samples produced by ball-milled powder that are pressed-and-sintered [3,9].

Summarizing, according to microstructural analysis, the effects of process parameters are the following:

1. Excessively high energy density increases pore size and results in accumulation of materials on the top surface corners;
2. Most of the parameter sets lead to coarse porosity located at the outer surface, especially in high VED conditions. As energy decreases porosity is more homogeneously distributed in the sample;
3. High energy results in coarse and homogeneous phase distribution;
4. Low VED samples are more affected by hot-cracking.

Therefore, the best conditions, i.e., minimum number of pores and cracks are in the middle-right of the parameter matrix (see Table 1), are for parameter sets E, C, F, and I, since these process parameter sets have intermediate VED, balancing the effects of high and low VED.

4.2. Lattice Structures

Lattice structures were obtained by LPBF and proved to keep their shape almost unchanged after 100 thermal cycles across the solid/liquid transition of the Sn phase. Cracks were observed on as-built lattice surfaces only on horizontal trusses and not on vertical ones. Vertical beams are thin enough to avoid detrimentally high thermal stresses and, so, to prevent vertical crack formation. On the other hand, horizontal segments, show cracks with spacing comparable with that of bulk sample produced with the same process parameter combination (I2). This means that the designer can act both on process parameters and part geometry to reduce or avoid hot cracks.

After thermal cycling, Sn leaked out from the lattice surface. As previously seen for ball-milled and compressed samples [8,9], a fine microstructure without coarse interconnected particles, can help to reduce the risk of significant Sn losses. Nevertheless, the significance of this phenomenon depends on the service condition of the material. Indeed, a feature of interest can be the number of times the transition is activated in component life, i.e., only once (e.g., for safety device) or cyclically, leading to the functional fatigue of the material. Another feature to be considered is the environment where the Al-Sn component works, since Sn leakage could or could not damage other structures in the system.

5. Conclusions

The present work analyzed the effect of LPBF process parameters on Al-20%vol Sn alloy properties. Process parameters affect phase distribution, presence of discontinuities, and geometrical features of samples, while they did not change hardness significantly. To optimize each of these features, an intermediate VED with low hatch distance appears to give the best results, reducing the risk of pore and crack formation.

Furthermore, a lattice structure was successfully produced and proved to be relatively stable even after thermal cycling across Sn melting temperature. Such kind of metal PCM structure could potentially replace homogeneous Al-alloy lattice, providing a "safety function" to the part if temperature increases excessively. It could be inserted for instance in a more complex thermal storage device where a low melting organic PCM (e.g., a paraffin or a fatty acid) fills the Al-Sn alloy lattice, providing also mechanical strength and thermal conductivity.

Considerations on LPBF of Al-Sn alloy and thermal cycling of lattice structures could be extended to other miscibility gap alloys.

Author Contributions: Conceptualization, E.G.; data curation, C.C.; formal analysis, C.C.; investigation, C.C. and R.C.; resources, E.G.; visualization, C.C.; writing—original draft, C.C.; writing—review & editing, C.C., R.C. and E.G. All authors have read and agreed to the published version of the manuscript.

Funding: This research received no external funding.

Institutional Review Board Statement: Not applicable.

Informed Consent Statement: Not applicable.

Data Availability Statement: The raw data required to reproduce these findings cannot be shared at this time as the data also form part of an ongoing study. The processed data required to reproduce these findings cannot be shared at this time as the data also form part of an ongoing study.

Acknowledgments: The Italian Ministry of Education, University and Research is acknowledged for the support through the Project "Department of Excellence LIS4.0—Lightweight and Smart Structures for Industry 4.0.

Conflicts of Interest: The authors declare no conflict of interest.

References

1. Liu, X.; Zeng, M.; Ma, Y.; Zhu, M. Promoting the high load-carrying capability of Al–20wt%Sn bearing alloys through creating nanocomposite structure by mechanical alloying. *Wear* **2012**, *294–295*, 387–394. [CrossRef]
2. Sugo, H.; Kisi, E.; Cuskelly, D. Miscibility gap alloys with inverse microstructures and high thermal conductivity for high energy density thermal storage applications. *Appl. Therm. Eng.* **2013**, *51*, 1345–1350. [CrossRef]
3. Confalonieri, C.; Perrin, M.; Gariboldi, E. Combined powder metallurgy routes to improve thermal and mechanical response of Al—Sn composite phase change materials. *Trans. Nonferrous Met. Soc. China* **2020**, *30*, 3226–3239. [CrossRef]
4. Zhai, W.; Hu, L.; Geng, D.; Wei, B. Thermodynamic properties and microstructure evolution of ternary Al–10%Cu–x%Sn immiscible alloys. *J. Alloys Compd.* **2015**, *627*, 402–409. [CrossRef]
5. Liu, X.; Zeng, M.; Ma, Y.; Zhu, M. Wear behavior of Al–Sn alloys with different distribution of Sn dispersoids manipulated by mechanical alloying and sintering. *Wear* **2008**, *265*, 1857–1863. [CrossRef]
6. Lu, Z.; Zeng, M.; Gao, Y.; Zhu, M. Significant improvement of wear properties by creating micro/nano dual-scale structure in Al–Sn alloys. *Wear* **2012**, *296*, 469–478. [CrossRef]
7. Liu, X.; Zeng, M.; Ma, Y.; Zhu, M. Melting behavior and the correlation of Sn distribution on hardness in a nanostructured Al–Sn alloy. *Mater. Sci. Eng. A* **2009**, *506*, 1–7. [CrossRef]
8. Confalonieri, C.; Grimaldi, A.T.; Gariboldi, E. Ball-milled Al–Sn alloy as composite Phase Change Material. *Mater. Today Energy* **2020**, *17*, 100456. [CrossRef]
9. Confalonieri, C.; Bassani, P.; Gariboldi, E. Microstructural and thermal response evolution of metallic form-stable phase change materials produced from ball-milled powders. *J. Therm. Anal.* **2020**, *142*, 85–96. [CrossRef]
10. Makhatha, M.E.; Fatoba, O.S.; Akinlabi, E.T. Effects of rapid solidification on the microstructure and surface analyses of laser-deposited Al-Sn coatings on AISI 1015 steel. *Int. J. Adv. Manuf. Technol.* **2018**, *94*, 773–787. [CrossRef]
11. Marrocco, T.; Driver, L.C.; Harris, S.J.; McCartney, D.G.; Mc Cartney, G. Microstructure and Properties of Thermally Sprayed Al-Sn-Based Alloys for Plain Bearing Applications. *J. Therm. Spray Technol.* **2006**, *15*, 634–639. [CrossRef]
12. Lucchetta, M.C.; Saporiti, F.; Audebert, F. Improvement of surface properties of an Al–Sn–Cu plain bearing alloy produced by rapid solidification. *J. Alloys Compd.* **2019**, *805*, 709–717. [CrossRef]
13. Kim, W.T.; Cantor, B. Solidification of tin droplets embedded in an aluminium matrix. *J. Mater. Sci.* **1991**, *26*, 2868–2878. [CrossRef]
14. Zhang, W.; Zhao, B.; Zhai, Q.; Gao, Y. Application of Fast Scanning Calorimetry in the Rapid Solidification of Tin Particles Embedded in Al Matrix. In *TMS2013 Supplemental Proceedings*; Wiley: Hoboken, NJ, USA, 2013; pp. 477–484.
15. Zhang, Z.; Wang, Y.; Bian, X.; Wang, W. Orientation of nanocrystals in rapidly solidified Al-based alloys and its correlation to the compound-forming tendency of alloys. *J. Cryst. Growth* **2005**, *281*, 646–653. [CrossRef]
16. Confalonieri, C.; Gariboldi, E. Al-Sn Miscibility Gap Alloy produced by Power Bed Laser Melting for application as Phase Change Material. *J. Alloys Compd.* **2021**, *881*, 160596. [CrossRef]
17. DebRoy, T.; Wei, H.; Zuback, J.; Mukherjee, T.; Elmer, J.; Milewski, J.; Beese, A.; Wilson-Heid, A.; De, A.; Zhang, W. Additive manufacturing of metallic components – Process, structure and properties. *Prog. Mater. Sci.* **2018**, *92*, 112–224. [CrossRef]
18. Kim, W.R.; Bang, G.B.; Park, J.H.; Lee, T.W.; Lee, B.-S.; Yang, S.-M.; Kim, G.-H.; Lee, K.; Kim, H.G. Microstructural study on a Fe-10Cu alloy fabricated by selective laser melting for defect-free process optimization based on the energy density. *J. Mater. Res. Technol.* **2020**, *9*, 12834–12839. [CrossRef]

19. Zafari, A.; Xia, K. Nano/ultrafine grained immiscible Fe-Cu alloy with ultrahigh strength produced by selective laser melting. *Mater. Res. Lett.* **2021**, *9*, 247–254. [CrossRef]
20. Hubert, R.; Matar, O.B.; Foncin, J.; Coquet, P.; Tan, D.; Li, H.; Teo, E.H.T.; Merlet, T.; Pernod, P. An effective thermal conductivity model for architected phase change material enhancer: Theoretical and experimental investigations. *Int. J. Heat Mass Transf.* **2021**, *176*, 121364. [CrossRef]
21. Li, Z.; Gariboldi, E. On the use of effective thermophysical properties to predict the melting process of composite phase change materials with coarse structures. *Int. J. Heat Mass Transf.* **2021**, *180*, 121765. [CrossRef]
22. Vakhshouri, A.R. Paraffin as Phase Change Material. In *Paraffin—An Overview*; IntechOpen: London, UK, 2020.
23. Li, Z.; Gariboldi, E. Modelling the conditions for natural convection onset in open-cell porous Al/paraffin composite phase change materials: Effects of temperature, paraffin type and metallic structure geometry. *Int. J. Heat Mass Transf.* **2021**, *173*, 121279. [CrossRef]
24. Casati, R.; Vedani, M. Aging Response of an A357 Al Alloy Processed by Selective Laser Melting. *Adv. Eng. Mater.* **2019**, *21*, 1800406. [CrossRef]
25. Rasband, W.S. ImageJ. 2018. Available online: https://imagej.net/Welcome (accessed on 20 March 2022).
26. Ferreira, T.; Rasband, W. ImageJ User Guide. 2012. Available online: https://imagej.nih.gov/ij/docs/guide/146.html (accessed on 25 November 2019).
27. Takashimizu, Y.; Iiyoshi, M. New parameter of roundness R: Circularity corrected by aspect ratio. *Prog. Earth Planet. Sci.* **2016**, *3*, 2. [CrossRef]
28. Russ, J.C. *The Image Processing Handbook*; CRC Press: Boca Raton, FL, USA, 2006.
29. Ferro, P.; Meneghello, R.; Savio, G.; Berto, F. A modified volumetric energy density–based approach for porosity assessment in additive manufacturing process design. *Int. J. Adv. Manuf. Technol.* **2020**, *110*, 1–11. [CrossRef]
30. Zhang, J.; Song, B.; Wei, Q.; Bourell, D.; Shi, Y. A review of selective laser melting of aluminum alloys: Processing, microstructure, property and developing trends. *J. Mater. Sci. Technol.* **2019**, *35*, 270–284. [CrossRef]
31. Weingarten, C.; Buchbinder, D.; Pirch, N.; Meiners, W.; Wissenbach, K.; Poprawe, R. Formation and reduction of hydrogen porosity during selective laser melting of AlSi10Mg. *J. Mater. Process. Technol.* **2015**, *221*, 112–120. [CrossRef]
32. Wang, Z.; Ummethala, R.; Singh, N.; Tang, S.; Suryanarayana, C.; Eckert, J.; Prashanth, K.G. Selective Laser Melting of Aluminum and Its Alloys. *Materials* **2020**, *13*, 4564. [CrossRef]
33. Yap, C.Y.; Chua, C.K.; Dong, Z.L. Preliminary investigation on selective laser melting of pure tin. *Proc. Int. Conf. Prog. Addit. Manuf.* **2016**, *1290*, 409–414.
34. Gariboldi, E.; Perrin, M. Metallic Composites as Form-Stable Phase Change Alloys. *Mater. Sci. Forum* **2018**, *941*, 1966–1971. [CrossRef]

quantum beam science

MDPI

Article

Use of 3D Laser Scanning and Additive Technologies for Reconstruction of Damaged and Destroyed Cultural Heritage Objects

Vadim Parfenov [1,*], Sergei Igoshin [2], Dmitriy Masaylo [2], Alexey Orlov [2] and Dzmitry Kuliashou [3]

[1] Department of Photonic, Faculty of Electronics, St. Petersburg Electrotechnical University, 197376 St. Petersburg, Russia

[2] Institute of Mechanical Engineering, Materials and Transport, Peter the Great St. Petersburg Polytechnic University, 195251 St. Petersburg, Russia; sergei.igosshin@gmail.com (S.I.); dmasaylo@gmail.com (D.M.); orlov_alexey88@mail.ru (A.O.)

[3] Center of Prototyping, 197376 St. Petersburg, Russia; sdimasik1102@gmail.com

* Correspondence: vaparfenov@etu.ru

Abstract: Three-dimensional laser scanning is a novel measurement technique that is frequently used for the documentation of cultural heritage (CH) objects. In the process of 3D scanning, one can obtain computing 3D models of artworks to be documented. It allows one to produce detailed digitized archives of important CH objects. Moreover, the use of 3D scanning enables the digital reconstruction of architectural fragments, sculptures, and other artworks. One more important application of this technique relates to the creation of molds and replicas for replacements of outdoor CH objects in case their preservation requirements do not allow them to remain in their original place due to the influence of environmental factors. One of the most effective ways of creating replicas is the use of laser additive technologies. Therefore, the combination of 3D scanning and additive technologies is a very promising way of preservation of CH. This paper describes several case studies concerned with the combined usage of 3D laser scanning and additive technologies for digital reconstruction and replication and of outdoor sculptures in St. Petersburg city. One of them is the reconstruction of the zinc sculpture "Eva at the fountain" (XIX century, England), which was destroyed during WWII. Its replica was created by means of laser stereolithography. Eventually, one more project is related to the reconstruction of the fragment of the sufficiently damaged cast-iron XIX century monument. This object was reconstructed using two laser technologies: direct metal laser sintering (DMLS), and laser cladding (LC).

Keywords: laser additive technologies; 3D printing; 3D scanning; cultural heritage object; restoration; reconstruction; end-to-end technologies

1. Introduction

In recent decades, one of the most serious challenges in the preservation of cultural and historical heritage has been the rapid decay of exterior monuments due to environmental deterioration, especially in large industrial megapolises. However, in addition to poor environmental conditions, sculptures and other cultural heritage objects also suffer from natural disasters and vandal attacks, which also result in damage and sometimes total loss.

In this context, the question on the need to reconstruct damaged CH objects or to gradually replace them with copies with subsequent transfer of originals to closed museum premises was on the agenda. According to the world practice, today, it is the only opportunity to preserve the most important monuments of the past for descendants, at least their most valuable ones. Although the idea of replacing originals with copies has always caused and still causes an ambiguous attitude in society and even among the museum community, unfortunately, there is no other way to save CH objects from destruction nowadays. It should be noted that the idea of the replication of monuments is not new. Michelangelo's masterpiece, the famous marble sculpture of David, which has remained for almost 370 years in Piazza della Signoria in Florence, was copied in 1873 when the original David was moved for eternal storage in the Gallery of Academy of Fine Arts in the city.

However, nowadays, when museum curators, art experts, and restorers gradually come to an agreement on the need for copying monuments in principle, the question arises of what technologies may be used (and most importantly, are acceptable) when creating copies. Over the years, copies of sculptural monuments were created from different materials. In the 1980s, natural marble was used, and copies were made by "manual" cutting of sculptures and bas-reliefs of stone blocks. Later, cement with marble powder was used, but now various types of synthetic materials are used instead of cement. Such a composition is called "artificial stone". However, this approach, which has been widely adopted in recent years, has many serious shortcomings. The most important of them is that copies made of artificial stone are obtained as a result of forming the original sculpture, and this inevitably leads to a significant physical and chemical impact on its surface. Molding can lead to mechanical damages in the form of fractures and broken small parts of monuments occurring during the mold removal. In addition, the impact of chemical reactions of molding materials with the monument substrate can also be significant.

Now, there is a very attractive alternative to the above-mentioned approach. Innovative 3D laser scanning technology in combination with stone milling machines with numerical software control (CNC) is attractive way of replicating cultural heritage objects. This allows copying sculptural monuments made of natural stone (marble, limestone, granite, etc.). The main advantage of this method is that it is contactless and does not have any negative impact on the original monument. Thanks to this, laser-based contactless copying technology is now widespread in some European countries [1–3].

Ultimately, copying CH objects using natural stone is expensive, and it is not always advisable to use this approach. A different approach can be used to replicate ordinary artifacts and to create copies of lost fragments of works of art for modeling restoration work. Such tasks can be resolved by means of using laser additive technologies. In recent years, several research groups reported case studies where different 3D printing techniques were used, but all known works are not systematic [4–6]. The purpose of this work is to demonstrate the principal possibility of the application and benefits of the use of end-to-end 3D scanning technologies and the reproduction of scan results using CNC and 3D printers with a laser source for repairing and reconstructing cultural heritage objects. In this paper, we describe the results of cases studies on the reconstruction of CH objects in the city of St. Petersburg.

2. Replication and Reconstruction of Sculptures

For the first time in Russia, the non-contact copying of sculptural monuments was carried out by the scientists of St. Petersburg Electrotechnical University (ETU) in collaboration with Italian colleagues in 2008–2010. It was the project on the replication of the XVIII century Italian marble bust "Primavera" from the State-museum preserve "Tsarskoye Selo" collection. This work began with the creation of a 3D computer model of the sculpture obtained using 3D laser scanning. Then, the 3D model was forwarded to our colleagues in Carrara in Italy, who have years of experience in the creation of replicas of historical objects from natural marble using CNC machines. Firstly, they converted 3D model into CAD model requiring for operation of CNC robotic machines. After that, they manufactured a precise copy of the sculpture "Primavera" from a block of white Carrara marble by using a CNC milling robotic machine. The detailed description of this project is given in [3,7], and in Figure 1, one can see photos of the original, the process of carving the marble block, and replica placed in the location of the original sculpture.

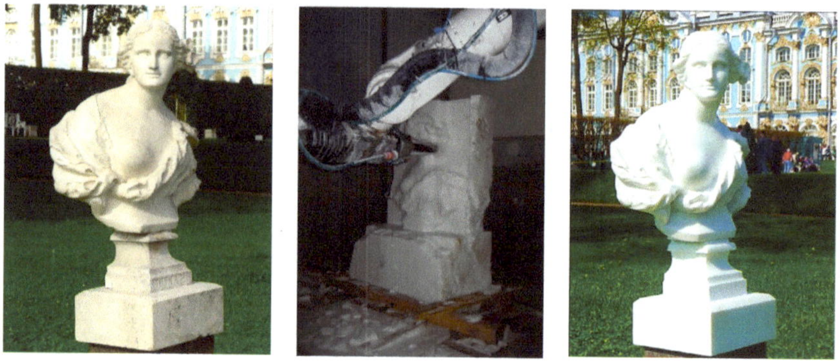

(a) (b) (c)

Figure 1. Marble sculpture "Primavera": general view of original, June 2009 (**a**); process of manufacturing the replica by CNC machine (**b**); general view of replica, June 2010 (**c**).

One more project was conducted by the scientific group of the ETU in 2017 when a copy of marble bust of XIX century of the Russian Emperor Peter the Great from the State-museum preserve "Peterhof" collection marble bust was created. This sculpture was given by Russian sponsoring organizations as a present to the French Academy of Sciences in Paris in 2017 on the occasion of the 300th anniversary of the Peter the Great visit to France. During the implementation of this project, 3D scanning of Peter's bust was carried out in the storage facility of the museum "Peterhof", and then, the same as "Primavera", its copy was made of a marble block in Carrara, Italy by using a CNC machine (Figure 2) [8].

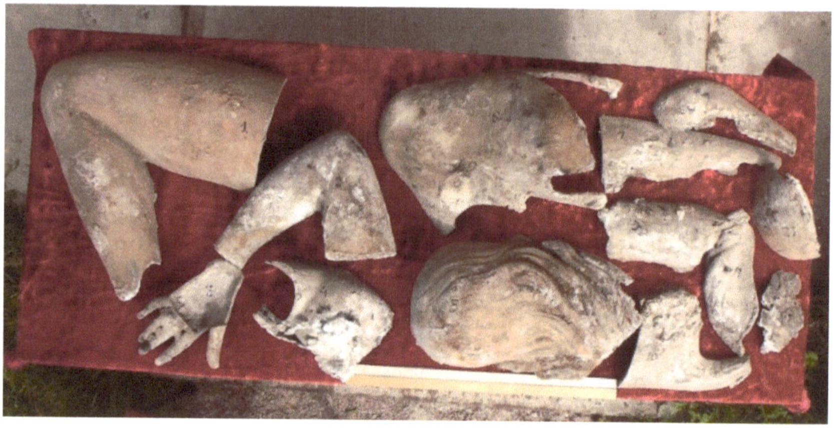

Figure 2. Fragments of sculpture "Eve".

The results of the projects on copying marble sculptures of Peter I and Primavera provide a convincing demonstration of the high efficiency of the contactless method for creating physical copies of sculptural monuments made of stone. Its relatively low cost, speed of execution and the full preservation of the original in the process are of such significance that it will inevitably lead to its wide application in museum practice soon.

3. Reconstruction of Damaged Cultural Heritage Objects

Another interesting perspective in modern museum work is connected with the use of 3D scanning for the reconstruction of damaged and even completely destroyed monuments.

3.1. Case Study of Zinc Sculpture "Eve"

One of the case studies of such works is the reconstruction of a totally lost sculpture from the former estate Sergievka in the suburbs of St. Petersburg, which in the XIX century was the country residence of the Duke of Leuchtenberg, the stepson of Napoleon Bonaparte. The Duke of Leichtenberg collected antiquities and possessed the richest collection of masterpieces. Unfortunately, almost all the items of this unique collection were lost during the Great Fatherland War, as Sergievka was in the epicenter of combat activities. Among the many lost masterpieces was a 19th-century zinc sculpture "Eve at the water spring", the fragments of which were discovered underground during construction works in 2007 (Figure 2).

They represented a pile of scattered fragments that did not allow carrying out the reconstruction of this monument by traditional methods of the museum work. However, the use of 3D laser scanning technology, computer simulation, and 3D printing made possible creating a replica of this sculpture, allowing us to judge what the original monument was like (Figure 3). The replica was created from polymer material using additive technology FDM (fused deposition modeling).

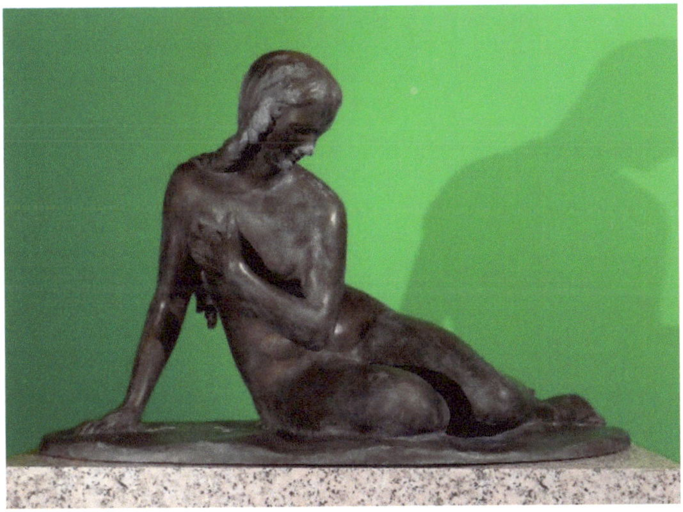

Figure 3. Replica of sculpture "Eve".

The results of this project are described in the work [5], but it is worth mentioning that the replication and reconstruction of works of art puts a serious issue on the agenda—what is the accuracy of creating the physical copies of objects? In other words, how precise is the correspondence between surfaces of the same object in its 3D model and replica obtained using additive technologies? This issue is very important from point of view of authenticity of any original CH object and its replica, but it is not considered in the scientific literature in the papers devoted to the replication of sculptures.

We carried out an experimental study on the evaluation of the accuracy of the replication of the sculpture "Eve". In those experiments, we used a laser scanner Surphaser 25SHX (scanning accuracy—2.5 microns) and did find that deviations in the surfaces of the original 3D model and replica were in the range of ± 0.7 mm. During a detailed analysis of the 3D model of the replica, a "cellular structure" (resembling honeycomb) was clearly visible on its surface, especially pronounced in the area of the sculpture's back (see Figure 4, where one can see the result of "overlapping" of 3D model of replica and 3D model that was used for the creation of replica).

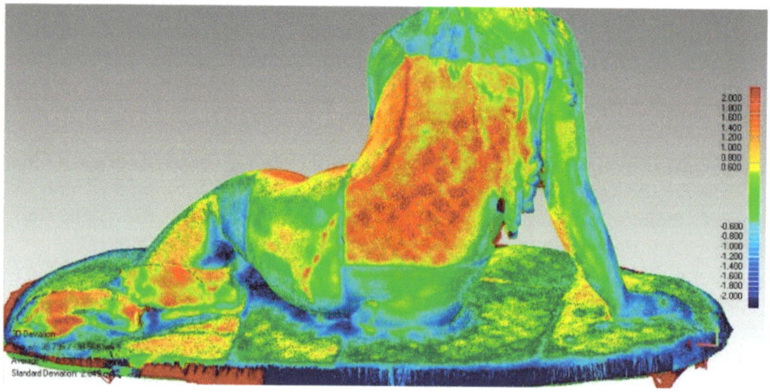

Figure 4. The result of comparing the replica's 3D model and the 3D model that was used to create the replica.

This may be a consequence of the 3D printing technique used, in which, to reduce the cost of replication, we decided to save used material (PLA plastic) by having the sculpture be hollow inside (the volume filling was 10%). Because of this, local "minima" (deflections) of the sculpture surface are observed in the places where the surface layer of the sculpture is attached to the stiffeners, while the sagging areas correspond to local maxima. It was these deformations that were detected by laser scanning.

Thus, the accuracy of reproduction of the sculpture "Eve" can be considered good, but it must be borne in mind that when replicating sculptural monuments, distortions of their geometric shape are possible.

3.2. *Case Study of Cast-Iron Star*

One of our most recent works relates to the reconstruction of CH objects created from cast-iron. Nowadays, it is a typical conservation problem in CH preservation. There are sculptures, objects of decorative art, grids around historical buildings, parks, and gardens as well as just decorative elements on the facades of buildings. Many of them are highly deteriorated and usually have severely damaged and lost parts (see Figure 5a). Until recently, experts in the field of CH did not attach much importance to such items, and as they fell into complete disrepair, they were replaced with copies. However, in recent years, there has been a reassessment of values, and a new trend has emerged in the work of restorers, which requires the reconstruction of objects damaged by corrosion instead of replacing them with copies.

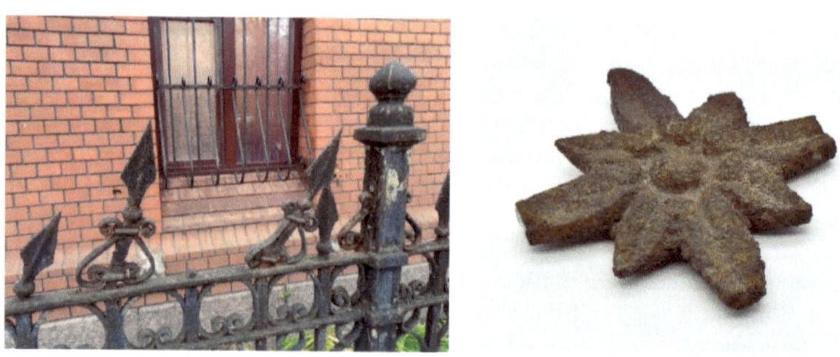

(**a**) (**b**)

Figure 5. (**a**)—An example of a damaged cast-iron fence; (**b**)—cast-iron star for repairing.

The authors of this article understand this problem and proposed its technical solution based on the use of laser powder coating technology. In our work, we demonstrated the principal possibility of the realization of such an approach.

The object of our studies was a small (10 cm) iron star that is a decorative element of a XIX century cast-iron tombstone fence of the Alexander Nevsky monastery in St. Petersburg. This object is highly deteriorated due to corrosion and has losses of some small elements (see Figure 5b).

The main idea of our project was to recreate the losses of individual elements of the star using a combination of 3D scanning technology, direct metal laser sintering (DMLS), and laser cladding.

Firstly, we analyzed the chemical composition of the star using X-ray fluorescence using XL3t-32280 equipment. The analysis results are shown in Table 1.

Table 1. The result of the chemical analysis of the part.

Element	Fe	Si	Co	Mn	P	Zn	Pb	Ti	Ag	Other
Content, wt. %	91.05	6.38	0.79	0.45	0.34	0.24	0.22	0.17	0.13	0.24

We did find that the main chemical element is Fe (its concentration is of about 91%). Additionally, there are permanent impurities typical for gray cast-iron (the total concentration is only about 7.2%).

Secondly, we removed the corrosion from the star surface. For the removal of corroded layers, we tried to use different treatment techniques: laser cleaning, sand blasting and chemical treatment; the latter gave the best result (see Figure 6a).

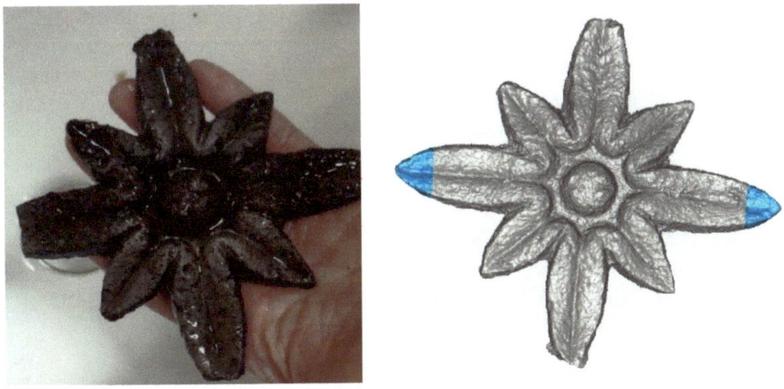

(a) (b)

Figure 6. (**a**)—star after chemical treatment; (**b**)—3D model with added rays.

Then, we carried out 3D scanning of the star using laser triangular scanner Konica Minolta V-910 and created its 3D model. The next stage of our work was the computer modeling. The missing ray of the cast-iron star was modeled with the Zbrush software. The main distinguishing feature of this software is the ability to "sculpt" 3D objects. The surviving cones were projected, processed, and "glued" to the main body of the star in the parts where there were losses (see Figure 6b), where blue ends are reconstructed lost parts of the star.

It was decided to separate those experiments into two stages: firstly, we created one of the star rays, which we proposed to join with the star; the second stage of reconstruction will be based on a reconstruction of the lost end of another star ray by direct metal deposition. It is obvious that such a method of reconstruction is more complicated since the very precise movement of a laser beam is needed, and such a task can be solved by means of the development of specialized software.

A separate ray of the star was grown by the DMLS method according to the CAD model. We used a CW fiber Ytterbium laser with an output power of up to 80 W. Stainless-steel powder 316 L20 (manufacturer—Hoganas, Belgium) with a granule size of 53 μm was used for printing. The result of creating this piece can be seen in Figure 7a.

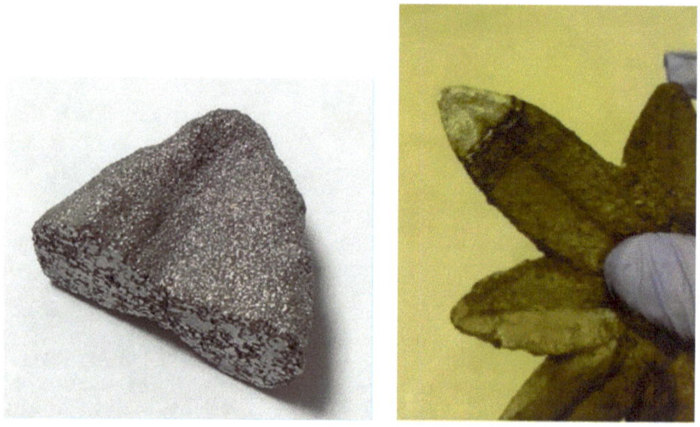

(**a**) (**b**)

Figure 7. (**a**)—DMLS printed star ray; (**b**)—welded star ray.

We then applied direct laser deposition (DLD) [9,10] using the OKTA-Printer machine developed at the Peter the Great St. Petersburg Polytechnic University (see Figure 8). The essence of the DLD method is to directly feed a metal powder or composite powder mixture into a molten bath formed by a laser beam [11–13]. The local action of heating the laser beam, the selective effect, as well as the high accuracy of modern robotic manipulators allow using this technology as an advanced and modern method for repairing and restoring products. The main parts of the OKTA-Printer are the powder cladding head and the CAMAU robot. For joining, we used a nickel alloy powder Inconel 625 (manufacturer—Hoganas, Belgium) with a particle size distribution of 50–150 μm. It is one of the most popular alloys in laser cladding and DLD [14,15]. To connect the two pieces, they were glued to each other with glue, then welded in one pass on each side. The following parameters were used for welding: laser spot width 1.5 mm, laser power 700 W, robot movement speed 1500 mm/s, and powder feed 20 g/min. The result of the stage of the star reconstruction is shown in Figure 7b.

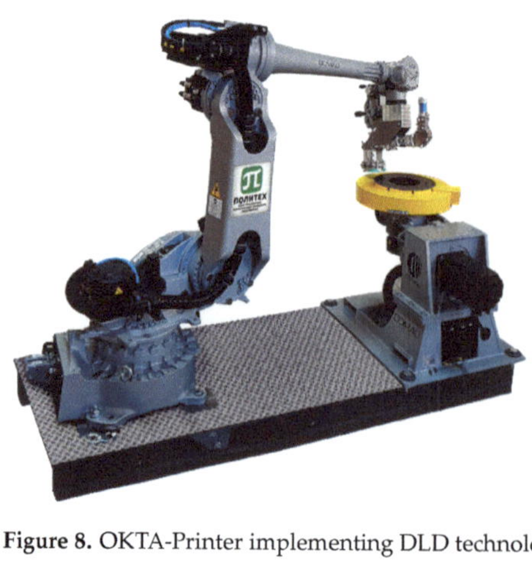

Figure 8. OKTA-Printer implementing DLD technology.

Using the DLD printer, an attempt was made to deposit the missing part of the star's ray on the material from which it is made. For this, a parallel piece was cut off and deposited on it from the same Inconel 625 that was used for welding. As a result of the cladding, an excessive absorption of laser radiation by the star material was detected, which leads to melting and a geometry change in the substrate along the edges, even with a relatively low heat input.

Furthermore, to assess the thermal effect on the structure of the star material, a materials science study of the initial structure and structure after laser cladding was carried out, and the transition zone was also investigated. Additionally, the microhardness was measured at a load of 0.3 kgf with the same step of 200 μm to evaluate the change in metal properties from the nickel alloy overlay to the cast-iron from which the star is made (see Figure 9).

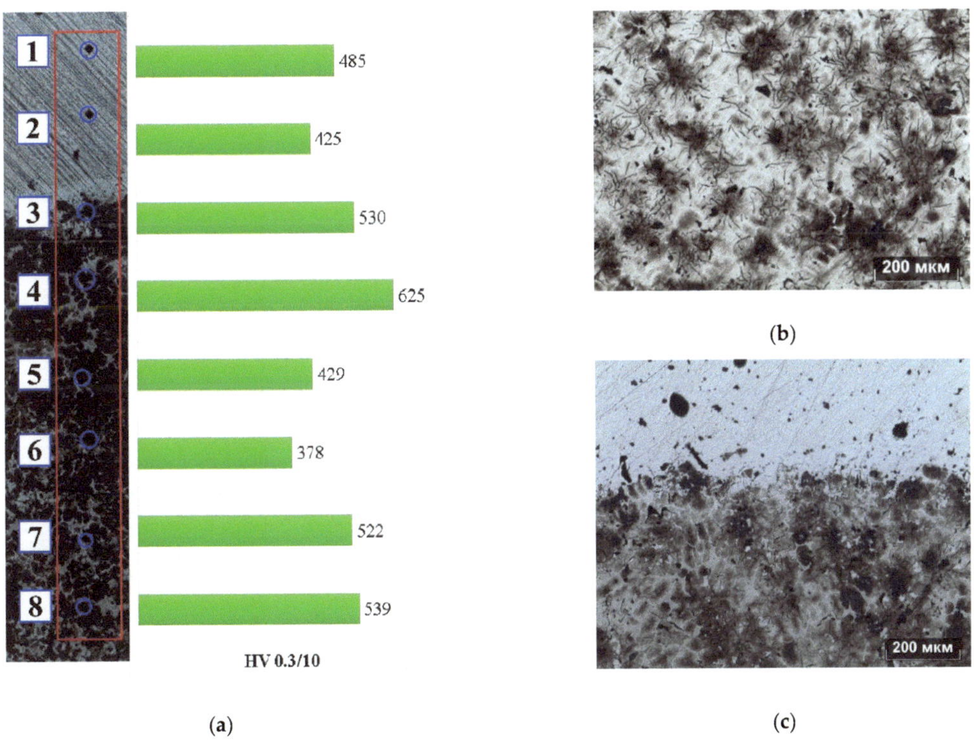

Figure 9. (**a**)—hardness measurement in HV from cladding to cast-iron with a step of 200 μm, the structure of the material was investigated using a Leica optical microscope: (**b**)—structure of cast-iron-before cladding; (**c**)—structure of cast-iron with cladding.

Separate hardness measurements were made at four to five points for each area of interest: cast-iron without surfacing is 240 ± 60 HV, with weld overlay 467 ± 76 HV, hardness of deposited Inconel 625 corresponds to 462 ± 26 HV, hardness in the transition zone is 601 ± 134 HV. Examination of the state of the interface on an optical microscope (Figure 9c) showed a strong metallic bond of the cladding with the star material: there were no cracks or pores at the interface.

Since there are no data on the percentage of carbon in the composition of the studied cast-iron, we assume that the initial microstructure of the star material corresponds to the structure of gray cast-iron on a ferrite base with lamellar-free graphite. Due to the thermal effect of the laser beam, the hardness of cast-iron increased significantly, which can be associated with rapid heating followed by rapid cooling, which leads to the formation of a pearlite structure, as well as the accumulation of thermal stresses. It was noted that at more than 1 mm from the surfacing, the hardness of the cast-iron base was significantly higher than the hardness of the same cast-iron without cladding. This indicates a large heat-affected zone that is not typical for standard cladding materials. Usually, this area is no more than 0.5 mm. This is most likely due to the size of the substrate itself and the low heat-dissipation. For the experiment on direct restoration of the missing part, a substrate with an area of 2 cm^2 was used, whereas the substrates for cladding and DLD are usually at least 100 cm^2.

4. Conclusions

This article describes several case studies concerned with the reconstruction and replication of CH objects in the city of St. Petersburg. It was shown that such tasks can be effectively achieved by means of the combined use of 3D scanning technologies, CNC milling, and laser additive technologies.

It should be noted that, as far as we know, our work on the reconstruction of the cast-iron star was the first case study that demonstrated the principal possibility of the use of direct metal laser sintering and laser powder cladding technology for the conservation of cast-iron CH objects. Therefore, the combined use of 3D scanning, DMLS, and laser cladding technologies has great potential for exact copying of the texture of metal monuments. The main advantage of this approach is a slight thermal effect on the restoration object at the joining of the reconstructed elements with a damaged object itself by laser cladding. Direct reconstruction of damaged CH objects by the DLD method directly on the object of restoration looks preferable, but it is much more complicated due to the unsuitability of cast iron as a substrate, from which many CH objects are made. Nevertheless, it is no doubt an interesting field for further scientific work, and the authors plan to continue their studies.

Author Contributions: Conceptualization, V.P.; methodology, V.P.; software, D.M.; validation, V.P. and S.I.; formal analysis, V.P.; investigation, V.P., S.I. and D.K.; resources, V.P. and S.I.; data curation, S.I.; writing—original draft preparation, V.P. and D.K.; writing—review and editing, V.P., S.I.; visualization, V.P., D.K. and S.I.; supervision, V.P.; project administration, V.P., A.O.; funding acquisition, V.P. and D.M. All authors have read and agreed to the published version of the manuscript.

Funding: This research received no external funding.

Institutional Review Board Statement: Not applicable.

Informed Consent Statement: Not applicable.

Data Availability Statement: By request to authors.

Acknowledgments: The authors would like to acknowledge Vitaly Tishkin and Anton Zhuravlev for taking part in the experimental studies.

Conflicts of Interest: The authors declare no conflict of interest. The funders had no role in the design of the study; in the collection, analyses, or interpretation of data; in the writing of the manuscript, or in the decision to publish the results.

References

1. Fowles, P.S. The Garden Temple at Ince Blundell: A Case Study in the Recording and Non-Contact Replication of Decayed Sculpture. *J. Cult. Herit.* **2000**, *1*, S89–S91. [CrossRef]
2. la Pensée, A.; Parsons, J.; Cooper, M.; Broadbent, S.; Bingham, R. The Use of 3D Laser Scanning and 3D Modelling in the Realisation of an Artistic Vision; Production of Large Scale Public Art in Tudor Square, Sheffield. In Proceedings of the International Archives of Photogrammetry, Remote Sensing and Spatial Information Sciences, Newcastle upon Tyne, UK, 21–24 June 2010; Volume XXXVIII, pp. 375–380.
3. Parfenov, V.A. Non-Contact Replication of Marble Sculptures Using Laser Technology. In *Sculpture of XVIII-XIX Centuries in Out-Door Environment;* St. Petersburg's Museum of Urban Sculpture Publishing House: St. Petersburg, Russia, 2010; pp. 66–69.
4. Skarlatos, D.; Theodoridou, S.; Hennings, D.; Ville, S. Replication of Marble Exhibits Using Photogrammetry and Laser Scanning (or How to Forge Exhibits). In Proceedings of the XIXth CIPA Symposium, Antalya, Turkey, 30 September–4 October 2003.

5. Wachowiak, M.J.; Karas, B.V. 3d Scanning and Replication for Museum and Cultural Heritage Applications. *J. Am. Inst. Conserv.* **2009**, *48*, 141–158. [CrossRef]
6. Cekus, D.; Kwiatoń, P.; Nadolski, M.; Sokół, K. Quality Assessment of a Manufactured Bell Using a 3D Scanning Process. *Sensors* **2020**, *20*, 7057. [CrossRef] [PubMed]
7. Parfenov, V.A. Laser Techniques in Artworks Conservation in St.Petersburg. *Rev. Cuba. Fis.* **2016**, *33*, E29–E31.
8. Parfenov, V.A. Use of Laser Technologies for Restoration, Documentation and Replication of Sculptural Monuments in Saint Petersburg. *Insight Non-Destr. Test. Cond. Monit.* **2020**, *62*, 129–133. [CrossRef]
9. Thompson, S.M.; Bian, L.; Shamsaei, N.; Yadollahi, A. An Overview of Direct Laser Deposition for Additive Manufacturing; Part I: Transport Phenomena, Modeling and Diagnostics. *Addit. Manuf.* **2015**, *8*, 36–62. [CrossRef]
10. Masaylo, D.V.; Orlov, A.V.; Igoshin, S.D. Effect of Heat Treatment on the Structure and Phase Composition of a High-Temperature Nickel Alloy Obtained by Laser Cladding. *Met. Sci. Heat Treat.* **2019**, *60*, 728–733. [CrossRef]
11. Masaylo, D.V.; Popovich, A.A.; Sufiyarov, V.S.; Orlov, A.V.; Shamshurin, A.I. A Study of Structural Features of a Gradient Material from a Heat-Resistant Nickel Alloy Produced by Laser Cladding. *Met. Sci. Heat Treat.* **2019**, *60*, 739–744. [CrossRef]
12. Schwendner, K.I.; Banerjee, R.; Collins, P.C.; Brice, C.A.; Fraser, H.L. Direct Laser Deposition of Alloys from Elemental Powder Blends. *Scr. Mater.* **2001**, *45*, 1123–1129. [CrossRef]
13. Leyens, C.; Beyer, E. Innovations in Laser Cladding and Direct Laser Metal Deposition. In *Laser Surface Engineering*; Elsevier: Amsterdam, The Netherlands, 2015; pp. 181–192.
14. Todaro, C.J.; Easton, M.A.; Qiu, D.; Zhang, D.; Bermingham, M.J.; Lui, E.W.; Brandt, M.; StJohn, D.H.; Qian, M. Grain Structure Control during Metal 3D Printing by High-Intensity Ultrasound. *Nat. Commun.* **2020**, *11*, 142. [CrossRef] [PubMed]
15. Abioye, T.E.; Folkes, J.; Clare, A.T. A Parametric Study of Inconel 625 Wire Laser Deposition. *J. Mater. Process. Technol.* **2013**, *213*, 2145–2151. [CrossRef]

quantum beam science

MDPI

Article

Laser Treatment as a New Approach to the Passivation of Iron-Based Historical Monuments

Iuliia Ruzankina [1,2,*], Vadim Parfenov [3], Oleg Vasiliev [4], Oleg Zotov [5] and Alexandra Zotova [5]

1 Department of Mathematics and Physics, Univesita Cattolica del Sacro Cuore, I-25121 Brescia, Italy
2 Department of Chemistry, KU Leuven, Celestijnenlaan 200D, 3001 Leuven, Belgium
3 Department of Photonics, St. Petersburg Electrotechnical University, 197376 Saint Petersburg, Russia; vaparfenov@etu.ru
4 LLC 'Laser Center', 195176 Saint Petersburg, Russia; tesla_90@mail.ru
5 Laboratory of Synthesis New Materials and Structures, Peter the Great St. Petersburg Polytechnic University, 195251 Saint Petersburg, Russia; zog-58@mail.ru (O.Z.); zotova_ao@spbstu.ru (A.Z.)
* Correspondence: ruzankinajulia@gmail.com

Abstract: This article is devoted to the study of the possibility of the passivation of iron-based metallic materials. The experimental results obtained for the laser treatment of carbon steel model samples by the radiation of repetitively pulsed and continuous-wave 1.064 μm Nd:YAG lasers are described. It is shown that the laser treatment allows the formation of dense protection films, 62–77 microns thick, on the steel surface. The films enhance the anticorrosion properties of the metal. Exposure to laser radiation reduces the surface roughness (from $R_a = 0.53$ μm to $R_a = 0.38$ μm). Laser radiation power densities of 10.2×10^5 W/cm^2 and 10.7×10^5 W/cm^2 for these two laser generating modes, respectively, correspond to the optimum (in terms of the degree of corrosion resistance) modes of steel treatment. The conducted studies show that the application of Nd: YAG lasers is a promising method for the surface passivation of artworks created from steel and cast iron. One of the most promising applications of the proposed method for the anticorrosion protection of iron is the passivation of the surface of iron-based historical monuments.

Keywords: laser passivation; Nd:YAG laser; anticorrosion coating; steel; cultural heritage; historical monument; artworks; restoration

check for updates

Citation: Ruzankina, I.; Parfenov, V.; Vasiliev, O.; Zotov, O.; Zotova, A. Laser Treatment as a New Approach to the Passivation of Iron-Based Historical Monuments. *Quantum Beam Sci.* **2022**, *6*, 9. https://doi.org/10.3390/qubs6010009

Academic Editors: Swee Leong Sing and Wai Yee Yeong

Received: 20 January 2022
Accepted: 14 February 2022
Published: 16 February 2022

Publisher's Note: MDPI stays neutral with regard to jurisdictional claims in published maps and institutional affiliations.

1. Introduction

One of the most important practical tasks in modern museum work is the passivation of the surface of cultural heritage (CH) objects made of iron, steel, and cast iron. In the conservation of such objects, restorers frequently have to deal with the removal of corrosion products. This is a very difficult task in itself, since the corrosion layer thickness of many monuments (primarily archaeological objects) can be significant (up to 1 cm). However, this problem is aggravated by the fact that the reoccurring formation of the foci of corrosion on the surface of such objects is possible after the completion of the restoration process. This puts the task of developing effective technologies for creating inhibitory (protective) coatings on the surface of monuments on the agenda.

Corrosion inhibitors are the substances that, when in a corrosive environment in sufficient concentrations, dramatically slow down or even stop the corrosive degradation of metal. There are several different types of inhibitors; however, in terms of restoration-related tasks, the most relevant is the application of coatings which enhance the resistance of museum objects to the effects of atmospheric corrosion. Most often, wax and various types of lacquers are used as inhibitors in the conservation of CH objects; but in recent years special protective materials have emerged, including those made of inorganic materials [1].

According to the mechanism of action, inhibitors can be divided into two types: passivating and adsorption. Adsorption-based corrosion inhibitors are adsorbed on the surface of a protected artifact, forming a film, and inhibit electrochemical reactions (sometimes forming a thin monomolecular film is sufficient for this). Adsorption inhibitors are most often surface-active agents, as well as organic compounds which, owing to their impact on the artifact, additionally enhance the protective properties of the oxide film. The presence of oxygen in a corrosive environment contributes to enhancing the protective effect of adsorption corrosion inhibitors. If the oxide film is unstable, then the adsorption of the inhibitor on the metal surface will be hampered, with the oxygen having no additional impact.

Passivating corrosion inhibitors play an important role in the formation of a protective film on the metal surface. Most often, passivators are inorganic compounds with oxidising properties (nitrites, molybdates, and chromates). Passivating compounds are considered more effective than most non-passivating ones. Thus, the passivation of metals involves the transition of the metal surface into an inactive, passive state, which is associated with the formation of thin surface layers of chemical compounds that prevent corrosion.

In modern technology, passivation refers to methods used to protect metals from corrosion through chemical treatments or technological processes leading to the creation of an oxide film on the treated surface. One of the most advanced approaches for the creation of passivating coatings in industry is the laser treatment of metal surfaces. In particular, from the scientific literature, the possibility of protecting metals from corrosion as a result of the creation of patterned micro- and nanostructures on their surface under the influence of radiation from solid-state lasers with pico- and femtosecond pulse duration has been reported [2,3]. Such a pulse duration can be achieved in the so-called mode-locking generation regime of lasers. However, the laser passivation of metals is still not applied in the restoration of CH objects. One of the possible reasons for this is the fact that pico- and femtosecond laser systems are very expensive, and only highly qualified professionals are able to work with them.

In order to further develop methods for the laser restoration of metals in museums, a study was conducted on the possibility of creating anticorrosive coatings on the surface of iron objects using laser treatment. In this case, unlike in the above-mentioned works, the authors of this article proposed and experimentally proved the possibility of using continuous-wave and repetitively pulsed Nd:YAG lasers for this purpose [2,3]. Lasers operating in such generation regimes are much cheaper than mode-locked laser systems and can be easily exploited even by professional restorers who do not have an engineering background.

It should be noted that research on the possibility of the passivation of metal monuments using pulsed Nd:YAG lasers is also currently being carried out by the scientific group of S. Siano et al. [4,5]. In the works by S. Siano, experiments were carried out focusing on the treatment of iron surfaces using a Nd:YAG laser that generated pulses at a fundamental wavelength of 1.064 μm and operated in three different generating modes: Q-switched mode, long Q-switched mode (LQS—Q-switched mode with increased pulse duration), and Short Free Running mode (SFR—free-running mode with shortened pulse duration). The treatment of the metal was performed using single laser pulses.

Even S. Siano et al. [4,5] themselves consider their results as preliminary, since they explored the task of iron passivation only in relation to model samples and certain types of historical monuments with the foci of corrosion on their surfaces. As a result of the treatment of corroded areas by radiation from a laser operating in SFR mode (with a pulse duration of 20 μs) and heating, the phase transformation of iron oxides occurred—iron oxide (FeO) was converted to magnetite (Fe_3O_4). Although magnetite is a stable iron compound that is affected by corrosion, such an approach to the problem of the passivation of monuments seems to be rather controversial [6]. Firstly, it does not solve the problem of the anticorrosive protection of "clean" (i.e., without foci of corrosion) surfaces. Secondly, the formation of magnetite leads to the appearance of a grey-black colour on the laser-treated surface areas, which may be unacceptable in terms of the aesthetic properties of CH objects.

The approach suggested by the authors of this article is more universal, since it allows the formation of protective anticorrosion layers on "clean" surfaces of monuments made of iron and steel. In addition, in terms of the effect achieved, CW and nanosecond Nd:YAG lasers are alternatives to the above-mentioned pico- and femtosecond laser systems but are simpler to operate and maintain; this is very important from the perspective of routine museum work. It should also be noted that the results obtained in this work are a further development of research on the laser anticorrosion treatment of metals in general, which the authors have devoted themselves to during the last few years [7–11]. This means that the proposed approach is also very useful for iron treatment in industry.

2. Materials and Methods

In order to test the technology involved in the laser passivation of historical monuments made of iron, small carbon steel plates were selected as the model samples (with areas up to 5 cm^2 and thicknesses of 3–5 mm). With electron microscopy, the following chemical composition data were obtained: iron (Fe)—83.4%; carbon (C)—13.5%; silicon (Si)—0.7%; manganese (Mn)—0.5%. In addition to these elements, alloying elements such as nickel (Ni), chromium (Cr), copper (Cu), and cobalt (Co) were also present in the samples in low concentrations. In Russia, a steel grade with such a chemical composition is called Steel20. This steel was chosen for use in experimental studies due to the fact that many historical monuments were created of ferrous metals, which are close to Steel20 in terms of their chemical composition.

Our samples were treated using a Nd:YAG laser at a wavelength of λ = 1064 µm in repetitively pulsed and continuously pulsed modes (Figure 1). A laboratory model developed in the research institute "Polyus" (Moscow) was used in the experiments.

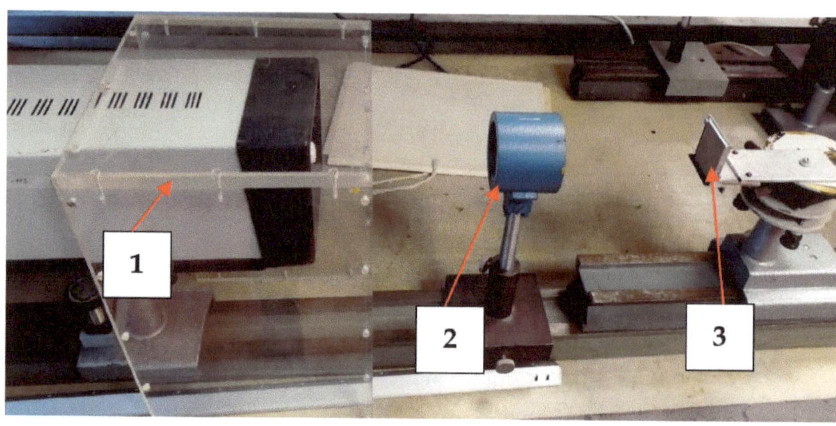

Figure 1. Photo of the optical layout of the Nd:YAG laser experimental setup: (**1**) Nd:YAG laser with a wavelength of 1064 µm, (**2**) focusing lens, and (**3**) sample surface. The laser focuses a 1064 µm beam onto the steel sample.

Laser radiation was focused on the surface of the samples using a special focusing system. The beam was moved across the sample's surface using a high-speed scanning system based on galvanometer mirrors. The maximum output power of the laser in the pulse-periodic treatment mode varied in the range of 3–20 W (which corresponds to a radiation power density of about 1.5×10^5–11.2×10^5 W/cm^2 and an energy density of about 48–152 J/cm^2) and in the continuous treatment mode varied in the range of 21–22 W (which corresponds to a radiation power density of about 10.7×10^5–11.2×10^5 W/cm^2 and an energy density of about 0.03–0.1 J/cm^2).

The sample processing time was 1–5 s. The metal surface treatment took place at room temperature (23 °C) and 55% relative humidity.

According to the calculations (as seen in Table 1), the average temperature on the sample surface in the laser treatment zone was: 300.3 °C (for a laser operating in a repetitively pulsed mode) and 308.1 °C (for a continuously pulsed laser). The speed of the laser beam was 0.05 m/s in repetitively pulsed mode and from 0.01 m/s to 0.05 m/s in CW mood. The laser spot diameter was 50 μm for both regimes.

Table 1. Nd:YAG laser parameters used to calculate the temperature.

Processing Mode	Power Density, W/cm^2	Temperature, °C	V, m/s
Periodically pulsed laser radiation treatment	1.5×10^5	294.4	0.05
	9.7×10^5	301.8	
	10.2×10^5	302.2	
	11.2×10^5	303.1	
Continuously pulsed laser radiation treatment	10.2×10^5	313.6	0.01
	10.7×10^5	306.7	0.01
		302.7	0.025
	11.2×10^5	315.7	0.01
		307.3	0.025
		303.1	0.05

When a body is heated by laser radiation, various processes are activated. When determining the main parameters of this process, it is sufficient to estimate the threshold radiation power density q_0 (or threshold power P_n, threshold energy W_n). The threshold radiation power density shows the value at which the specified changes begin to occur in the irradiated material. The theoretical value q_n is defined as the value of the incident radiation power density, q_0, at which the maximum temperature of the processed material reaches the value T* corresponding to the beginning of this process. Threshold characteristics can be determined from an expression that determines the temperature on the surface of the body in the centre of the irradiated area in the form of a circle with a radius r_0 at the end of the exposure period. For irradiation in the volume absorption mode, these expressions are presented in Equations (1) and (2). In the presented technological process of laser processing, the treated surface is scanned with a laser beam. The results of thermal exposure depend on the scanning speed used.

The temperature was calculated for the repetitively pulsed and continuously pulsed treatment modes according to Equations (1) and (2):

$$T = \frac{2q_0 A\sqrt{D\tau}}{k\sqrt{\pi}} + T_i, \quad (1)$$

$$T = \frac{2}{\sqrt{\pi}} \frac{q_0(1-R)}{K} \frac{\sqrt{2Dr_0}}{V_{sp}} + T_i, \quad (2)$$

where: q_0—laser radiation power density; K—thermal conductivity coefficient; D—temperature conductivity; r_0—spot radius; R—metal surface reflectance coefficient; k—thermal conductivity; τ—duration of exposure; T_i—initial temperature; V_{sp}—speed of the laser beam movement relative to the sample surface (scanning speed); A—absorptive capacity of the material.

The values of all the variables used in the calculations are given in Table 2.

Table 2. Carbon steel parameters used to calculate the temperature on the surface.

R	D, m^2/s	K, W/m·K	r_0, cm	T_0, K
0.63	1.172×10^5	50	0.0025	293

Using a JSM-5610 LV scanning electron microscope (Japan) equipped with the EDX JED-2201 chemical analysis system, SEM images of the treated steel surface were obtained and the elemental composition of the samples was determined.

The change in the surface roughness of the metal was recorded using the contact microprofilometer HOMMEL TESTER T8000 (produced by Hommelwerke GmbH, Germany), and a 3D model of the structure surface was obtained using the stylus profilometer KLA Tencor: P-7 (produced by KLA-Tencor, Milpitas, CA, USA).

In addition, the microstructure of the material surface was examined using an optical light microscope Leica DMI 5000 (produced by Leica Microsystems, Wetzlar, Germany).

3. Results

Figure 2 shows an image of the steel surface before treatment with a laser beam, which was recorded using a scanning electron microscope JSM-5610 LV.

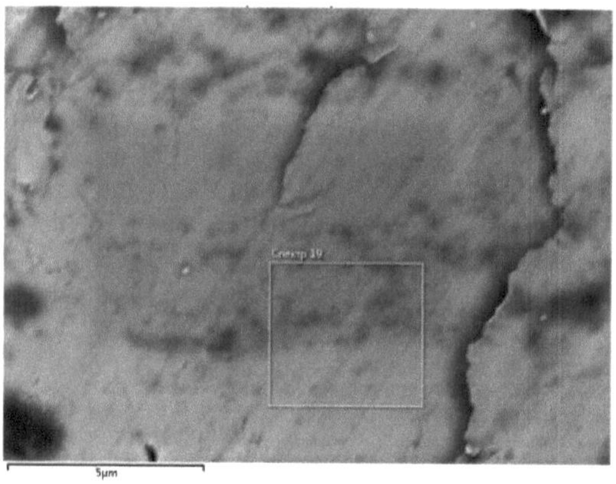

(a)

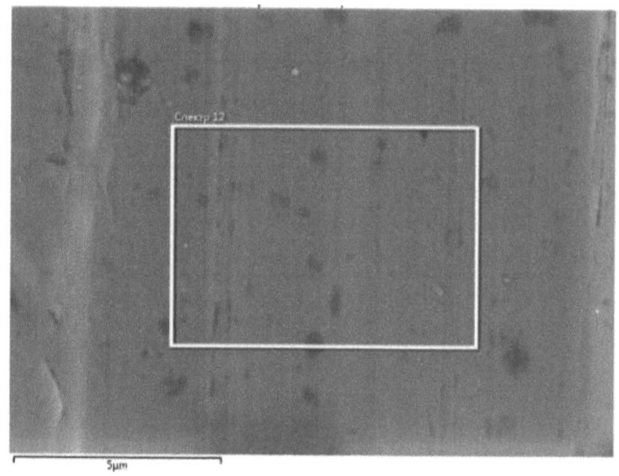

(b)

Figure 2. SEM image of the surface steel (**a**) before laser treatment and (**b**) after laser treatment (before connection with chemical reagent).

Under the impact of a laser, anticorrosion layers were formed on the steel surface as a result of the microstructure of a thin surface layer of the steel. Figure 2b shows an image of the steel surface after the laser treatment obtained under a microscope. The effect of laser radiation on the surface of Steel 20 contributed to a slight change in the chemical composition. It was found that the laser treatment resulted in a local redistribution of iron and carbon in the surface layer of the steel, leading to the formation of iron carbide (Fe_3C). This effect can be associated with the significant heating of the metal surface.

The changes in the surface roughness of the metal are presented in Table 3. The results obtained allow us to conclude that a significant decrease in the surface roughness of the steel under the influence of a Nd:YAG laser can be obtained using only continuous laser radiation. In Table 3, the samples in which a decrease in surface roughness was observed (from value R_a = 0.53 μm to R_a = 0.38 μm) are highlighted in green; the best result was obtained for No. 7.

In Table 3, the values R_a and R_z are the arithmetic averages of the absolute values of the deviations of the surface profile within the base length and the sum of the average absolute values of the heights of the five largest profile protrusions and the five largest profile dips within the base length, respectively.

Additionally, the microstructure of the surface of the model samples obtained using an optical light microscope was examined. For metallographic studies, only these samples were selected, the surface roughness of which significantly decreased as a result of laser treatment (in Table 3, they are highlighted in green). For this purpose, the microspecimens used for the qualitative and quantitative analyses of the structure of carbon steel were created. The microspecimens were etched in a 5% solution of nitric acid with the addition of water. Figure 3 shows a general view of the etched surface, and it can be concluded that the steel under examination had a ferrite-pearlite structure.

Table 3. The surface roughness of the model samples before and after laser treatment by Nd:YAG laser.

№	Processing Mood	Treated Material	
		R_a, µm	R_z, µm
1	Treatment with pulsed-periodic laser radiation	1.22	7.20
2	Continuous laser radiation treatment	0.47	2.86
3	Continuous laser radiation treatment	0.44	2.80
4	Treatment with pulsed-periodic laser radiation	1.40	9.05
5	Continuous laser radiation treatment	0.61	4.10
6	Continuous laser radiation treatment	0.60	3.71
7	Continuous laser radiation treatment	0.49	2.76
8	Treatment with pulsed-periodic laser radiation	1.12	7.65
9	Continuous laser radiation treatment	0.38	3.17
10	Continuous laser radiation treatment	0.51	3.62
11	Treatment with pulsed-periodic laser radiation	0.70	5.85
12	Continuous laser radiation treatment	0.40	2.72
	Raw material	0.53	3.66

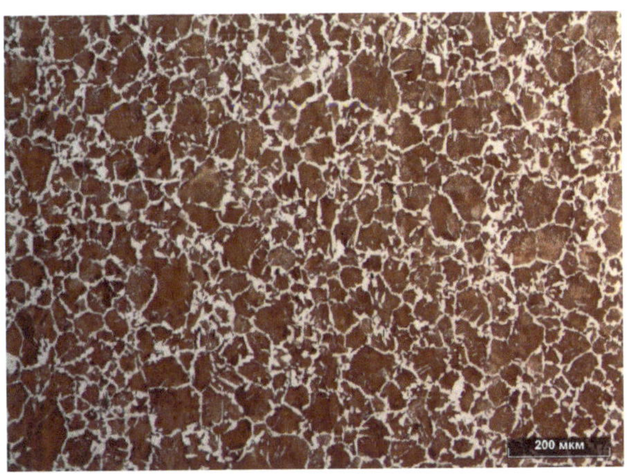

Figure 3. The surface of the etched micro-sections under a microscope at 100× magnification.

Among the analysed samples (Table 3), the best results were shown by samples No. 7 and No. 12.

Figures 4 and 5 show the microstructure of the steel surface treated with an Nd:YAG laser. At the edge of the macrophotography in the cross-section of the micro specimen in Figures 4 and 5, we can clearly see a white stripe, which is a corrosion-resistant layer of steel formed as a result of laser treatment. The best results were obtained with strong carbon diffusion.

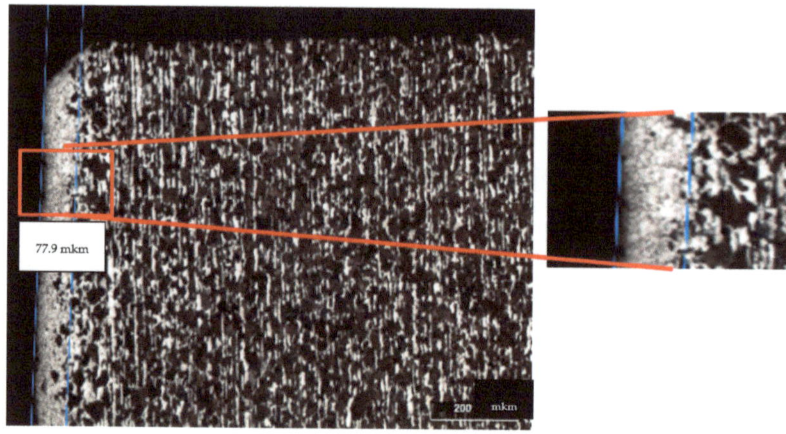

Figure 4. An image of the transverse structure of the microscope of the Nd:YAG laser-treated steel surface obtained with an optical microscope. Sample No. 7.

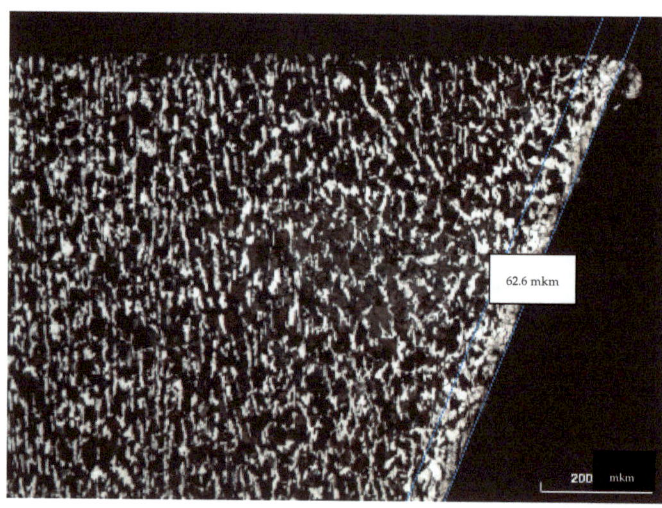

Figure 5. An image of the transverse structure of the microscope of the Nd:YAG laser-treated steel surface obtained with an optical microscope. Sample No. 12.

Sample No. 7 distinguishes itself by a pronounced dense protective layer with an h = 77.9 μm thickness. A decrease and compaction of the grains is evident, which is a positive result and indicates the high quality of the layer and its high corrosion resistance. The disadvantages of this treatment mode (power density $q = 10.2 \times 10^5$ W/cm^2) include the uneven temperature distribution across the sample; as a result, in some places, a decrease in thickness to h = 31.5 μm and a porous structure are observed.

Sample No. 12 is distinguished by a uniformly distributed protective layer with an h = 62.5 μm thickness. A decrease and compaction of the grains can be seen, which is a positive result, as in sample No. 7. The disadvantages of this treatment mode (power density $q = 10.7 \times 10^5$ W/cm^2) include the insufficiently dense anticorrosion coating structure, similar to that of sample No. 7.

Samples with the best treatment results were subjected to corrosion testing. The following solutions were chosen as the electrolyte for the electrochemical method used for determining the corrosion rate: 3% NaCl and 3% Na_2SO_4. These solutions were chosen due to the fact that they simulate the occurrence of real aggressive conditions in the natural environment during the storage and operation of historical monuments. The samples prepared for testing were coated with a layer of hot adhesive compound made of rosin with wax, leaving the untreated area of about 0.54 cm^2, and afterwards were placed into the abovementioned saline solutions. Figure 6 shows the results obtained from measuring the electric potential over time on a steel surface not treated with a laser, which were adopted as standard. The measurements were carried out using the IPC-Pro M potentiostat. As a result of testing in both solutions, an active release of iron (Fe) into the environment was observed, leading to active corrosion processes.

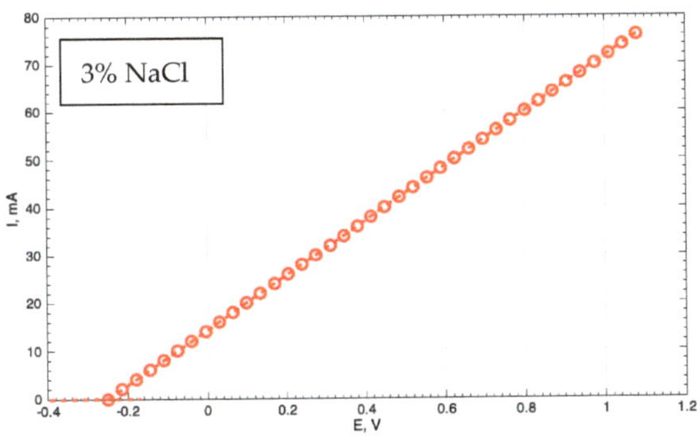

(a)

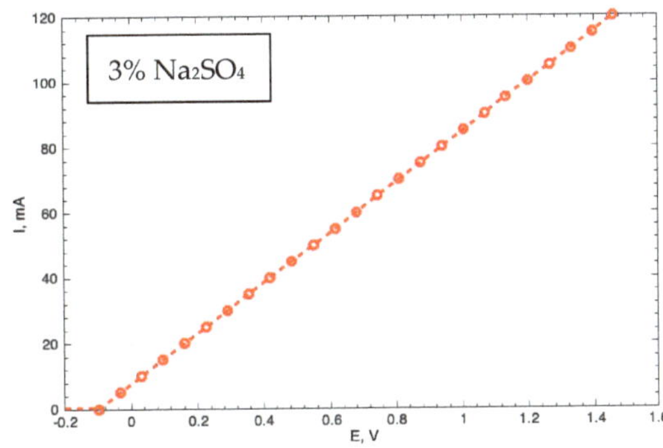

(b)

Figure 6. Potentiostatic polarisation curves on the untreated laser surface of steel in (**a**) 3% NaCl and (**b**) 3% Na_2SO_4.

It is impossible to create potentiostatic polarisation curves for the samples with protective coatings. However, as a result of these corrosion studies, it was found that the coatings formed on the surface of the steel samples using an Nd:YAG laser do not transmit electric current, and this confirms the fact that the obtained anticorrosion coatings have high protective properties. This is an important advantage of the anticorrosion coatings obtained by laser treatment.

4. Discussion

The conducted studies have shown the potential of enhancing the corrosion resistance of steel through treatment with continuous and repetitively pulsed Nd:YAG laser radiation generated at a wavelength of 1.064 μm. As a result of these experiments, the optimal operating modes of the laser treatment were determined, including the level of radiation power density at which the formation of a protective anticorrosion layer takes place. This is around 10.2×10^5 W/cm^2 and 10.7×10^5 W/cm^2 for the continuous and repetitive laser generating modes, respectively. Under such conditions, a protective anticorrosion coating with a thickness of about 62–77 μm was obtained on the steel surface.

It should be noted that in the experiments an interesting effect was observed. As a result of the laser processing of steel, various colour shades (including blue and light-blue colours) sometimes appeared on its surface; see Figure 7.

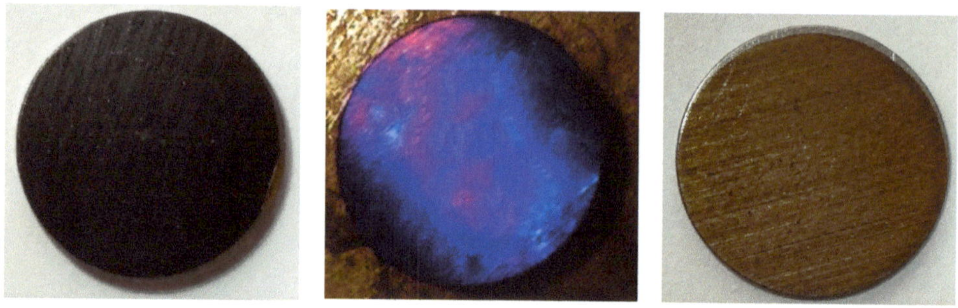

(**a**) (**b**) (**c**)

Figure 7. Colour shades on the steel surface after laser treatment: (**a**) black; (**b**) blue; (**c**) gold.

This opens up possibilities for the use of Nd:YAG lasers to restore the artistic finishing (colour appearance) of decorative art objects made of steel. The possibility of carrying out this restoration task with the help of laser treatment has been discussed previously in one of our articles [12].

Regarding the results obtained in this work, the main conclusion that can be drawn on the basis of the experimental studies conducted lies in the fact that the laser treatment of iron-based metallic materials using continuous-wave and repetitively pulsed Nd:YAG lasers generated at a wavelength of 1.064 μm allows the problem of the passivation of the surface of such materials to be solved. Therefore, the approach proposed in this article may be considered as a promising way to passivate the surface of CH objects created from iron, steel, and cast iron. However, it should be noted that this conclusion is preliminary and needs experimental validation. Since, in these experiments, we used only model samples in order to make our conclusions more general, it is necessary to conduct experiments on the laser passivation of authentic historical artifacts, the surfaces of which are inhomogeneous as a result of weathering and the removal of corrosion layers in the course of conservation works. The authors do plan to carry out such studies in the near future in collaboration with professional restorers.

Meanwhile, it is without doubt that laser treatment allows one to defend newly created metallic artworks against corrosion.

5. Conclusions

The experimental results obtained regarding the laser treatment of carbon steel model samples by the radiation of repetitively pulsed and continuous-wave 1.064 μm Nd:YAG lasers are described in the present article. We can conclude that the laser treatment allows the formation of dense protection films on the steel surface, which enhance the anticorrosion properties of the metal. The application of Nd:YAG lasers is a promising means for the surface passivation of artworks created from steel and cast iron. One possible explanation for this may be that laser treatment results in the local redistribution of iron and carbon in the surface layer of the steel, which leads to the formation of iron carbide (Fe_3C). This effect can be associated with the significant heating of the metal surface. It is known from the scientific literature [13] that, under a temperature change in steel in the range of 600–100 °C (which fits our case), the elements iron (Fe), cobalt (Co) and nickel (Ni) can form carbide iron (Fe_3C) due to chemical reactions with carbon. The specified microstructuring of the steel surface can increase its corrosion resistance. The iron pillar of Delhi is an example of steel with a high percentage of Fe being saved from corrosion.

Author Contributions: Conceptualisation, I.R. and V.P.; methodology, I.R., V.P. and O.V.; validation, I.R., V.P. and O.V.; formal analysis, O.Z.; investigation, O.Z. and A.Z.; resources, O.V.; data curation, I.R.; writing—original draft preparation, I.R.; writing—review and editing, V.P.; visualisation, I.R.; supervision, V.P.; project administration, I.R. All authors have read and agreed to the published version of the manuscript.

Funding: This research received no external funding.

Institutional Review Board Statement: Not applicable.

Informed Consent Statement: Not applicable.

Data Availability Statement: The data supporting the findings of this study are available from the corresponding author upon reasonable request.

Acknowledgments: The authors would like to thank V.G. Bondarenko and S.R. Rustamov (both are with the R&D Institute "Polyus", Moscow) for their assistance in experiments using Nd:YAG lasers.

Conflicts of Interest: The authors declare no financial or commercial conflict of interest.

References

1. Nikitin, M.K.; Melnikova, E.P. *Chemistry in Restoration*; Khimiya: Leningrad, Russia, 1990.
2. Emelyanenko, A.M.; Shagieva, A.G.; Domantovsky, A.G.; Boinovich, L.B. Nanosecond laser micro- and nanotexturing for the design of a superhydrophobic coating robust against long-term contact with water, cavitation, and abrasion. *Appl. Surf. Sci.* **2015**, *332*, 513. [CrossRef]
3. Vorobyev, A.Y.; Ghunlei, G. Multifunctional surfaces produced by femtosecond laser pulses. *J. Appl. Phys.* **2015**, *117*, 3. [CrossRef]
4. Osticioli, I.; Siano, S. Dependence of Nd: YAG laser derusting and passivation of iron artifacts on pulse duration. In Proceedings of the SPIE 9065, Fundamentals of Laser-Assisted Micro- and Nanotechnologies, St. Petersburg, Russia, 24–28 June 2013; p. 906513.
5. Siano, S.; Agresti, J.; Cacciari, I.; Ciofini, D.; Mascalchi, M.; Osticioli, I.; Mencaglia, A.A. Laser cleaning in conservation of stone, metal, and painted artifacts: State of the art and new insights on the use of the Nd: YAG lasers. *Appl. Phys. A* **2012**, *106*, 419. [CrossRef]
6. Tareen, J.; Krishnamurthy, K.V. Hydrothermal stability of hematite and magnetite. *Bull. Mater. Sci.* **1981**, *3*, 9. [CrossRef]
7. Vasiliev, O.V.; Veiko, V.P.; Gornyi, S.G.; Ruzankina, Y.S. Laser apparatus for microstructuring a metal surface, using a fiber laser. *J. Opt. Technol.* **2015**, *82*, 831. [CrossRef]
8. Ruzankina, J.S.; Parfenov, V.A.; Vasiliev, O.S. Anti-corrosion prevention of carbon steel by means of laser treatment. *Laser Phys.* **2019**, *29*, 015203. [CrossRef]
9. Iakovlev, A.; Ruzankina, J.; Kasheev, S.; Vasilyev, O.; Parfenov, V.; Grishkanich, A. Laser anti-corrosion treatment of metal surfaces. In Proceedings of the SPIE 10097, High-Power Laser Materials Processing: Applications, Diagnostics, and Systems VI, San Francisco, CA, USA, 28 January–2 February 2017; p. 100970S.
10. Ruzankina, J.S.; Vasiliev, O.S. Study on possibility for the improvement of corrosion resistance of metals using laser-formed oxide surface structure. *J. Phys. Conf. Ser.* **2016**, *735*, 012050. [CrossRef]
11. Ruzankina, J.S.; Vasiliev, O.S.; Parfenov, V.A. Anti-corrosion treatment of metal surfaces based on photonics methods. *J. Phys. Conf. Ser.* **2017**, *917*, 062039. [CrossRef]
12. Gerashenko, M.D.; Parfenov, V.A. Formation of non-ferrous oxide films on the surface of metals under the influence of laser radiation. *Bull. St. Petersburg State Electrotech. Univ. LETI* **2011**, *3*, 68.
13. Glinka, N.K. *Nauka*; Khimiya: Moscow, Russia, 2017; p. 752.

quantum beam science

MDPI

Article

Laser Peening Analysis of Aluminum 5083: A Finite Element Study

Ali Tajyar [1], Noah Holtham [1], Nicholas Brooks [1], Lloyd Hackel [2], Vincent Sherman [2], Ali Beheshti [3] and Keivan Davami [1,*]

1 Department of Mechanical Engineering, The University of Alabama, Tuscaloosa, AL 35487, USA; atajyar@ua.edu (A.T.); nholtham@crimson.ua.edu (N.H.); nabrooks1@crimson.ua.edu (N.B.)
2 Curtiss Wright Surface Technologies, Metal Improvement Company, Livermore, CA 94551, USA; Lloyd.Hackel@cwst.com (L.H.); Vincent.Sherman@cwst.com (V.S.)
3 Department of Mechanical Engineering, George Mason University, Fairfield, VA 22030, USA; abehesh@gmu.edu
* Correspondence: kdavami@eng.ua.edu

Abstract: In this research, a finite element (FE) technique was used to predict the residual stresses in laser-peened aluminum 5083 at different power densities. A dynamic pressure profile was used to create the pressure wave in an explicit model, and the stress results were extracted once the solution was stabilized. It is shown that as power density increases from 0.5 to 4 GW/cm^2, the induced residual stresses develop monotonically deeper from 0.42 to 1.40 mm. However, with an increase in the power density, the maximum magnitude of the sub-surface stresses increases only up to a certain threshold (1 GW/cm^2 for aluminum 5083). Above this threshold, a complex interaction of the elastic and plastic waves occurring at peak pressures above ≈2.5 Hugoniot Elastic Limit (HEL) results in decreased surface stresses. The FE results are corroborated with physical experiments and observations.

Keywords: laser peening; finite element method; residual stress; Al5083

1. Introduction

Laser technology has been used excessively utilized in material processing and manufacturing techniques such as forming [1], peening [2], additive manufacturing [3], cladding [4], and welding [5]. Among them, laser peening (LP) is an innovative post-processing technique used in the industry to mitigate surface-related failures such as corrosion, fatigue, fretting fatigue, corrosion–fatigue, etc. This versatile technique is also used to form complex shapes and structures [6]. Compared to other similar surface engineering methods such as shot peening [7], water jet peening [8], and ultrasonic peening [9], LP is advantageous as it generates deeper residual stresses with increased thermal stability that is attributed to the lower amount of cold work [10]. However, to achieve the full potential of this technique, a precise understanding of the peening process along with the effects of different process parameters are required [11].

Many experimental studies have focused on parameter optimization of the LP process and the effects of LP on the mechanical properties and material performance [12–15]. However, far fewer attempts have been made to fundamentally understand the wave propagation and corresponding residual stress distribution [16]. This is, of course, anticipated as in situ monitoring of the residual stress distribution during peening is extremely challenging if not impossible [11]. Thus, a hybrid experimental and simulation approach enables an improved understanding of how adjusting various peening parameters affects the pressure wave as it propagates through the material as well as the final state of residual stresses.

The literature contains several studies focused on the numerical simulation of the LP process. Braisted et al. [17] used a combination of explicit and implicit dynamic analysis algorithms in ABAQUS to study the residual stresses induced by the LP process in Ti-6Al-4V as well as 35 CD4. Ding et al. [18] expanded their approach from 2D to 3D and implemented an HEL plastic model to study different LP processing conditions in different metal alloys. Peyre et al. [19] also applied a finite element method (FEM) along with the Johnson–Cook plasticity model to simulate the LP process through 2D axisymmetric FE models for martensitic stainless steel and 7075 aluminum. These studies, among others [20–23], provided improved insight into the LP process and contributed immensely to the process optimization.

In this research, the effects of power density on the magnitude and distribution of the residual stresses in the LPed Al 5083 were studied. Al 5083 is an emerging material of choice for applications in aerospace and marine industries due to its high strength-to-weight ratio as well as other outstanding attributes [24]. While this alloy is widely used in different sectors, the literature has few experimental studies on LP of Al 5083, which are mainly focused on its corrosion cracking behaviors [24,25]. However, no analytical effort has been attempted to quantitatively understand the effect of the LP process on the Al 5083 state of residual stress. This work provides the first combined experimental and numerical analysis on the LP of Al 5083, with new insights on how the laser power density affects the magnitude, depth, and distribution of the induced residual stresses in the alloy.

2. 3D Simulation of the Laser Peening Process

A 3D FE model was created using ABAQUS software to investigate the impact of a single layer LP with different power densities on Al5083 specimens. The overall dimensions of the specimen were modeled to be 12 mm × 12 mm × 7 mm, where an axisymmetric quarter of the block was only considered (Figure 1). Following the experimental conditions discussed later, the simulations were carried out with four power densities of 0.5, 1, 2, and 4 GW/cm^2, which produce peak pressures (P_{Peak}) of 0.72, 1.02, 1.44, and 2.44 GPa. Pressure loading condition was estimated based on the methodology developed by Fabbro et al. [26–28]. Detailed explanation of the method is provided in supplementary materials—Supplementary Information (SI), Section S1.1.

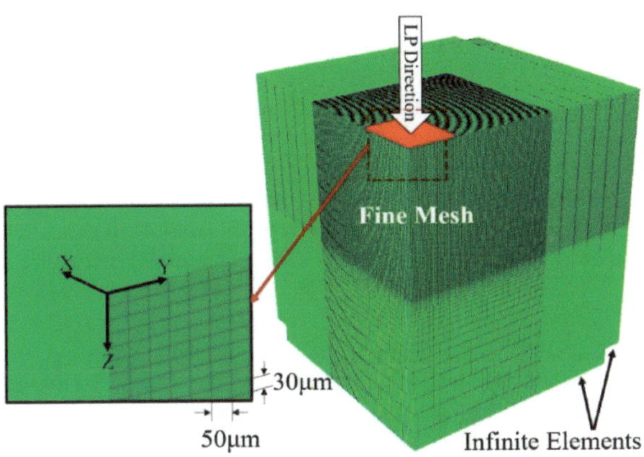

Figure 1. A three-dimensional model used in the FE simulation of the LP process.

The target material was assumed to be initially stress free and considered to be elastic–plastic, homogeneous, and isotropic. It is known that in the LP process, the material becomes deformed at an extremely high strain rate (up to 10^7 s^{-1}); therefore, the constitutive relations obtained from quasi-static conditions are not valid. As a result, herein, the Johnson–Cook (JC) model, being capable of predicting the material response to high strain rates and large deformations, was selected for the simulation. The JC model relates the strain hardening, the strain rate effects, and thermal effects to the flow stress in material expressed as:

$$\sigma = \left[A + B\varepsilon_p^n\right]\left[1 + Cln\frac{\dot{\varepsilon}}{\dot{\varepsilon}_0}\right]\left[1 - \left(\frac{T - T_0}{T_m - T_0}\right)^m\right] \quad (1)$$

where A, B, n, C, and m are the material constants; ε_p represents the equivalent plastic strain; $\dot{\varepsilon}$ and $\dot{\varepsilon}_0$ are the plastic strain rate and the reference plastic strain rate, respectively. A is defined as the yield strength; B denotes the strain-hardening modulus; n is the strain-hardening exponent; and C accounts for the strain rate-hardening effect. T is the temperature in Kelvin and T_0, T_m, and m are the room temperature, the melting point of material, and the power of thermal softening, respectively. Since in the LP technique, the thermal effect of the process is negligible compared to the mechanical effects, the temperature term in the JC model could be eliminated. The properties of Al 5083 used here were adopted from Refs. [29,30] for the dynamic response of Al 5083 and are listed in Table 1.

Table 1. Material properties and Johnson–Cook parameters of Al 5083 [29,30].

Material Properties	
Density, ρ (kg/mm^3)	2.7×10^{-6}
Young's modulus, E (GPa)	70
Poisson's ratio, ν	0.3
Hugoniot elastic limit (*HEL*), (GPa)	0.57
Johnson–Cook parameters	
A (MPa)	167
B (MPa)	596
C	0.001
m	0.859
n	0.551
$\dot{\varepsilon}_0$	1

To enhance the accuracy of the model as well as facilitate obtaining a converged plastic strain distribution, a finer mesh was used in and around the pulse area where elements of 0.05 mm × 0.05 mm × 0.03 mm were chosen (Figure 1). C3D8R, a continuum solid eight-node reduced integration element, was chosen as the element type. To reduce the analysis time, a coarser mesh was implemented outside of the critical region. Stress waves reflected from the back and bottom surfaces can lead to an error in the analysis; hence, to mitigate this problem, infinite elements (CIN3D8) were implemented along the back and bottom surfaces (Figure 1) so that the stress waves were able to pass through. The numbers of finite and infinite elements in the model were 873,375 and 26,925, respectively.

Each simulation included two steps. In the first step and following the experimental procedure, a square laser spot (3 mm × 3 mm) with a very high pressure was applied on the top surface of the specimen in a short time. In the second step, to assure obtaining a stabilized solution, the stress results were given sufficient time to relax. ABAQUS/Explicit was used for the analysis of both first and second steps. While previously a combination of dynamic explicit analysis and static analysis has been typically used in the literature [16,31–33], it has been also shown that a pure explicit model can be also utilized for both steps if the proper solution time is considered for each step [10,21,34,35]. Further information about the calculation of solution times for step one (to ensure the occurrence of all the plastic deformation in the material), and step two (to obtain the equilibrium of stresses in the material) is provided in SI (Section S1.2).

3. Experiments

3.1. LP Process

A Q-switched Nd:YLF laser was employed to do the laser peening on the AL5083 specimens. The spots had a square shape with dimensions of 3 mm × 3 mm. Specimens were moved using a robotic arm for placing laser impact spots with 100 micron accuracy. A de-ionized (15 M ohm resistance) water layer of ≈1 mm thickness acting as a plasma tamper was flowed over the specimen to be peened. The laser energy passes through the water layer, forms a plasma during the first nanosecond of the pulse, and heats the plasma approximately to 13,000 K. By controlling the distance between the specimen surface and the final imaging lens, the power density was adjusted to achieve a plasma pressure, which was confined by the tamping layer that rises in pressure to above the HEL of the material. It should be added that here, the laser spot was not focused on to the target, so there is no issue of inexact focusing. In addition, breakdown in the current system with the relay imaging was tested where water breakdown only occurred above a power density of 12 GW/cm^2, which is much higher than the power density values used in this study. In this study, four power densities of 0.5, 1, 2, and 4 GW/cm^2 with 18 ns laser pulse duration were selected for the experiments. It is worth noting that given the laser pulse properties and since the heat capacity of the metal is sufficiently high, only a few dozens of microns of the metal experience the heating in the LP process.

3.2. Residual Stress Measurement

A portable X-ray diffraction (XRD) analyzer, Pulstec μ-X360 (Pulstec Industrial Co., Ltd., Hamamatsu, Japan) using the cosα method (detailed information of method are described in the SI, Section S2) was utilized to characterize the surface and in-depth residual stress. A low-intensity Cr $K\alpha$ source was employed to irradiate a 2 mm diameter spot for 30 s, while an image plate was positioned normal to the incident beam at a sample-to-detector distance of ≈39 mm collecting diffracted X-rays. The X-ray incidence angle was set to 25° and the X-ray tube voltage and current were 30 kV and 1.50 mA, respectively. Since the XRD techniques are only able to measure the surface-level stress, material was removed from the surface by an electrolytic polishing machine (Proto, Proto 8818-V3, Proto Manufacturing Inc., Taylor, MI, USA) and a saline electrolyte (Proto Electrolyte A, Proto Manufacturing Inc., Taylor, MI, USA) for in-depth residual stress measurements. The material was carefully etched in four separate regions on each sample corresponding to four different depths of ≈50, 100, 150, and 200 μm, which created circular areas (5 mm diameter) suitable for XRD measurement (Section S2, Figure 2). The precise depth measurement was performed on etched regions with a stylus profilometer (Alpha-Step D-500, KLA-Tencor, Milpitas, CA, USA).

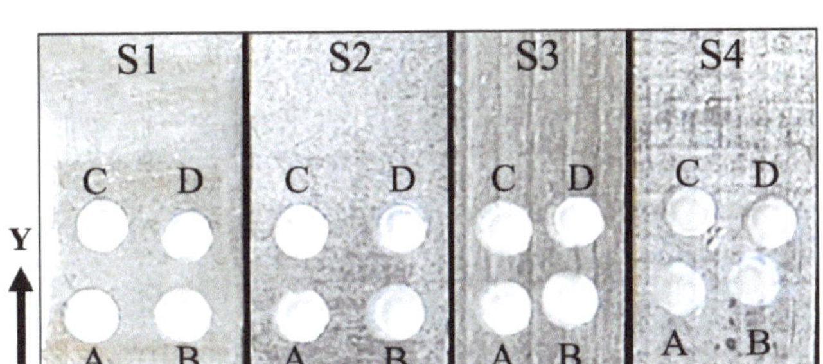

Figure 2. The circular etched regions (A–D) used for residual stress measurement on the four different laser-peened samples (Samples S1–S4 were laser peened with power densities of 0.5, 1, 2, and 4 GW/cm^2, respectively).

4. Results and Discussion

Figure 3 compares the numerical simulation results for the residual stresses along with their experimentally obtained values. The stresses were measured at different depths up to 200 μm. The experimental residual stress values for each point can be considered as the average residual stress within the measured area that is exposed to the X-ray beam. The simulation results were obtained from the average of the residual stress values of nodes along a path from the center to the edge of a peened spot.

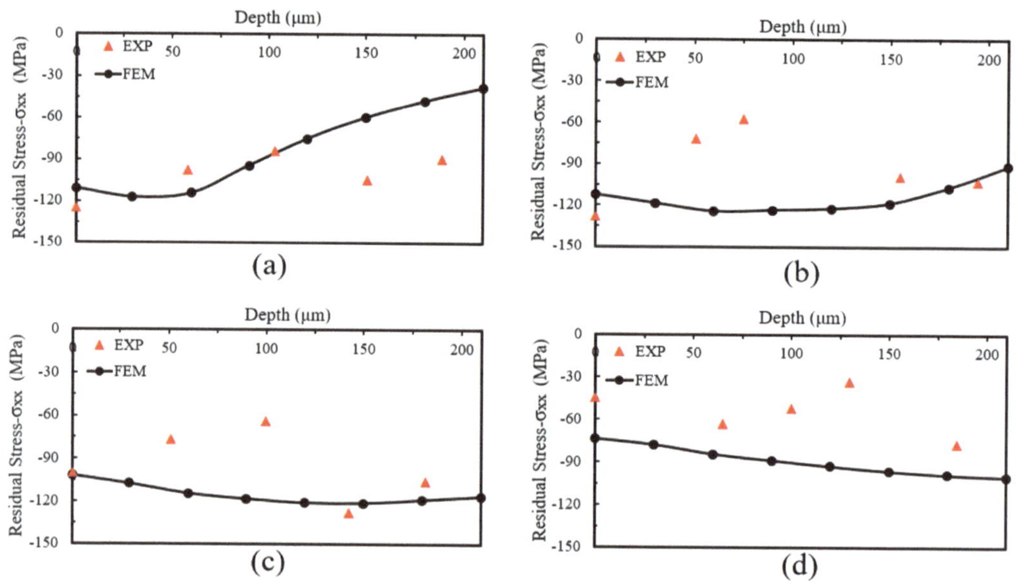

Figure 3. Comparison of residual stresses versus distance (in depth) from the LP face between simulation and experiment for different power densities: (**a**) 0.5 GW/cm^2, (**b**) 1 GW/cm^2, (**c**) 2 GW/cm^2, and (**d**) 4 GW/cm^2.

As shown in Figure 3, only a slight difference in the compressive residual stresses is observed with an increase in power density from 0.5 to 2 GW/cm^2. However, at a power density of 4 GW/cm^2, a considerable decrease in the compressive residual stress values is observed for both simulation and experimental results with a majority of the points having a value less than −90 MPa. While FE analysis is able to successfully predict general experimental trends, there are differences between stress values. The differences might be attributed to couple of factors. The main factor could be that the μXRD patterns might not perfectly represent the global aluminum diffraction constants, since it was mostly obtained from regions inside grains on very small diffracting crystallites [21]. In addition, the experimental residual stress values were calculated from the whole surface of a peened spot, but the simulated residual stress values were obtained from a line (from the center to the outer edge of the spot). Additionally, for aluminum with a relatively low yield strength, XRD measurements might result in even higher errors since the magnitude of the measured stresses are generally low. Another minor contributing factor is the JC model and its sensitivity on several constants. While material properties were obtained directly from the available data in the literature for Al 5083 that was modeled here, inevitable slight differences may exist between current material constants and those of the reported in the literature that might affect the FE results [10,17].

Figure 4a shows the 3D distribution of σ_{xx} residual stresses with a power density of 2 GW/cm^2. It can be seen that compressive and tensile residual stresses have been developed inside and in the neighboring area of the peened spot, respectively. Figure 4b,c show the distribution of σ_{xx} on the surface with different laser power densities along the x (at y = z = 0) and y (at x = z = 0) axes, respectively. The residual stresses in the peened spot are compressive in both x and y directions. This indicates that all four power densities, 0.5 GW/cm^2, 1 GW/cm^2, 2 GW/cm^2, and 4 GW/cm^2, are able to generate peak pressures that exceed the dynamic yield strength of the material and consequently cause plastic deformation that results in the formation of compressive residual stresses [36].

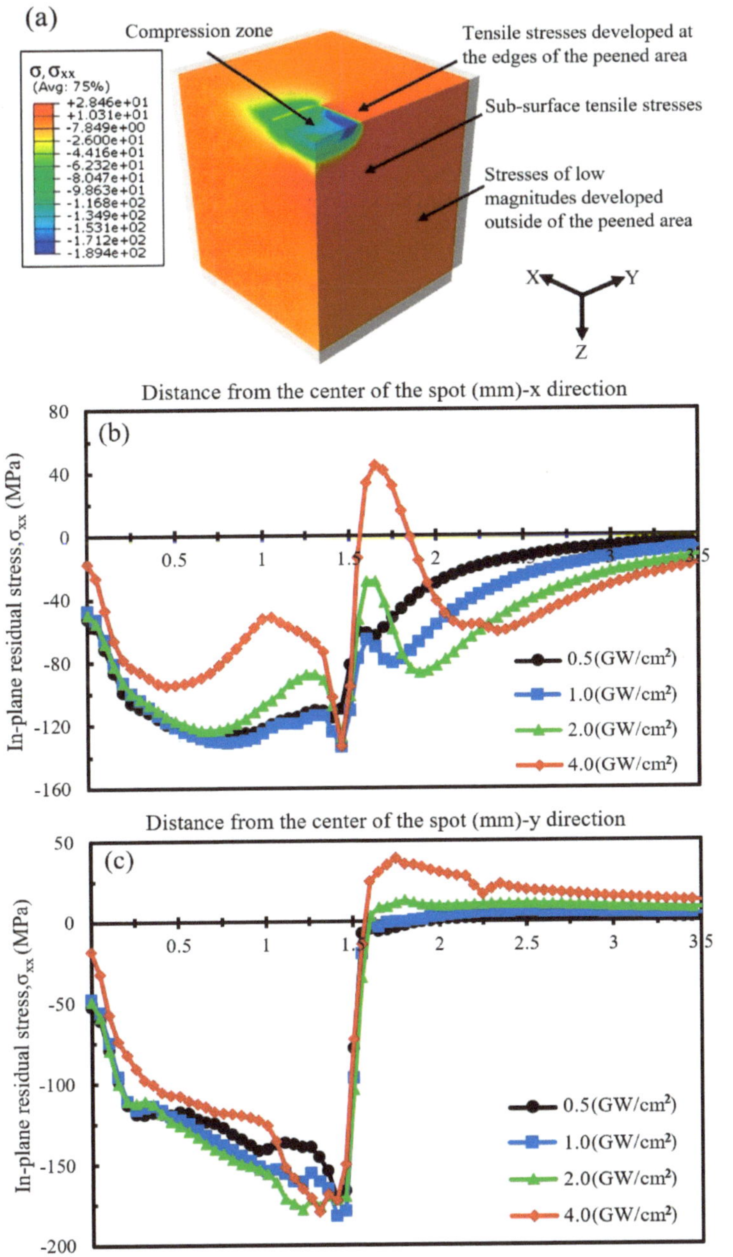

Figure 4. (**a**) In-plane residual stress (σ_{xx}) distribution for specimen with a power density of 2 GW/cm^2, (**b**,**c**) Distribution of σ_{xx} along the x and y axes at the surface for different power densities.

Surprisingly, the maximum value of the residual stresses is not predicted to be at the center of the laser spot (Figure 4a–c). This phenomenon, called residual stress hole (or "stress empty"), was reported for both square and circular spots [37,38]. The residual stress hole may in large part be due to the concentration of the rarefaction waves that are generated by the edges of the peened area at the spot center and reverse plastic deformation. Li et al. [39] explained this phenomenon in a similar way where they attributed the formation of the stress hole to the removal of the compressive stresses at the center of the spot due to the large pulses generated from the surface waves expanding radially to the center of the spot. It was reported that there is a relationship between the magnitude of the stresses in the residual stress hole on the surface and the wave peak pressure, P_{Peak}.

As depicted in Figure 4b, there are spatially abrupt changes in the stress values at the edge of the spot ($x = \approx 1.5$ mm), which are more pronounced when the power density increased from 0.5 to 4 GW/cm^2. It is notable that the residual stresses for the power density of 4 GW/cm^2 in the x direction transition from compressive to tensile to compressive when moving from the spot center to the outside edge. Additionally, the magnitude of surface residual stresses for 4 GW/cm^2 is lower than that for other power densities (Figure 4b). However, along the y direction, more uniform residual stress profiles were observed for all power densities (Figure 4c). There is an intensified peak in compressive stresses around the boundaries of the pulse area, which is followed by a rapid reduction and conversion to tensile stress outside of the spot (Figure 4c). For the power density of 4 GW/cm^2 (P_{Peak} = 2.04 GPa), the residual stress drop at the center is more pronounced in comparison to the other three power densities in both the x and y directions.

Figure 5 shows the variation of σ_{xx} and σ_{yy} with the depth. In order to avoid the effect of the residual stress hole, a position with a distance of 0.75 mm from the center of the peened spot (x = 0.75 mm, y = 0) and located on the symmetry line was selected to collect residual stress variation in depth. It should be also noted that the magnitude of the stress at other locations with close proximity to the center is checked, and a negligible difference between the residual stress values was observed. It can be seen from Figure 5a that at a power density of 0.5 GW/cm^2, compressive stresses are formed up to a distance of $\approx$0.42 mm from the peened surface, and tensile stresses are generated beneath that ($0.42 < z < 3$ mm) to counter-balance the compressive stresses. With an increase in the power density from 0.5 to 4 GW/cm^2, the depth of the compressive residual stresses also increases (from 0.42 for 0.5 GW/cm^2 to 1.40 mm for 4 GW/cm^2). This was expected, as the depth of the compressive residual stresses in an LPed specimen is closely related to the plastically deformed area [40].

The value and depth of the maximum residual stresses for the power density of 0.5 GW/cm^2 are 135 MPa and $\approx$0.03 mm, respectively. The results show that σ_{xx} compressive residual stresses near the surface achieve magnitudes as high as 140 MPa with increasing power density to 1 GW/cm^2 (P_{Peak} = 1.02 GPa) at a depth of $\approx$0.06 mm (Figure 5a). With increasing the power density to 2 GW/cm^2, although the values of residual stresses decrease slightly, the residual stresses are almost constant (in the range of 119.6–125.4 MPa) to the depth of 0.29 mm. Interestingly, while the compressive residual stresses are observed at a greater distance from the surface for the power density of 4 GW/cm^2 compared with lower power densities, the magnitude of compressive residual stresses on the surface and sub-surface drops remarkably. Similar observations have been reported for A356-T6 alloy as well as Steel 1045 previously [38,41]. As shown in Figure 5b, similar results were observed for the σ_{yy} in-plane residual stress.

The observation here agrees well with the model developed by Peyre et al. [41] where the plastic deformation rises linearly when the peak pressure increases from 1 HEL to 2 HEL and its maximum limit is attained at around 2 to 2.5 HEL. Above that, the surface release waves focus and intensify from the edges of the impacts, and this phenomenon leads to the modification of the residual stress field. Therefore, while a power density of 4 GW/cm^2 (P_{Peak} = 2.04 GPa > 2.5 HEL_{Al5083}) generates deeper residual stresses, its magnitudes are smaller remarkably in comparison to those that the power densities of 1 and 2 GW/cm^2 (P_{Peak} = 1.02 and 1.44 G $\cong$ (2 to 2.5) $\times$ HEL_{Al5083}) can generate. This is in agreement with the previously reported findings that materials can be optimally treated with P_{Peak} in (2 to 2.5) $\times$ HEL range [37,41].

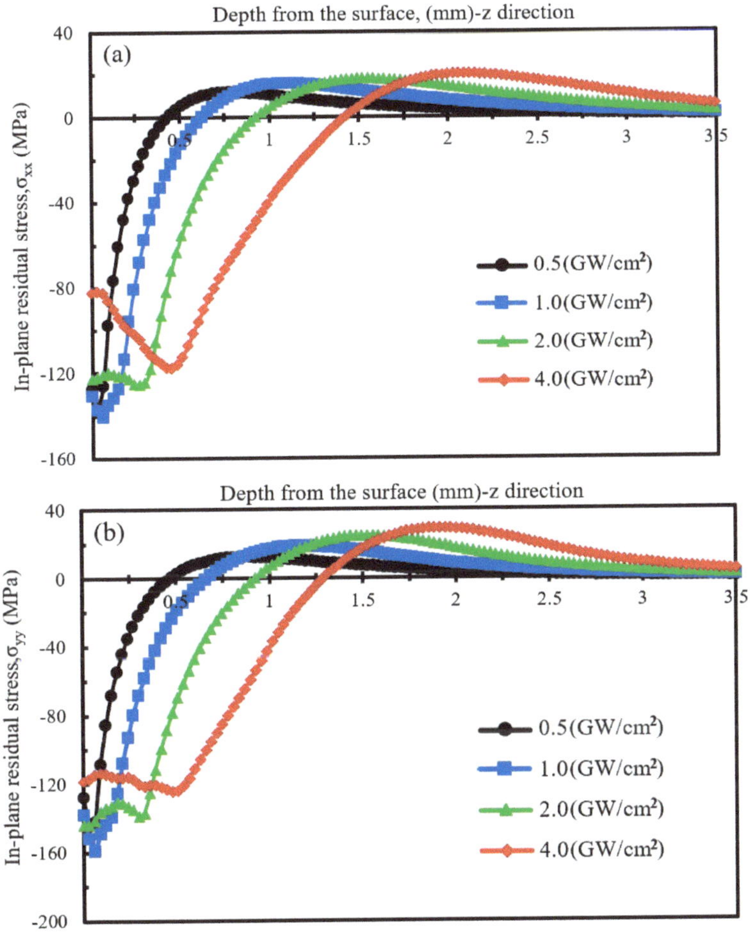

Figure 5. Variation of in-plane residual stress with depth (x = 0.75 mm, y = 0), (**a**) σ_{xx}, (**b**) σ_{yy}.

5. Conclusions

Herein, an explicit model was used to study the effects of four different power densities on the laser peening of aluminum 5083. The magnitude of the generated residual stresses up to a depth of 200 µm was compared with the experimental results. Simulations show a residual stress hole in the middle of the peened spot due to a plastic unloading wave. It was shown that with an increase in the power density from 0.5 to 4 GW/cm^2, residual stresses are generated deeper into the workpiece. At a power density of 4 GW/cm^2, the resulting peak pressure above 2.5 HEL reduced the near surface residual stresses.

Supplementary Materials: The following are available online at https://www.mdpi.com/2412-382X/5/4/34/s1, Figure S1: Temporal pressure profile, Figure S2: (a) History of the internal energy, elastically stored energy, plastically dissipated energy and artificial strain energy during the first step (b) In-plane stress profiles (σxx) versus distance from the center of spot at different calculation times during the second step (A dynamic state towards a residual state). It can be concluded that a quasi-equilibrium state is reached above 100,000 ns. Figure S3: Debye ring measurement schematic.

Author Contributions: Supervision & funding acquisition, K.D.; writing—original draft preparation, A.T.; Formal Analysis, K.D., A.T, N.H., N.B. and A.B.; Methodology, A.T. and K.D.; Review and editing, A.B., L.H., V.S. All authors have read and agreed to the published version of the manuscript.

Funding: Advanced Manufacturing program of the National Science Foundation, award CMMI-AM #2029059.

Institutional Review Board Statement: Not applicable.

Informed Consent Statement: Not applicable.

Data Availability Statement: All the raw data is available upon request.

Acknowledgments: The authors would like to thank Pulstec USA, Inc. and Toshi Suzuki (KLA) for the help with the residual stress measurements. The authors, Russell Rowe and Keivan Davami, extend gratitude to the Alabama Transportation Institute (ATI) for their support of the graduate student involved in this work. Keivan Davami acknowledges the support of the Advanced Manufacturing program of the National Science Foundation, award CMMI-AM #2029059.

Conflicts of Interest: The authors declare no conflict of interest.

References

1. Bachmann, A.L.; Dickey, M.D.; Lazarus, N. Making Light Work of Metal Bending: Laser Forming in Rapid Prototyping. *Quantum Beam Sci.* **2020**, *4*, 44. [CrossRef]
2. Gujba, A.K.; Medraj, M. Laser Peening Process and Its Impact on Materials Properties in Comparison with Shot Peening and Ultrasonic Impact Peening. *Materials* **2014**, *7*, 7925–7974. [CrossRef]
3. Thiede, T.; Mishurova, T.; Evsevleev, S.; Serrano-Munoz, I.; Gollwitzer, C.; Bruno, G. 3D Shape Analysis of Powder for Laser Beam Melting by Synchrotron X-ray CT. *Quantum Beam Sci.* **2019**, *3*, 3. [CrossRef]
4. Zhu, L.; Xue, P.; Lan, Q.; Meng, G.; Ren, Y.; Yang, Z.; Xu, P.; Liu, Z. Recent research and development status of laser cladding: A review. *Opt. Laser Technol.* **2021**, *138*, 106915. [CrossRef]
5. Shobu, T.; Shiro, A.; Kono, F.; Muramatsu, T.; Yamada, T.; Naganuma, M.; Ozawa, T. Internal Strain Distribution of Laser Lap Joints in Steel under Loading Studied by High-Energy Synchrotron Radiation X-rays. *Quantum Beam Sci.* **2021**, *5*, 17. [CrossRef]
6. Munther, M.; Martin, T.; Tajyar, A.; Hackel, L.; Beheshti, A.; Davami, K. Laser shock peening and its effects on microstructure and properties of additively manufactured metal alloys: A review. *Eng. Res. Express* **2020**, *2*, 022001. [CrossRef]
7. Bagheri, S.; Guagliano, M. Review of shot peening processes to obtain nanocrystalline surfaces in metal alloys. *Surf. Eng.* **2009**, *25*, 3–14. [CrossRef]
8. Hayashi, M.; Okido, S.; Suzuki, H. Residual Stress Distribution in Water Jet Peened Type 304 Stainless Steel. *Quantum Beam Sci.* **2020**, *4*, 18. [CrossRef]
9. Malaki, M.; Ding, H. A review of ultrasonic peening treatment. *Mater. Des.* **2015**, *87*, 1072–1086. [CrossRef]
10. Peyre, P.; Chaieb, I.; Braham, C. FEM calculation of residual stresses induced by laser shock processing in stainless steels. *Model. Simul. Mater. Sci. Eng.* **2007**, *15*, 205–221. [CrossRef]
11. Yang, C.; Hodgson, P.D.; Liu, Q.; Ye, L. Geometrical effects on residual stresses in 7050-T7451 aluminum alloy rods subject to laser shock peening. *J. Mater. Process. Technol.* **2008**, *201*, 303–309. [CrossRef]
12. Chupakhin, S.; Klusemann, B.; Huber, N.; Kashaev, N. Application of design of experiments for laser shock peening process optimization. *Int. J. Adv. Manuf. Technol.* **2019**, *102*, 1567–1581. [CrossRef]
13. Palma, T.; Munther, M.; Sharma, M.; Hackel, L.; Beheshti, A.; Davami, K. Nanomechanical Characterization of Laser Peened Additively Manufactured Inconel 718 Superalloy. *Adv. Eng. Mater.* **2019**, *21*, 1900499. [CrossRef]
14. Ren, X.; Chen, B.; Jiao, J.; Yang, Y.; Zhou, W.; Tong, Z. Fatigue behavior of double-sided laser shock peened Ti-6Al-4V thin blade subjected to foreign object damage. *Opt. Laser Technol.* **2020**, *121*, 105784. [CrossRef]
15. Kalainathan, S.; Prabhakaran, S. Recent development and future perspectives of low energy laser shock peening. *Opt. Laser Technol.* **2016**, *81*, 137–144. [CrossRef]
16. Hu, Y.; Yao, Z.; Hu, J. 3-D FEM simulation of laser shock processing. *Surf. Coat. Technol.* **2006**, *201*, 1426–1435. [CrossRef]
17. Braisted, W.; Brockman, R. Finite element simulation of laser shock peening. *Int. J. Fatigue* **1999**, *21*, 719–724. [CrossRef]
18. Ding, K.; Ye, L. FEM simulation of two sided laser shock peening of thin sections of Ti-6Al-4V alloy. *Surf. Eng.* **2003**, *19*, 127–133. [CrossRef]
19. Peyre, P.; Sollier, A.; Chaieb, I.; Berthe, L.; Bartnicki, E.; Braham, C.; Fabbro, R. FEM simulation of residual stresses induced by laser Peening. *Eur. Phys. J. Appl. Phys.* **2003**, *23*, 83–88. [CrossRef]
20. Xiao, Y. Effect of laser shock peening on bending fatigue performance of AISI 9310 steel spur gear. *Opt. Laser Technol.* **2017**, *94*, 15–24. [CrossRef]
21. Hfaiedh, N.; Peyre, P.; Song, H.; Popa, I.; Ji, V.; Vignal, V. Finite element analysis of laser shock peening of 2050-T8 aluminum alloy. *Int. J. Fatigue* **2015**, *70*, 480–489. [CrossRef]
22. Zhou, W.; Ren, X.; Yang, Y.; Tong, Z.; Asuako Larson, E. Finite element analysis of laser shock peening induced near-surface deformation in engineering metals. *Opt. Laser Technol.* **2019**, *119*, 105608. [CrossRef]
23. Cao, Y.; Shin, Y.C.; Wu, B. Parametric study on single shot and overlapping laser shock peening on various metals via modeling and experiments. *J. Manuf. Sci. Eng. Trans. ASME* **2010**, *132*, 0610101–06101010. [CrossRef]

24. Yang, Y.; Zhou, W.; Tong, Z.; Chen, L.; Yang, X.; Larson, E.A.; Ren, X. Electrochemical Corrosion Behavior of 5083 Aluminum Alloy Subjected to Laser Shock Peening. *J. Mater. Eng. Perform.* **2019**, *28*, 6081–6091. [CrossRef]
25. Sun, S. Laser Shock Peening Process to Prevent Stress Corrosion Cracking of 5xxx Aluminum Alloys. Embargoed Master's Thesis, University of Nebraska-Lincoln, Lincoln, NE, USA, April 2018.
26. Ballard, P.; Fournier, J.; Fabbro, R.; Frelat, J. Residual Stresses Induced By Laser-Shocks. *J. Phys. IV* **1991**, *1*, C3-487–C3-494. [CrossRef]
27. Fabbro, R.; Fournier, J.; Ballard, P.; Devaux, D.; Virmont, J. Physical study of laser-produced plasma in confined geometry. *J. Appl. Phys.* **1990**, *68*, 775–784. [CrossRef]
28. Peyre, P.; Fabbro, R. Laser shock processing: A review of the physics and applications. *Opt. Quantum Electron.* **1995**, *27*, 1213–1229. [CrossRef]
29. Elwasli, F.; Zemzemi, F.; Mkaddem, A.; Mzali, S.; Mezlini, S. A 3D multi-scratch test model for characterizing material removal regimes in 5083-Al alloy. *Mater. Des.* **2015**, *87*, 352–362. [CrossRef]
30. Boteler, J.M.; Dandekar, D.P. Dynamic response of two strain-hardened aluminum alloys. *J. Appl. Phys.* **2006**, *100*, 054902. [CrossRef]
31. Wei, X.L.; Ling, X. Numerical modeling of residual stress induced by laser shock processing. *Appl. Surf. Sci.* **2014**, *301*, 557–563. [CrossRef]
32. Kim, J.H.; Kim, Y.J.; Lee, J.W.; Yoo, S.H. Study on effect of time parameters of laser shock peening on residual stresses using FE simulation. *J. Mech. Sci. Technol.* **2014**, *28*, 1803–1810. [CrossRef]
33. Ding, K. Three-dimensional dynamic finite element analysis of multiple laser shock peening processes. *Surf. Eng.* **2003**, *19*, 351–358. [CrossRef]
34. Bikdeloo, R.; Farrahi, G.H.; Mehmanparast, A.; Mahdavi, S.M. Multiple laser shock peening effects on residual stress distribution and fatigue crack growth behaviour of 316 L stainless steel. *Theor. Appl. Fract. Mech.* **2020**, *105*, 102429. [CrossRef]
35. Sealy, M.P.; Guo, Y.B. Surface integrity and process mechanics of laser shock peening of novel biodegradable magnesium-calcium (Mg-Ca) alloy. *J. Mech. Behav. Biomed. Mater.* **2010**, *3*, 488–496. [CrossRef]
36. Sun, R.; Li, L.; Zhu, Y.; Zhang, L.; Guo, W.; Peng, P.; Li, B.; Guo, C.; Liu, L.; Che, Z.; et al. Dynamic response and residual stress fields of Ti6Al4V alloy under shock wave induced by laser shock peening. *Model. Simul. Mater. Sci. Eng.* **2017**, *25*, 065016. [CrossRef]
37. Kim, J.H.; Kim, Y.J.; Kim, J.S. Effects of simulation parameters on residual stresses for laser shock peening finite element analysis. *J. Mech. Sci. Technol.* **2013**, *27*, 2025–2034. [CrossRef]
38. Hu, Y.; Gong, C.; Yao, Z.; Hu, J. Investigation on the non-homogeneity of residual stress field induced by laser shock peening. *Surf. Coat. Technol.* **2009**, *203*, 3503–3508. [CrossRef]
39. Li, P.; Huang, S.; Xu, H.; Li, Y.; Hou, X.; Wang, Q.; Fu, W.; Fang, Y. Numerical simulation and experiments of titanium alloy engine blades based on laser shock processing. *Aerosp. Sci. Technol.* **2015**, *40*, 164–170. [CrossRef]
40. Achintha, M.; Nowell, D. Eigenstrain modelling of residual stresses generated by laser shock peening. *J. Mater. Process. Technol.* **2011**, *211*, 1091–1101. [CrossRef]
41. Peyre, P.; Fabbro, R.; Merrien, P.; Lieurade, H.P. Laser shock processing of aluminium alloys. Application to high cycle fatigue behaviour. *Mater. Sci. Eng. A* **1996**, *210*, 102–113. [CrossRef]

quantum beam science

MDPI

Review

A Survey of Process Monitoring Using Computer-Aided Inspection in Laser-Welded Blanks of Light Metals Based on the Digital Twins Concept

Ahmad Aminzadeh [1], Sasan Sattarpanah Karganroudi [1,2,*], Mohammad Saleh Meiabadi [3], Dhanesh G. Mohan [4] and Kadiata Ba [5]

1 Département de Mathématique, Informatique et Génie, Université du Québec à Rimouski, Rimouski, QC G56 3A1, Canada; ahmad.aminzadeh@uqar.ca
2 Department of Mechanical Engineering, Université du Québec à Trois-Rivières, Trois-Rivieres, QC G8Z 4M3, Canada
3 Department of Mechanical Engineering, École de Technologie Supérieure, 1100 Notre Dame West, Montreal, QC H3C 1K3, Canada; mohammadsaleh.sheikhmohammadmeiabadi.1@ens.etsmtl.ca
4 Institute of Materials Joining, Shandong University, Jinan 250061, China; dhanesh@sdu.edu.cn
5 Applied Sciences Department, Université du Québec à Chicoutimi, 555 boul. Université, Chicoutimi, QC G7H 2B1, Canada; kadiata_ba@uqac.ca
* Correspondence: sattarpa@uqtr.ca

Abstract: The benefits of laser welding include higher production values, deeper penetration, higher welding speeds, adaptability, and higher power density. These characteristics make laser welding a superior process. Many industries are aware of the benefits of switching to lasers. For example, metal-joining is migrating to modern industrial laser technology due to improved yields, design flexibility, and energy efficiency. However, for an industrial process to be optimized for intelligent manufacturing in the era of Industry 4.0, it must be captured online using high-quality data. Laser welding of aluminum alloys presents a daunting challenge, mainly because aluminum is a less reliable material for welding than other commercial metals such as steel, primarily because of its physical properties: high thermal conductivity, high reflectivity, and low viscosity. The welding plates were fixed by a special welding fixture, to validate alignments and improve measurement accuracy, and a Computer-Aided Inspection (CAI) using 3D scanning was adopted. Certain literature has suggested real-time monitoring of intelligent techniques as a solution to the critical problems associated with aluminum laser welding. Real-time monitoring technologies are essential to improving welding efficiency and guaranteeing product quality. This paper critically reviews the research findings and advances for real-time monitoring of laser welding during the last 10 years. In the present work, a specific methodology originating from process monitoring using Computer-Aided Inspection in laser-welded blanks is reviewed as a candidate technology for a digital twin. Moreover, a novel digital model based on CAI and cloud manufacturing is proposed.

Keywords: real-time monitoring; Computer-Aided Inspection (CAI); laser welded blanks (LWBs); digital twin (DT); Industry 4.0

1. Introduction

The transportation industry has dedicated a lot of engineering effort and innovative research into reducing the weight of its products. Air pollution and emission of greenhouse gases from the transportation sector have had detrimental environmental and health effects for decades. For this reason, governments have enacted restrictive regulations on automotive industries to prevent and control the spread of vehicular emissions. Strict regulations have led car manufacturers to look for different solutions and new technologies to solve the problem. One of the strategies that has been adopted in this field is to reduce the weight of cars, leading to fuel consumption and carbon dioxide emission reduction.

Given that the body and other exterior components are a large portion of the car's weight, using light metal structures such as aluminum alloys in automobiles is an effective way to lessen the overall car weight. Aluminum alloys are known for their superior properties, such as strength-to-weight ratio, heat resistance, and corrosion resistance. Laser welding is an effective method of joining materials with high accuracy, good flexibility, and low distortion [1]. However, laser welding of aluminum structures is associated with a range of difficulties due to excessive heat dissipation, the hydrogen solubility of molten aluminum, and an oxide layer inclusion. Manufacturers are motivated by Computer-Aided Inspection (CAI) to ensure high product quality and avoid production defects, which requires automated, rapid, and accurate inspection [2]. CAI commonly refers to automated inspection, among other computer-aided applications extensively used in different industries [3]. By using manufacturing standards and geometric dimensioning and tolerancing (GD&T) criteria, CAI is not only able to detect laser welding defects but also to compensate for these shortcomings. Advances in scanning technology, digital cameras, and controllers have led to a significant increase in real-time monitoring of laser welding processes. A digital twin (DT) aims to build a digital replica of a physical system in a virtual space, such that the digital replica represents the same elements and the same dynamics of a physical system. DT systems can be very helpful for understanding, analyzing, and improving a product, service system, or production [4]. DT systems can also be used to inspect the process, to enable visualization of the impact of variations [5]. Integration of real-time monitoring and real-time simulation in a laser welding process ultimately leads to adopting a DT in laser welding processes. To communicate data, information technology advancements, like the Internet of Things (IoT) and Augmented Reality (AR), can be implemented to link the physical system and its digital twin [6]. Real-time data collection, data analysis, and physics-based simulation are basic phases in defect detection aimed at avoiding the occurrence of defects, and improving the quality of this cutting-edge technology. Thus, a critical review of monitoring technology for the laser welding process is provided. Kong, et al. [7] utilized spectrographic monitoring to control the laser welding process of galvanized high strength steel in two cases, with zinc coating and without zinc coating, in a lap joint configuration. Considering zinc vapor signals as the process feedback, welding defects were identified by the presence of spatters induced by zinc vapor at the faying surface. A series of experiments were conducted to investigate the effects of laser welding parameters on the keyhole dynamics and weld pool, using a high-speed charge-coupled device (CCD) camera with a green laser as an illumination source. The results revealed that welding quality strongly depends on zinc vapor at the faying surface; a higher depth of penetration was also observed in the case of removing the zinc coating. Sebestova, et al. [8] monitored Nd: YAG laser welding by measuring plasma spectral emission lines to calculate the plasma electron temperature. They found a relationship between electron temperature and depth of penetration, which can be used as a controller to identify welding defects and achieve desired penetration depth. Liu, et al. [9] studied laser hot-wire welding of butt joints to assess the molten pool dynamics and the stability of the welding process. A high-speed CCD camera and a spectrometer were used for real-time monitoring of the process through visualization of the molten pool and calculation of the electron temperature according to the Boltzmann plot method. Research established that the contribution of a hot wire facilitates the formation of a molten pool, though laser beams were not able to make the molten pool in butt joints with a large gap. Harooni, et al. [10] conducted real-time spectroscopic monitoring of laser welding of AZ31B magnesium alloy in lap joint configuration. Spectroscopic analysis was performed to study the correlation of the oxide layer on welding sheets and the generation of defects in the interface of overlapped sheets. In addition, a high-speed CCD camera, assisted with a green laser as an illumination source, was employed to monitor the molten pool and the keyhole dynamics due to the oxide layer. The results confirmed that the existing oxide layer on magnesium sheets leads to the generation of pores in the interface area. Blecher, et al. [11] utilized inline coherent imaging for real-time monitoring of keyhole depth in five different alloys. A comparison of real-time keyhole depth measurements and metallographic depth measurements proved that the proposed method was capable of time measurement of keyhole depth except for aluminum alloys. Luo, et al. [12] improvised the acoustic signal monitoring of laser welding by offering a plane microphone array with a time delay recognition. They concluded that the welding process could be monitored and justified using the suggested method even with background noises in the working environment, which had been an obstacle to traditional acoustic signal monitoring. Mirapeix, et al. [13] proposed plasma optical spectroscopy to identify aluminum in the laser welding of Usibor1500 tailor-welded blanks. The estimation of aluminum was done by the line-to-continuum method in real-time. A correlation was identified between aluminum content in real-time monitoring and off-line tests like macrographs or tensile tests. However, the correlation found in the tensile specimen test at lower aluminum contents was not clear because it was affected by other parameters like seam geometry. Recently, our research team developed a new automatic technique to address the distortion in real-time monitoring of aluminum laser-welded blanks [14,15]. The research also provided experimental and numerical investigation of different types of key process parameters and their impact on production quality in automobile applications [16–19]. Wang, et al. [20] developed a real-time monitoring system for disk laser welding based on the feature selection method for pattern recognition, and the Support Vector Machine (SVM) and Back-Propagation (BP) neural network for pattern classification. Images of the plume and spatters were processed, and a sequential forward floating selection (SFFS) algorithm was used for detecting the optimal feature subset. The classification accuracy of BP and SVM were very close to one other; however, the accuracy of SVM reached the maximum of 98.43 using 10 features. It should be noted that the overall processing time remained a challenge for the proposed method. In another study, Wang, et al. [21] used a combination of a Support Vector Machine and a Pearson product-moment correlation coefficient to characterize disk laser welding quality. High-speed photography was employed for image processing, and the area of the plume, the number of spatters, and the horizontal coordinate of the plume centroid were selected among six features to establish an SVM model with 93.58% classification accuracy. The authors concluded that the proposed monitoring system could be used for real-time monitoring of high-power laser welding. De Bono, et al. [22] evaluated two different monitoring methods of laser welding: optical-based and laser interferometry monitoring methods. The optical-based method investigated photodiodes signals of butt welding, and the laser interferometry monitoring took advantage of the In-Process Depth Meter (IDM) sensor from Precitec in stake welding. Photodiode data obtained at the wavelengths between 600 and 850 nm deduced defects correlated to laser power and joint contamination and gap. However, for detecting defects like porosities and cracks, photodiode data need to be decomposed by orthogonal empirical mode decomposition (OEMD) theory. The data acquired by the IDM sensor established a correlation between the IDM signal and the keyhole depth. Chen, et al. [23] employed an SVM model for real-time monitoring in high-power disk laser welding using 15 features of the metal vapor plume and spatters. A high-speed camera was used to capture laser-induced metal vapor for image processing. SVM classification using seven features reached a remarkably accurate 95.93% by 10-fold cross-validation. The authors suggested that the centroid, perimeter, average grayscale value, and quantity of the spatters were critical to improving welding quality. Pasinetti, et al. [24] proposed in-line monitoring of the laser welding process by a smart vision system based on the Industrial Internet of Things (IIoT) approach, to make an interconnection and remotely control the process. Two different setups were used to fulfill two goals. The first setup, called seam tracking, was targeted to keep the laser welding in an optimal position. The second setup, called the keyhole monitor, aimed to detect incomplete keyhole penetration. The researchers suggested that the architecture used enables remote monitoring of multiple welding units from a central unit. Lei, et al. [25] developed a multi-information fused modeling system for predicting weld waist width and the weld back width by a combination of Principal Component Analysis (PCA), genetic algorithm (GA), and neural networks (NN). Images were acquired by a modified optical fiber laser coaxial monitoring system, and pre-processed by the PCA algorithm to effectively remove the redundancy of extracted information. Two morphological features, in addition to laser power and welding speed, were selected as input parameters of the NN. GA was used to optimize the architecture of the NN. Considering the low errors of the developed model, and the short processing time of less than 90 m, the authors proposed that it could be used for real-time monitoring of the laser welding process. Zhang, et al. [26] employed a multiple-optical-sensor system to integrate with a Deep Belief Network (DBN) that was optimized by a genetic algorithm for online monitoring of the high-power disc laser welding process. The multiple-optical-sensor system was able to deliver effectively a thorough insight into the laser welding process. A deep learning model based on the DBN demonstrated more than 10% higher average accuracy compared to the back-propagation neural network (BPNN) model. Haubold [27] offered a monitoring system for remote laser welding using two parallel processing algorithms customized for identifying spatter number and size. The reproducibility of spatter formation was investigated at four different settings of process parameters for ten repetitions. Although a correlation between spatter number and the corresponding standard deviation was established, no resolution for reduction of spatter size and number was made. Shevchik, et al. [28] developed a hybrid monitoring system for data acquisition and processing applied to titanium laser welding. The monitoring system included optical and acoustic sensors combined with machine learning (ML) techniques. M-band wavelets transformation was utilized to decompose optical and acoustic signals, and the normalized energy of the frequency bands was extracted. The Laplacian graph Support Vector Machine (LapSVM) was used to correlate the extracted features with welding quality. The proposed method displayed more than 85.9% classification accuracy, which is notable given the low cost of data preparation. Accordingly, the researchers claimed that the hybrid monitoring system could be used for the industrialization of laser welding monitoring, and they also raised some concerns about sensors selection rather than sensors combination. Zhang, et al. [29] put forward a vision-based monitoring system for laser welding of tailor rolled blanks (TRB) through coaxial visual monitoring and Convolution Neural Network (CNN) processing algorithms. The monitoring system was dedicated to evaluating the penetration quality of the laser welding of TRB. Four statuses for the penetration state were considered for the creation of an image dataset to train and validate the CNN. They advised that with the 2 ms latency of the CNN for TRB, the proposed monitoring system could be effectively employed for real-time monitoring applications. Gonzalez, et al. [30] introduced ConvLBM to monitor laser deposition and welding processes based on medium wavelength infrared (MWIR) imaging. ConvLBM employed a Convolution Neural Network (CNN) to obtain features from MWIR. ConvLBM estimated dilution for the laser deposition process due to its significance on the quality of the process. Defect characterization was also achieved for the laser welding process by ConvLBM for three different materials, proving the adaptability of the monitoring method for different applications. Kaewprachum, et al. [31] employed an infrared camera for real-time monitoring of the laser welding process to apprehend fast dynamic heating phenomena. The images were captured and analyzed to reveal the effects of laser power and welding speed on the average molten pool temperature and the width of the molten pool. Infrared camera measurements were validated by microscopic measurements, and a good correspondence was observed, especially at high powers. Papacharalampopoulos, et al. [32] employed a methodology as a candidate for process-level digital twins (DTs) in laser welding. A simplified laser welding paradigm capable of displaying temperature profiles was studied to assess the employed methodology. The proposed digital twin approach consisted of decomposing spatial domains, adaptation to accuracy, adaptation to measurements, and estimation of inner state, providing intuitiveness to the operator, and real-time function. The methodology was adopted to solve linear partial differential equations, and was validated following measures ensuring the operational performance of a DT.

To the best of the authors' knowledge, the present work is the most comprehensive attempt to present a DT for laser-welded blanks. A virtual system of the physical laser welding system has been developed using CAI to monitor, quality control, and optimize the laser welding process. The developed DT resides in the cloud, and it continuously communicates with physical and virtual systems to provide appropriate commands to operating processes and machines in real-time. In this DT, an evaluation of different aspects of laser welding qualities has been made in order to give a product license to laser-welded blanks.

2. Quality Control Based on 3D Geometrical Inspection

For developing a DT, the raw data of a physical system is collected to extract inspection features and analyze the physical system in real-time. Computer-Aided Inspection (CAI) can help to identify defects and abnormalities occurring in the geometry of a physical system. A 3D scan measurement is one of the CAI tools which provides non-contact, non-destructive, and accurate measurements of a physical system. In other words, it is a 3D geometric inspection technology using data acquisition and data pre-processing to obtain the size and shape of a physical part to display the part in digital space in three dimensions. The 3D scanning provides an opportunity to immediately detect where the digital replica does not match with the 3D CAD model. Three-dimensional scanning is a viable option for the quality control of geometrical features of special welding jigs and fixtures. Using 3D scanning, it is possible to identify where deviations occur, and to measure them instantly. To better understand Geometric Dimensioning and Tolerancing (GD&T), manufacturing standards such as ASME Y14.5 and ISO-GPS have been developed in the era of automation. In addition, as part of its standards and requirements, the American Society of Mechanical Engineers (ASME) also established rules, definitions, defaults, and recommended practices. According to the ASME, parts and workpieces should be evaluated in a free state. Therefore, it is necessary to consider the compliance and deformation of non-rigid parts during the inspection. In response, definitions for geometric dimensioning and tolerancing of non-rigid parts have been developed, based on the ASME Y14.5 and ISO standards. Figure 1 presents the types and tools of CAI algorithms. In fact, inspection 4.0 aims at intelligent inspection by illustrating the basic work that can be implemented. Based on the compliance behavior and inspection parameters, a digital inspection protocol can be implemented onto the cloud, and the appropriate machine and inspection method will be selected. This novel aspect will be presented in the upcoming parts of this article. Generally, components are designed to fit into the right material and mechanical properties based on rigid and non-rigid concepts in computer-aided modeling.

Regarding the compliance behavior of parts, rigid and non-rigid parts, CAI algorithms are developed. CAI is primarily used for comparing the reference geometry, computer-assisted design (CAD), with measured data, scan models [34]. Due to gravity and/or residual stress, some mechanical components often have different shapes in the free-state position compared to the state-of-use position. To make it possible to inspect different types of parts, different registration methods have been developed to classify workpieces into rigid and non-rigid ones. Furthermore, rigid registration is the primary step in computer-assisted inspections of non-rigid parts. In conventional CAI software, it is assumed by default that any data entered into the software is from a rigid part. Therefore, any deviation between the input data and the nominal CAD model should be considered a potential manufacturing defect [35]. Rigid registration has the primary goal of bringing CAD and scan models into a common coordinate system without deforming either model. The model is translated and rotated using an optimal transformation matrix without affecting its shape [36]. Initial CAI approaches were introduced using a rigid registration algorithm with Iterative Close Points (ICP) [37]. The ICP algorithm is known as one of the most robust and efficient rigid registration approaches. Although various methods have been developed over the years—including those described by researchers [38,39]—in different domains, such as aeronautic inspections, the ICP algorithm remains a widely used registration approach [40], thanks to its statistically robust and reliable method of registering. A CAD and a scan of a workpiece that is not presented in the same coordinate systems are shown in Figure 2a, and the ICP algorithm applies the best geometrical fit in Figure 2b. In this regard, the closest point in the reference set (CAD) is first identified for every point the point cloud set contains. The transformation matrix (rotation and translation) is then calculated, to move the CAD model towards scan data. This iteration is repeated until the best geometrical fit is obtained.

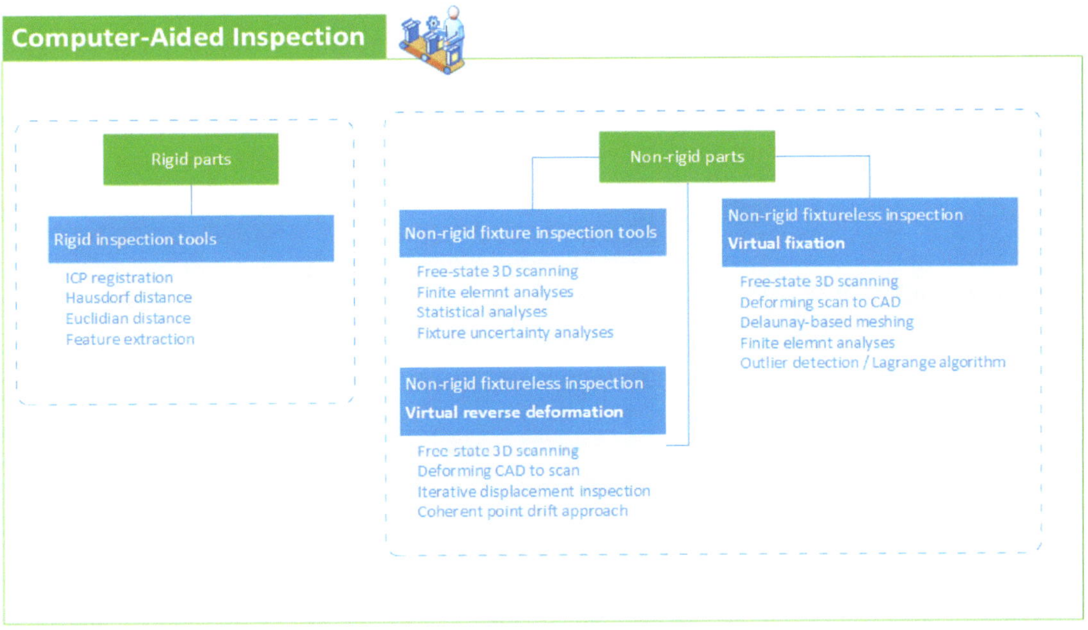

Figure 1. Computer-Aided Inspection methods and tools [33].

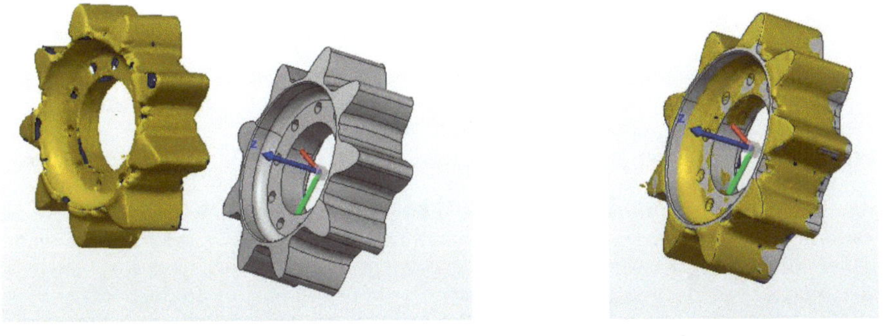

(**a**) (**b**)

Figure 2. CAD and scanned models (**a**) before registration (**b**) after rigid registration using ICP algorithm [33].

Each iteration of the ICP registration minimizes the distance between the two models by estimating and computing the transformation matrix that combines translation and rotation. The Hausdorff distance is the main tool in this algorithm [41]. A distance measure is taken between the CAD mesh and the point cloud data acquired by scanning. In other words, it is the maximum distance between every point of a non-empty set and some point of another non-empty set. Equation (1) illustrates this, where d_H (X, Y) is the Hausdorff distance and (X, Y) are the two non-empty subsets.

$$d_H(X,\ Y) = \max\{sup_{x\in X}inf_{y\in Y}d(x,y), sup_{y\in Y}inf_{x\in X}d(x,y)\} \quad (1)$$

The ICP algorithm has undergone a lot of improvements and upgrades, as it is one of the most powerful and widely used algorithms. The ICP algorithm was also modified and developed to decrease calculation time [42]. This method proposes a robust solution by applying random sampling to the point clouds. The algorithm also knew the minimization strategy [43] or measured the transformation in a way that minimizes its error. By using the corresponding points in previous iterations of the ICP algorithm, and searching only in the immediate neighborhood of those points, the closest points search was significantly improved in terms of speed [44]. In addition, some techniques have been used to improve the efficiency and speed of the registration process [45]. A variation of the algorithm has also been implemented to enhance the conversion of the sets by taking color information from the workpieces. Even though not all scanners are able to capture the color information from workpieces, this algorithm can still be used. There have been many variants of the algorithm explored and many improvements made by the ICP algorithm [43].

Since non-rigid workpieces have so much more parameters to consider, rigid registration needs to be accompanied by non-rigid algorithms, to take into consideration the part's deviation in its free state [46]. Scanning models cannot be compared to CAD models due to the flexible deformation of parts in a free state. CAI methods can resolve this problem for non-rigid parts where defects (e.g., geometric deviations from the CAD model) are separated from the deformations caused by the compliance or flexible deformation of non-rigid parts. Typically, non-rigid parts are dimensioned and inspected with over-constrained inspection fixtures to compensate for the flexible nature of these components and to ensure that the measurement setup accurately reflects the part's assembly functionality.

3. Verification and Validation of the Methods in CAI

All Computer-Aided Inspection methods cited are based on scan data and computational calculations. It follows that verification and validation of the calculations are imperative due to this aspect of the methods. Both rigid and non-rigid inspection methods are prone to uncertainty in computational simulations and measurement errors due to inaccuracies in data acquisition devices. Due to the technical limitations of devices, optical effects (such as light fraction and reflectivity of surfaces), or the inaccessible features of some parts, scanners are inaccurate. The results of CAI are influenced by these noisy data. Simulation models can be assessed for accuracy, reliability, and robustness by applying verification and validation (V&V) approaches [47]. Validation evaluates the consistency of computed simulation results compared to the actual ones, while verification measures the accuracy of the solution to a problem using a computational model. All numerical methods, including CAI methods, must be thoroughly verified and validated because of various sources of uncertainty in computer codes and simulations. Validating the result of a numerical approach concerning input noise aims at evaluating a computational model's robustness. An effective computational model should be able to produce satisfactory results despite the presence of noises in the input. A robust approach can still produce acceptable results for noise-containing input data compared with noise-free input data. Typically, the input noise in CAI methods comes from measurement noise that is inherent to measuring data acquisition devices. Thus, it is necessary to study the robustness of CAI methods, given the noise generated by scanning devices. A first development model will be generated based on the CAI method, and real feedback will be received during the production process. Furthermore, by combining the concepts of physical and simulation, the human and machine interface theory can make a powerful and self-learning device.

This smart connected modeling is the trigger for Industry 4.0 and intelligent manufacturing by developing a digital twin model.

4. Digital Twins (DT)

Industry 4.0 is the latest revolution in the industrial era, and refers to the digitization of manufacturing by merging physical and virtual (digital) worlds. Digital twins (DTs) are a strategy within Industry 4.0, operating on the virtualization principle [48]. DTs are digitalized integrated systems to monitor, analyze, and simulate the behavior of a physical system. DTs are composed of three main components: the physical system, the virtual system, and the communication layer that connects these two systems. The communication layer is a linkage for data storage, data processing, and data mapping functionalities [49]. The data from the physical and virtual systems must be stored and processed in the communication layer. In this regard, the communication layer needs to be capable of transmitting a big amount of data (big data) in addition to easy fault detection characteristics. Internet of Things (IoT) technology can be used to make interactions between different layers of the integrated systems for real-time data transmission. IoT effectively maintains two-way synchronization of physical and virtual systems, to keep the virtual system updated and to provide real-time control commands for the physical system. The physical system changes are reflected in the virtual system; in other words, the virtual system is updated by employing feedback from the physical system. Real-time control commands are made based on the past and present conditions of the physical system to take care of the consistency of the manufacturing process and the quality of manufactured parts [50]. The constant synchronization between physical and virtual systems through the communication layer ends up in a real-time quality control platform which is also supported and updated by the physical system. As illustrated in Figure 3, all sorts of information originating from physical and virtual systems—GD&T standards, historical data, customer feedback, and fabrication protocols—are communicating with the cloud network to provide enough material to make decisions. Continuous and online communication between different physical and virtual data providers is only made possible by the ability of IoT [51] to transmit large volumes of data.

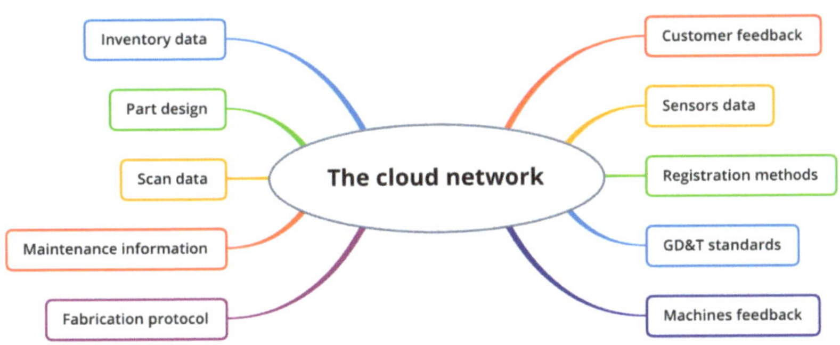

Figure 3. The cloud network in a 4.0 manufacturing factory.

Smart welding is heading inevitably toward the Industry 4.0 paradigm. A schematic of the DT model designed for intelligent laser welding leading to a product license for laser-welded blanks is presented in Figure 4. In this DT, all data from the physical system, including seam tracking, in-process depth meter, and weld inspect data, are communicating with the cloud to update and support the cloud. There is a two-way network of interactions between consequent stages of physical and virtual twins, to transfer and update information, guaranteeing high-quality laser seam according to standards, process command, and specifications defined in the cloud. The application of DTs might facilitate the provision of production licenses for parts manufactured in different production sites, with no need to re-inspect the parts.

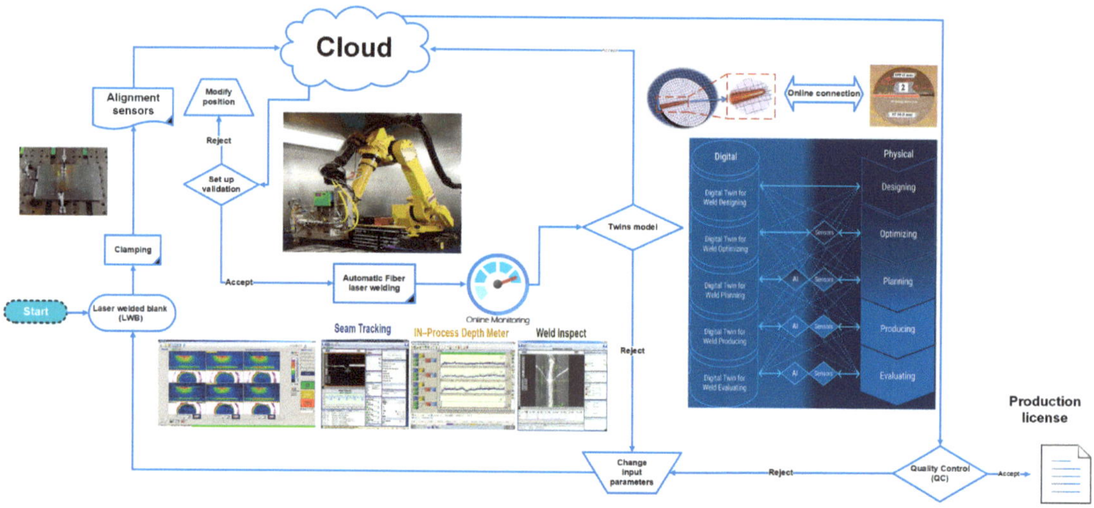

Figure 4. Digital twins model for Inspection 4.0 of laser-welded blanks.

In general, digital twins are efficient platforms for predicting every machine and device's performance, due to their intelligent data processing capability. In a virtual model or DT, physical models of machine operations will be combined with sensor data collected and processed from real assets during real-world operations. In this regard, operators of laser welding machines will benefit from being able to predict structural failure and to plan maintenance activities more effectively. This strategy will result in reduced maintenance costs and operational downtime during welding. As shown in the following model, aluminum sheets are prepared before welding to ensure there is no contamination on the surface. Then, the clamping procedure is adjusted to apply an equivalent force on the surface of the plates. To do so, alignment sensors are used to define the error, and the results are sent to the cloud for future action. By using the validation method, all the process parameters are set, and acceptance/rejection outcomes will be considered, to make a cloud-based smart decision based on the DG&T criteria. If the alignment has been accepted, automatic laser welding will start, and real-time monitoring will be done (seam tracking, in-process depth penetration, weld inspection, etc.). Using sensors and artificial intelligence, digital platforms and physical operations communicate data simultaneously. A cloud platform should be able to process big data and refine it based on pass/fail production criteria. Finally, a license will be issued for the quality assessment of each production. It is worth mentioning that this model can be used in mass production as well as remote manufacturing platforms in any location throughout the world. Thus, this model can be considered the first step toward cloud manufacturing and connected production which can be remotely accessible anytime.

5. Summary and Future Scopes

Investigation of the digital twins market reflects the challenges that have hindered cost-efficient application of digital twins (DTs) in manufacturing. Some of these challenges are due to the complex physics of manufacturing processes and production uncertainties, which in turn leads to difficulties in capturing physical phenomena by a virtual replica. The desire is to set up data-driven digital twins based on a hierarchical structure without any conflict between the physical and virtual systems, which entails appropriate communication and collaboration between them. However, the development of digital twins is still costly due to the restrictions of communication platforms. The ability to predict, prevent and resolve problems and faults also requires the proper implementation of data analysis, decision making, and problem-solving techniques.

In this regard, an overview of computer-aided process monitoring was reviewed, based on the digital twins concept for lightweight laser-welded metals. Different types of 3D geometric inspection, Computer-Aided Inspection (CAI) methods, and tools in the manufacturing industry, are presented and compared in this paper. CAI approaches address automated inspection challenges and requirements for different types of manufactured parts. The development of this process is essential in the production cycle of a part, and therefore should not be ignored. In addition, as moving further toward Industry 4.0, its concepts ought to be incorporated into geometric inspections allowing a comparison between nominal data (CAD model) with respect to a manufactured part, to determine whether it meets specifications without having to apply human judgment. An automated cloud-based Inspection 4.0 is therefore applied. Another objective is to propose an automated production cycle that does not require human intervention. This survey presents an agile approach allowing automation of the laser-welded blanks process. Applying CAI, the process is automated along with the implementation of its DTs. This original model allows remote monitoring of the process, increasing its precision by removing human intervention, increasing productivity, and providing a proper decision-making tool. The challenge now is to integrate artificial intelligence to delegate all redundant work to the machines, and have them provide feedback and auto-maintenance at some point. More research is also needed to develop cost-effective digital twins so that these solutions can meet Industry 4.0 requirements.

Author Contributions: Conceptualization, A.A., S.S.K. and M.S.M.; methodology, S.S.K., D.G.M. and K.B.; validation, S.S.K., M.S.M. and D.G.M.; formal analysis, A.A., S.S.K. and K.B.; investigation, A.A., S.S.K. and M.S.M.; resources, S.S.K. and D.G.M.; data curation, M.S.M. and K.B.; writing—original draft preparation, A.A., S.S.K. and M.S.M.; writing—review and editing, S.S.K., A.A., D.G.M., K.B. and M.S.M.; visualization, A.A., D.G.M. and K.B., supervision and project administration, S.S.K. All authors have read and agreed to the published version of the manuscript.

Funding: We acknowledge the support of the Fonds Québécois de la Recherche sur la Nature et les Technologies (FRQNT) [funding reference number 06351].

Institutional Review Board Statement: This article does not involve human or animal participation or data, therefore ethics approval is not applicable.

Informed Consent Statement: Not applicable.

Data Availability Statement: All data, material, and codes used in this paper are available.

Conflicts of Interest: The authors declare no conflict of interest.

References

1. Katayama, S. *Handbook of Laser Welding Technologies;* Elsevier: Amsterdam, The Netherlands, 2013.
2. Zhao, F.; Xu, X.; Xie, S.Q. Computer-Aided Inspection Planning-The state of the art. *Comput. Ind.* **2009**, *60*, 453–466. [CrossRef]
3. Minetola, P.; Iuliano, L.; Calignano, F. A customer oriented methodology for reverse engineering software selection in the computer aided inspection scenario. *Comput. Ind.* **2015**, *67*, 54–71. [CrossRef]
4. Zhang, L.; Chen, X.; Zhou, W.; Cheng, T.; Chen, L.; Guo, Z. Digital Twins for Additive Manufacturing: A State-of-the-Art Review. *Appl. Sci.* **2020**, *10*, 8350. [CrossRef]
5. Gaha, R.; Durupt, A.; Eynard, B. Towards the implementation of the Digital Twin in CMM inspection process: Opportunities, challenges and proposals. *Procedia Manuf.* **2020**, *54*, 216–221. [CrossRef]
6. Papacharalampopoulos, A.; Michail, C.; Stavropoulos, P. Manufacturing Process Control through a Digital Twin: Encoding Issues. In Proceedings of the TESConf 2020—9th International Conference Through-Life Engineering Services, Cranfield, Bedfordshire, UK, 3–4 November 2020. [CrossRef]
7. Kong, F.; Ma, J.; Carlson, B.; Kovacevic, R. Real-time monitoring of laser welding of galvanized high strength steel in lap joint configuration. *Opt. Laser Technol.* **2012**, *44*, 2186–2196. [CrossRef]
8. Sebestova, H.; Chmelickova, H.; Nozka, L.; Moudry, J. Non-destructive real time monitoring of the laser welding process. *J. Mater. Eng. Perform.* **2012**, *21*, 764–769. [CrossRef]

9. Liu, W.; Liu, S.; Ma, J.; Kovacevic, R. Real-time monitoring of the laser hot-wire welding process. *Opt. Laser Technol.* **2014**, *57*, 66–76. [CrossRef]
10. Harooni, M.; Carlson, B.; Kovacevic, R. Detection of defects in laser welding of AZ31B magnesium alloy in zero-gap lap joint configuration by a real-time spectroscopic analysis. *Opt. Lasers Eng.* **2014**, *56*, 54–66. [CrossRef]
11. Blecher, J.J.; Galbraith, C.M.; Van Vlack, C.; Palmer, T.A.; Fraser, J.M.; Webster, P.J.L.; DebRoy, T. Real time monitoring of laser beam welding keyhole depth by laser interferometry. *Sci. Technol. Weld. Join.* **2014**, *19*, 560–564. [CrossRef]
12. Luo, Z.; Liu, W.; Wang, Z.; Ao, S. Monitoring of laser welding using source localization and tracking processing by microphone array. *Int. J. Adv. Manuf. Technol.* **2016**, *86*, 21–28. [CrossRef]
13. Mirapeix, J.; Vila, E.; Valdiande, J.J.; Riquelme, A.; Garcia, M.; Cobo, A. Real-time detection of the aluminium contribution during laser welding of Usibor1500 tailor-welded blanks. *J. Mater. Process. Technol.* **2016**, *235*, 106–113. [CrossRef]
14. Aminzadeh, A.; Karganroudi, S.S.; Barka, N.; El Ouafi, A. A real-time 3D scanning of aluminum 5052-H32 laser welded blanks; geometrical and welding characterization. *Mater. Lett.* **2021**, *296*, 129883. [CrossRef]
15. Aminzadeh, A.; Karganroudi, S.S.; Barka, N. A novel approach of residual stress prediction in ST-14/ST-44 laser welded blanks; mechanical characterization and experimental validation. *Mater. Lett.* **2021**, *285*, 129193. [CrossRef]
16. Aminzadeh, A.; Nasiri, N.; Barka, N.; Parvizi, A.; Abrinia, K.; Moradi, M.; Sattarpanah Karganroudi, S. Statistical Analysis of Laser-Welded Blanks in Deep Drawing Process: Response Surface Modeling. *J. Mater. Eng. Perform.* **2022**, *31*, 2240–2256. [CrossRef]
17. Aminzadeh, A.; Sattarpanah Karganroudi, S.; Barka, N. Experimental and numerical investigation of forming defects and stress analysis in laser-welded blanks during deep drawing process. *Int. J. Adv. Manuf. Technol.* **2021**, *117*, 1193–1207. [CrossRef]
18. Aminzadeh, A.; Parvizi, A.; Moradi, M. Multi-objective topology optimization of deep drawing dissimilar tailor laser welded blanks; experimental and finite element investigation. *Opt. Laser Technol.* **2020**, *125*, 106029. [CrossRef]
19. Aminzadeh, A.; Parvizi, A.; Safdarian, R.; Rahmatabadi, D. Comparison between laser beam and gas tungsten arc tailored welded blanks via deep drawing. *Proc. Inst. Mech. Eng. Part B J. Eng. Manuf.* **2020**, *235*, 673–688. [CrossRef]
20. Wang, T.; Chen, J.; Gao, X.; Qin, Y. Real-time monitoring for disk laser welding based on feature selection and SVM. *Appl. Sci.* **2017**, *7*, 884. [CrossRef]
21. Wang, T.; Chen, J.; Gao, X.; Li, W. Quality monitoring for laser welding based on high-speed photography and support vector machine. *Appl. Sci.* **2017**, *7*, 299. [CrossRef]
22. De Bono, P.; Allen, C.; D'Angelo, G.; Cisi, A. Investigation of optical sensor approaches for real-time monitoring during fibre laser welding. *J. Laser Appl.* **2017**, *29*, 022417. [CrossRef]
23. Chen, J.; Wang, T.; Gao, X.; Wei, L. Real-time monitoring of high-power disk laser welding based on support vector machine. *Comput. Ind.* **2018**, *94*, 75–81. [CrossRef]
24. Pasinetti, S.; Sansoni, G.; Docchio, F. In-Line Monitoring of Laser Welding Using a Smart Vision System. In Proceedings of the IEEE Metrology for Industry 4.0 and IoT, Brescia, Italy, 16–18 April 2018; pp. 134–139. [CrossRef]
25. Lei, Z.; Shen, J.; Wang, Q.; Chen, Y. Real-time weld geometry prediction based on multi-information using neural network optimized by PCA and GA during thin-plate laser welding. *J. Manuf. Process.* **2019**, *43*, 207–217. [CrossRef]
26. Zhang, Y.; You, D.; Gao, X.; Katayama, S. Online Monitoring of Welding Status Based on a DBN Model During Laser Welding. *Engineering* **2019**, *5*, 671–678. [CrossRef]
27. Haubold, M.W.; Zäh, M.F. Real-time spatter detection in laser welding with beam oscillation. *Procedia CIRP* **2019**, *79*, 159–164. [CrossRef]
28. Shevchik, S.A.; Le-Quang, T.; Farahani, F.V.; Faivre, N.; Meylan, B.; Zanoli, S.; Wasmer, K. Laser welding quality monitoring via graph support vector machine with data adaptive kernel. *IEEE Access* **2019**, *7*, 93108–93122. [CrossRef]
29. Zhang, Z.; Li, B.; Zhang, W.; Lu, R.; Wada, S.; Zhang, Y. Real-time penetration state monitoring using convolutional neural network for laser welding of tailor rolled blanks. *J. Manuf. Syst.* **2020**, *54*, 348–360. [CrossRef]
30. Gonzalez-Val, C.; Pallas, A.; Panadeiro, V.; Rodriguez, A. A convolutional approach to quality monitoring for laser manufacturing. *J. Intell. Manuf.* **2020**, *31*, 789–795. [CrossRef]
31. Keawprachum, B.; Srisungsitthisunti, P. Real-time process monitoring of laser welding by infrared camera and image processing. *Key Eng. Mater.* **2020**, *856*, 160–168. [CrossRef]
32. Papacharalampopoulos, A.; Stavropoulos, P.; Petrides, D. Towards a digital twin for manufacturing processes: Applicability on on laser laser welding. *Procedia CIRP* **2019**, *88*, 110–115. [CrossRef]
33. Sattarpanah Karganroudi, S. *Contribution à L'inspection Automatique des Pièces Flexibles à L'état Libre Sans Gabarit de Conformation*; Université du Québec à Trois-Rivières: Trois-Rivières, QC, Canada, 2017.
34. Sabri, V.; Sattarpanah, S.; Tahan, S.A.; Cuillière, J.C.; François, V.; Pham, X.T. A robust and automated FE-based method for fixtureless dimensional metrology of non-rigid parts using an improved numerical inspection fixture. *Int. J. Adv. Manuf. Technol.* **2017**, *92*, 2411–2423. [CrossRef]
35. Babanezhad, K.; Aidibe, A.; Foucault, G.; Tahan, A.; Bigeon, J. Improved Bi-Criterion flexible registration for fixtureless inspection of compliant parts. *Precis. Eng.* **2020**, *65*, 116–129. [CrossRef]
36. Sattarpanah Karganroudi, S.; Cuillière, J.-C.; François, V.; Tahan, S.-A. "What-if" scenarios towards virtual assembly-state mounting for non-rigid parts inspection using permissible loads. *Int. J. Adv. Manuf. Technol.* **2018**, *97*, 353–373. [CrossRef]

37. Besl, P.J.; McKay, N.D. Method for registration of 3-D shapes. In *Sensor Fusion IV: Control Paradigms and Data Structures*; SPIE: Bellingham, WA, USA, 1992; Volume 1611, pp. 586–606.
38. Li, Y.; Gu, P. Free-form surface inspection techniques state of the art review. *Comput. Des.* **2004**, *36*, 1395–1417. [CrossRef]
39. Savio, E.; Chiffre, L.D.; Schmittc, R. Metrology of freeform shaped parts. *CIRP Ann.* **2007**, *56*, 810–835. [CrossRef]
40. Ravishankar, S.; Dutt, H.; Gurumoorthy, B. Automated inspection of aircraft parts using a modified ICP algorithm. *Int. J. Adv. Manuf. Technol.* **2010**, *46*, 227–236. [CrossRef]
41. Henrikson, J. Completeness and total boundedness of the Hausdorff metric. *MIT Undergrad. J. Math.* **1999**, *1*, 10.
42. Masuda, T.; Yokoya, N. A robust method for registration and segmentation of multiple range images. *Comput. Vis. Image Underst.* **1995**, *61*, 295–307. [CrossRef]
43. Rusinkiewicz, S.; Levoy, M. Efficient variants of the ICP algorithm. In Proceedings of the Third International Conference on 3-D Digital Imaging and Modeling, Quebec City, QC, Canada, 28 May–1 June 2001; pp. 145–152.
44. Greenspan, M.; Godin, G. A nearest neighbor method for efficient ICP. In Proceedings of the Third International Conference on 3-D Digital Imaging and Modeling, Quebec City, QC, Canada, 28 May–1 June 2001; pp. 161–168.
45. Zhu, L.; Barhak, J.; Srivatsan, V.; Katz, R. Efficient registration for precision inspection of free-form surfaces. *Int. J. Adv. Manuf. Technol.* **2007**, *32*, 505–515. [CrossRef]
46. Sattarpanah Karganroudi, S.; Cuillière, J.-C.; Francois, V.; Tahan, S.-A. Automatic fixtureless inspection of non-rigid parts based on filtering registration points. *Int. J. Adv. Manuf. Technol.* **2016**, *87*, 687–712. [CrossRef]
47. Schwer, L.E. An overview of the PTC 60/V&V 10: Guide for verification and validation in computational solid mechanics. *Eng. Comput.* **2007**, *23*, 245–252.
48. Roy, R.B.; Mishra, D.; Pal, S.K.; Chakravarty, T.; Panda, S.; Chandra, M.G.; Pal, A.; Misra, P.; Chakravarty, D.; Misra, S. Digital twin: Current scenario and a case study on a manufacturing process. *Int. J. Adv. Manuf. Technol.* **2020**, *107*, 3691–3714. [CrossRef]
49. Zheng, Y.; Yang, S.; Cheng, H. An application framework of digital twin and its case study. *J. Ambient. Intell. Humaniz. Comput.* **2019**, *10*, 1141–1153. [CrossRef]
50. Mohan, D.G.; Tomków, J.; Sattarpanah Karganroudi, S. Laser Welding of UNS S33207 Hyper-Duplex Stainless Steel to 6061 Aluminum Alloy Using High Entropy Alloy as a Filler Material. *Appl. Sci.* **2022**, *12*, 2849. [CrossRef]
51. Duriagina, Z.; Holyaka, R.; Tepla, T.; Kulyk, V.; Arras, P.; Eyngorn, E. Identification of Fe3O4 nanoparticles biomedical purpose by magnetometric methods. In *Biomaterials in Regenerative Medicine*; InTech: Rijeka, Croatia, 2018; p. 448. [CrossRef]

quantum beam science

MDPI

Review

Femtosecond Laser-Based Additive Manufacturing: Current Status and Perspectives

Atiq Basha Kaligar [1,2], Hemnath Anandan Kumar [3], Asghar Ali [2], Wael Abuzaid [2,4], Mehmet Egilmez [1,2], Maen Alkhader [2,4], Farid Abed [2,5] and Ali Sami Alnaser [1,2,*]

1 Department of Physics, American University of Sharjah, Sharjah 26666, United Arab Emirates; b00090888@aus.edu (A.B.K.); megilmez@aus.edu (M.E.)
2 Materials Science and Engineering Program, College of Arts and Sciences, American University of Sharjah, Sharjah 26666, United Arab Emirates; aasghar@aus.edu (A.A.); wabuzaid@aus.edu (W.A.); malkhader@aus.edu (M.A.); fabed@aus.edu (F.A.)
3 Department of Mechanical Engineering, Indian Institute of Information Technology, Design and Manufacturing, Kancheepuram, Chennai 600127, India; hemnathceg@gmail.com
4 Department of Mechanical Engineering, American University of Sharjah, Sharjah 26666, United Arab Emirates
5 Department of Civil Engineering, American University of Sharjah, Sharjah 26666, United Arab Emirates
* Correspondence: aalnaser@aus.edu

Abstract: The ever-growing interest in additive manufacturing (AM) is evidenced by its extensive utilisation to manufacture a broad spectrum of products across a range of industries such as defence, medical, aerospace, automotive, and electronics. Today, most laser-based AM is carried out by employing continuous-wave (CW) and long-pulsed lasers. The CW and long-pulsed lasers have the downside in that the thermal energy imparted by the laser diffuses around the irradiated spot and often leads to the creation of heat-affected zones (HAZs). Heat-affected zones may degrade the material strength by producing micro-cracks, porous structures and residual stresses. To address these issues, currently, attempts are being made to employ ultrafast laser sources, such as femtosecond (fs) lasers, in AM processes. Femtosecond lasers with pulse durations in the order of 10^{-15} s limit the destructive laser–material interaction and, thus, minimise the probability of the HAZs. This review summarises the current advancements in the field of femtosecond laser-based AM of metals and alloys. It also reports on the comparison of CW laser, nanosecond (ns)/picosecond (ps) lasers with fs laser-based AM in the context of heat-affected zones, substrate damage, microstructural changes and thermomechanical properties. To shed light on the principal mechanisms ruling the manufacturing processes, numerical predictions are discussed and compared with the experimental results. To the best of the authors' knowledge, this review is the first of its kind to encompass the current status, challenges and opportunities of employing fs lasers in additive manufacturing.

Keywords: femtosecond lasers; additive manufacturing; 3D printing; heat-affected zone; powder bed fusion; direct writing; selective laser sintering

1. Introduction

Additive manufacturing (AM—commonly referred to as 3D printing) has already revolutionised industry and is positioned to make a notable impact across a wide range of sectors [1,2]. This is primarily induced by the significant simplifications and freedom in the design process combined with the adaptability of 3D printing to an impressively wide range of materials not shared by any other manufacturing technique [3]. Although the potential benefits of 3D printing can be exploited in a wide range of applications and industries, including aerospace [4–9], automotive [7,10], defence sectors [11], jewellery making [12], construction [13], electronics [14], food [15], health care [10,16,17], footwear [18], clothing [19], sports [20] and others [21], utilisation in the biomedical is of special interest due to the relatively complex requirements and intricate designs commonly encountered in these fields. The interest in AM continues to grow, and current research and development efforts span across almost all relevant aspects such as the utilised materials, 3D printing technology, post-processing treatments, and optimisation of processing parameters in terms of design and fabrication. One of the major advantages of 3D printing is the ability to adapt and optimise this manufacturing technique to all materials including polymers, ceramics, metals, and composites [1]. Such versatility is not shared by any other manufacturing technique. AM of metals is of particular importance due to the fact of their desirable properties in many applications (e.g., load-carrying capacity). Steel, titanium, aluminium, nickel-based superalloys, iron, copper, gold, and silver have all been successfully processed, even at an industrial scale in some cases [22–24]. Such efforts are no longer limited to lab-scale specimens as adoption by industry continues to grow. The aerospace industry was among the first to adopt AM technology for large-scale production. For example, GE aviation employed AM to print nozzles for its LEAP engines. In addition to reducing the total parts count from 20 to 5, durability was also found to be enhanced by a factor of five [25,26]. Similarly, Boeing is saving millions per plane through the use of AM. As of now, more than 70,000 AM parts fly through Boeing programs [27].

Although various techniques have been developed over the years for AM-based synthesis, including material extrusion (ME), direct energy deposition (DED), powder bed fusion (PBF), fused deposition modelling (FDM), sheet lamination (SL) and binder jetting (BJ) [28], the methods that rely on the utilisation of metal powders have been more widely adopted by industry (i.e., PBF, DED and BJ processes). The metal AM systems are usually composed of a powder delivery system and an energy delivery system [29]. In PBF systems, selective laser melting (SLM) or selective laser sintering (SLS) are key processes. In SLM or SLS, the material will heat up and subsequently melt utilising a laser source. At present, metal AM technologies are predominantly reliant on long-pulsed lasers or CW lasers to process materials [30,31]. In general, CW lasers are utilised for fabricating larger parts, whereas pulsed lasers are considered when fabricating precise and thin parts [32]. In the case of CW laser-based AM, there are certain important process parameters that influence the quality of the produced parts using SLM. This includes hatch spacing, scanning speed, laser power and layer thickness [33,34]. In any SLM process, along with these parameters, the light absorptance and the laser energy density play vital roles in melting and sintering. Despite the significant progress made, there are certain challenges that must be overcome such as accuracy and reduced materials usage [35]. In addition, some materials continue to pose challenges and are difficult to process using AM. For example, some ceramics and refractory metals, due to the fact of their high melting temperatures and high thermal conductivity [36], are still difficult to process using CW or long-pulsed laser-based AM technologies. To process such materials, novel technologies and new processes must be developed to reach very high temperatures while causing minimal heat-affected zones (HAZs), along with good precision and accuracy at sub-micron levels. In this regard, ultrafast lasers (i.e., picosecond (ps) and femtosecond (fs) lasers) are well suited for lifting the shortcomings of the existing additive manufacturing techniques, especially in situations where high melting point materials are involved or extreme precision and reproducibility are required [7,37]. Although AM via ultrafast lasers is a relatively new area, recent works have already highlighted its huge potential and advantages over the use of CW lasers [38]. In short, the main advantages of ultrashort pulsed lasers over CW lasers are increased part resolution [39,40], rapid cooling rate, reduced residual stresses, reduced oxidation effect, lower substrate damage compared to CW laser, suitable to process dielectrics and better wettability [41]. These aspects will be discussed in further detail throughout this article.

The use of ultrafast lasers as a manufacturing tool is gaining notable momentum across various industries. In a recent study, the global ultrafast lasers market was predicted to cross USD 1.43 billion by 2020, a number that is further expected to reach the USD 3.31 billion milestone by 2026 with an estimated compound annual growth rate (CAGR) of 16.6% between 2021 and 2026 [42]. Though the initial investment is high for such laser technologies, the significant advantages (e.g., precise manufacturing and reduced HAZs) provide justification for their use in medical, aerospace and military applications. As noted above, fs lasers are being explored for precise material processing due to the ultrashort pulse duration in the range of a few hundred fs that produces lower laser–matter interaction times and reduces HAZs. In addition to pulse duration, the scanning speed and pulse repetition rate are also major deciding factors for precise AM. Fs laser sources produce higher peak intensities compared to CW lasers or long-pulsed lasers. This allows for rapid energy delivery into the material and paves the way to achieve localised heating [43]. Apart from this, fs lasers have high penetration depth in a short range of time. It is because of these attributes that fs lasers can accurately remove a material, sinter it and can change its properties in a highly localised and controlled manner [44]. Over the past few years, various types of fs lasers, such as fibre laser and solid-state laser systems, have been used in the material processing field. They are capable of producing pulse energies in millijoules and output powers in kilowatts, pulse durations up to 100 s femtosecond and pulse repetition rate can be up to100 MHz [44,45]. With such properties, many applications have already been developed relying on this relatively new technology. Examples include their use in cataract surgeries in the health care sector and in material processing. As fs laser sources are capable of producing precise features at the micro and nano levels in a highly localised and controlled manner, applications at the nanomanufacturing processes [30], and micro fabrications (e.g., fabrication of micro-needles for medical applications [46]) are among the most commonly explored in the literature [47,48]. In addition, various works have explored the potential use of fs lasers for post-processing of 3D printed metallic components (i.e., utilising the associated heat to alter the microstructure) [49,50]. Further, fs laser sources were utilised to modify the flexural strength and surface morphology of materials such as translucent monolithic zirconia (for dental restoration) [51].

Apart from the machining and surface structuring processes, fs laser sources have been explored for the precise 3D printing of various materials such as copper [52–54], silver [55,56], iron [57], tungsten [7,44,58], aluminium alloys [59,60], YSZ [61] and functional ceramics [62]. Some examples include the utilisation of fs lasers in micro sintering to fabricate components at the microscale (e.g., micro engines with materials such as steel, nickel and titanium). Unlike bulk engines, micro engines must be sized down to a few mm, up to a cm, and must be manufactured with remarkable precision at the micro level. Using a CW laser in such a microfabrication process generates HAZs, which limits the process resolution and the finishing quality of the part [46]. In such cases, apart from single-material fabrication, ultrafast laser sources have been utilised in multi-material processing. For example, 12Cr2Si and 9Cr1Mo were reported to give excellent bimetallic structure following fs laser AM. The resulting bimetallic structure between the 12Cr2Si steel and 9Cr1Mo steel exhibited a smooth phase transition between interfaces, which led to excellent strength between the dissimilar metals [63]. Femtosecond laser-based AM is still in its infancy. This review is an attempt to highlight some of the fs laser-based research endeavours, identify the intended industrial applications and outline future prospects of the fs laser AM. We specifically focused on fs laser-assisted sintering and melting of powders, especially metals. We begin with the role of lasers in AM and the important parameters that affect the process. This is followed by a brief discussion on the simulations and models used to elucidate ultrafast laser–material interactions. Subsequently, an account for the role and importance of fs laser powder bed fusion (PBF) and multi-material layered structuring is presented. The reported parameters for sintering different materials are summarised. The review is concluded by spotlighting the future scope and prospects of fs laser AM [64,65].

2. Lasers in Metal Additive Manufacturing

Initially, lasers were employed in cutting and other subtractive manufacturing processes such as milling. Later applications considered the use of laser systems in surface modification and functionalisation. The laser-based AM processes or material deposition became feasible to use only when lasers with increased spatial control of the laser energy input were introduced. This was because these lasers had a high beam quality and enhanced beam delivery [66]. Different AM technologies use lasers as a source to process materials and fabricate complex 3D printed components. Such processes include SLS [22,67,68], SLM [22,69], direct metal deposition (DMD) [22], direct writing (DW) [70] and stereolithography (SLA) [69,70]. All of these, except for the SLA process, are executable with metallic materials [25]. Nowadays, different types of laser sources are being employed in AM. These include diode lasers, Nd:YAG lasers, CO_2 lasers, Yb-doped fibre lasers and excimer lasers [10,29]. The CO_2 lasers, which can run at relatively high power (kilowatt) levels, were widely utilised in metal additive manufacturing and welding processes at the beginning of the AM era. They were followed by Nd:YAG lasers, which are commonly employed as pulsed laser sources. Particularly for metal AM, diode lasers have longer lifetimes and higher efficiency. With relatively compact sizes, high reliability and low maintenance and operation costs, fibre-based lasers attracted significant attention by the AM community, especially for the fabrication and functionalisation of metallic structures [71]. A few commercially available AM machines and their laser systems are listed in Table 1.

Table 1. Commercially available laser-based metal AM machines [72].

Category	Manufacturing Systems	Laser
Direct energy deposition (DED)	Trumpf GmbH: TruLaser series	TruDiode diode laser, up to 6 kW (600 nm)
	Meltio	1200 W diode laser
	BeAM: Modulo series	500–2000 W fibre laser
	Oerlikon Metco Group: MetcoClad systems	1–6 kW diode laser
	InssTek: Fab series	Maximum 2000 W fibre laser
	Optomec Inc.: LENS series	400–1000 W fibre laser
Powder bed fusion (PBF)	Renishaw: AM250	200 or 400 W fibre laser
	SLM Solutions GmbH: SLM systems	400–1000 W fibre laser (for metals)
	EOS GmbH: EOSINT, EOS M and PRECIOUS M machines	30, 70 or 2 × 50 W CO_2 lasers (for thermoplastics) 200 W–1 kW fibre laser (for metals)
	3D Systems Inc.: ProX, sPro and ProX SLM systems	30–200 W CO_2 laser (for thermoplastics) 50–500 W fibre laser (for metals)
	Concept Laser	400–1000 W fibre laser (for metals)
	Aconity ONE	400–1000 W fibre laser
	Trumpf: Truprint 5000	500 W fibre laser

Across industries, many of the aforementioned AM technologies have been utilised for custom and mass production of various components. A summary highlighting the need for AM-based processing in different industrial sectors and the utilised processes are summarised in Table 2.

Table 2. Laser-based AM and its applications in various fields [73,74].

Industry	Trend/Goal	Laser-Based AM Process
Aerospace [12,29]	Demand for lightweight structures	DMD, SLS and SLM
	Rapid tooling, fixturing	DMD and SLS
	Fuel reduction	DMD, SLS and SLM
	Organic features	SLM, SLS and DMD
Automotive [10]	Demand for lightweight structures	SLS, SLM and DMD
Medical (dental, implants) [75]	Minimally invasive surgery	SMS and SLM
	Replication of anatomic structures	SLA and SLS
	Biomaterial manufacturing	SLS and SLA
Electronics [76]	Smart microsystems	SLA and Micro-SLS
	Miniaturisation	SLA and Micro-SLS
	Accelerated product development	SLA and Micro-SLS

Laser Parameters Used in AM

High throughput in manufacturing can be achieved with higher laser absorptivity [74]. In SLM, melting takes place due to the absorption of the thermal energy resulting from the laser–matter interaction. Specific heat capacity and latent heat vary from one material to another and may affect the final product's quality [75]. In some cases, the provision of insufficient energy affects the material build quality, thus leading to detrimental structural impacts. A number of factors, such as laser power, layer thickness, scanning speed and hatch spacing, can be tuned to determine the energy input. An extremely high laser power can result in excessive evaporation of molten material that causes a keyhole effect. In addition, if there is more vaporisation of material in SLM, the vapours may condense and result in laser power disruption [76]. In metal AM, better absorptivity is achieved by shorter wavelengths. CO_2 laser sources have relatively long wavelengths and, hence, lower throughput compared to Nd:YAG lasers. The resolution of the manufacturing method is highly dependent on the focusing ability of the laser source which is dependent on the operating wavelength [77–81].

Energy density is a critical parameter in laser-based AM, as it is closely associated with the occurrence of the underlying physical phenomena, whether it be sintering, melting or solidification [82]. Additionally, some materials that possess high thermal diffusivity and high reflectivity are influenced by energy densities. These energy densities are directly affected by laser power, which serves as the base for determining the build rate. Extremely high laser powers may also worsen the fabrication of parts. Hence, the optimum combination of processing parameters should be chosen to achieve good-quality part fabrication [83,84]. The beam spot size is one important parameter that determines the precision and manufacturing resolution. To calculate the beam quality, AM processes usually use the beam parameter product (BPP), which helps to identify the energy confinement at a point. BPP is usually calculated by the product of the half-angle of beam divergence and beam waist radius [29]. For CW laser-based SLM, the main process parameters, divided into powder-related, powder-bed related and laser related, are detailed in Figure 1 [41].

Different laser sources are classified based on the mode of operation as discussed in an earlier section. The most commonly used laser sources in AM processes, such as SLM, SLS and LENS, are CO_2, Nd:YAG and Yb-fibre lasers. Each laser source has a different wavelength and pulse duration that range from milliseconds ms to ns. On the other hand, ultrafast lasers operate in the range of fs–ps. When it comes to ultrafast laser-based AM, there are several other laser-related parameters that come into the picture such as laser wavelength, pulse duration, pulse energy, repetition rate, spectral bandwidth, average power, beam quality, beam diameter and power stability. Some laser parameters are more critical than the others, for they may greatly affect the finish and quality of the part produced. Some of these critical parameters are average power, pulse energy density, beam quality, spot size and pulse duration. The laser-related parameters and properties are crucial in a CW laser-based SLM process. The laser power source is the main element that provides sufficient energy to melt the powder particles. As discussed earlier, the laser source can be operated at different energy levels, which is denoted by the laser power. If the laser power is not sufficient, powders will not melt properly, and if the laser power is very high, improper melting occurs. The laser spot diameter also plays a major role in determining the energy transfer to melt the powder material [85]. Hatch spacing is the amount of overlap that is present between the adjacent tracks for the layer to improve the bonding [86]. Larger hatch spacing provides insufficient boding between adjacent layers [87]. In any SLM process, the laser moves with a particular velocity in a certain pattern, called a hatch pattern or a scan pattern, that helps to fill in the contours of the particular layer with laser-melted tracks [88]. A summary of the operational parameters specific to different lasers is presented in Table 3.

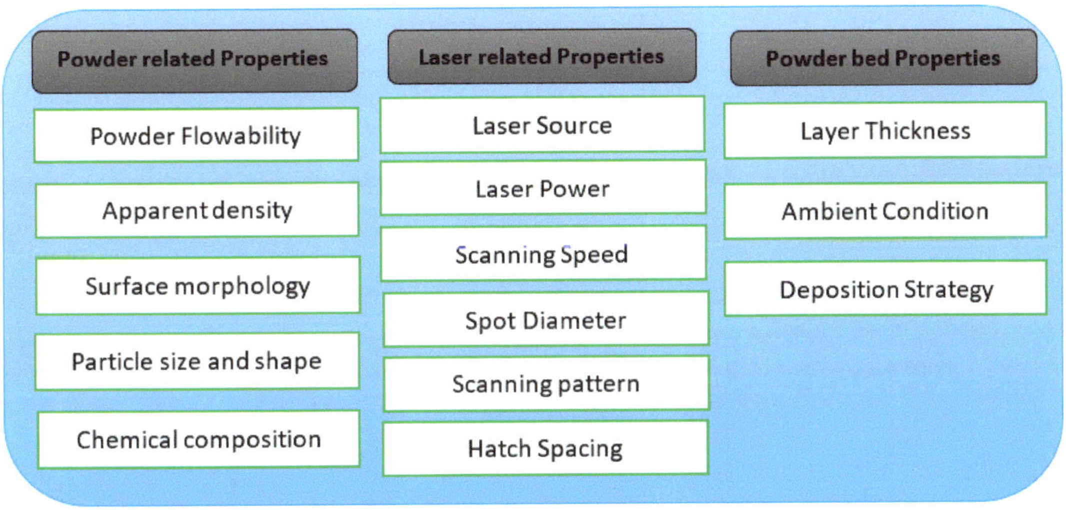

Figure 1. Summary of CW-based SLM process parameters [41].

Table 3. Types of lasers and related parameters used in AM processes [77].

Laser Type	CO_2 Laser	Yb-Fibre Laser	Nd:YAG Laser	Excimer Laser
Type of laser	Pulsed and CW	Pulsed and CW	Pulsed and CW	Pulsed
AM process	SLA, SLM, SLS and LENS	SLS, SLM and LENS	SLS, SLM and LENS	SLA
Wavelength	9.4 and 10.6 µm	1.07 µm	1.06 µm	193, 248 and 308 nm
Output power (CW)	Up to 20 kW	Up to 10 kW	Up to 16 kW	300 W (average)
Pulse duration	100–10 s ns	10 s ns to 10 s ms	Few ns to 10 s ms	10 s ns
Efficiency	5–20%	10–30%	10–20%	1–4%
Beam quality (mm.mrad)	3–5	0–4	0.4–20	0.5–2

Apart from the laser-related properties, powder-related properties are also equally important in determining the quality of the part. The particle size and shape should be within a specific range so that the part quality and surface finish can be assured [89]. The various process response characteristics of laser-based sintered parts are part resolution, surface finish, mechanical properties, microstructure, density and residual stresses, which are important for determining the quality of a 3D printed part [41]. Generated defects, such as cracks, swelling, residual stresses, substrate warping and melt ball formation, reduce the quality of the 3D printed part and should be investigated once the part has been 3D printed [33].

3. Femtosecond Lasers and Laser–Material Interaction

3.1. A Brief History of Ultrafast Laser Development

It is widely accepted that Theodore Maiman demonstrated the first short pulsed laser (i.e., ruby lasers) in the 1960s [64]. In the 1960s and 1970s, revolutionary mode locking research on organic dye lasers and solid-state lasers was published, encompassing both experimental [90,91] and theoretical investigations [92]. With the introduction of fibre amplifiers and fibre lasers in the 1980s, ultrafast fibre lasers became a new class of technology for ultrafast laser sources [93]. Further, Strickland and Mourou developed chirped pulse amplification (CPA) in 1985 that allowed researchers to make ultrashort, ultrahigh intensity laser pulses [66]. During the 1990s, D.E Spence developed a self-mode locked Ti:sapphire laser to produce pulses with pulse durations up to 60 fs, which was a turning point in ultrafast laser development [17,94]. With significant advancements during the 1990s, pulse durations as low as 6.5 fs were achieved [95]. Today's commercial fs fibre lasers can easily deliver pulses of durations less than 100 fs, repetition rates in MHz, and average power in the kW regime. Previously, ultrashort pulse lasers with pulse energy in nanojoules and operating in MHz were mostly reported for communication and information transmission. AM, on the other hand, requires tunable but high pulse energies to process materials [65]. The potential to produce ultrashort pulses with lower HAZs and high peak powers makes fs lasers desirable in industrial applications.

3.2. Mechanisms of Ultrafast Laser–Matter Interaction

Ultrafast lasers are distinguished mainly by three factors: extremely short pulse duration, high intensity and a broad spectral bandwidth [96,97]. In laser–materials interactions, fs lasers allow for rapid energy delivery into the material (in ps) that is significantly faster than plasma expansion time (from ns to μs), causing the local temperature to rapidly rise to temperatures as high as 6000 °C [44]. These factors enable the use of ultrafast lasers in high-quality manufacturing processes with minimal heat dissipation in the surrounding environment. This is a huge advantage compared to nanosecond lasers in which the melted material at the laser focus has time to heat up and diffuse heat into the surroundings, generating large craters with off stoichiometric compositions. Furthermore, during long-pulsed laser processing, micro droplets are generated as a result of the ejected vaporised material, leaving the remaining material to resolidify, which leads to poor processing and generates HAZs, microcracks, dross and recast [64]. For pulse durations in the range of nanoseconds, the absorption of the laser pulse is governed by the linear optical absorption depth of the laser, which causes energy dissipation by heat conduction into the substance [45]. In general, for CW and long-pulsed lasers, the processing would include melting of material, reflow and solidification [64]. Figure 2 shows the comparison of CW, ns and fs-pulsed lasers (i.e., high and low power, respectively) and their material absorption characteristics [57].

When ultrashort pulsed lasers with high laser fluence are applied, ablation of heated matter occurs in a few tens of ps after absorption [47]. In the case of metals interacting with ultrashort lasers, the electron gas absorbs the laser and heats up in less than a hundred fs, whereas the lattice heats up with a delay of 1–100 ps [98,99]. Additionally, HAZ can be less than 5 μm, and for plastic materials, it can be up to 30–50 μm [47]. On the other hand, the penetration depth per pulse for ultrashort pulses is typically between 20 and 100 nm for metals, polymers, and semiconductors but up to 500 nm for glass and transparent materials. Therefore, as the pulse duration decreases, the ablation rate increases, which is also dependent on the laser wavelength, i.e., the absorption spectrum of the material [45,47]. For example, Table 4 shows the maximum ablation rate at 400 fs of pulse duration and 1035 nm wavelength of laser. Generally, with the decrease in pulse duration, the energy and ablation depth increases, while thermal diffusion length become shorter (Figure 3) [47]. Such trends can be advantageous for precise material processing [45].

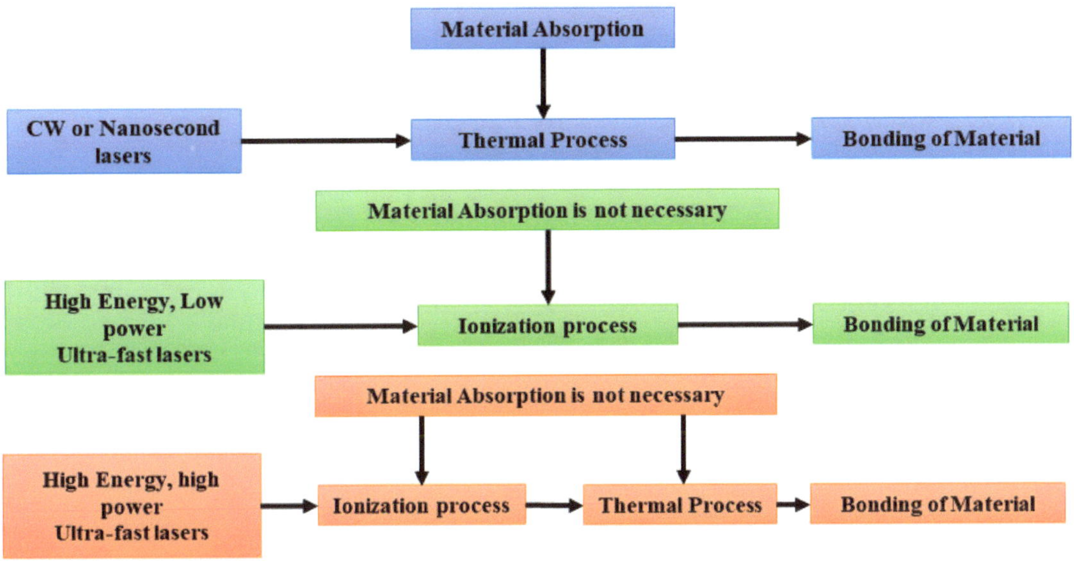

Figure 2. Comparison of CW, ns and fs laser material absorption processes [57].

Table 4. Different maximum ablation rates for various material processes [96].

Material	Optimum Avgerage Fluence at 400 fs and 1035 nm (J/cm^2)	Maximum Ablation Rate at 400 fs and 1035 nm (mm^3/W min)
Steel	0.35	0.22
Nitinol	0.6	0.21
Aluminium	1	0.3
Copper	1.7	0.16
Si	1.3	0.16
SiC	0.7	0.13
PET	0.7	8
Fused silica	3	0.4
Sapphire	4	0.3

The data in Table 4 are included in [44] as a basis for estimating ablation rates, which may be useful for micromachining, structuring and other industrial applications. However, in the case of SLS, ablation of the material may be unfavourable for additive manufacturing, because it requires melting or partial fusing of particles to print layer by layer. Therefore, by appropriately tuning the fs laser parameters and utilising the most important characteristics of fs laser sintering (i.e., generating reduced HAZs and lower heat dissipation), it was possible to print different materials such as copper [52,53], iron [100], silver [55,56], tungsten [7,44,101] and aluminium [38,60]. Additive manufacturing of parts utilising fs lasers is complex and comprises various factors/parameters as shown in Table 5.

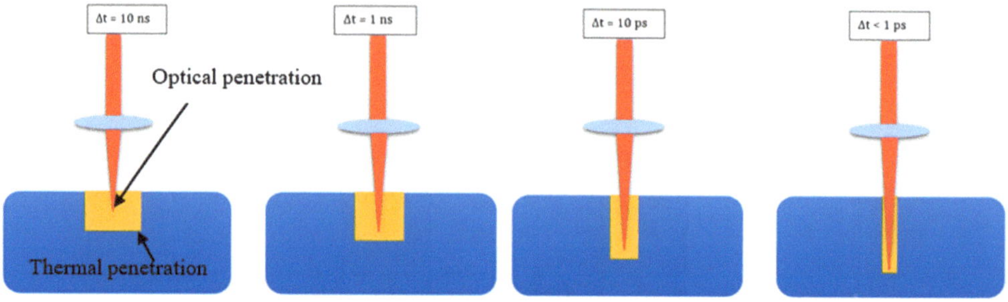

Figure 3. Energy penetration (red) and volume heated via heat conduction (yellow) or different pulse durations [47].

Table 5. Various factors that influence fs laser material processing [44].

Various Factors	Description
Pulse energy	Depends on the average output power and pulse repetition rate
Pulse width	Called pulse duration also and, in general, varies a few hundred femtoseconds in the case of fs laser material processing
Average power	Total average output power utilised in material processing
Pulse repetition rate	Number of pulses per second, in general, between kHz and a few MHz will be utilised during material processing
Peak power	Maximum peak power attained by a single pulse
Focus spot area/volume	The laser spot area or volume is the exposed area/volume, which is important to consider during precise processing
Hatch spacing	The spacing between each line exposed during area-wise material processing
Scanning velocity	The scan velocity is the speed of the laser travelling during processing; it is the most critical parameter to control because the exposure time depends on this parameter
Operation mode	The environment during processing
Wavelength	The laser operating wavelength
Powder particle size	The powder size is important to consider, depending on the application
Shape of the powder particle	In general, for SLS/M spherical powder particles are considered
Powder morphology	The uniformity of powder size distribution

Pulsed lasers produce discrete pulses of laser energy at a specified repetition rate. In Table 5, pulse energy is defined as the energy per each pulse, which is proportional to the average power and inversely proportional to the repetition rate of the laser. The full width at half maximum (FWHM) in the laser's optical power vs. time plot is defined as the laser pulse duration, or pulse width. The average power of a pulsed laser is calculated as the energy of the pulse divided by the pulse duration. The number of pulses released per second is defined as the pulse repetition rate. Higher repetition rates result in less thermal relaxation time at the surfaces, which leads to more rapid material heating. The maximum laser power that a single pulse attains is known as laser peak power. The laser spot at the focal plane of a focusing lens is described by the spot size of a focused laser beam [102]. In general, the goal of many applications, such as materials processing, is having a minimum spot size. In materials processing, different materials will have different wavelength-dependent absorption characteristics, resulting in distinct interactions with the substance. The operation mode relates to the laser processing environment; in many situations, argon or nitrogen gas purging has been used to avoid oxidation issues [89,103]. It is also necessary to consider and monitor the powder quality and size distribution before processing. The powder quality depends upon the size and shape of the powder. The powder size distribution is crucial in facilitating the sintering of powder particles and, as such, the powder particles should be of uniform shape, because dissimilar-shaped powder particles will lead to poor melting and will affect the quality of the fabricated part [104,105]. Both powder size and laser spot diameters determine the precision of 3D printed parts generated by fs laser-based 3D printing [77].

As for metallurgical aspects, melting in general refers to particle–particle fusion during fs laser melting or sintering. Phase change refers to change in phase during sintering process. This is dependent on the uniform cooling that happens in the process and on the material's thermo-physical properties. Cracking and residual stresses, in general referred to as defects generated in the printed parts, need to be analysed once the part is fabricated. Thermal diffusion depends on the material property, i.e., thermal conductivity. For example, due to the fact of its high thermal conductivity, when copper interacts with the laser, a large amount of heat is dissipated into the surroundings.

A simplified illustration of the temporal evolution of the fs-laser-based AM process was developed by Shaung et al. [44]. As shown in Figure 4, fs laser ablation causes ionisation of materials and the development of new grains and microstructures during cooling and solidification, which occur on a ps–µs time scale. When the pulse duration is at the lowest pulse duration (i.e., at the start and less than ps), the laser–matter interaction is mainly dominated by ionisation of materials, ablation and plasma formation. When the pulse duration is, in general, between fs and ns, the local temperature may exceed 10,000 K. Similarly, as the pulse duration increases, there will be thermal energy dominance. Finally, correlation between the pulse number and temperature shows that it is possible to reach higher temperatures with higher pulse repetition rates.

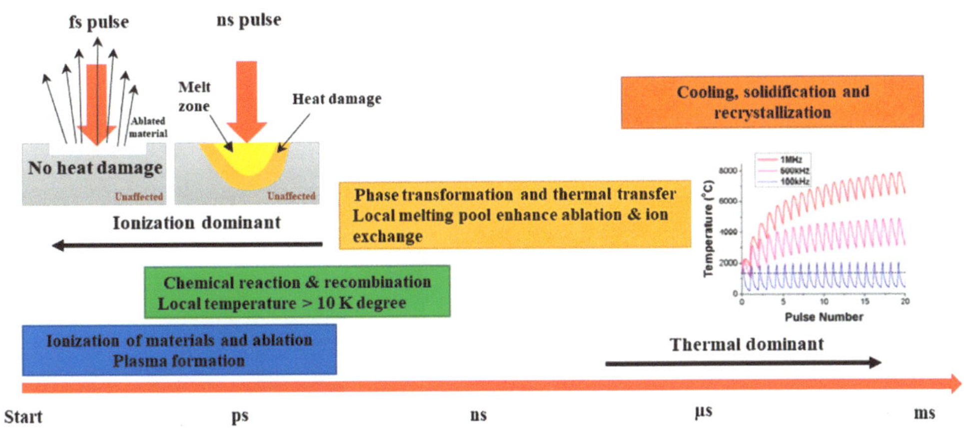

Figure 4. Temporal evolution of an fs-laser-based AM process [44]. The inset shows the correlation between pulse number and temperature for different repetition rates.

3.3. Modelling and Numerical Analysis of Laser-Based AM

To better understand the principal physical interactions and the governing mechanisms of a manufacturing process, it is essential to develop numerical-based models that capture the underlying physical phenomena of the process. Such models, for instance, can provide details about the temporal and spatial distribution of the temperature, deformation and stress fields resulting from the material–tool (e.g., laser or cutting tool) interaction during the manufacturing process. These fields are difficult and often impossible to obtain experimentally; however, they allow for realising a better understanding of the processes' underlying physical interactions and their effects on the quality of the manufactured part. The latter is needed to optimise the manufacturing process (e.g., increase its sustainability, throughput or reduce its cost) and improve the quality of the manufactured parts (e.g., enhance their surface finish and mechanical properties).

Developing an accurate physically informed numerical model of a manufacturing process requires identifying and including the physical laws and equations that describe the evolution, interaction and equilibrium of the physical parameters pertaining to the physical phenomena associated with the manufacturing process. Applying this to laser-based material processing techniques proved challenging as they are intrinsically multi-physical problems and involve complex coupled governing equations. Thus, different strategies for modelling laser-based material processing were developed. The different strategies, which are overviewed in the following, included different assumptions and used different numerical schemes (e.g., finite element and molecular dynamics). Most importantly, each approach was designed to investigate a certain aspect of laser-based material processing.

The mostly used strategy to model laser-based processing of materials simplifies the modelling process by modelling the laser–material interaction as an intense heat source. Subsequently, the response of the material to the intense heat source is modelled using thermo-mechanical equilibrium and constitutive equations that compute the temperature and deformation fields in the vicinity of the heat source. Later, temperature and deformation fields are used to determine the processed material microstructure (e.g., grain size and dislocation density). This approach, which was mostly used to model CW laser-based processing, was applied successfully to model laser welding [106], DED [107] and SLM [108].

The aforementioned thermo-mechanical approach was extended to model fs laser processing of metals. The extension involved emphasising more on the heat and mass transfer and applying the analysis at two length scales: one at the microscale and another at the nanoscale. Modelling heat transfer and temperature distributions at small scales (i.e., nano and micro) is of great importance, as the fabrication process is highly dependent on phenomena occurring at those small scales. However, at the microscale level and below, additional challenges arise. Using fundamental and phenomenological laws, such as Fourier's law of heat conduction, become highly challenging as the heat transfer time characteristics vary for various heat carriers, which may align with the energy excitation time [109]. In addition, modelling heat transfer at the microscale is computationally challenging, as it requires considering micro time steps, which increases the computational costs. Even with the aforementioned challenges, many preliminary modelling-based studies have been conducted over the past two decades to analyse the capability of fs lasers to precisely cut materials. These showed that fs lasers can be used to precisely cut materials [110,111] and produce "precise cuts" with minimal damage [112]. In addition, models showed that the HAZ and the rate of heat can be precisely controlled in fs laser processing in comparison with the processing of materials using long-pulsed lasers [113].

Developing more capable thermo-mechanical models that better describe the interaction of fs lasers with the processed material necessitated representing the fs-laser induced energy and heat transfer process more accurately. During fs laser processing of materials, three different types of heat transfer regimes exist [114] and should be accounted for in the models. In the primary stage, the energy from the laser is absorbed by the electrons of the processed material. At this stage, the excited electrons are in a state of thermal non-equilibrium. In the second stage, the electrons gradually attain a state of thermal equilibrium, and fermi distribution can be used to represent the density of the existing states. But the lattice and electrons will be at two different states of temperature regimes. During the second stage, heat transfer mainly occurs due to the diffusion of hot electrons. In the third and final stage, the lattice and electrons reach a state of thermal equilibrium.

In this stage, the energy is carried into the bulk through a normal thermal diffusion process [115]. In general, when an fs laser interacts with any metal, the electron subsystem absorbs the laser pulse energy, which increases the electrons' temperature to very high temperatures in the range of thousands of degrees kelvin. However, during irradiation, the lattice temperature lags behind that of the electrons, and the lag remains for the next few ps. Eventually, the laser energy transferred to the electron subsystem is carried to the lattice subsystem. Models that account for the aforementioned three stages have been developed and used to describe fs laser–material interaction during the processing of copper [116].

Specialised models were also developed to investigate specific physical mechanisms pertaining to laser–material interaction. For instance, to better understand and predict fs–laser–induced ablation during fs-laser-based processing of materials, numerical and theoretical models were developed. These included molecular dynamics [117,118] and hydrodynamics models [119,120] (continuous thermodynamics model). Predicted ablation depth, using a hydrodynamics model, for copper and aluminium subjected to an fs laser is shown in Figure 5. This figure shows a relatively good correlation between the experimental and numerical results, underscoring the importance of numerical models. The molecular dynamics models include the kinematic equations of each atom present in the ablation entity. Whereas the hydrodynamics model uses a set of equations in a Lagrangian form that represent hydrodynamics along with the multiphase equation of the state. Though these models are able to represent the underlying physics of the process, they are complex and consume large amounts of computational time.

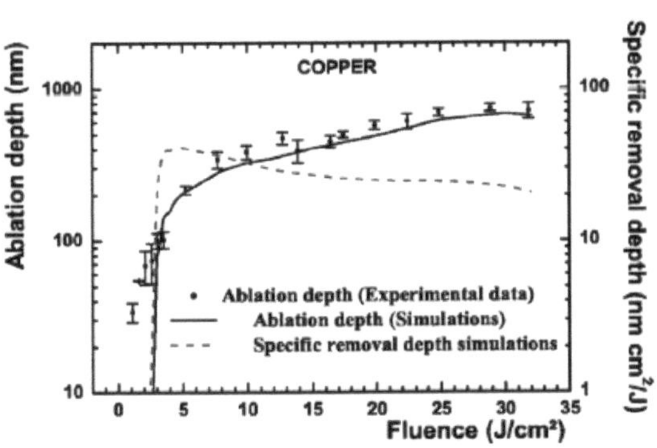

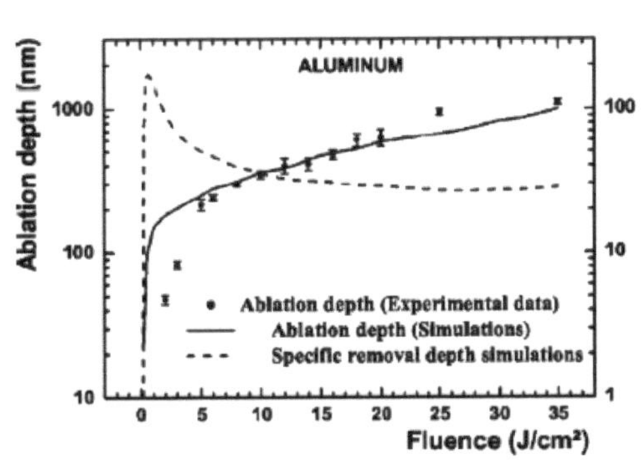

Figure 5. Experimental and numerical results of ablation depth as a function of laser fluence using a hydrodynamics model for (**a**) copper and (**b**) aluminium with a 170 fs laser pulse (Adapted from reference [119]).

To study the complex process of ablation and to predict the non-equilibrium temperature distribution between the lattice and electrons regime, while avoiding the computational complexities of hydrodynamics and molecular dynamics models, a two-temperature numerical model was developed by Anisimov et al. [121]. Due to the fact of their computational efficiency, two-temperature models (TTMs) are widely used to model fs laser processing of metals [99,122]. The two-temperature model was developed from the Boltzmann equation and is composed of the following coupled PDEs (partial differential equations) [123]:

$$C_e(T_e)\frac{\partial T_e}{\partial t} = K_e\nabla^2 T_e - G(T_e - T_l) + Q(r,t) \quad (1)$$

$$C_l\frac{\partial T_l}{\partial t} = K_l\nabla^2 T_l + G(T_e - T_l) \quad (2)$$

where C_e is the electron heat capacity, C_l is the lattice heat capacity, K_l is the lattice thermal conductivity, K_e is the electron thermal conductivity, $Q(r,t)$ is the laser energy density absorbed per unit time, and G is the electron–phonon coupling constant. In these equations, the temperature-dependent variables are G, K_e, and C_e. Equations (1) and (2) represent the mechanics of heat transfer in the electron and lattice reservoirs, respectively, and they are composed of the diffusion equations for both reservoirs and the coupling term that represents the temperature difference between the two (i.e., electrons and lattices). Accordingly, these are the energy balance equations that represent the absorption of the laser pulse by the metal. The basic TTM, represented by Equations (1) and (2), has been subjected to various modifications and adaptations, to increase its accuracy or investigate a particular physical interaction.

TTM was adapted to account for additional physical properties. For instance, Ahmed et al. [124] developed a numerical model to simulate fs laser ablation of copper. In this effort, a TTM model that accounts for the thermophysical and dynamic optical properties was used. The important process parameters considered in their work included pulse number, laser fluence and the time interval between pulses. The laser pulse chosen was Gaussian with the FWHM mode having a wavelength of 800 nm. In addition, electron temperature and lattice heat capacity were considered in calculating the dynamic thermal properties. For both single- and multi-pulse laser irradiation with varying process settings, numerical simulations were carried out. It was concluded that during ablation of copper, while keeping the fluence constant, the ablation depth increases with the increase in the number of pulses.

Attempts were made to implement TTMs in commercial modelling packages that could enable a wide range of users to model laser–material interactions. For instance, Lee et al. implemented a TTM in the finite-element-based commercial software ABAQUS [125,126]. Temperature predictions obtained by the implemented model were validated using analytical results of the linear two-temperature model. The low and high fluences were also validated using nonlinear simulations and data values taken from literature [123]. The overall research concluded that a pulse repetition rate in the range of 0.1–1 GHz aids in maximising ablation and reducing melt pool generation. The latter two conditions enabled a more precise metal cutting process [125,126]. Limitations and potential improvements to TTMs attracted the interest of the research community. For instance, Jian et al. analysed an existing TTM and found that it was limited only by low fluence, which is used for the estimation of important parameters such as electron heat capacity and reflectivity [127]. To improve the prediction of the existing TTM, some parameters, such as electron relaxation time, absorption coefficient, electron heat capacity, reflectivity and electron conductivity, were introduced. The modified model was used to predict the initiation of melting in gold metal and to study the effect of pulse duration on predicting the fluence threshold for initiation of damage [127]. Davydov et al. also attempted to improve the accuracy of TTMs using a semi-empirical equation for the state [128]. However, this approach was less efficient than Jian et al.'s model [127]. A TTM was also modified and used to investigate the effect of the angle of incidence. For studying the temperature and ablation depth during the ablation of copper at an oblique angle of incidence using an fs laser, a numerical simulation was developed by Dasallas et al. [129]. The used model was an improved model of the TTM. Improvements included accounting for laser spot size, laser fluence and the dynamic changes in the reflectivity of the target. Simulation results showed that threshold energy of ablation was highly dependent on the angle of polarisation and the polarisation of incident light. However, the model did not predict the topography of the crater ablation in detail. TTM-based simulations were found to be useful in studying rapid melting and solidification using laser-based processing. Kuo et al. used a TTM to study the melting and solidification of materials using ultrafast lasers and found that if pure conduction is considered, after turning off the laser pulse, melted layers near the heating surface will solidify [130]. Fischer et al. [131] and Konrad et al. [132] conducted similar investigations but for SLM of metal powders using ultrashort pulses. A one-dimensional TTM that considers the thermophysical properties and temperature-dependent material properties was developed by Cheng et al. to study and simulate fs-laser-induced melting of copper nanoparticles [133]. This model included the extended Drude model with dynamic optical properties. The model was successfully validated using experimental results [52]. Cheng et al. [133] also experimented with fs laser processing of silver nanoparticles and simulated the sintering process using TTM. Jia et al. developed another one-dimensional TTM and used it to investigate the dependence of ablation depth in gold, copper and aluminium on various process parameter settings [134]. In this model, the spatial temperature distribution of the lattice was used to determine the ablation depth. Both TTM- and molecular dynamics (MD)-based models have been used to model laser–material interaction for ultrafast and ultrashort pulsed lasers. However, each approach has its advantages and limitations [135]. For instance, MD better represents the underlying physical interactions, while TTM is less complex and computationally demanding, and it is more compatible with widely used modelling software. In order to overcome the individual limitations of each method, hybrid models that better represent the underlying physics of laser–material interactions were developed. Hybrid models comprising the advantages of both TTM and MD were used to study laser–material interactions for processes utilising ultrashort lasers [136,137].

4. Femtosecond Laser-Based Additive Manufacturing—Powder Bed Fusion

As mentioned previously, the use of ultrashort pulsed lasers in AM results in lower thermal damages to the surrounding environment due to the high peak intensities and short pulse duration. Those result in rapid transfer of energy into the material, causing ionisation that is much quicker than plasma expansion (in the range of ns) [44]. Fs lasers in AM have been employed mainly in two processes, namely, PBF and DW technology. The DW technology is explained in detail in Section 5, and Figure 6 shows the overall schematic of an fs laser source integrated with PBF, i.e., (SLS/M).

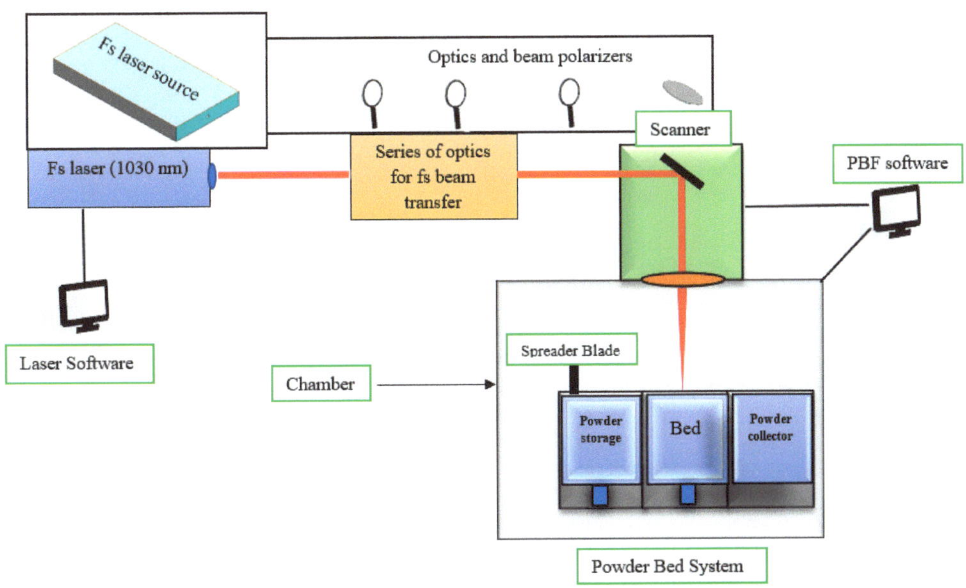

Figure 6. Schematic of the fs-laser-based selective laser sintering–powder bed fusion process.

The main heating or melting source element during fs laser processing is the fs laser source that is usually operated by the inbuilt laser software. Through this software, laser parameters, such as pulse duration, pulse repetition rate and beam profile, can easily be controlled. When laser parameters are set and the laser beam is allowed to pass through a series of optical elements, the beam is directed towards the scanner system. The required average output power is usually regulated by the beam polariser. The scanner software is utilised to set the scanning speed, hatch spacing, part geometry and the other aspects of the 2D drawing. The laser light is then focused through the scanner onto the powder bed system. The powder system consists of a spreader, powder bed, powder storage and powder collector. Before the laser light falls on the powder bed, the recoater mechanism spreads the powder on the powder bed with a set layer thickness. Then printing is conducted layer by layer. The PBF system could be enclosed in a chamber with an inert gas environment to eliminate oxidation issues. By employing further optimised parameters in fs laser AM, successful manufacturing of more precise functional parts for diverse applications, such as in the microelectronics, aerospace, automotive and biomedical industries, have already been demonstrated [130].

5. Femtosecond Laser Additive Manufactured Powder Materials, Print Qualities and Characterisation

As discussed earlier, laser-based AM has shown great potential in the last few decades for fabricating complex 3D geometries with diverse functional materials and with relative ease. Continuous wave laser-based 3D printing has been the industry standard in the field of laser additive manufacturing. However, and despite the significant advantages associated with the use of CW lasers, there still remain challenges related to heat affected zones and the development of cracks that tend to result in defective parts with poor quality. Many research and development efforts focus on optimising the CW laser processing parameters and conditions to address these issues. More recently, the use of ultrafast femtosecond lasers (pulse duration = 10^{-15} s) in SLS/SLM (PBF techniques) [54,138] and DW technology [52,53,139,140] is being considered. The use of short laser pulses reduces the developed thermal gradients and would, consequently, reduce the heat affected zones and limit thermal stress levels (associated with the development of cracks during printing). In addition, the smaller spot size in femtosecond lasers allows for a greater precision in the submicron range. Such accuracy and resolution are not typically offered by CW laser systems, which have spot sizes in the mm range. Some of the most recent developments in fs-based AM are discussed below. As different materials bring along different sets of challenges and requirements, this review is presented in sections based on the considered base metal for fabrication. Combined, the sections below provide a comprehensive review of relevant works on fs laser-based AM.

5.1. *Femtosecond Laser Sintering of Copper*

Copper and copper alloys are widely utilised in industry because of their remarkable properties such as thermal, electrical and corrosion resistance [141]. The utilisation of this metal in AM has diverse applications in various sectors including electronics [142], aerospace [143], automotive [141], heat exchangers [143] and MEMs [142]. Due to the high thermal conductivity of copper (i.e., 400 W/m·K), this material has historically been considered as one of the most difficult to print due to the large heat dissipation into the substrate [143], which prevents a sufficient temperature rise to melt the powders during printing. Additionally, sintering copper-based materials has been reported to be challenging with CW laser sources due to the fact of its high reflectivity that reduces effective energy deposition into the material [144]. Nevertheless, various attempts with certain levels of success have been reported in the literature for AM of Cu-based materials. For example, Pogson et al. [144] investigated the sintering of pure copper through PBF process utilising CW and ns lasers but failed to produce high-density parts [144]. Sciammarella et. al. [145] fabricated 12 cubic mm volume of C1100 copper onto a 4142-steel substrate utilising CW laser at a 900 W laser power [145]. NASA has also reported the successful fabrication of the first full-scale copper rocket part utilising AM methods and copper-based alloys [143]. NASA further fabricated combustion chamber liners, integral channels and closeouts with a high conductive and high-strength copper-alloy i.e., GRCop-42 (copper–chrome–niobium) utilising the PBF (SLM) process [143,146]. Cu–Cr–Zr–Ti alloy powders were also used in the SLM process to produce parts that have applications in the combustion chamber liner of a rocket engine and as heat sinks of the components of the first wall and diverter of the international thermonuclear experimental reactor (ITER) [147]. In addition, Colopi et al. [148] utilised a 1 kW CW laser to fabricate a heat exchanger consisting of complex geometries and fine critical features, where the use of high power was meant to overcome the limitation of poor laser absorptivity [148].

In the current era of the fourth industrial revolution, and with the growing demand for functionality and performance in MEMs devices, an increasing number of transistors must be packed and interconnected on electronic boards, resulting in smaller chips and interconnects [141,148]. To fabricate transistors and interconnects, traditional manufacturing techniques have been utilised. However, the fabrication of miniaturised features using such traditional techniques is limited [142]. Currently available macroscale metal AM techniques, such as PBF utilising CW lasers, are reported to produce a minimum feature with sizes up to 100 μm, which is still too large. The minimum feature size of a back-end-of-line (BEOL) wafer interconnect is in the range of 15–20 μm [149]. To address this issue, nowadays, a new technique called microscale AM is being employed to fabricate parts at the micro- and nanoscales. The DW process is a widely used AM technology for such microfabrication of conductive micropatterns using Ag, Au and Cu metals [150,151]. Among these, Cu is considered to be the key material for low-cost printing [152]. Further, the ultrafast lasers, such as ns and fs lasers, are preferred over CW lasers in micro-level fabrication because of the smaller spot sizes, lower HAZs, and less substrate damage [149,153]. Copper has been most widely in fs laser sintering due to the fact of its wide range of applications in MEMS [116], microsensors [53], complex cooling structures [138], among others. Cheng et al. [52] demonstrated experimentally and theoretically the sintering of copper nanoparticles (NPs) utilising a femtosecond laser. The fs laser sintering was carried out on a copper-coated substrate with a pulse repetition rate of 80 MHz, pulse width of 100 fs and a wavelength of 800 nm. Figure 7 shows SEM images of copper patterns generated at two average powers of 195 and 210 mW, and a scanning speed of 0.1 mm/s [52]. The experimental and theoretical results for copper nanoparticles sintered by fs laser reported by Cheng et al. were found to be in good agreement demonstrating the great potential of this technique in the field of micro- and nanoscale manufacturing.

N Roy et al. (2017) utilised microscale SLS techniques to investigate and compare the processing capabilities of CW, ns, and fs lasers to achieve miniaturised features of 1 μm sized interconnect transistors [142,149,150]. The oxidation issues were reported to be more severe in CW laser sintered parts compared to the ns and fs laser sintered parts. The HAZs were also minimal and there was lower substrate damage for the ns and fs lasers compared to CW laser sintering [142]. Mizoshiri [53,152] utilised an fs-laser-based DW additive manufacturing process to fabricate copper-based microsensors for temperature sensing. This was achieved through reductive sintering of CuO. In this experiment, Cu_2O-rich sensing parts and Cu-rich electrodes were 3D printed. Though laser reductive sintered metal oxide NPs were reported to have higher resistivity than laser sintered metal NPs, their absorption of irradiated light was higher [152]. Figure 8 shows the Cu NPs spin-coated substrate irradiated with a femtosecond laser to form Cu- and Cu_2O-rich micropatterns. The film was spun-coated at 7000 rpm on a substrate with a thickness of 1 mm with different materials, i.e., CuO NPs at 60 wt%, ethylene glycol at approximately 27 wt% and PVP solution at approximately 13 wt%, respectively. Later, the unsintered part was removed by ethylene glycol and ethanol.

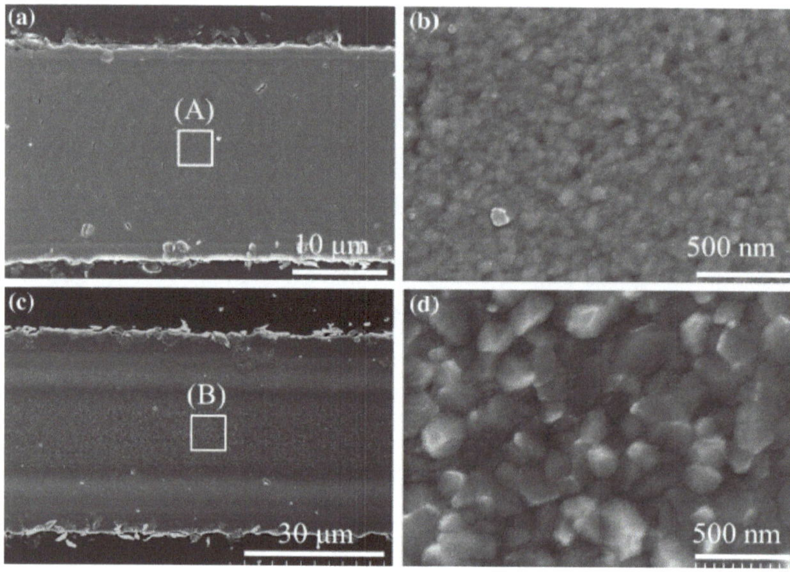

Figure 7. SEM images of Cu line patterns at a constant speed of 0.1 mm/s and laser fluences of (**a**) 12.8 mJ/cm^2 at 195 mW; (**c**) 13.8 mJ/cm^2 at 210 mW where (**b**,**d**) are magnified images of regions (**A**) and (**B**) (Adapted from reference [52]).

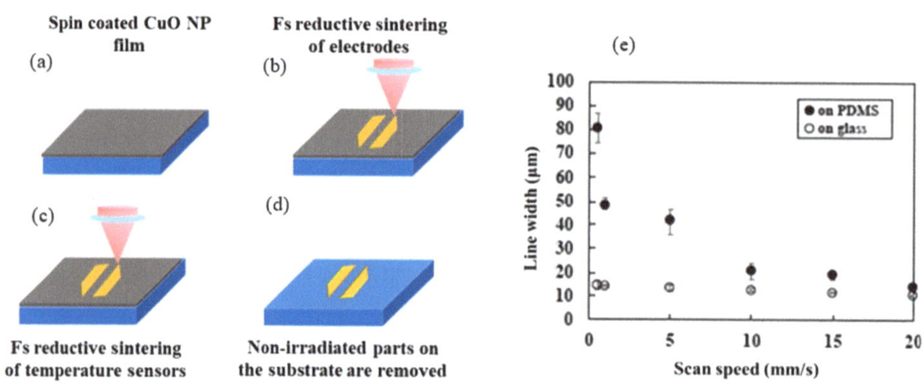

Figure 8. (**a**) Spin-coated CuO NP film; femtosecond reductive sintering of (**b**) electrodes, (**c**) temperature sensors and (**d**) non-irradiated parts on the substrate were removed; (**e**) fs laser reductive sintered line width on PDMS vs. glass as a function of the scanning speed [53].

As for the laser processing parameters, a pulse repetition rate of 80 MHz, pulse duration of 120 fs and a max pulse energy up to 0.62 nanojoules, operating at an 800 nm wavelength, were used [53]. It is evident from Figure 8e, that in the case of both the glass and the PDMS substrates, the width of the printed lines decreased with the increase in the scanning speed. In addition, the authors noted that at a particular scanning speed, the line width on the PDMS substrate was broader than on glass. This was due to the higher thermal conductivity in the case of the PDMS substrate. Cu, Cu_2O and CuO were present in all of the sintered micropatterns. The micropatterns, characterised using XRD, showed that the Cu peak was stronger at a 5 mm/s scanning speed compared to a 1 mm/s. The ratio of Cu_2O to CuO peak intensities in the XRD spectra of the sintered sample was considered to evaluate Cu_2O generation. According to the XRD spectra, the maximum

Cu_2O generation occurred at a scanning speed of 1 mm/s. Therefore, the Cu_2O-rich sensing part of the micro-temperature sensors has been demonstrated in this paper under these conditions. Therefore, in the aforementioned work, Cu-rich and Cu_2O-rich micropatterns were selectively fabricated by optimising the laser parameters [53]. This work paves a new way for better manufacturing techniques utilising fs laser reductive patterning for the manufacturing of microdevices. Mizoshiri et al. [154] further investigated the effect of various parameters, such as scanning speed and laser fluence, during fs laser reductive sintering of NiO and CuO mixtures on heat accumulation during sintering. It was identified that short pulsed laser irradiation at higher fluence reduces the metal oxide content in the fabricated pattern. Further, n-type and p-type thermoelectric micropatterns were fabricated using fs sintering, which may serve as metal electrodes in flexible displays.

Figure 9 depicts the surface morphologies of the micropatterns sintered at various scanning speeds while keeping fluence constant at 0.059 J/cm^2. At lower scanning speeds, more pronounced ablation was observed. Furthermore, at scanning speeds of 5 mm/s, instead of full melting, the powder particles were properly sintered. It was discovered that even when the fluence was kept constant, the scanning speed could affect the content of the Ni and Cu percentages in the sintered micropatterns. It was further mentioned that Cu converts to CuO when temperatures rise above 673 K [154]. When compared to the single exposed sintered sample, the double-exposed sintered sample contained more metal oxides. The heat accumulation and thermal history (single or multiple times exposed) during sintering are important in determining the composition and thermoelectric properties of the sintered sample [155]. Similarly, by utilising near-infrared fs laser pulses, three-dimensional copper-based microstructures were fabricated [156–158]. Mizoshiri et al. [158] expanded their research and printed Cu-based micropatterns inside Cu_2O nanosphere films using a femtosecond laser. To minimise the thermal diffusion, the line width was maintained to be the same as the diameter of the laser spot, i.e., 0.7 μm. Copper-based microstructures were printed via thermochemical reduction of Cu_2O by varying the focal plane along the z-axis, and the laser spot was focused inside the Cu_2O film (Figure 10). Different micropatterns have been demonstrated by varying the focus spot in the z-direction as shown in Figure 10. The laser peak intensity was set at 204 GW/cm^2 and the scanning speed was 0.01 mm/s [158]. Square micropatterns of a size 1.8×1.8 mm^2 were fabricated at a laser peak intensity of 163 GW/cm^2 and a scanning speed of 100 m/s.

Mizoshiri et al. [152] carried out laser-reduced sintering patterning in an inert gas (N_2/Ar) environment and were able to produce lower copper oxide (CuO/Cu_2O) generation in the fabricated sample. They used a pulse duration of 120 fs, a laser wavelength of ~780 nm, a scanning speed from 5 to 10 mm/s, a pulse energy of 0.74 nJ and a pulse repetition rate of 80 MHz [152]. Their investigations revealed that as the injection rate of inert gases (N_2 and Ar) increased, lower metal oxides were produced, but the fabricated samples had lower surface densities. The XRD results show that the fabricated pattern was greatly reduced (i.e., Cu rich) and the degree of reduction was maximised at a scanning speed of 8 mm/s. Furthermore, the Cu generation in the composition of the fabricated pattern increased with the rate of gas injection, while the degree of reduction was unaffected by the type of gas (N_2/Ar). However, as the gas injection rate increased (i.e., higher than 100 mL/min), the porosity in the patterns increased. Using fs laser reductive sintering, the copper micropatterns could be fabricated with a much lower pulse energy of approximately 0.5 nJ and a lower average power of approximately 50 mW, but, in the case of CW and nanosecond pulse lasers, a minimum of 0.2 W would be needed.

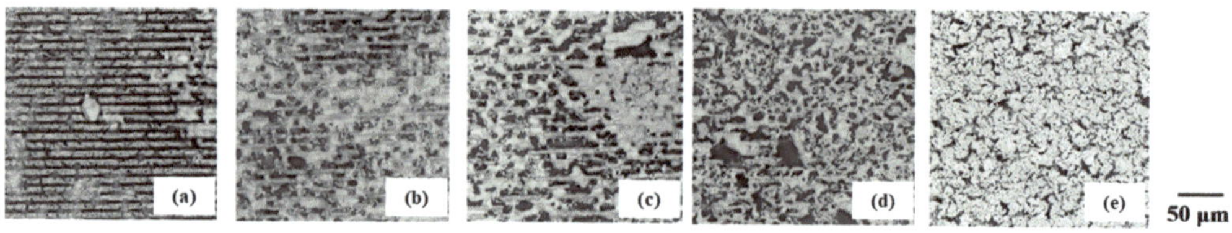

Figure 9. SEM images of sintered CuO–NiO NP micropatterns at different scanning speeds: (**a**) 0.1; (**b**) 0.5; (**c**) 1; (**d**) 3; (**e**) 5 mm/s [154].

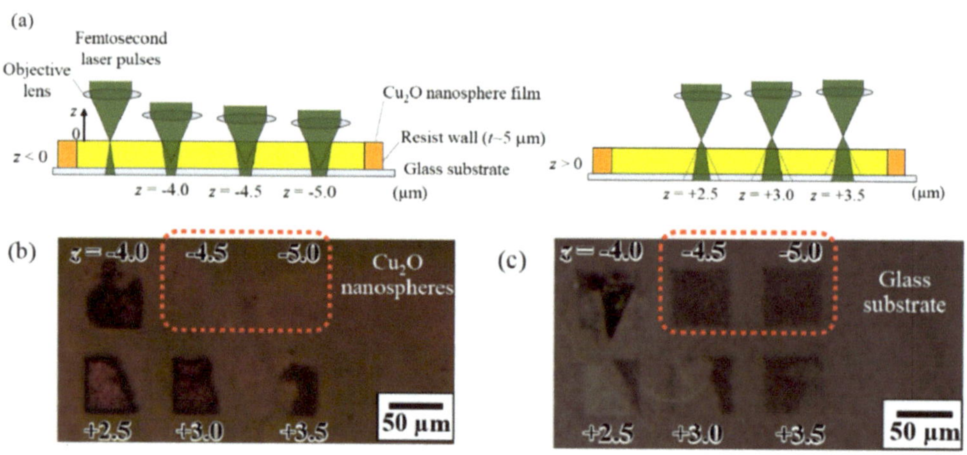

Figure 10. (**a**) Schematic of microfabrication of Cu-based patterns within a Cu_2O film. Microscopic images of (**b**) sintered patterns and (**c**) after Cu_2O nanosphere film removal (Adapted from reference [158]).

Although DW technology has been successful in producing Cu micropatterns using the fs laser sintering technique, the process appears to be time-consuming, requiring the preparation of film coated on substrate, sintering and, finally, removing the unsintered area from the substrate. However, in the PBF process, using layer-by-layer sintering, 3D structures can be produced that could have applications in cooling structures and heat exchangers. Kaden et al. [54] demonstrated printing of copper by PBF process, i.e., printing layer by layer utilising an fs laser with a 1030 nm wavelength and a focal spot of 35 µm [54]. The experiment was carried out in a nitrogen gas environment. Powder layer thickness was maintained manually at approximately 30 micrometres using a squeegee. The results were benchmarked and compared with different repetition rates utilising the energy per unit length (line energy) given by:

$$\text{Line Energy (El)} = \frac{P_{avg}}{V_{scan}} = \frac{E_{pulse} \times F_{rep}}{V_{scan}}$$

where El is the energy per unit length, P_{avg} is the average power, V_{scan} is the scanning speed, E_{pulse} is the pulse energy and F_{rep} is the repetition rate.

In general, with lower repetition rates, insufficient melting occurs, resulting in poor fusion of the metal particles to the substrate. By increasing the pulse repetition rate to 20 MHz and maintaining the pulse energy to 1 µJ, proper bonding of the copper powder to the substrate has been demonstrated [54]. Blasting and ablation effects were reported when the pulse energy increased by more than 1.5 µJ. It was also found that the thermal accumulation effect could be responsible for successful fusing of metal particles to the substrate at higher repetition rates. The line energy also had an impact on the resulting print quality. Further, printing of thin-walled web-like structures at a scanning speed of 666 mm/s and a pulse energy of 1 microjoule was reported. These thin walls were reported to have an aspect ratio of approximately 15:1 and a thickness of less than 100 μm. Figures 11 and 12 show samples fabricated using fs sintering of copper particles with ultrashort laser pulses. At higher line energies, the HAZ increased significantly which, consequently, negatively impacted the local precision. As a result, the line energy was reported to be kept below 100 J/m in their subsequent experiments [138].

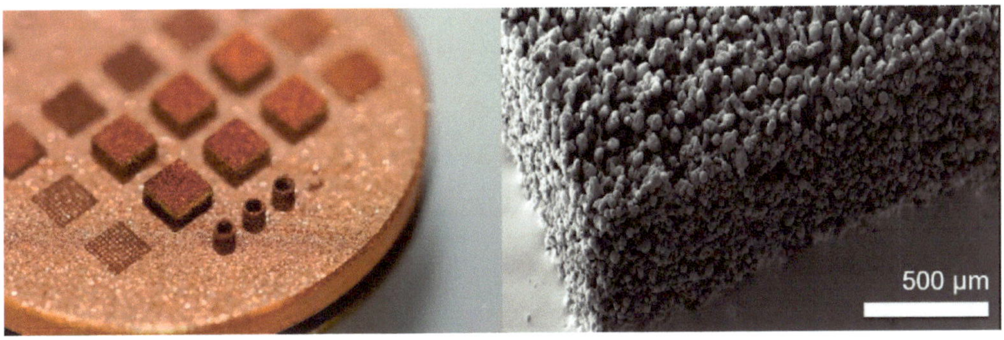

(a) (b)

Figure 11. (**a**) The samples fabricated with cuboids of a 2 × 2 mm^2 size, and total height of 1.4 mm; (**b**) SEM images of the sample (Adapted from reference [54]).

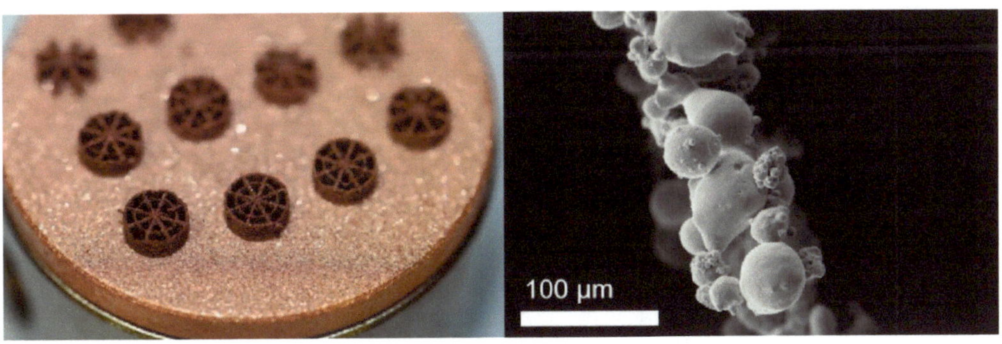

(a) (b)

Figure 12. (**a**) Thin-walled circular samples; (**b**) SEM image of a single wall (Adapted from reference [54]).

5.2. Femtosecond Laser Sintering of Iron and Tungsten

Tungsten and its alloys have diverse applications in various fields such as lighting engineering, aerospace, electronics, medical, nuclear and military [159,160]. This refractory material possesses exceptional intrinsic properties such as high tensile strength, high hardness, high melting temperature, high density, high thermal conductivity, high recrystallisation temperature and low thermal expansion [159–161]. These properties make tungsten ideal for high-temperature, high heat flux applications in radiation environments such as collimators, radiation shields in imaging systems (CT, SPECT, MRI and X-ray) [162], plasma-facing components (PFCs) in future nuclear fusion devices, such as the International Thermonuclear Experimental Reactor (ITER), and high-performance rocket nozzles [159–161,163,164]. However, tungsten's main disadvantage is its lack of room-temperature ductility that restricts its machinability and limits its use as a structural material. The brittle-to-ductile (BDT) transition temperature of tungsten, which is typically between 200 and 400 °C, limits its fabricability [162]. Because of this BDT transition temperature, tungsten products are conventionally manufactured by chemical vapour deposition (CVD), spark plasma sintering (SPS), powder metallurgy (PM) and hot isostatic pressing (HIP). These techniques, however, have limitations when it comes to complex internal and external structures [159]. SLM/S was used to overcome these limitations. Though it was not an easy process in the early stages, since the AM of tungsten is hindered by almost all of the difficult challenges in metal SLM/S processing such as high melting point, high thermal conductivity, affinity for oxygen at high temperatures, high viscosity, and brittle nature at room temperature, resulting in cracks and porous microstructures of fabricated parts [161].

Despite the listed challenges with processing tungsten, successful examples are reported in the literature. For example, Ghosh et al. [165] utilised a pulsed Nd:YAG laser with a pulse duration of approximately 1000 ns to investigate SLS of tungsten carbide and cobalt powder alloys. Porous samples were produced in this experiment. Dianzheng et al. [166] utilised CW laser-based SLM to fabricate pure tungsten material parts with densities of up to 96 percent; however, this was accompanied by some microcracks in the printed components. Chaolin et al. (2018) utilised CW laser to fabricate pure tungsten samples by SLS processes. The produced parts possessed dense microstructures without balling but a few microcracks still existed [159]. Muller et al. (2019) carried out experiments to fabricate pure tungsten powder parts utilising CW laser-based PBF with laser power up to 400 W and by preheating the substrate up to 1000 °C. The produced parts had a relative density of up to 98 percent, and cracks were minimised but not eliminated completely. The same research team also fabricated honeycomb-like structures with tungsten–copper composite materials, which were utilised as heat sink materials for PFCs with high heat loads [164]. Li et al. (2020) investigated various process parameters in CW laser-based SLS, such as scanning speed, hatch spacing and laser power, and their effect on the surface microstructure, densification and morphology of fabricated tungsten samples. With the optimum parameters of a scanning speed of 400 mm/s, hatch spacing of 0.08 mm and laser power of 300 W, the produced tungsten samples had densities of up to 98.31 percent [160]. As noted from the aforementioned studies considering CW laser-based AM of tungsten, and despite the reported success, shortcomings in terms of cracking still represent a challenge. The studies utilising fs lasers aimed to improve the relative density, hardness and strength of SLS/M-produced tungsten parts. The high peak power and the ultrashort pulse duration of fs lasers make them an emerging technology in melting/sintering high-temperature metals such as tungsten [7,44,58,101]. Due to the phenomena of fast cooling, localised heating, lower HAZs and greater precision in the submicron range, these ultrafast lasers have many advantages over CW and long-pulsed lasers. 3D printing of such high-temperature metals would benefit industries, including the automotive, biomedical and aerospace, that require high-temperature materials with outstanding mechanical qualities and accuracy [7].

In an early study, Ebert et al. (2012) initially investigated fs laser processing of tungsten powder and was able to report sintered structures. In these experiments, the fs laser used had an operating wavelength of 1030 nm and 180 fs pulse duration. The laser repetition rate was tuned from 0.125 to 1 MHz, and the laser spot diameter was ~36 microns. The layer thickness was reported to be maintained around 1 mm and was irradiated from 1 to 50 times. The experiments were carried out in vacuum at 0.05 Pa, with helium used as a residual gas during the sintering process [101]. It was reported that when the line spacing was at approximately 0.01 mm, the sintering of continuous surfaces was possible, and the sintered structures were in the range of 1 to 10 μm. The SEM images of the sintered part under different processing settings are shown in Figure 13a–d. These results demonstrate some sintering phenomena utilising fs lasers but do not provide precise and optimum laser parameters on the quality of the sintered structures.

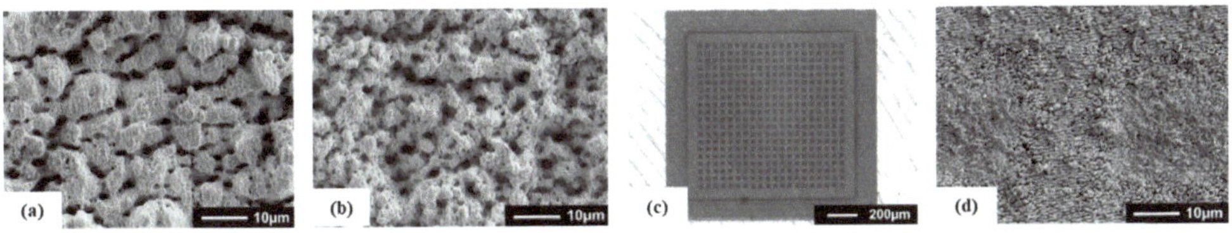

Figure 13. (**a**) SEM image of sintered samples, operated at max intensity = 6.74×10^{12} W/cm^2, energy per unit length = 0.7 J/m, scanning speed = 1250 m m/s, line spacing = 10 μm and pulse repetition rate = 125 kHz, 10 scans; (**b**) SEM image of sintered samples, operated at max intensity = 6.74×10^{12} W/cm^2, energy per unit length = 0.23 J/m, scanning speed = 3750 m m/s, line spacing = 10 μm and pulse repetition rate = 125 kHz, 10 scans; (**c**) optical image of sintered grid-like structures, operated at max intensity = 1.77×10^{12} W/cm^2, energy per unit length = 3 J/m, scanning speed = 600 m m/s, line spacing = 10 μm, and pulse repetition rate = 1 MHz, 6 scans; (**d**) SEM image of sintered grid-like structure sample (Adapted from reference [101]).

Furthermore, Huan Huang (2015) [7] carried out fs laser sintering/melting experiments with tungsten and iron powders to produce 3D structures fused to the substrate. To compare the mechanical properties and microstructure of fs-laser-fabricated samples, similar 3D structures were fabricated using a CW laser source while maintaining the same average power of 50 W, and the scanning speeds for both the CW and fs pulse lasers operated at 80 MHz. The particle sizes of the iron and tungsten powders were in the range of 1–5 μm. For analysing the properties of the printed structures, the 3D printed samples were vertically cut as shown in Figure 14.

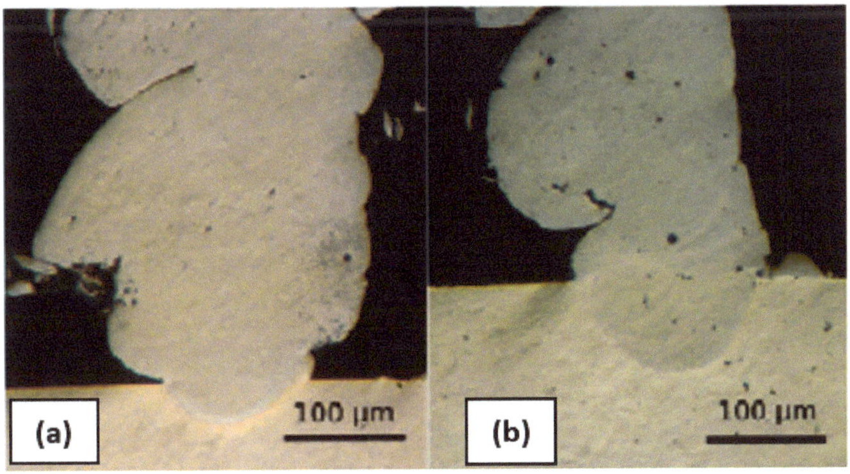

Figure 14. Iron rings fabricated by (**a**) an 80 MHz fs laser; (**b**) a CW laser (Adapted from reference [7]).

The penetration depth of the fs-laser-fabricated iron-powder sintered sample was approximately 30 μm, while the penetration depth of the CW fabricated sample was 75 μm. This difference was attributed to the smaller HAZ in the case of fs laser-based 3D printing. Using the same 50 layer printing, the size of the sample fabricated using an fs laser was 0.8 mm tall, with a wall thickness of 300 μm, and the sample size fabricated using a CW laser was 1.03 mm tall with a wall thickness of 380 μm. This paper demonstrated how localised heating in an fs laser can result in the precision printing of 3D structures. Furthermore, the microhardness of the fs-laser-fabricated iron sample was higher than that of the CW-laser-fabricated sample, because the average grain size in the fs-laser-fabricated sample was smaller at all heights compared to the CW laser 3D printed samples. This is due to the well-known fact that hardness increases as grain size decreases. The grains in CW-laser-fabricated samples were reported to be slightly bigger due to the lower cooling rates and greater HAZs [57]. The next challenging material, tungsten, was fabricated in cube structures by the same research group [7]. With tungsten's higher melting temperature compared to iron, 1 MHz pulse repetitions at 45 W, a pulse duration of 400 fs, a layer thickness of 15 μm and scanning at a speed of 25 mm/s yielded strongly fabricated parts fused to the substrate (Figure 15). On the other hand, 80 MHz fs laser and CW laser operating at higher power failed to completely melt and fuse tungsten powder to the substrate.

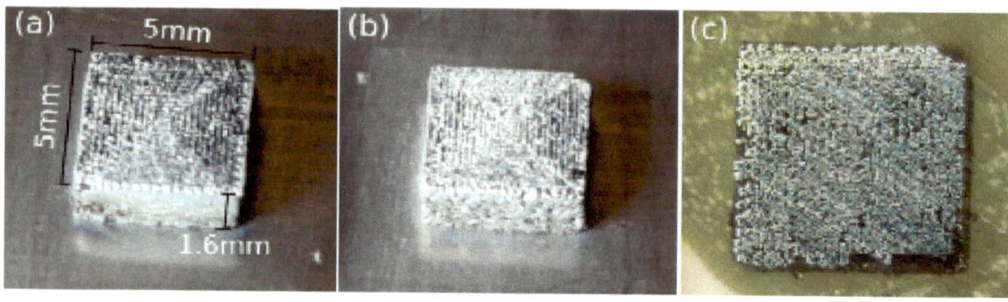

Figure 15. (**a**,**b**) The fs laser 3D printed tungsten cube with fs laser viewed from different angles; (**c**) polished top surface (Adapted from reference [7]).

The mechanical properties, such as average ultimate tensile strength (388.4 MPa), were determined from three sample locations. However, because of the porosity and potential oxidation during 3D printing, the microhardness values were reported to be unsatisfactory. Further, three-dimensional structures utilizing tungsten material were fabricated [44]. Different tungsten samples, including 100 μm thin walls, were 3D printed using fs laser source as shown in Figure 16 [44].

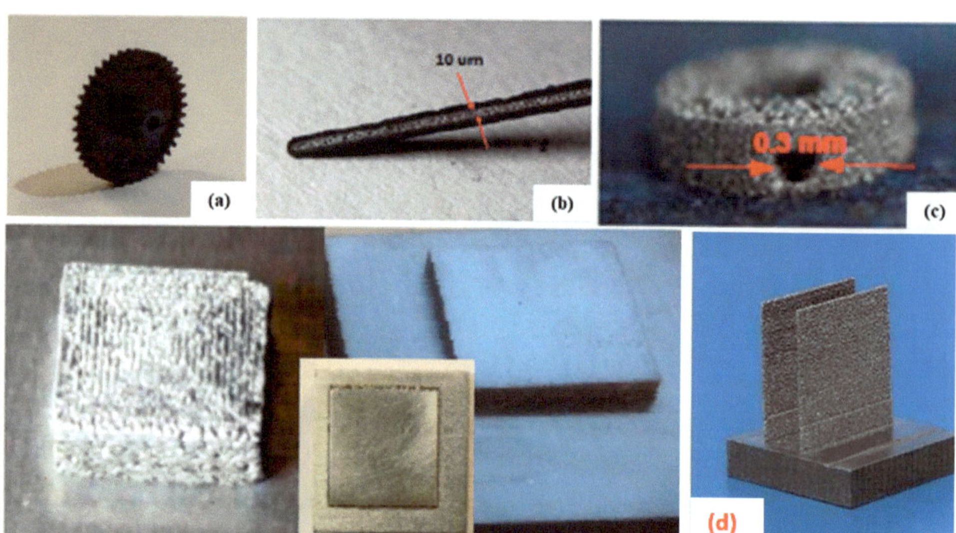

Figure 16. (**a**) A gear a half-inch in diameter 3D printed by fs laser; (**b**) fs sintered tungsten feature; (**c**) fs sintered tungsten with a small circular feature with a hole; (**d**) 3D printed thin wall of a 100 microns (Adapted from reference [44]).

For comparison, 20 ps and 200 ps pulsed lasers as well as a 750 fs laser and a CW laser system were employed in the 3D printing of tungsten [44] while keeping all other parameters similar. Figure 17 shows the average grain area versus pulse duration for fs, 20 ps, 200 ps and CW laser sintered samples, where the left is for the top surface and the right is for the cross-section. Comparing the microhardness in the case of pulsed lasers at different durations with the CW laser showed that fs-laser-based AM had the highest hardness as displayed in Table 6.

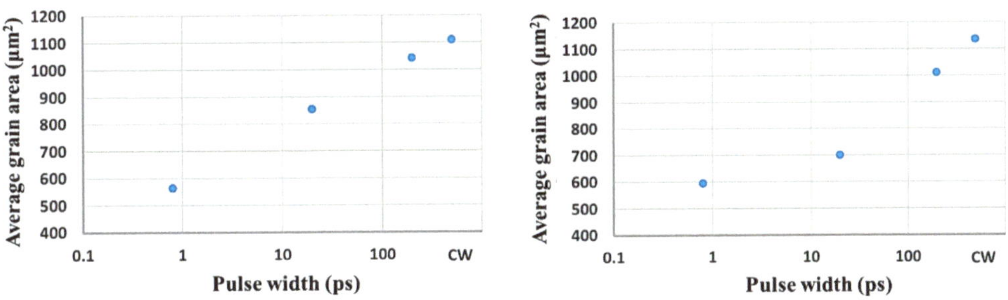

Figure 17. Average grain size area as a function of pulse width (Adapted from reference [44]).

Table 6. Hardness values for the tungsten sample processed with different lasers [44].

Hardness (HRC)	Fs Sample	CW Sample	20 ps Sample	200 ps Sample	Tungsten Sample
Cross-section	47.7	44.7	41.8	45.1	45.8
Top	45.4	44.9	44.1	42.4	44.9

The aforementioned work also revealed that the fs laser sintered samples had lower cracks and defects compared to the other laser printed samples. Similarly, fs laser sintering of iron powder coated on a glass substrate was demonstrated by Liu et al. (2016) [100]. Melting and fusing both (i.e., iron and glass) materials is challenging because of the glass' brittleness and the different thermal expansion coefficients of iron and glass. In this study, the fs laser was utilised to overcome this issue, because of its localised heating, high temperature generated in a shorter time and quick cooling rate, The sintering parameters, such as average power of 37 W, powder layer thickness of 40 μm and 20 μm line spacing were used during the sintering process at various scanning speeds [100]. The reflectance was measured for the fabricated samples at different values of the laser power and scanning speeds. It was found that at lower scanning speeds, the reflectance was reduced, while noting that glass was prone to breaking at lower scanning speeds. The reported findings suggest that fs laser AM could be a new way to achieve an excellent blackening effect with a reflectance of less than 1%, rendering it useful for applications in stray light reduction.

5.3. Femtosecond Laser Sintering of Silver

Nowadays, electronics has seen substantial improvements in the field of sensors, printed electronic components and flexible electronics. These flexible sensors are rapidly evolving, where they can be used in many applications [167]. In the medical sector, these flexible electronics have a large impact, as they can be low-cost, tactile, low-weight and non-pervasive wearable systems; in addition, they can be used as monitors to observe patients' health conditions on a regular basis. Hence, there is an existing special need to manufacture such flexible devices using appropriate manufacturing technology. This can be facilitated by using AM technologies, such as SLS, that can process metal NPs and also in direct writing technology. Initially, the SLS process was used for NPs of noble metals like silver and gold, but later it was also expanded to more cost-effective materials such as copper and nickel [151]. Silver material has been utilised by inkjet technology-based AM process for fabrication of temperature sensors [168–170]. Hong et al. processed silver particles via a laser sintering process to fabricate a large and flexible transparent conductor based on microgrid structures that can be used in touch screen panels and optoelectronic devices [171]. In 2011, using direct writing technology, Lee et al. fabricated conductive metal films made out of silver nanoparticles. Femtosecond laser characteristics aid in the fabrication of metal conductors with submicron-sized features and high conductivity. Due to the fact of its reduced HAZ, femtosecond laser-based metal patterns on transparent and flexible polymer substrates has garnered special attention owing to its several practical applications in photonic devices and flexible electronics [41,56,167,172]. Fs laser has also been utilised to fabricate SERS (surface enhanced Raman scattering) substrates [172]. SERS is an analytical tool for detecting molecular fingerprints and integrating them into microfluidic platforms that allow for liquid sample analysis for biological and medical diagnosis. Traditionally, lithographic techniques have been used to produce SERS substrates with significant Raman enhancements. However, fabricating them, on the other hand, entails a number of time-consuming steps. Furthermore, using lithographic techniques to achieve ordered arrays of nanostructures of arbitrary size can be expensive [56], challenging [56], hazardous and incompatible with sensitive substrates [172]. To address these issues, fs lasers have been used to fabricate SERS substrates sintered with silver nanoparticles [56]. Based on the process parameter set and the layer thickness, sintering of nanoparticles may lead to three different phenomena: surface necking, full melting of silver particles and balling. Kurnoothala et al. [56] sintered silver nanoparticles on a silica-based microfluidic channel via the surface necking phenomenon using an fs laser source to fabricate the SERS substrate. The width of the fabricated lines at various laser powers and scanning speeds were reported [56] and are shown in Figure 18. The utilised fs laser system operated at a wavelength of 1030 nm, a 370 fs pulse duration and had a pulse repetition rate of 1 MHz.

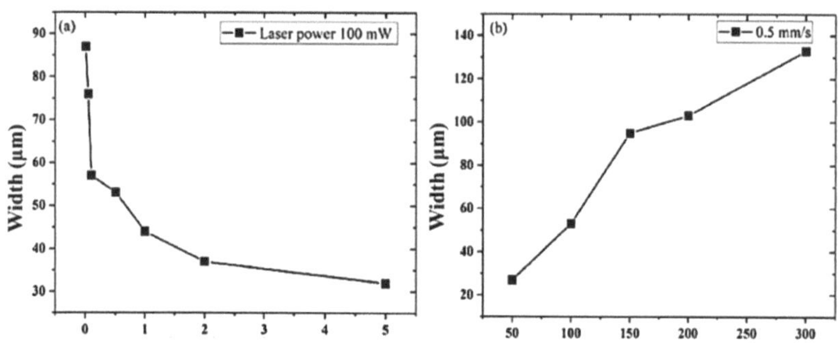

Figure 18. (**a**) Track width as a function of varying scan speeds with a constant laser power of 100 mW; (**b**) track width as a function of varying laser powers with a constant scan speed of 0.5 mm/s (Adapted from reference [56]).

Due to the ultrashort pulse durations in fs laser sintering, the thermal diffusion effect is suppressed, and sintering of metal nanoparticles can be restricted to the laser focal spot. This largely reduces the heat-affected zone and enables the fabrication of submicron-sized metal patterns on flexible substrates [55]. Noh et. al. [173] utilised a Ti:sapphire laser system operating at an 800 nm wavelength, a 50 fs pulse duration and a pulse repetition rate of 1 kHz to fabricate silver NPs on a flexible substrate. The laser fluence and effective pulse number were 10–120 mJ/cm^2 and 1000–10,000, respectively. The scanning speed, V, varied between 20 and 200 µm/s, and the beam size was 200 µm. The hatch space between the scanning lines was set to 200 µm [173]. The reported SEM images of sintered microstructures of the Ag NPs on the PET substrates after fs laser irradiation are shown in Figure 19 [173]. Noha et. al. also compared the results obtained with a KrF excimer nanosecond laser operating at a 248 nm wavelength, a 25 ns pulse duration and a repetition rate of 10 Hz. The experiments were carried out with a fluence = 10–40 mJ/cm^2 and a pulse number of 1–1000. The effective pulse number was varied by varying scanning speeds in the 0.015–15 mm/s range at f = 10 Hz and d = 1.5 mm [41].

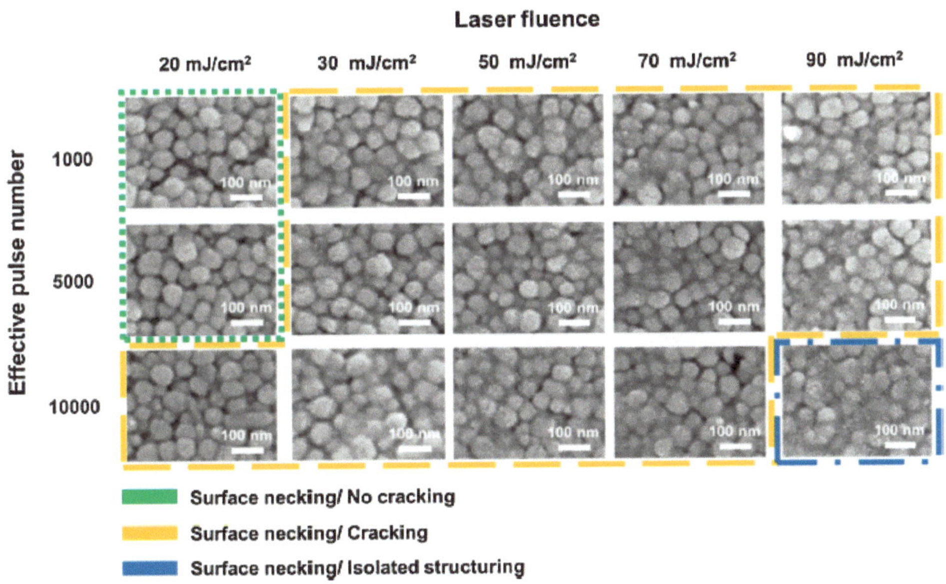

Figure 19. SEM images of fs Ag NPs sintered at various laser fluences (Adapted from reference [173]).

For the entire fluence range reported in [173], fs laser irradiation sintered the Ag NPs without completely melting them, instead creating necks between the particles by solid-state diffusion. As the fluence increased, the significant neck growth arose by grain boundary and volume diffusion. At fluence = 20 mJ/cm^2 and an effective pulse number = 1000, the Ag NPs were reported to form necks with an average neck diameter of 12 $\pm$ 2 nm. At fluence = 90 mJ/cm^2 and an effective pulse number = 10,000, the average neck diameter increased to 36 $\pm$ 3 nm. The increased neck formation was reported to reduce the porosity by blocking open pores in the particle bed [173]. As depicted in Figure 20, with the increasing fluence and EPN (effective pulse number), the fraction of the exposed area rose to 40%. This study showed that EPN was less significant in film cracking than laser fluence [173]. It also suggests that the formation of the interparticle necking after laser sintering greatly decreases the electrical resistance. The resistance decreased as fluence and EPN increased until the fluence = 40 mJ/cm^2. At a fluence = 30 mJ/cm^2 and an EPN = 1000, the lowest resistance was reported as shown in Figure 20c. The mechanical properties of fs laser sintered Ag particles were also examined in this paper for interfacial characteristics between Ag NPs and the PET substrate. The cross-sectional SEM images are also presented as shown in Figure 21 [173].

The aforementioned work reported that fs laser irradiation resulted in substantial embedding of the Ag NPs into the PET layer, which led to an increase in the contact area (Figure 21b) and would significantly improve the adhesion strength [173]. At fluence of 90 mJ/cm^2, the embedded depth was found to be approximately half the particle size. Additionally, the reported comparative results of the fs and ns laser-sintered samples showed that due to the low substrate damage and fewer film cracks, fs-laser-generated films were of higher electrical conductivity compared to the ones generated with an ns laser [173]. The surface topography AFM analysis results showed that in the case of ns laser sintering, the average affected spot was 1.2 μm wide and 500 nm deep, whereas in case of fs laser sintering, the average affected spot was 200 wide and 90 nm deep [173].

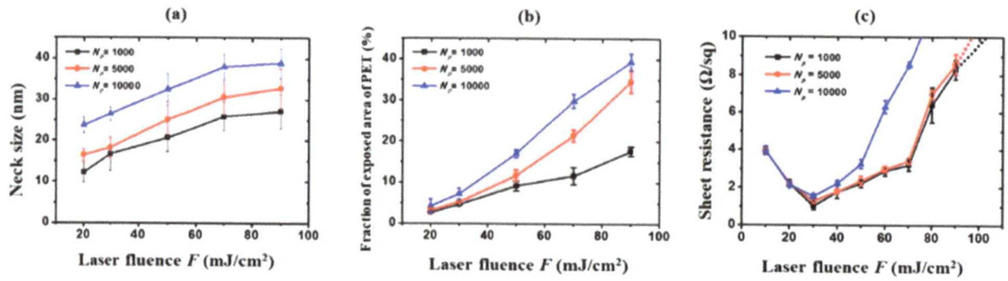

Figure 20. (**a**) Neck size; (**b**) fraction of the exposed area of the PET substrate after fs laser sintering; (**c**) sheet resistances of the fs laser sintered Ag particles [173].

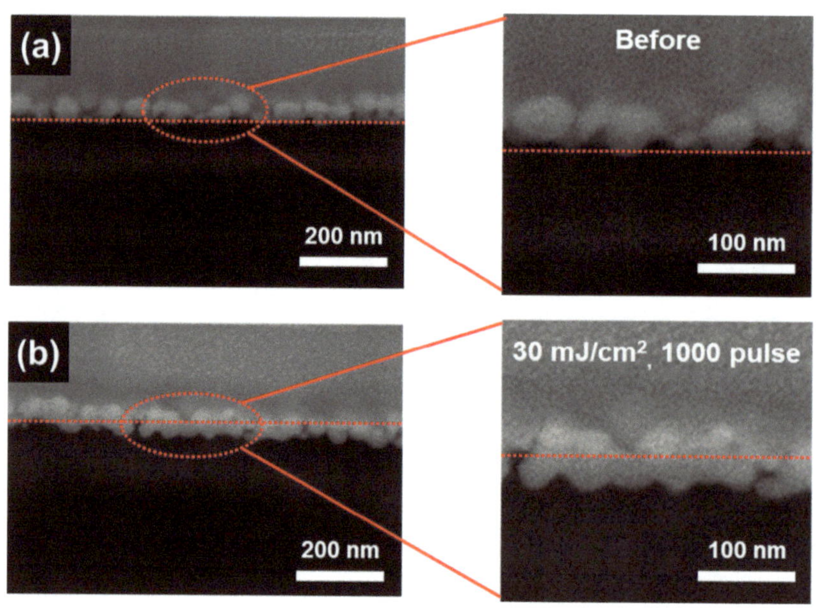

Figure 21. Cross-sectional SEM images (**a**) before fs laser sintering and (**b**) after fs laser sintering (F = 30 mJ/cm^2, effective pulse number = 1000) (Adapted from reference [173]).

Noh et al. further investigated the correlation between different process parameters and the conductivity, microstructure and adhesion strength of the sintered films [172]. Melting, interparticle necking, balling and film cracking were analysed by varying the EPN, fluence and layer thickness. It was found that both adhesion strength and electrical conductivity increased by increasing the fluence up to the maxim when melting of particles began [174]. By varying the spin-coated layer's thickness from 350, 200 and to 100 nm, different conclusions were drawn from this study. For the 350 nm layer thickness, short thermal penetration helped in the fabrication of thin-film samples. In the case of the 200 nm layer thickness, the highest thermal conductivity was reported when melting just began in NPs. Whereas with the 100 nm layer thickness, complete melting of particles deteriorated the conductivity due to the capillary instability of the molten film and, therefore, the highest conductivity was reported just before melting started as shown in Figure 22b,c [172]. Moreover, fine patterns of a few hundred nanometre line widths utilising ultrashort lasers were fabricated in other sequel studies [175]. Microstructure formation by varying the sintering parameters of Ag NPs utilising ultrashort pulses was presented and revealed that the fs laser sintering process was similar to typical thermal sintering processes.

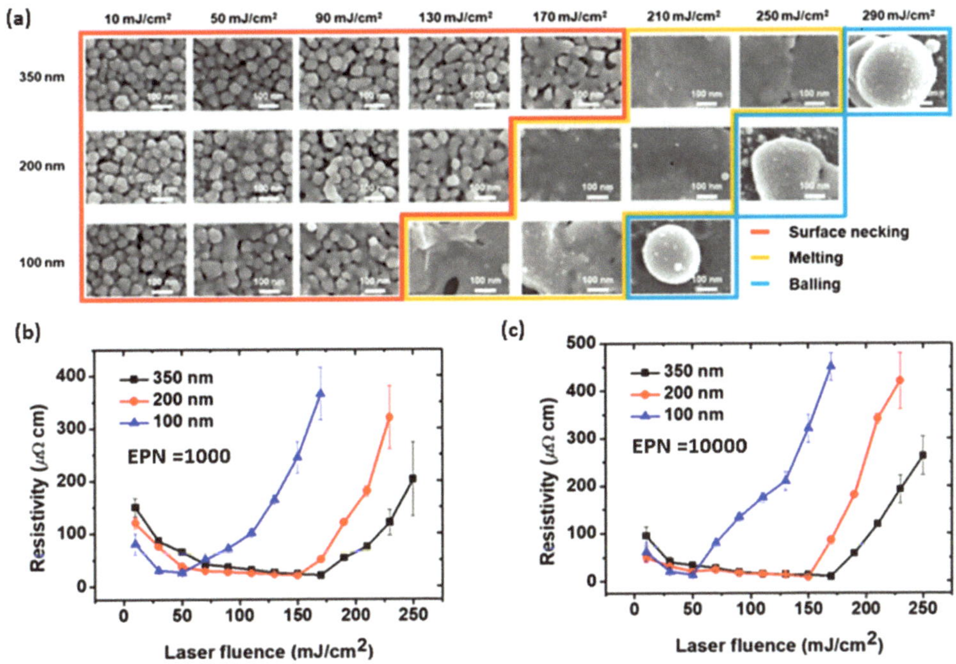

Figure 22. (**a**) Microstructures of fs sintered Ag particles during surface necking and melting stages. Variations in the resistivity of sintered Ag films as a function of fluence; (**b**) Np = 1000; (**c**) Np = 10,000 (Adapted from reference [172]).

5.4. Femtosecond Laser Sintering of Aluminium Alloy

Aluminium is one of the lightest materials that is used for many burgeoning applications such as in automotive parts, electricity lines, defence and aerospace, and food and beverages containers. Conventional manufacturing processes are capable of processing pure aluminium while processing them using SLM is quite difficult. This is because of challenges such as high reflectivity of the laser beam, oxidation and flowability. In addition, pure aluminium has high thermal conductivity compared to its alloys, making it more challenging to fabricate in the SLM process. Additive manufacturing of Al and its alloys has various applications in the automotive and aerospace fields, where fabricating light-weight structures with complex geometries is challenging using other traditional methods [59]. SLM processing of Al and its alloys has been found to be beneficial for hard-to-machine materials. To make Al fabrication possible through PBF process, additives were included [80,176]. Using one of aluminium's common alloys, AlSi10Mg, parts were fabricated using SLM process. This alloy has a very good hardness and strength and, hence, it is suitable for parts containing thin walls subjected to high loads, especially in aerospace applications [177]. AM-made Al parts are actively used in consumer products [178]. Various Al alloys were processed using the SLM technique including Al6061 and AA2024, among others [179]. These alloys possess good fatigue resistance as well as resistance to stress, corrosion and cracking. In 2010, AlSi12 alloy was processed using the SLM technique to achieve a denser part, but there were oxidation issues [180]. Micromechanical models were developed to quantitatively link aluminium material fracture properties, to microstructure features at multiple lengths scales, and manufacturing conditions [181]. An attempt was made by adding Cu to the Al powders to reduce oxidation, and the control was better when compared to conventional processes [179]. Al–Li alloys are reported to have great potential in light-weight construction, as the lithium content in the alloy significantly increases the stiffness at a lower mass, and the elastic modulus rises dramatically as the lithium concentration increases [59]. However, in traditional casting processes, a maximum Li fraction, up to 2 wt.%, has been reported due to the precipitation of the brittle δ-Al–Li [8]. Recently, it was reported that an ultrashort pulsed laser with a 500 fs pulse duration was used to 3D print the binary element Al–Li with Li content up to 4 wt.% [60]. The high content of Li generated during fs laser 3D printing of Al–Li alloys could be attributed to the high cooling rate within the melt pool during fs laser sintering, which has much shorter laser–matter interaction times. This also, in turn, supresses excessive Li evaporation during sintering. As the Li content increases in the Al–Li alloy, a significant increase in elasticity was found as depicted in Figure 23.

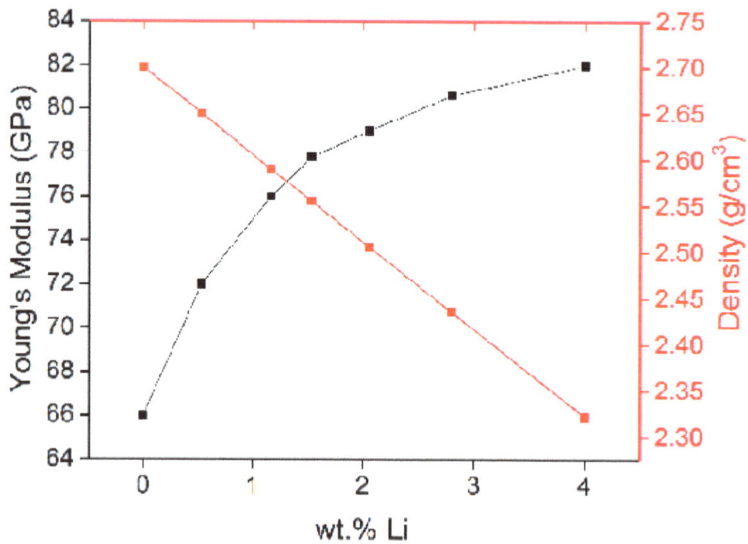

Figure 23. Lithium content versus density and Young's modulus in Al–Li alloys [60].

Furthermore, Al 3D parts were printed with an fs laser operating at a 20 MHz repetition rate and a pulse energy of 1.5 μJ at four different scanning speeds (Figure 24). The layer thickness during fabrication was reported to be 40 μm, and the hatching spacing was 30 μm. Complex gear wheels were fabricated by the same research group to prove the feasibility of the fs laser sintering process as shown in Figure 25.

Further, Ullsperger (2017) [38] utilised an fs laser operating at a 1030 nm wavelength, a pulse duration of 500 fs, an average power of 30 W at a pulse repetition ratio of 20 MHz to 3D print AlSi40 alloys. Higher concentrations of Si in AlSi40 served to primarily reinforce the material and to reduce thermal expansion during sintering. Previously, a CW laser was used in additive manufacturing of AlSi40. However, when the CW laser additively manufactures hypereutectic alloys, such as AlSi40, low cooling rates cause decomposition due to the low Si solubility in Al and poor precision due to the larger melting zone. To achieve minimal structural sizes, single tracks fabricated by CW laser were reported to be up to 150 μm [182]. To address these challenges, researchers utilised ultrafast laser sources of picosecond and femtosecond pulse durations to fabricate these alloys with reduced HAZs. The 3D printing process was carried out in a nitrogen gas environment to avoid oxidation issues, such that the oxygen concentration in the chamber was below 0.5 percent. The powder bed fusion technique has been utilised, and the powder layer-by-layer spreading was conducted manually with a rubber blade with the layer height maintained between 25 and 50 μm. In the sub-picosecond regime, the single pulse ablation threshold for Al–Si alloy operating at a 1030 nm wavelength was reported to be 0.12 J/cm^2 [38]. Ullsperger et al. found that for a layer thickness of 30 μm and at fluence greater than 0.13 J/cm^2, the powder layer was blasted from the substrate, indicating possible limitations due to the effect of higher pulse energies. By increasing the pulse repetition rate, the blasting effect was slightly reduced, and sintering and melting were found to start with a laser fluence below 0.13 J/cm^2. The experiments were carried out at a 20 MHz pulse repetition rate, initially single tracks were fabricated with a laser power ranging from 3 to 30 W, corresponding to the energy per unit length of 50–1000 J/m [38] as shown in Figure 26.

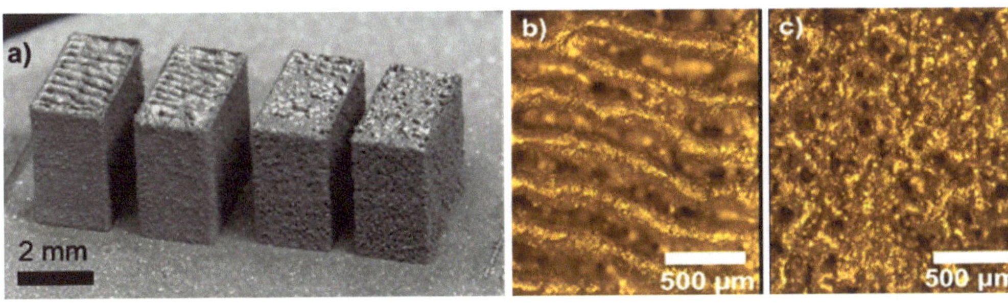

Figure 24. (**a**) Samples fabricated at different scan velocities (0.2, 0.3, 0.5 and 0.7 m/s, from left to right); Printed structure's microscopic images with a scan velocity of (**b**) 0.3 m/s and (**c**) 0.7 m/s [60].

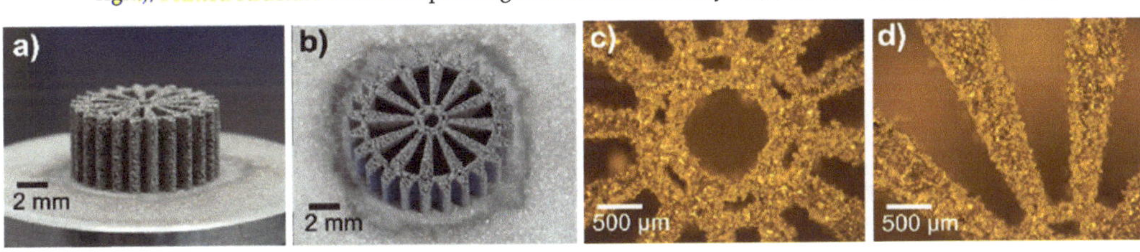

Figure 25. (**a**,**b**) Figures of a gear wheel fabricated at a scanning speed of 0.7 m/s, pulse energy of 1.5 μJ and 20 MHz pulse repetition rate; (**c**,**d**) light microscope images at different locations on the gear [60].

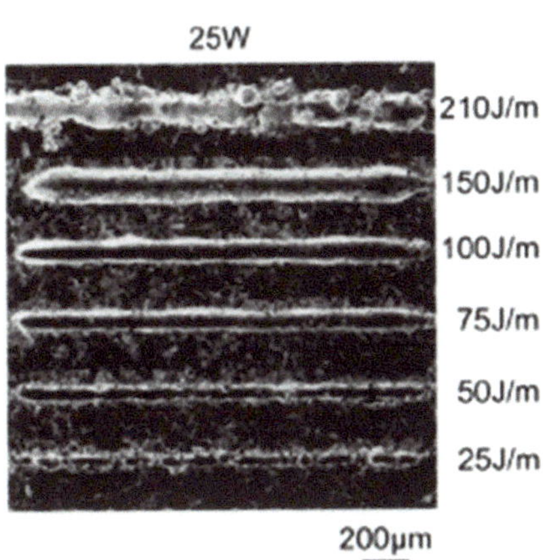

Figure 26. SEM images of single tracks at different parameters at a pulse energy of 1.25 μJ (Adapted from reference [38]).

The reported results in [38] showed that at lower scanning speeds (i.e., less than 120 mm/s (>210 J/m)) the fs laser sintering resulted in melt warps and extensive HAZs were observed with line widths in the range of 150–250 microns. Whereas at higher scanning speeds (i.e., more than 800 mm/s (<30 J/m)), irregular tracks with droplets were formed. Furthermore, with laser powers lower than 6 W, only a surface sintering effect was reported, with no fully formed melt pools. Good structures with lower roughness were formed when the laser power was set to be from 12 to 25 W with an energy per unit length from 40 to 170 J/m. With stable and reproducible single rings of 1.5 mm in diameter with 50 layers, each layer was fabricated with a thickness of 30 microns. The wall thickness produced was 54 μm with an average laser power of 12 W, whereas a 95 μm thickness was produced with a laser power of 25 W [38]. Based on these studies, light-weight 3D structures were demonstrated with a laser power of 25 W at a scanning speed of 200 mm/s as shown in Figure 27. These 3D structures fabricated were 8 mm in diameter, consisting of 120 layers with 30 microns for each layer thickness and a final wall thickness of 100 microns [38].

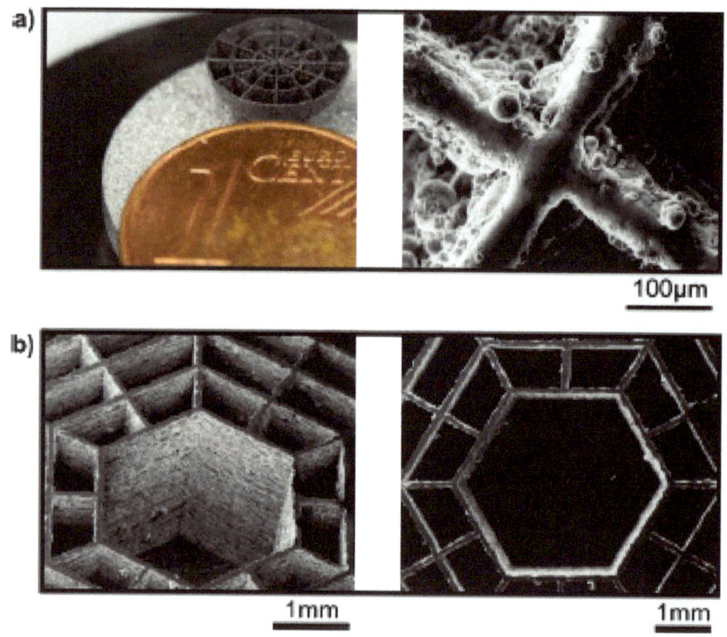

Figure 27. (**a**) Hollow thin-walled structure fabricated using fs-based AM; (**b**) hexagonal structure fabricated to a height of 5 mm (Adapted from reference [38]).

Moreover, Ullsperger et al. [183] carried out comparative studies on laser-assisted powder bed fusion of Al–40Si (40 percent Si by weight). They utilised an fs laser source operating at a 1030 nm wavelength with a repetition rate between 6 and 20 MHz as well as a CW laser operating at a 1070 nm wavelength. The laser spot diameter was approximately 50 microns, the average power around 25 W, the layer height was 15 μm and a scanning speed of 200 mm/s were set for the fs laser additive manufactured parts 1 mm height (Figure 28). The experiments were reported by setting the layer thickness to 30 μm at different pulse durations, i.e., 500 fs, 20 ps and 800 ps. It was reported that generating a stable melt pool on a thin powder layer requires an average power of more than 10 W and a pulse repetition rate of more than 1 MHz as shown in Figure 29. Higher ablation has been reported with a fluence greater than 0.4 J/cm^2. With ultrafast laser pulses of 500 fs and 20 ps operating at 20 MHz, the lowest melting pool width of 70 μm was formed, and enhanced fabricated parts with higher hardness were reported [183].

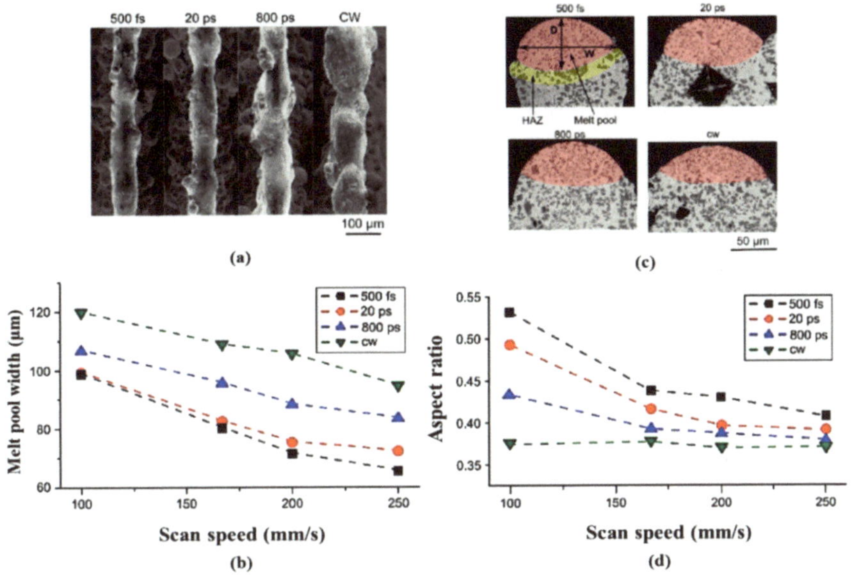

Figure 28. (**a**) SEM images of the walls (top view) above the parameters and a layer thickness of 15 microns; (**b**) scan speed versus melt pool width for different lasers; (**c**) melt pool width at the tip of the wall captured by optical microscopy; (**d**) scan speed versus aspect ratio between melt pool depth and width (increases for shorter pulse duration) (Adapted from reference [183]).

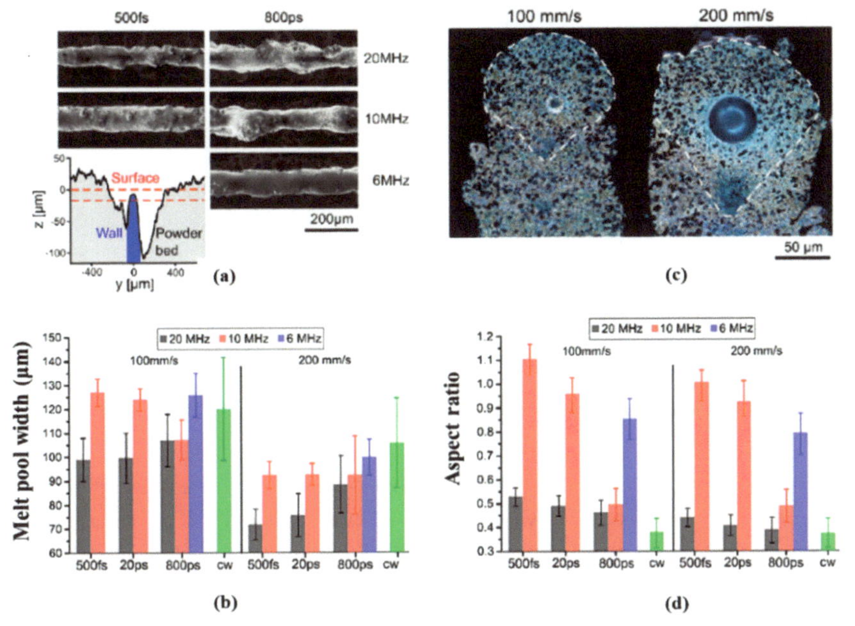

Figure 29. (**a**) SEM images of the tip of wall with a constant scanning speed of 200 mm/s; (**b**) different pulse durations versus melt pool width; (**c**) cross-section of two polished walls at 500 fs and 10 MHz repetition rate; (**d**) different scanning speeds versus aspect ratio [183].

5.5. Femtosecond-Pulsed-Laser Sintering in Hard Tissue Engineering

Tissue engineering and bone grafting have proven to be a promising approach in developing compatible tissues required at the repair site. There are different types of bone grafts that can be mainly divided into allografts (same species), autograft (same individual) and synthetic (alloplast). The latter is made of biomaterials (biocompatible polymers, ceramics, metals and composites) that are required to heal damaged or traumatised human body tissues [184]. However, there are significant drawbacks in the case of allografts and autografts such as the lack of prior donor tissue, lack of bioactivity and graft rejection. [185,186]. These issues could be resolved with alloplast-type bone grafting. In AM processes, SLS techniques have been employed for bone tissue repair using biopolymers, composites and ceramics [186]. Tan et al. (2003) utilised SLS of polyethereherketone–hydroxyapatite biocomposite blends to fabricate bone scaffolds [187]. SLS can also be used to fabricate scaffolds for the repair or regeneration of dental tissues in addition to bone tissue engineering scaffolds. SLS can be considered a versatile technology in biomaterials and tissue engineering for restoring and reconstructing tooth and bone deformities as well as for enhancing existing implants and scaffold coatings [62]. Fine powder composites formed by combining epoxy resin E-12 (as a binder) with K_2O–Al_2O_3–SiO_2 series dental glass–ceramic were used to fabricate dental restoration devices utilising SLS [186]. Sintering of hard tissues must be safe enough not to damage the delicate tissues nearby. However, there are few biomaterials that can undergo thermal effects during sintering. They include proteins, such as melanin and haemoglobin that are capable of absorbing UV spectra, and the hydroxyl group members that absorb infrared radiation [62]. Taking into account all of the aforementioned factors, it has been reported that sintering hard tissue requires a short pulsed laser with an emitted wavelength between the visible and infrared [62]. This range was selected to avoid the absorption properties of melanin (N700 nm) and haemoglobin (N600 nm) as well as water. Further, the smaller HAZs, lower irradiation time and shorter pulse durations with ultrashort lasers play key role in such fabrication.

A.D. Anastasiou et al. utilised femtosecond (100 fs) pulsed lasers operating at a wavelength of 1045 nm for sintering ceramic-based synthetic, i.e., calcium phosphate minerals such as brushite (DCPD: $CaHPO_4{\cdot}2H_2O$) and hydroxyapatite (HAP: $Ca_{10}(PO_4)6(OH)_2)$) [62]. The calcium phosphate minerals (i.e., brushite and hydroxyapatite) were further doped with iron (10%) to improve the sintering phenomenon with an fs laser [62]. It was reported that microstructural sintering and densification were observed when doping with Fe^{3+}-ions, and the laser absorption of the materials increased. After sintering, Fe^{3+}-doped brushite transformed to β-calcium pyrophosphate and Fe^{3+}-doped HAP transformed to calcium–iron–phosphate. It was observed that a temperature increase of 1000 °C occurred over a 30 μm diameter during irradiation; however, it was localised because it was estimated to decline to 40 degrees within 500 μm. From this work [62], it implies that soft tissues located more than 500 μm away from the irradiation zone are safe from thermal damage. Highly porous calcium pyrophosphate has been reported to have applications in bone regeneration, such as coatings or scaffold construction, and a dense layer of calcium–iron–phosphate might be used in acid eroded enamel restoration and for the treatment of tiny bone defects [62]. This shows a new way for alloplast grafting (i.e., synthetic bone grafting), which effectively lowers damage to the surrounding soft tissues, and the quality of sintering using fs lasers.

5.6. Femtosecond Laser-Based Additive Manufacturing Multi-Material Layered Structure

A solid oxide fuel cell (SOFC) is an electrochemical system that converts chemical energy from hydrogen fuel to electrical energy, in general, operating at high temperatures [188,189]. An anode, electrolyte and cathode are the three primary components of the SOFC. Currently, several traditional manufacturing techniques, such as chemical vapour deposition (CVD), tape casting, electrophoretic deposition (EPD), physical vapour deposition (PVD), screen printing, spray pyrolysis, sputtering and inkjet printing, were utilised to fabricate SOFCs [188,189]. Each of these processes has its own set of limitations such as tape casting's inability to produce layers thinner than 10 μm, in addition to the high cost (e.g., PVD, EPD and CVD). Furthermore, SOFCs' traditional fabrication methods involve a number of fabrication steps. A single-step fabrication approach that can provide reproducibility, flexibility and durability of SOFCs is much needed to address all of these limitations and further the commercialisation of SOFCs [188]. As a result, AM techniques have been recognised as a viable alternative that could address these shortcomings. Inkjet printing, stereolithography, aerosol jet printing, fused deposition modelling and SLS are among the AM techniques utilised in SOFC fabrication, with inkjet printing being the most prevalent because of its low-cost processing [188]. M. Lomberg et al. (2015) utilised CW laser-based SLS approach to produce SOFC electrodes with a laser power of 120 W and a scan speed of 400 mm/s. SOFCs with Ni powder as fuel electrodes, YSZ electrolyte, and LSCF-GDC air electrodes were successfully fabricated. The results reveal that the microcracks existed in SOFC electrodes manufactured using SLS [189]. Similarly, Arianna Pesce et al. (2020) used the SLA technique to fabricate the planar and conjugate LSM–YSZ/YSZ/Ni–YSZ SOFC layers. The results demonstrated that fully dense YSZ electrolytes with low cracks were produced [190]. Further, to overcome the limitations of CW laser-based SLS techniques, researchers utilised an fs laser-based SLS system to fabricate SOFCs. Bai et al. [191] utilised fs laser sintering to fabricate multilayer YSZ samples without the use of binders or heat treatment. The schematic of a multi-layered solid oxide fuel cell is shown in Figure 30. A high-power mode-locked Yb-doped fibre laser was employed with an average output power of 250 W, spot size of 25 μm, pulse duration of 800 fs, wavelength at 1030 nm and pulse repetition rate (PRR) of 80 MHz. The Ni-YSZ supporting layers were fabricated (Figure 31). High-density Ni-YSZ was fabricated when a scanning speed of 300 mm/s and laser power of 130 W were used. After first sintering of the Ni-YSZ supporting structure, a thin film of YSZ (powder or dye) was spread and laser-processed. Clear melting and fusing to the anode base were achieved, and the YSZ ink type had better uniformity. A thin coating of LSM (ink type) was put on top of the YSZ electrolyte layer and melted to act as the SOFC's cathode [191,192].

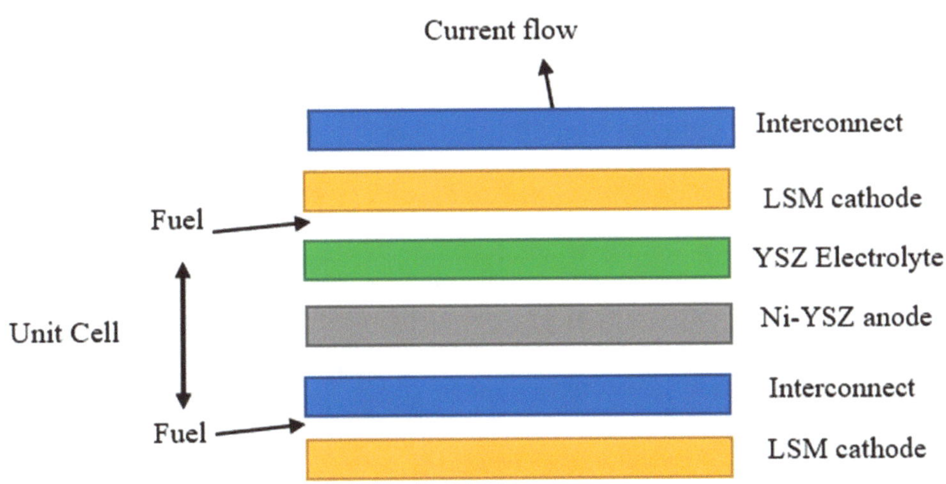

Figure 30. Schematic of a solid oxide fuel cell.

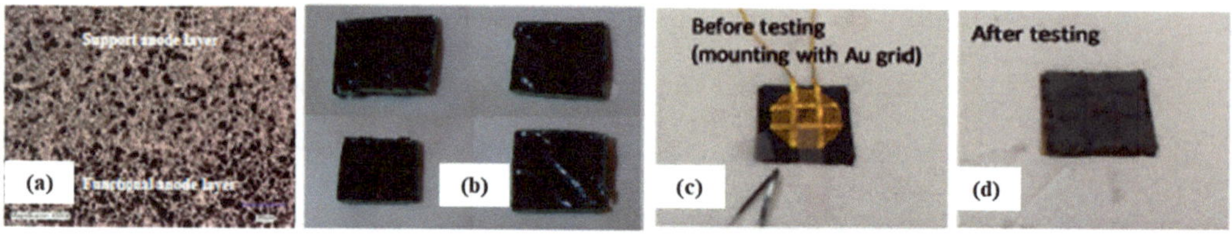

Figure 31. (**a**) Cross-section SEM image of the interface between the functional layer and support layer of an anode; (**b**) Ni-YSZ anode samples with the cell sample mounted on an Au grid for testing the I-V curve and EIS; (**c**) sample mounted on grid with Au before testing (**d**) cell sample after testing (Adapted from reference [191]).

5.7. Femtosecond Laser Processing of Titanium and Titanium Alloys

Titanium and its alloys have been widely utilised in automobile [193,194], biomedical [194,195], and aerospace [194,195] industries because of its key properties such as corrosion resistance [195], light weight [194,195], high strength [194,195], wear resistance [194] and high fracture toughness [195]. Further, because of its good biocompatibility, biostability, durability and mechanical properties, Ti has been widely used in dental and orthopaedic implants [196]. Several research studies have been carried out with pure titanium and its alloys (mainly Ti6Al4V) using CW laser-based SLM process [194,195,197]. Meanwhile, fs lasers have been mainly utilised in surface structuring and post-processing of 3D printed Ti parts. Surface treatment processes, meant to optimise surface roughness and dimensional accuracy, are of great importance in the field of AM to ensure that printed parts are useful for a large of number of applications. Post-processing techniques, such as CNC milling and polishing, can also be required to improve surface finishing [198]. However, these traditional processes may be challenging for thin walled, microscale and complex structures [49]. Further, the wettability behaviour of additive manufactured parts is also an important factor to consider, as it does impact the corrosion-resistance and water–material interaction [199]. To address these issues, researchers have been exploring ultrafast pulsed lasers (i.e., fs lasers), which enable efficient surface treatments or post-processing of additive manufactured parts. A.Y Vorobyev (2007) performed surface treatment of Ti utilising an fs laser, and they were able to produce a large variety of nanostructures on the surface of Ti material with sizes less than 20 nm [196]. Mingareev et al. (2013) also reported the utilisation of an fs laser to improve the surface quality of additive manufactured of Ti- and Ni-based alloy parts [49]. Jiao et al. (2018) observed that fs laser processing on Ti6Al4V material produced nanostructures that paved the way for AM part self-cleaning and hydrophobic properties [199]. Similarly, other research studies have been carried out utilising an fs laser to structure and treat Ti surfaces [200–202]. Yet, studies utilising femtosecond lasers to 3D print Ti parts are still scarce, which leaves a good room for exploration.

5.8. Femtosecond Laser Processing of Graphene

The unique properties of fs lasers make them attractive to be employed particularly in nano- and microfabrication. The applications of micro- and nanofabrication include microfluidic devices, medical and tissue engineering, metal micro- and nanostructures, photonic devices and micro and nano machining [203]. Fs lasers are also used in the fabrication of commonly used graphene products. Nowadays, many modern electronic devices have been developed that are flexible and smart electronics, have curved screens for mobiles and televisions, wearable displays, and electronic skins, making them particularly interesting for many researchers [204–206]. To produce such flexible electronics, materials such as graphene have unique and favourable properties. Graphene, a thin layer of carbon material, has numerous unique properties that make them suitable for many advanced electronic applications. Some of the unique properties include biocompatibility, mechanical strength, carrier mobility, conductivity and flexibility. There are different methods in which graphene can be processed and produced. Those methods include chemical vapour deposition (CVD), electron beam lithography, chemical synthesis and solvent exfoliation of graphene. Though these technologies exist, they are still in the early stage. Apart from these, AM technology has been successfully employed in the development of two-dimensional graphene structures. Yet, the development of graphene 3D structures remains a challenge. Direct writing and photolithography are two common AM technologies that are employed in the graphene development [207]. Attempts have been made by Chen et al., in 2018, to produce a composite from graphene oxide (GO), thermoplastic polyurethane and lactic acid [208]. These composites exhibited good biocompatibility and carrier mobility. Additionally, CW and pulsed lasers have been used to effectively process graphene materials [209]. The combined technology of an fs laser and DW technology was proposed by Bi et al., where they successfully fabricated varieties of complex micro-organic light-emitting diodes (OLEDs) [210]. As an application of electronic skins, based on the femtosecond laser-reduced graphene oxides (LRGOs), An et al. developed a graphene-based non-contact humidity sensor [211]. These LRGOs were also used in the development of strain sensors having a gauge factor greater than 400 by Wang et al. in 2016 [212]. Followed by this research, Qiao et al. fabricated an ultra-high gauge factored strain sensor which can be used to detect finger bends, pulse and respirational signals [213]. Fs laser-induced graphene (LIG) is another electronic skin similar to LRGOs. These LIGs were used in the fabrication of gas permeable temperature sensors as well as the throat sensors which are used in fabrication of artificial throats. These aforementioned findings on femtosecond laser-reduced LIGs and LRGOs demonstrate the great potential of fs lasers when employed in the electronic and health care industries.

5.9. A summary of the fs Laser AM Parameter Sets for Various Materials

The above discussions revealed that fs parameters play a crucial role in AM. It is evident that each set of parameters is specific to each material and the intended application. The various process parameters involved in fs laser AM, such as the wavelength, pulse duration, pulse repetition rate, laser power, scan speed, focus spot diameter, layer thickness, line spacing, pulse energy, fluence and energy density, were retrieved from the above discussed studies and are detailed in Table 7. These values can be used as a guide when planning fs laser-based AM with different materials:

Table 7. Showing materials processed through femtosecond lasers with different process settings.

Sample Number	Material	Wavelength (nm)	Pulse Duration (fs)	Pulse Repetition Rate (MHz)	Power (W)	Scan Speed (mm/s)	Spot Diameter (microns)	Layer Thickness (microns)	Line Spacing (µm)	Pulse Energy (J) (or) Fluence (J/cm^2) (or) Energy Density (W/cm^2)	Reference
1	Al–40Si	1030	500	6–20 MHz	25	200	50	15 to 30	-	<0.4 J/cm^2	[183]
2	Al–Li Alloy	1030	500	10–20 MHz	30	100–700	35	20 to 40	-	1.5–3 µJ	[60]
3	AlSi4O (40 microns)	1030	500	20 MHz	12 to 25	200	50	35 to 50	-	40–170 J/m	[38]
4	Calcium Phosphate	1045	130–190	1000	0.4	0.1	30	-	-	0.4 nJ	[62]
5	Copper (10 nm)	800	100	80 MHz	0.195–0.210	0.1	6.97	-	-	12.8–13.8 mJ/cm^2	[52]
6	Copper (35 microns)	1030		200–20 MHz	-	833 and 666	35	30	15	1, 1.25 µJ, 100 J/m	[54,138]
7	Copper (CuO)	780	120	81 MHz	-	0.5–20	-	1000	-	0.54 nJ	[53]
8	Cu_2O	780	120	83 MHz	-	100	0.7		-	163 GW/cm^2	[158]
9	CuO and NiO	780	120	82 MHz	-	0.1–5	1.3	10	-	0.059 J/cm^2	[154]
10	CuO/Cu_2O	780	120	84 MHz	-	10	-		-	0.74 nJ	[152]
11	Iron (1–5 microns)	1030	350	80 MHz	50	50	-		-	-	[7]
12	Iron on glass	1060	800	80 MHz	37 and 53	300 and 400	-	40	-	-	[100]
13	Monolithic zirconia	1030	400	200 kHz	5		-	-	-	25 µJ	[51]
14	Silver (Ag) NP	1030	370	1 MHz	0.05–0.3	0.01–5	-	-	-	-	[56]
15	Silver (Ag) NP	780	100	80 MHz	0.1–0.4	0.1–0.6	-	-	-	-	[174]
16	Silver (Ag) NP	800	50	1 kHz	-	0.02–4	-	-	-	10–300 m J/cm^2	[172]
17	Silver (Ag) NP	800	50	1 kHz	-	0.02–0.2	-	-	200	10–120 m J/cm^2	[173]
18	Silver (Ag) NP	780	100	1 kHz	0.5, 0.6	0.1–0.6	-	-	-	-	[55]
19	SS 316 L	793	150–200	1 kHz	0.15	-	-	-	-	-	[46]
20	Tungsten	1030	180	0.125–1 MHz	0.4 to 0.875	100–5000	36	-	10	0.4–7.5 µJ, 0.07–1.3 J/cm^2	[101]
21	Tungsten	1030	400	1 MHz	35	20	20	25–50	-	22.5 µJ	[58]
22	Tungsten	1030	750	100 kHz to 100 MHz	Maximum 1 kW	-	-	-	-	maximum 500 J	[44]
23	Tungsten	1030	400	1 MHz	45	25	-	-	-	-	[7]
24	YSZ, Ni-YSZ	1030	800	80 MHz	130	300	25	5–600	-	-	[191]

6. Summary

AM, one of the most rapidly evolving advanced manufacturing technologies is outpacing all other non-traditional manufacturing techniques, and it is positioned to make a major positive impact across all industries. This highly versatile technology represents one of the major enablers in the ongoing transformation of the fourth industrial revolution. The extreme flexibility and design freedom offered by AM, along with the wide selection of suitable materials (polymers, metals, ceramics and composites) and synthesis techniques positions 3D printing as the fabrication method of choice for an impressively wide range of applications. The fabrication of metallic parts is obviously of huge practical significance due to the fact of their desirable mechanical, electrical, thermal and magnetic properties. The development of various processing methods, metallic alloy compositions and optimising parameters for desirable properties are all active areas of research and development. Among the many recently developed AM techniques, selective laser sintering/melting represents one of the most promising methods capable of producing standard quality parts for various applications. The majority of current research efforts considering the SLM/S process has been carried out with CW and long-pulsed lasers to produce quality components. The process capabilities of SLS/M utilising different lasers sources, such as CW and pulsed lasers, were discussed in detail. The use of ultrafast lasers (picosecond and femtosecond lasers in particular), however, represents a major deviation and paves the way towards further enhancements by capitalising on shorter pulses, smaller HAZs, and superior resolution through significantly smaller spot sizes and shorter interaction times offered by fs lasers. Currently available commercial machines that utilise CW or pulsed lasers were compared to fs laser-based ones to highlight the benefits and shortcomings. Further, the main advantages of pulsed lasers over CW lasers were listed, which helps in orienting the research scope towards fs laser-based AM process. Though CW lasers have been proven to produce quality parts with various materials, there are still limitations such as HAZs, residual stresses, substrate damage, not being suitable for micro- and nanoscale parts, difficulty in processing materials with high thermal and melting points such as copper and tungsten. To address the issues mentioned in the case of CW and long-pulsed lasers, researchers utilised ultrashort pulsed lasers such as fs lasers in SLS/M.

***Fs laser science*:** To clearly understand the science behind these ultrafast lasers (i.e., fs lasers), a brief history, the fundamentals and fs laser–matter interaction were thoroughly discussed. In comparison with CW and ns lasers, fs lasers produce minimal HAZs, lower residual stresses and can produce miniaturised parts. Further, the fs laser-based AM and its different essential parameters affecting the AM parts were discussed. The ultrafast laser–material interaction studied by various researchers was consolidated and presented. Various numerical modelling approaches, such as the two-temperature model, molecular dynamics model, hydrodynamics model, hybrid model combining TTM and MD models and modified TTM models, were discussed to study the process in detail. In this review article, two major SLS/M techniques (i.e., powder bed fusion and direct writing) were utilised for fs laser-based AM. In the direct-writing technique, a pre-coated substrate is selectively sintered using a laser source. Similarly, to better understand the process of fs laser powder bed fusion technique, a schematic with components of the fs laser-based selective laser sintering/melting method was discussed.

***Materials*:** An fs laser source has been utilised for processing various materials that were challenging with CW or long-pulsed lasers. The different materials that were processed utilising fs laser source included copper, silver, aluminium, iron, tungsten, biomaterials, and ceramics. Copper material has been used for fs laser-based SLS/M utilising both DW and PBF techniques. Copper has been challenging to print using traditional CW lasers due to its high thermal conductivity and high reflectivity. A limitation that was clearly alleviated through the use of fs laser sintering process. Mainly in the case of miniaturised electronic devices, CW and long-pulsed laser failed to achieve parts at the micron or submicron levels because of HAZs, beam size, residual stresses and substrate damage. It was also reported that oxidation issues are much more prevalent in CW laser sintering than ns and fs laser sintering. Fs laser-reductive sintering of copper oxide material using DW technique has been reported to produce functional parts for temperature sensors applications. Attempts have also been made to fabricate micropatterns using copper–nickel alloys. Further sintering of copper particles utilising the PBF technique reported that at lower repetition rates, there was low melting, resulting in poor fusing of metal particles to the substrate. By increasing the pulse repetition rate and maintaining the pulse energy, proper bonding of copper powder to the substrate was achieved, which could have major applications in microdevices, heat sinks, and others. Further Very high melting point materials such as tungsten was also processed utilising the fs laser based PBF technique. Tungsten has eye-catching major applications in the aerospace, medical and nuclear sectors, among others. A few years back, AM of tungsten was a major challenge because of its high melting point, high thermal conductivity, and low thermal expansion. Since 2015, researchers have started utilising high-power CW laser sources to fabricate tungsten material to meet specific applications. Though they succeeded in fabricating the tungsten parts with CW laser source, there were still issues related to lower relative density, and micro-cracks were still prevalent. Research group explored the fabrication of tungsten parts utilising the fs laser-based PBF technique to address these issues. They demonstrated how processing parameters, including pulse repetition rate, laser spot diameter and layer thickness, played a crucial role in sintering tungsten particles. The capability of producing fine features using fs-laser-based AM, thin walls of 100 microns, smaller gear shapes and circular features with holes were fabricated with good accuracy. Comparing fs laser sintered parts with CW laser sintered and ps laser sintered parts, it was found that the defects present in fs laser sintered samples were fewer compared to other types of lasers. Further fs laser produced greater hardness and higher density parts as compared to CW laser sintered parts. One of the special features of fs lasers is localised heating, which was used to fuse iron powder onto a glass substrate that possesses extremely different material properties.

Furthermore, other precious metals, such as silver, also have been processed using an fs laser for specific applications in photonic devices and flexible electronics. It is fascinating to note that the silver nanoparticles were fabricated on a silica-based microfluidic channel utilising an fs laser to fabricate the SERS substrate. Researchers have also utilised both ns and fs laser sources to fuse silver nanoparticles on a PET substrate and compared the results by varying the effective pulse number and fluence. The results showed that in the case of the fs laser source, because of the low substrate damage and less film cracking, the produced parts had a higher electrical conductivity than ns laser sintered parts. Similarly, other experiments utilising fs laser sintering of silver nanoparticles were dedicated to analysing the effect of process parameters and varying spin-coated layer thicknesses on conductivity, microstructure and adhesion strength.

Aluminium and its alloys which are utilised in lightweight structures in different fields like aerospace, automotive, etc., were also investigated by utilising fs laser-based AM. In the case of Al and Li alloys for aerospace application, as the Li content increases in Al–Li alloy, the stiffness increases significantly at a lower mass. It was reported that the traditional casting process of Al–Li could process up to a max of 2 percent due to the precipitation of brittle δ-Al–Li. To address these issues, researchers utilised key factors of high cooling rates in fs laser-based technique to fabricate Al–Li alloy and produce Al–Li alloy with higher Li content. Similarly, other alloys such as AlSi4O, Al–40Si were also reported to fabricate parts utilising the fs laser-based AM technique. It is reported that in the case of AlSi4O, by properly optimising the process parameters, the minimum feature size of 50 μm was achieved utilising fs laser processing.

Fs laser based AM poses great potential in biomedical and tissue engineering to effectively fabricate hard tissues, which could have major dental and bone repair applications. The most important factors of fs laser sintering are the lower HAZs, lower irradiation time and localised heating, which play critical roles in fabricating or repairing the damaged tissues without affecting the surrounding area. The fs laser-based AM technique has also been utilised in the fabrication of multi-material SOFCs, which has solved a few limitations, such as microcracks that occur in CW laser-based-fabricated SOFCs. By utilising fs lasers, sintering of dense multi-material SOFCs was reported.

7. Conclusions

Fs laser-based sintering processes enhance the material processing library of conventional techniques based on CW or long-pulsed lasers by adding full control over the processing parameters. In particular, challenging materials, such as copper, silver, YSZ and tungsten, were reported to produce standard functional parts meeting the requirements of many applications. The fs laser sintering of copper has proven to have significant applications in the fabrication of micropatterns for interconnects on transistor IC chips. Further, the oxides of copper and nickel were utilised by the fs reductive sintering process to produce micropatterns that are sensitive to temperature and which could find applications in micro-sensing devices. Similarly, pure copper powder has also been investigated utilising fs lasers, which could have applications in heat sinks or cooling devices used in micro-robotic engines. Yet, this is still in the early stage because, as such, no quality parts have been fabricated utilising an fs laser source. Fs laser sintering of tungsten material has been reported to produce dense parts that could have significant applications in rocket parts, plasma-facing components in nuclear fusion reactors and radiation shielding in imaging systems. However, only a single research group has claimed to produce such dense parts with higher hardness, strength, etc. But the process parameters are not much evident, and there is a need to develop optimum process conditions to fabricate fs laser-based tungsten parts because tungsten material has much scope and applications in most emerging fields. In the case of aluminium and its alloys, Al–Li and AlSi4O, the reported results are encouraging. However, as these materials are utilised for structural applications in aerospace and automobile, the large-scale production may or may not be possible with the current research in fs laser sintering. Moreover, in the case of ceramics, which have significant applications in challenging tissue fabrication, fs laser sintering could be ideal, as it does not cause damage to the surrounding soft tissues during fabrication. Yet, more research is needed to identify the proper equipment and techniques that need to be developed to be able to commercialise the fabricated ceramic parts. For SOFCs, while inkjet printing process and other traditional manufacturing techniques are mainly employed to develop them at cheaper costs, the need for much more miniaturised parts with higher efficiency necessitates the application of fs laser sintering.

Author Contributions: Conceptualization, A.S.A.; investigation, A.A., H.A.K. and A.S.A.; validation, M.A., M.E., W.A. and A.S.A.; writing—original draft preparation A.B.K. and H.A.K.; writing—review and editing, M.A., M.E., W.A., F.A. and A.S.A.; Supervision, A.S.A. All authors have read and agreed to the published version of the manuscript.

Funding: This work was supported by the American University of Sharjah through FRG grant #FRG19-L-S61.

Institutional Review Board Statement: Not applicable.

Informed Consent Statement: Not applicable.

Data Availability Statement: Data underlying the results presented in this paper are not publicly available at this time but may be obtained from the corresponding authors upon reasonable request.

Conflicts of Interest: The authors declare no conflict of interest.

References

1. Gibson, I.; Rosen, D. *Additive Manufacturing Technologies*, 17th ed.; Springer: New York, NY, USA, 2014.
2. Dilberoglu, U.M.; Gharehpapagh, B.; Yaman, U.; Dolen, M. The Role of Additive Manufacturing in the Era of Industry 4.0. *Procedia Manuf.* **2017**, *11*, 545–554. [CrossRef]

3. Thompson, M.K.; Moroni, G.; Vaneker, T.; Fadel, G.; Campbell, R.I.; Gibson, I.; Bernard, A.; Schulz, J.; Graf, P.; Ahuja, B.; et al. Design for Additive Manufacturing: Trends, opportunities, considerations, and constraints. *CIRP Ann.* **2016**, *65*, 737–760. [CrossRef]
4. Barroqueiro, B.; Andrade-Campos, A.; Valente, R.; Neto, V. Metal Additive Manufacturing Cycle in Aerospace Industry: A Comprehensive Review. *J. Manuf. Mater. Process.* **2019**, *3*, 52. [CrossRef]
5. Katz-Demyanetz, A.; Popov, V.V.; Kovalevsky, A.; Safranchik, D.; Koptyug, A. Powder-bed additive manufacturing for aerospace application: Techniques, metallic and metal/ceramic composite materials and trends. *Manuf. Rev.* **2019**, *6*, 5. [CrossRef]
6. Mohanavel, V.; Ali, K.A.; Ranganathan, K.; Jeffrey, J.A.; Ravikumar, M.M.; Rajkumar, S. The roles and applications of additive manufacturing in the aerospace and automobile sector. *Mater. Today Proc.* **2021**, *47*, 405–409. [CrossRef]
7. Huang, H.; Nie, B.; Wan, P.; Yang, L.-M.; Bai, S.; Liu, J. Femtosecond fiber laser additive manufacturing and welding for 3D manufacturing. In *Laser 3D Manufacturing II*; Proc. SPIE: San Francisco, CA, USA, 2015; Volume 9353, p. 93530A. [CrossRef]
8. Rioja, R.J.; Liu, J. The Evolution of Al-Li Base Products for Aerospace and Space Applications. *Metall. Mater. Trans. A* **2012**, *43*, 3325–3337. [CrossRef]
9. Byskov-Nielsen, J.; Savolainen, J.-M.; Christensen, M.S.; Balling, P. Ultra-short pulse laser ablation of metals: Threshold fluence, incubation coefficient and ablation rates. *Appl. Phys. A* **2010**, *101*, 97–101. [CrossRef]
10. Chua, C.K.; Matham, M.V.; Kim, Y.-J. *Lasers in 3D Printing and Manufacturing*; World Scientific Publishing Company: Singapore, 2017. [CrossRef]
11. Dordlofva, C. A Design for Qualification Framework for the Development of Additive Manufacturing Components—A Case Study from the Space Industry. *Aerospace* **2020**, *7*, 25. [CrossRef]
12. Pinkerton, A.J. [INVITED] Lasers in additive manufacturing. *Opt. Laser Technol.* **2016**, *78*, 25–32. [CrossRef]
13. Paolini, A.; Kollmannsberger, S.; Rank, E. Additive manufacturing in construction: A review on processes, applications, and digital planning methods. *Addit. Manuf.* **2019**, *30*, 100894. [CrossRef]
14. Saengchairat, N.; Tran, T.; Chua, C.-K. A review: Additive manufacturing for active electronic components. *Virtual Phys. Prototyp.* **2017**, *12*, 31–46. [CrossRef]
15. Godoi, F.C.; Prakash, S.; Bhandari, B.R. 3d printing technologies applied for food design: Status and prospects. *J. Food Eng.* **2016**, *179*, 44–54. [CrossRef]
16. Huang, S.H.; Liu, P.; Mokasdar, A.; Hou, L. Additive manufacturing and its societal impact: A literature review. *Int. J. Adv. Manuf. Technol.* **2013**, *67*, 1191–1203. [CrossRef]
17. Sibbett, W.; Lagatsky, A.A.; Brown, C.T.A. The development and application of femtosecond laser systems. *Opt. Express* **2012**, *20*, 6989–7001. [CrossRef]
18. Application Spotlight: 3D Printing for Footwear, AMFG. 2019. Available online: https://amfg.ai/2019/09/18/application-spotlight-3d-printing-for-footwear/ (accessed on 30 October 2021).
19. Wong, K.V.; Hernandez, A. A Review of Additive Manufacturing. *ISRN Mech. Eng.* **2012**, *2012*, 208760. [CrossRef]
20. Meier, M.; Tan, K.H.; Lim, M.K.; Chung, L. Unlocking innovation in the sport industry through additive manufacturing. *Bus. Process. Manag. J.* **2019**, *25*, 456–475. [CrossRef]
21. Wimpenny, D.I.; Pandey, P.M.; Kumar, L.J. (Eds.) *Advances in 3D Printing & Additive Manufacturing Technologies*; Springer: Singapore, 2017; pp. 9–28. [CrossRef]
22. Das, S.; Bourell, D.L.; Babu, S. Metallic materials for 3D printing. *MRS Bull.* **2016**, *41*, 729–741. [CrossRef]
23. Frazier, W.E. Metal Additive Manufacturing: A Review. *J. Mater. Eng. Perform.* **2014**, *23*, 1917–1928. [CrossRef]
24. Herderick, E. Additive manufacturing of metals: A review. *Mater. Sci. Technol. Conf. Exhib.* **2011**, *2*, 1413–1425. Available online: http://www.scopus.com/inward/record.url?eid=2-s2.0-84856301323&partnerID=40&md5=e02018d10b2ca37a7e2ae1773e4fcaec (accessed on 30 November 2021).
25. Liu, R.; Wang, Z.; Sparks, T.; Liou, F.; Newkirk, J. Aerospace applications of laser additive manufacturing. In *Laser Additive Manufacturing: Materials, Design, Technologies, and Applications*; Woodhead Publishing: Sawston, UK, 2017; ISBN 9780081004340.
26. Najmon, J.C.; Raeisi, S.; Tovar, A. Review of additive manufacturing technologies and applications in the aerospace industry. In *Additive Manufacturing for the Aerospace Industry*; Elsevier: Amsterdam, The Netherlands, 2019; pp. 7–31.
27. Saracyakupoglu, T. The Qualification of the Additively Manufactured Parts in the Aviation Industry. *Am. J. Aerosp. Eng.* **2019**, *6*, 1. [CrossRef]
28. Vafadar, A.; Guzzomi, F.; Rassau, A.; Hayward, K. Advances in Metal Additive Manufacturing: A Review of Common Processes, Industrial Applications, and Current Challenges. *Appl. Sci.* **2021**, *11*, 1213. [CrossRef]
29. Lee, H.; Lim, C.H.J.; Low, M.J.; Tham, N.; Murukeshan, V.M.; Kim, Y.J. Lasers in additive manufacturing: A review. *Int. J. Precis. Eng. Manuf. Technol.* **2017**, *4*, 307–322. [CrossRef]
30. Deckers, J.; Meyers, S.; Kruth, J.; Vleugels, J. Direct Selective Laser Sintering/Melting of High Density Alumina Powder Layers at Elevated Temperatures. *Phys. Procedia* **2014**, *56*, 117–124. [CrossRef]
31. Kruth, J.; Froyen, L.; Van Vaerenbergh, J.; Mercelis, P.; Rombouts, M.; Lauwers, B. Selective laser melting of iron-based powder. *J. Mater. Process. Technol.* **2004**, *149*, 616–622. [CrossRef]
32. Biffi, C.; Fiocchi, J.; Bassani, P.; Tuissi, A. Continuous wave vs. pulsed wave laser emission in selective laser melting of AlSi10Mg parts with industrial optimized process parameters: Microstructure and mechanical behaviour. *Addit. Manuf.* **2018**, *24*, 639–646. [CrossRef]

33. Kumar, H.; Kumaraguru, S. Distortion in Metal Additive Manufactured Parts. In *3D Printing and Additive Manufacturing Technologies*; Springer: Berlin/Heidelberg, Germany, 2019; pp. 281–295.
34. Oliveira, J.P.; LaLonde, A.; Ma, J. Processing parameters in laser powder bed fusion metal additive manufacturing. *Mater. Des.* **2020**, *193*, 108762. [CrossRef]
35. Yeong, W.; Yap, C.; Mapar, M.; Chua, C. State-of-the-art review on selective laser melting of ceramics. In *High Value Manufacturing: Advanced Research in Virtual and Rapid Prototyping*; CRC Press: Boca Raton, FL, USA, 2013; pp. 65–70.
36. Lonergan, J.M.; Fahrenholtz, W.; Hilmas, G. Zirconium Diboride with High Thermal Conductivity. *J. Am. Ceram. Soc.* **2014**, *97*, 1689–1691. [CrossRef]
37. In't Veld, B.H.; Overmeyer, L.; Schmidt, M.; Wegener, K.; Malshe, A.; Bartolo, P. Micro additive manufacturing using ultra short laser pulses. *CIRP Ann.* **2015**, *64*, 701–724. [CrossRef]
38. Ullsperger, T.; Matthäus, G.; Kaden, L.; Rettenmayr, M.; Risse, S.; Tünnermann, A.; Nolte, S. Selective laser melting of AlSi40 using ultrashort laser pulses for additive manufacturing applications. In Proceedings of the Lasers in Manufacturing Conference 2017, Munich, Germany, 26–29 June 2017.
39. Neuenschwander, B.; Jaeggi, B.; Schmid, M.; Dommann, A.; Neels, A.; Bandi, T.; Hennig, G. Factors controlling the incubation in the application of ps laser pulses on copper and iron surfaces. In *Laser Applications in Microelectronic and Optoelectronic Manufacturing (LAMOM) XVIII*; Proc. of SPIE: San Francisco, CA, USA, 2013; Volume 8607, p. 86070D. [CrossRef]
40. Nedialkov, N.; Atanasov, P. Molecular dynamics simulation study of deep hole drilling in iron by ultrashort laser pulses. *Appl. Surf. Sci.* **2006**, *252*, 4411–4415. [CrossRef]
41. Nagarajan, B.; Hu, Z.; Song, X.; Zhai, W.; Wei, J. Development of Micro Selective Laser Melting: The State of the Art and Future Perspectives. *Engineering* **2019**, *5*, 702–720. [CrossRef]
42. Ultrafast Lasers Market-Growth, Trends, COVID-19 Impact, and Forecasts (2021–2026), Mordor Intell. 2020. Available online: https://www.mordorintelligence.com/industry-reports/ultrafast-lasers-market (accessed on 25 November 2021).
43. Eaton, S.M.; Zhang, H.; Herman, P.R.; Yoshino, F.; Shah, L.; Bovatsek, J.; Arai, A.Y. Heat accumulation effects in femtosecond laser-written waveguides with variable repetition rate. *Opt. Express* **2005**, *13*, 4708–4716. [CrossRef]
44. Bai, S.; Liu, J.; Yang, P.; Huang, H.; Yang, L.-M. Femtosecond fiber laser additive manufacturing of tungsten. In *Laser 3D Manufacturing III*; Proc. of SPIE: San Francisco, CA, USA, 2016; Volume 9738, p. 97380. [CrossRef]
45. Hodgson, N.O.R.M.A.N.; Laha, M.I.C.H.A.E.L.; Lee, T.S.; Steinkopff, A.L.B.R.E.C.H.T.; Heming, S.E.B.A.S.T.I.A.N. Industrial femtosecond lasers and material processing. In *Industrial Laser Solutions*; PennWell Publishing: Nashville, TN, USA, 2019.
46. Gieseke, M.; Senz, V.; Vehse, M.; Fiedler, S.; Irsig, R.; Hustedt, M.; Sternberg, K.; Nölke, C.; Kaierle, S.; Wesling, V.; et al. Additive Manufacturing of Drug Delivery Systems. *Biomed. Tech. Eng.* **2012**, *57*, 398–401. [CrossRef]
47. Birnbaum, M. Semiconductor Surface Damage Produced by Ruby Lasers. *J. Appl. Phys.* **1965**, *36*, 3688–3689. [CrossRef]
48. Hodgson, N.; Laha, M.; Lee, T.S.; Haloui, H.; Heming, S.; Steinkopff, A. Industrial Ultrafast Lasers–Systems, Processing Fundamentals, and Applications. In *CLEO: QELS_Fundamental Science*; Optical Society of America: San Jose, CA, USA, 2019. [CrossRef]
49. Mingareev, I.; Bonhoff, T.; El-Sherif, A.; Meiners, W.; Kelbassa, I.; Biermann, T.; Richardson, M. Femtosecond laser post-processing of metal parts produced by laser additive manufacturing. *J. Laser Appl.* **2013**, *25*, 052009. [CrossRef]
50. Mingareev, I.; Bonhoff, T.; El-Sherif, A.; Biermann, T.; Meiners, W.; Kelbassa, I.; Richardson, M. Ultrafast laser-based post-processing of parts produced by additive manufacturing. *Int. Congr. Appl. Lasers Electro-Opt.* **2013**, *2013*, 787. [CrossRef]
51. Liang, S.; Ye, H.; Yuan, F. Changes in Crystal Phase, Morphology, and Flexural Strength of As-Sintered Translucent Monolithic Zirconia Ceramic Modified by Femtosecond Laser. *Appl. Sci.* **2021**, *11*, 6925. [CrossRef]
52. Cheng, C.W.; Chen, J.K. Femtosecond laser sintering of copper nanoparticles. *Appl. Phys. A* **2016**, *122*, 1–8. [CrossRef]
53. Mizoshiri, M.; Hata, S. Direct Writing of Cu-based Micro-temperature Sensors onto Glass and Poly(dimethylsiloxane) Substrates Using Femtosecond Laser Reductive Patterning of CuO Nanoparticles. *Res. Rev. J. Mater. Sci.* **2016**, *4*, 47–54. [CrossRef]
54. Kaden, L.; Matthäus, G.; Ullsperger, T.; Engelhardt, H.; Rettenmayr, M.; Tünnermann, A.; Nolte, S. Selective laser melting of copper using ultrashort laser pulses. *Appl. Phys. A* **2017**, *123*, 596. [CrossRef]
55. Son, Y.; Yeo, J.; Ha, C.W.; Hong, S.; Ko, S.H.; Yang, D.Y. Fabrication of submicron-sized metal patterns on a flexible polymer substrate by femtosecond laser sintering of metal nanoparticles. *Int. J. Nanomanuf.* **2013**, *9*, 468. [CrossRef]
56. Kurnoothala, R.; Sai, M.V.; Vishnubhatla, K.C. Facile fabrication of integrated microfluidic SERS substrate by femtosecond laser sintering of silver nano particles. *Opt. Mater.* **2021**, *111*, 110518. [CrossRef]
57. Song, B.; Dong, S.; Deng, S.; Liao, H.; Coddet, C. Microstructure and tensile properties of iron parts fabricated by selective laser melting. *Opt. Laser Technol.* **2014**, *56*, 451–460. [CrossRef]
58. Nie, B.; Huang, H.; Bai, S.; Liu, J. Femtosecond laser melting and resolidifying of high-temperature powder materials. *Appl. Phys. A* **2014**, *118*, 37–41. [CrossRef]
59. Olakanmi, E.O.; Cochrane, R.; Dalgarno, K. A review on selective laser sintering/melting (SLS/SLM) of aluminium alloy powders: Processing, microstructure, and properties. *Prog. Mater. Sci.* **2015**, *74*, 401–477. [CrossRef]
60. Yürekli, B.; Schade, L.; Ullsperger, T.; Seyfarth, B.; Kohl, H.; Matthäus, G.; Liu, D.; Rettenmayr, M.; Nolte, S. Additive manufacturing of binary Al-Li alloys. *Procedia CIRP* **2020**, *94*, 69–73. [CrossRef]
61. Ferrage, L.; Bertrand, G.; Lenormand, P. Dense yttria-stabilized zirconia obtained by direct selective laser sintering. *Addit. Manuf.* **2018**, *21*, 472–478. [CrossRef]

62. Anastasiou, A.; Thomson, C.; Hussain, S.; Edwards, T.; Strafford, S.; Malinowski, M.; Mathieson, R.; Brown, C.; Brown, A.; Duggal, M.; et al. Sintering of calcium phosphates with a femtosecond pulsed laser for hard tissue engineering. *Mater. Des.* **2016**, *101*, 346–354. [CrossRef]
63. Bai, S.; Liu, J. Additive manufacturing of bimetallic structures. *SN Appl. Sci.* **2020**, *2*, 1152. [CrossRef]
64. Lei, S.; Zhao, X.; Yu, X.; Hu, A.; Vukelic, S.; Jun, M.B.G.; Joe, H.-E.; Yao, Y.L.; Shin, Y.C. Ultrafast Laser Applications in Manufacturing Processes: A State-of-the-Art Review. *J. Manuf. Sci. Eng.* **2020**, *142*, 031005. [CrossRef]
65. Mottay, E.; Liu, X.; Zhang, H.; Mazur, E.; Sanatinia, R.; Pfleging, W. Industrial applications of ultrafast laser processing. *MRS Bull.* **2016**, *41*, 984–992. [CrossRef]
66. Strickland, D.; Mourou, G. Compression of amplified chirped optical pulses. *Opt. Commun.* **1985**, *56*, 219–221. [CrossRef]
67. Bakshi, K. A Review on Selective Laser Sintering: A Rapid Prototyping Technology. *IOSR J. Mech. Civ. Eng.* **2016**, *4*, 53–57. [CrossRef]
68. Hong, S. Selective Laser Sintering of Nanoparticles. *Sinter. Funct. Mater.* **2018**, 147–164. [CrossRef]
69. Ruszaj, A. Additive methods in micro and nano manufacturing technologies. *Mechanik* **2019**, *92*, 386–390. [CrossRef]
70. Engstrøm, D.; Porter, B.; Pacios, M.; Bhaskaran, H. Additive nanomanufacturing–A review. *J. Mater. Res.* **2014**, *29*, 1792–1816. [CrossRef]
71. Milewski, J.O. *Lasers, Electron Beams, Plasma Arcs*; Springer: Singapore, 2017; pp. 85–97.
72. Jamie, D. A Comprehensive List of all the Metal 3D Printer Manufacturers, 3D Nativ. 2021. Available online: https://www.3dnatives.com/en/metal-3d-printer-manufacturers/#! (accessed on 13 November 2021).
73. Schmidt, M.; Merklein, M.; Bourell, D.; Dimitrov, D.; Hausotte, T.; Wegener, K.; Overmeyer, L.; Vollertsen, F.; Levy, G.N. Laser based additive manufacturing in industry and academia. *CIRP Ann.* **2017**, *66*, 561–583. [CrossRef]
74. Yap, C.Y.; Chua, C.K.; Dong, Z.L.; Liu, Z.H.; Zhang, D.Q.; Loh, L.E.; Sing, S.L. Review of selective laser melting: Materials and applications. *Appl. Phys. Rev.* **2015**, *2*, 041101. [CrossRef]
75. Mosadegh, B.; Xiong, G.; Dunham, S.; Min, J.K. Current progress in 3D printing for cardiovascular tissue engineering. *Biomed. Mater.* **2015**, *10*, 034002. [CrossRef]
76. Vaezi, M.; Seitz, H.; Yang, S. A review on 3D micro-additive manufacturing technologies. *Int. J. Adv. Manuf. Technol.* **2013**, *67*, 1721–1754. [CrossRef]
77. Majumdar, J.D.; Manna, I. *Laser-Assisted Fabrication of Materials*; Springer: Berlin, Germany, 2012.
78. Gu, D.; Meiners, W.; Wissenbach, K.; Poprawe, R. Laser additive manufacturing of metallic components: Materials, processes and mechanisms. *Int. Mater. Rev.* **2012**, *57*, 133–164. [CrossRef]
79. Mukherjee, T.; Zuback, J.S.; De, A.; Debroy, T. Printability of alloys for additive manufacturing. *Sci. Rep.* **2016**, *6*, 19717. [CrossRef] [PubMed]
80. Karia, M.C.; Popat, M.A.; Sangani, K.B. Selective laser melting of Inconel super alloy-a review. In *AIP Conference Proceedings*; AIP Publishing: Melville, NY, USA, 2017.
81. Garban-Labaune, C.; Fabre, E.; Max, C.E.; Fabbro, R.; Amiranoff, F.; Virmont, J.; Weinfeld, M.; Michard, A. Effect of Laser Wavelength and Pulse Duration on Laser-Light Absorption and Back Reflection. *Phys. Rev. Lett.* **1982**, *48*, 1018–1021. [CrossRef]
82. Buchbinder, D.; Schleifenbaum, J.H.; Heidrich, S.; Meiners, W.; Bültmann, J. High Power Selective Laser Melting (HP SLM) of Aluminum Parts. *Phys. Procedia* **2011**, *12*, 271–278. [CrossRef]
83. Sing, S.L.; Yeong, W.Y.; Wiria, F.E.; Tay, B.Y.; Zhao, Z.; Zhao, L.; Tian, Z.; Yang, S. Direct selective laser sintering and melting of ceramics: A review. *Rapid Prototyp. J.* **2017**, *23*, 611–623. [CrossRef]
84. Ke, L.; Zhu, H.; Yin, J.; Wang, X. Effects of peak laser power on laser micro sintering of nickel powder by pulsed Nd:YAG laser. *Rapid Prototyp. J.* **2014**, *20*, 328–335. [CrossRef]
85. Sufiiarov, V.; Popovich, A.; Borisov, E.; Polozov, I.; Masaylo, D.; Orlov, A. The Effect of Layer Thickness at Selective Laser Melting. *Procedia Eng.* **2017**, *174*, 126–134. [CrossRef]
86. Aboulkhair, N.T. Additive Manufacture of an Aluminium Alloy: Processing, Microstructure, and Mechanical Properties. Ph.D. Dissertation, University of Nottingham, Nottingham, UK, 2015.
87. Aboulkhair, N.T.; Everitt, N.; Ashcroft, I.; Tuck, C. Reducing porosity in AlSi10Mg parts processed by selective laser melting. *Addit. Manuf.* **2014**, *1–4*, 77–86. [CrossRef]
88. Thijs, L.; Kempen, K.; Kruth, J.-P.; Van Humbeeck, J. Fine-structured aluminium products with controllable texture by selective laser melting of pre-alloyed AlSi10Mg powder. *Acta Mater.* **2013**, *61*, 1809–1819. [CrossRef]
89. Aboulkhair, N.T.; Simonelli, M.; Parry, L.; Ashcroft, I.; Tuck, C.; Hague, R. 3D printing of Aluminium alloys: Additive Manufacturing of Aluminium alloys using selective laser melting. *Prog. Mater. Sci.* **2019**, *106*, 100578. [CrossRef]
90. DeMaria, A.J.; Stetser, D.A.; Heynau, H. Self mode-locking of lasers with saturable absorbers. *Appl. Phys. Lett.* **1966**, *8*, 174–176. [CrossRef]
91. Shank, C.V. Subpicosecond kilowatt pulses from a mode-locked cw dye laser. *Appl. Phys. Lett.* **1974**, *24*, 373. [CrossRef]
92. Haus, H.A. Theory of mode locking with a fast saturable absorber. *J. Appl. Phys.* **1975**, *46*, 3049–3058. [CrossRef]
93. Fermann, M.E.; Hartl, I. Ultrafast fibre lasers. *Nat. Photonics* **2013**, *7*, 868–874. [CrossRef]
94. Spence, D.E.; Kean, P.N.; Sibbett, W. 60-Femtosecond pulse generation from a self-mode-locked Ti:sapphire laser. *Opt. Lett.* **1991**, *16*, 42–44. [CrossRef] [PubMed]

95. Sutter, D.; Jung, I.; Kartner, F.; Matuschek, N.; Morier-Genoud, F.; Scheuer, V.; Tilsch, M.; Tschudi, T.; Keller, U. Self-starting 6.5-fs pulses from a Ti:sapphire laser using a semiconductor saturable absorber and double chirped mirrors. *IEEE J. Sel. Top. Quantum Electron.* **1998**, *4*, 169–178. [CrossRef]
96. Hamad, A.H. *Effects of Different Laser Pulse Regimes (Nanosecond, Picosecond and Femtosecond) on the Ablation of Materials for Production of Nanoparticles in Liquid Solution*; IntechOpen: London, UK, 2016.
97. Byskov-Nielsen, J. Short-Pulse Laser Ablation of Metals: Fundamentals and Applications for Micro-Mechanical Interlocking. Ph.D. Dissertation, University of Aarhus, Aarhus, Denmark, 2010.
98. Hu, A.; Li, R.; Bai, S.; Yu, Y.; Zhou, W.; Bridges, D.; Deng, Y.; Zhang, L. *Introduction to Laser Micro-to-Nano Manufacturing*; Springer: Singapore, 2020; pp. 1–74.
99. Wellershoff, S.-S.; Hohlfeld, J.; Güdde, J.; Matthias, E. The role of electron-phonon coupling in femtosecond laser damage of metals. *Appl. Phys. A* **1999**, *69*, S99–S107. [CrossRef]
100. Liu, J.; Deng, C.; Bai, S. Glass surface metal deposition with high-power femtosecond fiber laser. *Appl. Phys. A* **2016**, *122*, 1064. [CrossRef]
101. Ebert, R. Laser Processing of Tungsten Powder with Femtosecond Laser Radiation. *J. Laser Micro/Nanoeng.* **2012**, *7*, 38–43. [CrossRef]
102. Phillips, K.C.; Gandhi, H.H.; Mazur, E.; Sundaram, S.K. Ultrafast laser processing of materials: A review. *Adv. Opt. Photonics* **2015**, *7*, 684–712. [CrossRef]
103. Key Parameters of a Laser System, EDMUND Opt. (n.d.) Available online: https://www.edmundoptics.com/knowledge-center/application-notes/lasers/key-parameters-of-a-laser-system/ (accessed on 25 November 2021).
104. Zhang, B.; Li, Y.; Bai, Q. Defect Formation Mechanisms in Selective Laser Melting: A Review. *Chin. J. Mech. Eng.* **2017**, *30*, 515–527. [CrossRef]
105. Wang, L.; Wei, Q.; He, W.; Shi, Y. Influence of powder characteristic and process parameters on SLM formability. *J. HuaZhong Univ. Sci. Technol. (Nat. Sci. Ed.)* **2012**, *2*. [CrossRef]
106. Lindgren, L.-E.; Lundbäck, A. Approaches in computational welding mechanics applied to additive manufacturing: Review and outlook. *Comptes Rendus Mécanique* **2018**, *346*, 1033–1042. [CrossRef]
107. Francois, M.; Sun, A.; King, W.; Henson, N.; Tourret, D.; Bronkhorst, C.; Carlson, N.; Newman, C.; Haut, T.; Bakosi, J.; et al. Modeling of additive manufacturing processes for metals: Challenges and opportunities. *Curr. Opin. Solid State Mater. Sci.* **2017**, *21*, 198–206. [CrossRef]
108. Liu, J.; Jalalahmadi, B.; Guo, Y.; Sealy, M.P.; Bolander, N. A review of computational modeling in powder-based additive manufacturing for metallic part qualification. *Rapid Prototyp. J.* **2018**, *24*, 1245–1264. [CrossRef]
109. Wang, G.-X.; Prasad, V. Microscale heat and mass transfer and non-equilibrium phase change in rapid solidification. *Mater. Sci. Eng. A* **2000**, *292*, 142–148. [CrossRef]
110. Hopkins, J.-M.; Sibbett, W. Ultrashort-pulse lasers: Big payoffs in a flash. *Sci. Am.* **2000**, *283*, 72–79. [CrossRef]
111. Momma, C.; Chichkov, B.; Nolte, S.; von Alvensleben, F.; Tünnermann, A.; Welling, H.; Wellegehausen, B. Short-pulse laser ablation of solid targets. *Opt. Commun.* **1996**, *129*, 134–142. [CrossRef]
112. Zhang, Y.; Tzou, D.Y.; Chen, J.K. Micro-and nanoscale heat transfer in femtosecond laser processing of metals. *arXiv* **2015**, arXiv:1511.03566. Available online: https://arxiv.org/abs/1511.03566 (accessed on 25 November 2021).
113. Hirayama, Y.; Obara, M. Heat-affected zone of metals ablated with femtosecond laser pulses. In *Photon Processing in Microelectronics and Photonics II*; Proc. of SPIE: San Jose, CA, USA, 2003; pp. 417–425.
114. Hohlfeld, J.; Wellershoff, S.-S.; Güdde, J.; Conrad, U.; Jähnke, V.; Matthias, E. Electron and lattice dynamics following optical excitation of metals. *Chem. Phys.* **2000**, *251*, 237–258. [CrossRef]
115. Chowdhury, I.H.; Xu, X. Heat transfer in femtosecond laser processing of metal. *Numer. Heat Transf. Part A Appl.* **2003**, *44*, 219–232. [CrossRef]
116. Ji, P.; Zhang, Y. Multiscale modeling of femtosecond laser irradiation on a copper film with electron thermal conductivity from ab initio calculation. *Numer. Heat Transf. Part A Appl.* **2017**, *71*, 128–136. [CrossRef]
117. Povarnitsyn, M.; Fokin, V.B.; Levashov, P.R. Microscopic and macroscopic modeling of femtosecond laser ablation of metals. *Appl. Surf. Sci.* **2015**, *357*, 1150–1156. [CrossRef]
118. Perez, D.; Lewis, L.J. Molecular-dynamics study of ablation of solids under femtosecond laser pulses. *Phys. Rev. B* **2003**, *67*, 184102. [CrossRef]
119. Colombier, J.P.; Combis, P.; Bonneau, F.; Le Harzic, R.; Audouard, E. Hydrodynamic simulations of metal ablation by femtosecond laser irradiation. *Phys. Rev. B* **2005**, *71*, 165406. [CrossRef]
120. Rethfeld, B.; Ivanov, D.S.; E Garcia, M.; I Anisimov, S. Modelling ultrafast laser ablation. *J. Phys. D Appl. Phys.* **2017**, *50*, 193001. [CrossRef]
121. Anisimov, S.I.; Kapeliovich, B.L.; Perel-man, T.L. Electron emission from metal surfaces exposed to ultrashort laser pulses. *Zh. Eksp. Teor. Fiz* **1974**, *66*, 375–377.
122. Qiu, T.; Tien, C. Femtosecond laser heating of multi-layer metals—I. Analysis. *Int. J. Heat Mass Transf.* **1994**, *37*, 2789–2797. [CrossRef]
123. Qiu, T.Q.; Tien, C.L. Heat Transfer Mechanisms During Short-Pulse Laser Heating of Metals. *J. Heat Transf.* **1993**, *115*, 835–841. [CrossRef]

124. Abdelmalek, A.; Bedrane, Z.; Amara, E.-H.; Sotillo, B.; Bharadwaj, V.; Ramponi, R.; Eaton, S.M. Ablation of Copper Metal Films by Femtosecond Laser Multipulse Irradiation. *Appl. Sci.* **2018**, *8*, 1826. [CrossRef]
125. Lee, D.; Kannatey-Asibu, E. Numerical Analysis of Ultrashort Pulse Laser-Material Interaction Using ABAQUS. *J. Manuf. Sci. Eng.* **2009**, *131*, 021005. [CrossRef]
126. Lee, D.; Kannatey-Asibu, E. Numerical Analysis on the Feasibility of Laser Microwelding of Metals by Femtosecond Laser Pulses Using ABAQUS. *J. Manuf. Sci. Eng.* **2008**, *130*, 061014. [CrossRef]
127. Jiang, L.; Tsai, H.-L. An improved two-temperature model for metal thin film heating by femtosecond laser pulses. *Int. Congr. Appl. Lasers Electro-Opt.* **2004**, *2004*, M602. [CrossRef]
128. Davydov, R.; Antonov, V.; Angelina, M. Computer Simulation of Metal Ablation by Single and Multiple Ultrashort Laser Pulses. In *2018 IEEE International Conference on Electrical Engineering and Photonics (EExPolytech)*; IEEE: Piscataway, NJ, USA, 2018; pp. 236–239.
129. Dasallas, L.L.; Garcia, W.O. Numerical simulation of femtosecond pulsed laser ablation of copper for oblique angle of incidence through two-temperature model. *Mater. Res. Express* **2018**, *5*, 016518. [CrossRef]
130. Kuo, L.S.; Qiu, T. *Microscale Energy Transfer during Picosecond Laser Melting of Metal Films*; American Society of Mechanical Engineers: New York, NY, USA, 1996.
131. Fischer, P.; Karapatis, N.; Romano, V.; Glardon, R.; Weber, H. A model for the interaction of near-infrared laser pulses with metal powders in selective laser sintering. *Appl. Phys. A* **2002**, *74*, 467–474. [CrossRef]
132. Konrad, C.; Zhang, Y.; Shi, Y. Melting and resolidification of a subcooled metal powder particle subjected to nanosecond laser heating. *Int. J. Heat Mass Transf.* **2007**, *50*, 2236–2245. [CrossRef]
133. Cheng, C.-W.; Chang, C.-L.; Chen, J.-K.; Wang, B. Femtosecond laser melting of silver nanoparticles: Comparison of model simulations and experimental results. *Appl. Phys. A* **2018**, *124*, 371. [CrossRef]
134. Jia, X.; Zhao, X. Numerical study of material decomposition in ultrafast laser interaction with metals. *Appl. Surf. Sci.* **2019**, *463*, 781–790. [CrossRef]
135. Li, X.; Guan, Y. Theoretical fundamentals of short pulse laser–metal interaction: A review. *Nanotechnol. Precis. Eng.* **2020**, *3*, 105–125. [CrossRef]
136. Ji, P.; Zhang, Y. Melting and thermal ablation of a silver film induced by femtosecond laser heating: A multiscale modeling approach. *Appl. Phys. A* **2017**, *123*, 671. [CrossRef]
137. Wu, H.; Wu, C.; Zhang, N.; Zhu, X.; Ma, X.; Zhigilei, L.V. Experimental and computational study of the effect of 1 atm background gas on nanoparticle generation in femtosecond laser ablation of metals. *Appl. Surf. Sci.* **2018**, *435*, 1114–1119. [CrossRef]
138. Kaden, L.; Seyfarth, B.; Ullsperger, T.; Matthäus, G.; Nolte, S. Selective laser melting of copper using ultrashort laser pulses at different wavelengths. In *Laser 3D Manufacturing V*; Proc. of SPIE: San Francisco, CA, USA, 2018; Volume 10523, p. 1052312.
139. Paeng, D.; Lee, D.; Yeo, J.; Yoo, J.-H.; Allen, F.I.; Kim, E.; So, H.; Park, H.K.; Minor, A.M.; Grigoropoulos, C. Laser-Induced Reductive Sintering of Nickel Oxide Nanoparticles under Ambient Conditions. *J. Phys. Chem. C* **2015**, *119*, 6363–6372. [CrossRef]
140. Kang, B.; Han, S.; Kim, J.; Ko, S.; Yang, M. One-Step Fabrication of Copper Electrode by Laser-Induced Direct Local Reduction and Agglomeration of Copper Oxide Nanoparticle. *J. Phys. Chem. C* **2011**, *115*, 23664–23670. [CrossRef]
141. Jiang, Q.; Zhang, P.; Yu, Z.; Shi, H.; Wu, D.; Yan, H.; Ye, X.; Lu, Q.; Tian, Y. A Review on Additive Manufacturing of Pure Copper. *Coatings* **2021**, *11*, 740. [CrossRef]
142. Roy, N.; Dibua, O.; Foong, C.S.; Cullinan, M. Preliminary Results on the Fabrication of Interconnect Structures Using Microscale Selective Laser Sintering. In *ASME 2017 International Technical Conference and Exhibition on Packaging and Integration of Electronic and Photonic Microsystems*; American Society of Mechanical Engineers: New York, NY, USA, 2017.
143. Singer, F.; Deisenroth, D.C.; Hymas, D.M.; Ohadi, M.M. Additively manufactured copper components and composite structures for thermal management applications. In Proceedings of the 2017 16th IEEE Intersociety Conference on Thermal and Thermomechanical Phenomena in Electronic Systems (ITherm), Orlando, FL, USA, 30 May–2 June 2017; IEEE: Piscataway, NJ, USA, 2017; pp. 174–183.
144. Pogson, S.; Fox, P.; Sutcliffe, C.; O'Neill, W. The production of copper parts using DMLR. *Rapid Prototyp. J.* **2003**, *9*, 334–343. [CrossRef]
145. Sciammarella, F.; Gonser, M.J.; Styrcula, M. Laser Additive Manufacturing of Pure Copper. In Proceedings of the SME RAPID Conference and Exposition, Dearborn, MI, USA, 10–13 June 2013; Volume 71, pp. 1241–1248.
146. Gradl, P.R.; Protz, C.S.; Cooper, K.; Ellis, D.; Evans, L.J.; Garcia, C. GRCop-42 Development and Hot-fire Testing Using Additive Manufacturing Powder Bed Fusion for Channel-cooled Combustion Chambers. In Proceedings of the AIAA Propulsion and Energy 2019 Forum, Indianapolis, IN, USA, 19–22 August 2019. [CrossRef]
147. Polozov, I.A.; Borisov, E.V.; Sufiiarov, V.S.; Popovich, A.A. Selective laser melting of copper alloy. *Mater. Phys. Mech.* **2020**, *43*, 65–71. [CrossRef]
148. Colopi, M.; Caprio, L.; Demir, A.; Previtali, B. Selective laser melting of pure Cu with a 1 kW single mode fiber laser. *Procedia CIRP* **2018**, *74*, 59–63. [CrossRef]
149. Roy, N.; Jou, W.; Feng, H.; Jeong, J.; Wang, Y.; Cullinan, M. Laser Sintering of Copper Nanoparticles: A Simplified Model for Fluence Estimation and Validation. In *International Manufacturing Science and Engineering Conference*; American Society of Mechanical Engineers: New York, NY, USA, 2017.

150. Roy, N.K.; Dibua, O.G.; Jou, W.; He, F.; Jeong, J.; Wang, Y.; Cullinan, M.A. A Comprehensive Study of the Sintering of Copper Nanoparticles Using Femtosecond, Nanosecond, and Continuous Wave Lasers. *J. Micro Nano-Manuf.* **2017**, *6*, 010903. [CrossRef]
151. Lim, J.; Kim, Y.; Shin, J.; Lee, Y.; Shin, W.; Qu, W.; Hwang, E.; Park, S.; Hong, S. Continuous-Wave Laser-Induced Transfer of Metal Nanoparticles to Arbitrary Polymer Substrates. *Nanomaterials* **2020**, *10*, 701. [CrossRef]
152. Mizoshiri, M.; Yoshidomi, K. Cu Patterning Using Femtosecond Laser Reductive Sintering of CuO Nanoparticles under Inert Gas Injection. *Materials* **2021**, *14*, 3285. [CrossRef]
153. Le Harzic, R.; Huot, N.; Audouard, E.; Jonin, C.; Laporte, P.; Valette, S.; Fraczkiewicz, A.; Fortunier, R. Comparison of heat-affected zones due to nanosecond and femtosecond laser pulses using transmission electronic microscopy. *Appl. Phys. Lett.* **2002**, *80*, 3886–3888. [CrossRef]
154. Mizoshiri, M.; Nishitani, K.; Hata, S. Effect of Heat Accumulation on Femtosecond Laser Reductive Sintering of Mixed CuO/NiO Nanoparticles. *Micromachines* **2018**, *9*, 264. [CrossRef] [PubMed]
155. Constantin, L.; Wu, Z.; Li, N.; Fan, L.; Silvain, J.F.; Lu, Y.F. Laser 3D printing of complex copper structures. *Addit. Manuf.* **2020**, *35*, 101268. [CrossRef]
156. Mizoshiri, M.; Kondo, Y. Direct writing of Cu-based fine micropatterns using femtosecond laser pulse-induced sintering of Cu2O nanospheres. *Jpn. J. Appl. Phys.* **2019**, *58*, SDDF05. [CrossRef]
157. Mizoshiri, M.; Kondo, Y. Direct writing of two- and three-dimensional Cu-based microstructures by femtosecond laser reductive sintering of the Cu_2O nanospheres. *Opt. Mater. Express* **2019**, *9*, 2828–2837. [CrossRef]
158. Mizoshiri, M.; Tanokuchi, A. Direct writing of Cu-based micropatterns inside Cu_2O nanosphere films using green femtosecond laser reductive sintering. *Opt. Mater. Express* **2020**, *10*, 2533–2541. [CrossRef]
159. Tan, C.; Zhou, K.; Ma, W.; Attard, B.; Zhang, P.; Kuang, T. Selective laser melting of high-performance pure tungsten: Parameter design, densification behavior and mechanical properties. *Sci. Technol. Adv. Mater.* **2018**, *19*, 370–380. [CrossRef]
160. Li, J.; Wu, Y.; Zhou, B.; Wei, Z. Laser Powder Bed Fusion of Pure Tungsten: Effects of Process Parameters on Morphology, Densification, Microstructure. *Materials* **2020**, *14*, 165. [CrossRef]
161. Iveković, A.; Omidvari, N.; Vrancken, B.; Lietaert, K.; Thijs, L.; Vanmeensel, K.; Vleugels, J.; Kruth, J.-P. Selective laser melting of tungsten and tungsten alloys. *Int. J. Refract. Met. Hard Mater.* **2018**, *72*, 27–32. [CrossRef]
162. Selective Laser Melting (AM), Wolfmet. (n.d.) Available online: https://www.wolfmet.com/applications/slm/selective-laser-melting-tungsten/ (accessed on 25 November 2021).
163. Hirai, T.; Escourbiac, F.; Carpentier-Chouchana, S.; Fedosov, A.; Ferrand, L.; Jokinen, T.; Komarov, V.; Kukushkin, A.; Merola, M.; Mitteau, R.; et al. ITER tungsten divertor design development and qualification program. *Fusion Eng. Des.* **2013**, *88*, 1798–1801. [CrossRef]
164. Müller, A.V.; Schlick, G.; Neu, R.; Anstätt, C.; Klimkait, T.; Lee, J.; Pascher, B.; Schmitt, M.; Seidel, C. Additive manufacturing of pure tungsten by means of selective laser beam melting with substrate preheating temperatures up to 1000 °C. *Nucl. Mater. Energy* **2019**, *19*, 184–188. [CrossRef]
165. Ghosh, S.K.; Das, A.K.; Saha, P. Selective Laser Sintering: A Case Study of Tungsten Carbide and Cobalt Powder Sintering by Pulsed Nd:YAG Laser. *Funct. Graded Mater.* **2015**, 441–459. [CrossRef]
166. Wang, D.; Yu, C.; Zhou, X.; Ma, J.; Liu, W.; Shen, Z. Dense Pure Tungsten Fabricated by Selective Laser Melting. *Appl. Sci.* **2017**, *7*, 430. [CrossRef]
167. Zacharatos, F.; Theodorakos, I.; Karvounis, P.; Tuohy, S.; Braz, N.; Melamed, S.; Kabla, A.; De La Vega, F.; Andritsos, K.; Hatziapostolou, A.; et al. Selective Laser Sintering of Laser Printed Ag Nanoparticle Micropatterns at High Repetition Rates. *Materials* **2018**, *11*, 2142. [CrossRef] [PubMed]
168. Khosravani, M.R.; Reinicke, T. 3D-printed sensors: Current progress and future challenges. *Sens. Actuators A Phys.* **2020**, *305*, 111916. [CrossRef]
169. Courbat, J.; Kim, Y.; Briand, D.; De Rooij, N. Inkjet printing on paper for the realization of humidity and temperature sensors. In Proceedings of the 2011 16th International Solid-State Sensors, Actuators and Microsystems Conference, Beijing, China, 5–9 June 2011; pp. 1356–1359. [CrossRef]
170. Dankoco, M.; Tesfay, G.; Benevent, E.; Bendahan, M. Temperature sensor realized by inkjet printing process on flexible substrate. *Mater. Sci. Eng. B* **2016**, *205*, 1–5. [CrossRef]
171. Hong, S.; Yeo, J.; Kim, G.; Kim, D.; Lee, H.; Kwon, J.; Lee, H.; Lee, P.; Ko, S.H. Nonvacuum, Maskless Fabrication of a Flexible Metal Grid Transparent Conductor by Low-Temperature Selective Laser Sintering of Nanoparticle Ink. *ACS Nano* **2013**, *7*, 5024–5031. [CrossRef]
172. Noh, J.; Kim, D. Femtosecond laser sintering of silver nanoparticles for conductive thin-film fabrication. *Appl. Phys. A* **2020**, *126*, 1–7. [CrossRef]
173. Noh, J.; Ha, J.; Kim, D. Femtosecond and nanosecond laser sintering of silver nanoparticles on a flexible substrate. *Appl. Surf. Sci.* **2020**, *511*, 145574. [CrossRef]
174. Son, Y.; Lim, T.W.; Yeo, J.; Ko, S.H.; Yang, D.-Y. Fabrication of Nano-scale Conductors by Selective Femtosecond Laser Sintering of Metal Nanoparticles. In Proceedings of the 10th IEEE International Conference on Nanotechnology, Ilsan, Korea, 17–20 August 2010; IEEE: Piscataway, NJ, USA, 2010; pp. 390–393.
175. Son, Y.; Yeo, J.; Moon, H.; Lim, T.W.; Hong, S.; Nam, K.H.; Yoo, S.; Grigoropoulos, C.P.; Yang, D.-Y.; Ko, S.H. Nanoscale Electronics: Digital Fabrication by Direct Femtosecond Laser Processing of Metal Nanoparticles. *Adv. Mater.* **2011**, *23*, 3176–3181. [CrossRef]

176. Kimura, T.; Nakamoto, T. Thermal and Mechanical Properties of Commercial-Purity Aluminum Fabricated Using Selective Laser Melting. *Mater. Trans.* **2017**, *58*, 799–805. [CrossRef]
177. Manfredi, D.; Calignano, F.; Krishnan, M.; Canali, R.; Paola, E.; Biamino, S.; Ugues, D.; Pavese, M.; Fino, P. Additive Manufacturing of Al Alloys and Aluminium Matrix Composites (AMCs). In *Light Metal Alloys Applications*; InTech: Rijeka, Croatia, 2014.
178. DebRoy, T.; Wei, H.L.; Zuback, J.S.; Mukherjee, T.; Elmer, J.W.; Milewski, J.O.; Beese, A.M.; Wilson-Heid, A.; De, A.; Zhang, W. Additive manufacturing of metallic components–Process, structure and properties. *Prog. Mater. Sci.* **2018**, *92*, 112–224. [CrossRef]
179. Kannan, C.S.; Chandra, S.S.S.; Krishnan, G.P.; Raj, S.P. *A Review on Additive Manufacturing of AA2024 and AA6061 Alloys Using Powder Bed Fusion*; IOP Publishing: Bristol, UK, 2020; Volume 988, p. 012002.
180. Louvis, E.; Fox, P.; Sutcliffe, C.J. Selective laser melting of aluminium components. *J. Mater. Process. Technol.* **2011**, *211*, 275–284. [CrossRef]
181. Lassance, D.; Fabregue, D.; Delannay, F.; Pardoen, T. Micromechanics of room and high temperature fracture in 6xxx Al alloys. *Prog. Mater. Sci.* **2007**, *52*, 62–129. [CrossRef]
182. Grigoriev, S.N.; Tarasova, T.V.; Gvozdeva, G.O.; Nowotny, S. Structure Formation of Hypereutectic Al-Si-Alloys Produced by Laser Surface Treatment. *Stroj. Vestn.-J. Mech. Eng.* **2014**, *60*, 389–394. [CrossRef]
183. Ullsperger, T.; Liu, D.; Yürekli, B.; Matthäus, G.; Schade, L.; Seyfarth, B.; Kohl, H.; Ramm, R.; Rettenmayr, M.; Nolte, S. Ultra-short pulsed laser powder bed fusion of Al-Si alloys: Impact of pulse duration and energy in comparison to continuous wave excitation. *Addit. Manuf.* **2021**, *46*, 102085. [CrossRef]
184. Dinçel, Y.M. Bone Graft Types. In *Bone Grafting-Recent Advances with Special References to Cranio-Maxillofacial Surgery*; IntechOpen: London, UK, 2018; pp. 27–40.
185. Shivalkar, S.; Singh, S. Solid Freeform Techniques Application in Bone Tissue Engineering for Scaffold Fabrication. *Tissue Eng. Regen. Med.* **2017**, *14*, 187–200. [CrossRef]
186. Duan, B.; Wang, M. Selective laser sintering and its application in biomedical engineering. *MRS Bull.* **2011**, *36*, 998–1005. [CrossRef]
187. Tan, K.; Chua, C.; Leong, K.; Cheah, C.; Cheang, P.; Abu Bakar, M.; Cha, S. Scaffold development using selective laser sintering of polyetheretherketone–hydroxyapatite biocomposite blends. *Biomaterials* **2003**, *24*, 3115–3123. [CrossRef]
188. Masaud, Z.; Khan, M.Z.; Hussain, A.; Ishfaq, H.A.; Song, R.-H.; Lee, S.-B.; Joh, D.W.; Lim, T.-H. Recent Activities of Solid Oxide Fuel Cell Research in the 3D Printing Processes. *Trans. Korean Hydrog. New Energy Soc.* **2021**, *32*, 11–40. [CrossRef]
189. Tai, X.Y.; Zhakeyev, A.; Wang, H.; Jiao, K.; Zhang, H.; Xuan, J. Accelerating Fuel Cell Development with Additive Manufacturing Technologies: State of the Art, Opportunities and Challenges. *Fuel Cells* **2019**, *19*, 636–650. [CrossRef]
190. Pesce, A.; Hornés, A.; Núñez, M.; Morata, A.; Torrell, M.; Tarancón, A. 3D printing the next generation of enhanced solid oxide fuel and electrolysis cells. *J. Mater. Chem. A* **2020**, *8*, 16926–16932. [CrossRef]
191. Bai, S.; Liu, J. Femtosecond Laser Additive Manufacturing of Multi-Material Layered Structures. *Appl. Sci.* **2020**, *10*, 979. [CrossRef]
192. Liu, J.; Bai, S. Femtosecond laser additive manufacturing of YSZ. *Appl. Phys. A* **2017**, *123*, 293. [CrossRef]
193. Furuta, T. Automobile applications of titanium. In *Titanium for Consumer Applications*; Elsevier: Amsterdam, The Netherlands, 2019; pp. 77–90. [CrossRef]
194. Singh, N.; Hameed, P.; Ummethala, R.; Manivasagam, G.; Prashanth, K.; Eckert, J. Selective laser manufacturing of Ti-based alloys and composites: Impact of process parameters, application trends, and future prospects. *Mater. Today Adv.* **2020**, *8*, 100097. [CrossRef]
195. Agius, D.J.; Kourousis, K.I.; Wallbrink, C. A Review of the As-Built SLM Ti-6Al-4V Mechanical Properties towards Achieving Fatigue Resistant Designs. *Metals* **2018**, *8*, 75. [CrossRef]
196. Vorobyev, A.Y.; Guo, C. Femtosecond laser structuring of titanium implants. *Appl. Surf. Sci.* **2007**, *253*, 7272–7280. [CrossRef]
197. Löw, K.; Leong, K.F.; Sun, C. Review of Selective Laser Melting process parameters for Commercially Pure Titanium and Ti6Al4V. In *High Value Manufacturing: Advanced Research in Virtual and Rapid Prototyping*; CRC Press: Boca Raton, FL, USA, 2013; pp. 71–76.
198. Kumbhar, N.N.; Mulay, A.V. Post Processing Methods used to Improve Surface Finish of Products which are Manufactured by Additive Manufacturing Technologies: A Review. *J. Inst. Eng. India Ser. C* **2018**, *99*, 481–487. [CrossRef]
199. Jiao, L.; Chua, Z.Y.; Moon, S.K.; Song, J.; Bi, G.; Zheng, H. Femtosecond Laser Produced Hydrophobic Hierarchical Structures on Additive Manufacturing Parts. *Nanomaterials* **2018**, *8*, 601. [CrossRef]
200. Worts, N.; Jones, J.; Squier, J. Surface structure modification of additively manufactured titanium components via femtosecond laser micromachining. *Opt. Commun.* **2019**, *430*, 352–357. [CrossRef]
201. Cheng, C.W.; Huang, C.J.; Cheng, H.T.; Kuo, C.N. Fabrication of porous Ti structures with nanostructures from Ti powders by femtosecond laser pulses. *J. Laser Micro Nanoeng.* **2015**, *10*, 310. [CrossRef]
202. Hammouti, S.; Holybee, B.; Zhu, W.; Allain, J.P.; Jurczyk, B.; Ruzic, D.N. Titanium nitride formation by a dual-stage femtosecond laser process. *Appl. Phys. A* **2018**, *124*, 411. [CrossRef]
203. Sugioka, K.; Cheng, Y. Femtosecond laser three-dimensional micro- and nanofabrication. *Appl. Phys. Rev.* **2014**, *1*, 041303. [CrossRef]
204. Han, T.-H.; Kim, H.; Kwon, S.-J.; Lee, T.-W. Graphene-based flexible electronic devices. *Mater. Sci. Eng. R Rep.* **2017**, *118*, 1–43. [CrossRef]

205. You, R.; Liu, Y.; Hao, Y.; Han, D.; Zhang, Y.; You, Z. Laser Fabrication of Graphene-Based Flexible Electronics. *Adv. Mater.* **2020**, *32*, e1901981. [CrossRef]
206. Liu, Y.-Q.; Chen, Z.-D.; Mao, J.-W.; Han, D.-D.; Sun, X. Laser Fabrication of Graphene-Based Electronic Skin. *Front. Chem.* **2019**, *7*, 461. [CrossRef] [PubMed]
207. Li, Y.; Feng, Z.; Huang, L.; Essa, K.; Bilotti, E.; Zhang, H.; Peijs, T.; Hao, L. Additive manufacturing high performance graphene-based composites: A review. *Compos. Part A Appl. Sci. Manuf.* **2019**, *124*, 105483. [CrossRef]
208. Chen, Q.; Mangadlao, J.D.; Wallat, J.; De Leon, A.; Pokorski, J.K.; Advincula, R.C. 3D Printing Biocompatible Polyurethane/Poly(lactic acid)/Graphene Oxide Nanocomposites: Anisotropic Properties. *ACS Appl. Mater. Interfaces* **2017**, *9*, 4015–4023. [CrossRef] [PubMed]
209. Fu, X.-Y.; Chen, Z.-D.; Han, D.-D.; Zhang, Y.-L.; Xia, H.; Sun, H.-B. Laser fabrication of graphene-based supercapacitors. *Photonics Res.* **2020**, *8*, 577. [CrossRef]
210. Bi, Y.-G.; Feng, J.; Li, Y.-F.; Zhang, Y.-L.; Liu, Y.-S.; Chen, L.; Liu, Y.-F.; Guo, L.; Wei, S.; Sun, H.-B. Arbitrary Shape Designable Microscale Organic Light-Emitting Devices by Using Femtosecond Laser Reduced Graphene Oxide as a Patterned Electrode. *ACS Photonics* **2014**, *1*, 690–695. [CrossRef]
211. An, J.; Le, T.-S.D.; Huang, Y.; Zhan, Z.; Li, Y.; Zheng, L.; Huang, W.; Sun, G.; Kim, Y.-J. All-Graphene-Based Highly Flexible Noncontact Electronic Skin. *ACS Appl. Mater. Interfaces* **2017**, *9*, 44593–44601. [CrossRef]
212. Wang, D.-Y.; Tao, L.-Q.; Liu, Y.; Zhang, T.-Y.; Pang, Y.; Wang, Q.; Jiang, S.; Yang, Y.; Ren, T.-L. High performance flexible strain sensor based on self-locked overlapping graphene sheets. *Nanoscale* **2016**, *8*, 20090–20095. [CrossRef] [PubMed]
213. Qiao, Y.; Wang, Y.; Tian, H.; Li, M.; Jian, J.; Wei, Y.; Tian, Y.; Wang, D.-Y.; Pang, Y.; Geng, X.; et al. Multilayer Graphene Epidermal Electronic Skin. *ACS Nano* **2018**, *12*, 8839–8846. [CrossRef]

quantum beam science

Review

Making Light Work of Metal Bending: Laser Forming in Rapid Prototyping

Adam L. Bachmann [1,2], Michael D. Dickey [2] and Nathan Lazarus [3,*]

1 Fellowship Program at US Army Research Laboratory, Oak Ridge Associated Universities (ORAU), Adelphi, MD 20783, USA; abachma@ncsu.edu
2 Department of Chemical and Biomolecular Engineering, North Carolina State University, Raleigh, NC 27603, USA; mddickey@ncsu.edu
3 Sensors and Electron Devices Directorate, US Army Research Laboratory, Adelphi, MD 20783, USA
* Correspondence: nathan.lazarus2.civ@mail.mil

Received: 18 November 2020; Accepted: 10 December 2020; Published: 14 December 2020

Abstract: Lasers can be used to bend 2D metal sheets into complex 3D objects in a process called 'laser forming.' Laser forming bends metal sheets by locally heating the sheets to generate plastic strains and is an established metal bending technology in the shipbuilding industry. Recent studies have investigated the laser forming of thin metal parts as a complementary rapid prototyping technology to metal 3D printing. This review discusses the laser forming process, beginning with the mechanisms before covering various design considerations. Laser forming for the rapid manufacturing of metal parts is then reviewed, including the recent advances in process planning, before highlighting promising future research directions.

Keywords: laser forming; rapid prototyping; self-folding origami; metal bending

1. Introduction

Fabricating complex 3D structures is a difficult task, as many materials and processes are inherently 2D. Flat structures need to be carefully assembled to produce the desired 3D shape, whether a ship, an automobile, or a solar array. One of the oldest ways to produce 3D structures from flat objects is origami, the Japanese art of paper folding [1,2]. Origami principles can apply to other sheets of material, often with the goal of assembling the final 3D structure far from the point of production of the 2D pattern [3–5].

Researchers have developed algorithms to achieve complex 3D shapes from 2D fold patterns [6]. These algorithms are not limited to paper, although the algorithms typically neglect the effect of substrate thickness and, thus, work best on materials that are thin and inextensible, like paper. Oftentimes, the desired structures need to be made of materials that have a non-negligible thickness [7,8]. Folding rigid materials is typically done by attaching rigid facets with compliant hinges [9], but this places restrictions on what can be produced, a term called rigid foldability [10]. One of the most common rigid folding patterns is the Miura-ora pattern (Figure 1a,b), as it allows large area structures to be compactly stored before deployment, which is valuable for space applications [5,7,11,12]. In many applications, actuation (folding) is done manually (Figure 1c,d) [13]; however, researchers are exploring ways to create hinges that fold in response to external stimuli (e.g., light, electricity, heat, moisture), allowing for self-folding (Figure 1e) [3,14–17].

Origami manufacturing using computational design algorithms is a relatively new method for rapid prototyping. Rapid prototyping is defined as the direct translation of computer aided design (CAD) files into 3D objects, with 3D printing the most common approach [18]. Three-dimensional printing is a popular technology that additively builds objects through the layered deposition of material [19,20]. 3D printing allows highly customized metal parts to be fabricated with minimal waste (Figure 1f), making it an attractive technology for 'mass customization' [21]. Many metal 3D printing methods use a focused energy beam (laser or electron beam) to fuse metal powders together, building the part layer by layer, but the process is long and has a limited build volume [20,22,23] and metal 3D printers are also relatively expensive (to the order of hundreds of thousands of dollars for a commercial printer) [23]. The unfused powder acts a support, allowing pieces to be built with moderate overhangs, but sharp bends remain challenging [23], as well as thin shells [24]. Origami folding, which allows rapid and cheap creation of 3D shells of material, is therefore an important complementary technology, well-suited for many devices, such as antennas, waveguides, and other systems that rely on thin layers of metal. Thin metal sheets are easy to bend, and overhangs can be generated with almost any degree of bend angle, enabling the production of complex shapes with simple folds and cuts (Figure 1g).

Successful metal origami requires precise control over the bending of the sheets of metal. There are multiple ways to bend metal, the most common methods use expensive equipment, such as press brakes (Figure 2a), or roll formers (Figure 2b) [25–27]. Press brakes involves placing the sheet metal over a shaped die and then applying intense mechanical pressure to force the metal into the die. Roll forming involves the gradual bending of the sheet metal by passing through successively narrower rollers. Both processes rely on mechanically deforming the sheet, which leads to a spring-back effect that causes the final bend angle to differ from the dies and rollers, as a result of residual elastic strains after the mechanical pressure is removed [28–31]. Proper control for spring-break often involves extensive testing of how the brakes and substrates interact [29]. A change of design shape or material means this testing would need to be repeated, making this a poor choice for rapid prototyping.

Another method of metal bending involves thermal stress-induced bending called line heating [34]. Line heating uses a gas torch to carefully heat a piece of metal followed by cooling the part rapidly in water to generate plastic strains that bend the metal. This process, unlike press break forming, is highly labor intensive. Line heating also depends on the craftsmanship of the bender, since the gas torch is a diffuse heat source, which can lead to large heat-affected zones and degraded material properties [35]. Aiming to automate this process, researchers suggested replacing the skill of a bender and flame torches with the highly controllable heat of a laser [35]. The process is similar to line forming, but uses lasers to localize the heating. Thus, these early researchers called this process 'laser forming' [36,37].

Laser forming is defined as the use of a laser beam to locally heat and introduce thermal stresses to plastically deform a work piece [38]. The interaction of a laser beam and a substrate generates localized thermal gradients (Figure 2c) [36,37] that cause unequal material expansions. The thermal expansions generate stresses large enough to cause the heated material to yield, generating plastic response stresses [39,40]. As the piece cools, the scanned area returns to its normal size and stops straining the surrounding material, but the compressive stresses remain leading to a permanent deformation in the substrate without a spring-back effect [37]. Laser forming consists of several related mechanisms, and is most commonly used for bending but can also be used for shortening/adjusting a work piece [41,42].

While this review uses the term "laser forming" for thermal metal forming processes, as accepted in the related research community, we want to address potential confusion in terminology. Another technique also used for laser bending is laser peen forming (also known as laser shock forming). In laser peen forming (Figure 2d), a short-pulsed laser is focused on a sacrificial coating on top of the workpiece [43]. When the coating ablates, it generates a plasma plume that attempts to expand in all directions [43]. The laser peen forming setup confines this expanding plume, usually with a layer of water, and redirects this energy as a shockwave into the workpiece, leading to bending [43]. This process is entirely mechanical and, thus, susceptible to the similar drawbacks of more conventional fabrication. A recent review of the field can be found elsewhere [44], and this approach will not be covered further here. The term 'laser forming' has also been used by researchers in reference to other technologies based on producing (i.e., forming) a material with a laser, including powder bed fusion [45], or laser metal cladding (Figure 2e) [46]. Both techniques use a laser to selectively heat metal powders, causing them to coalesce, but 'laser forming' is not the preferred terminology in those fields.

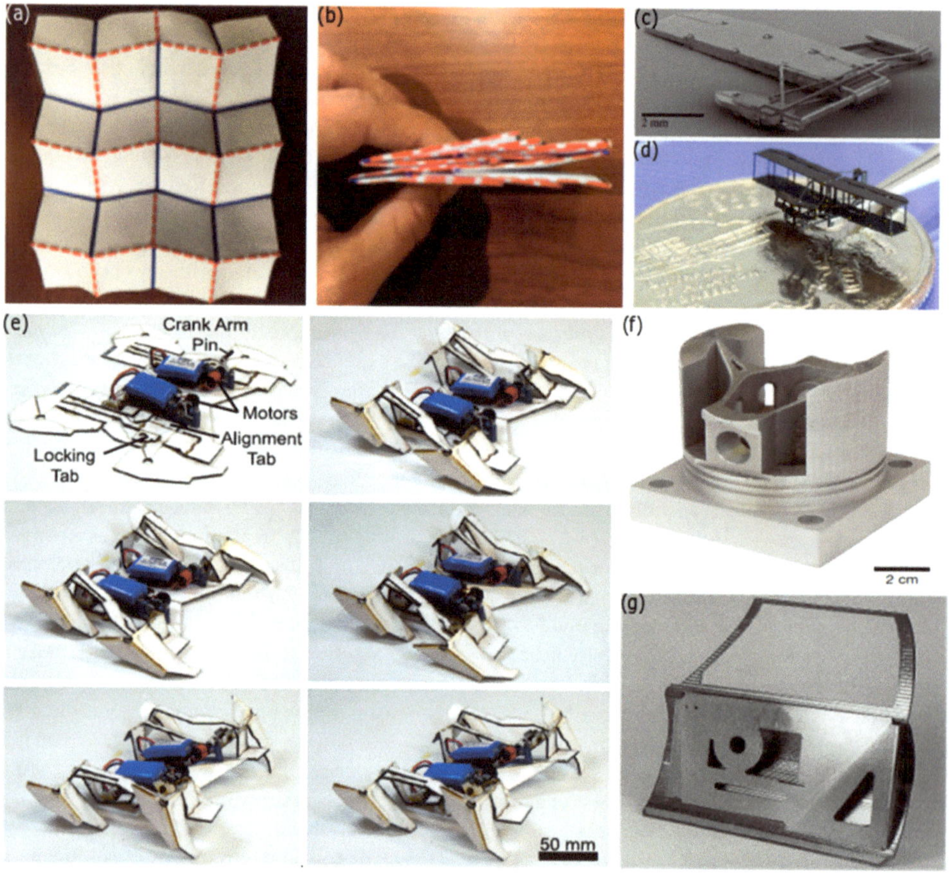

Figure 1. Complex 3D origami requires fold patterns such as the Miura-ori, which compresses a (**a**) large sheet in the unfolded sheet into a (**b**) compact folded state [1]. Copyright SAGE publications, 2016. Origami principles can be used to produce complex structures. A (**c**) folded microelectromechanical systems (MEMS) structure becomes a (**d**) scale replica of the Wright flyer once the unfolding is complete [13]. © IOP Publishing. Reproduced with permission. All rights reserved. Self-folding (**e**) has been used to produce crawling robots from flat sheets [3]. Reprinted with permission from AAAS. Rapid prototyping of metallic 3D structures can be done with (**f**) 3D printing [32]. Reprinted with permission from Springer Nature, copyright 2017. Metal products can also be formed by the (**g**) laser forming of sheet metal [33]. Reproduced with permission from Emerald Publishing, copyright 1997.

Laser forming was first developed in the 1980s [35], and much of the early research was focused on understanding the complex interaction between the laser and the material properties with a goal of developing formulas that can accurately predict the final bend angle [37,48,49]. A number of studies now exist on modelling of laser forming, including a notable review [38], so we refrain from focusing on these research efforts here. Instead, we aim to survey laser forming as a rapid prototyping strategy for developing 3D structures from flat substrates. The most recent review focusing on the manufacturing applications of laser forming is almost two decades old [50], and there have been many advances in the field since then.

This review of laser forming begins with a discussion of the three dominant sub-mechanisms of laser forming, before discussing how to select appropriate process parameters to achieve a desired bend shape. We then survey the application space of laser forming, from larger scale fabrication to smaller scale rapid prototyping and adjustment, before providing an outlook on current challenges and unresolved problems in the field.

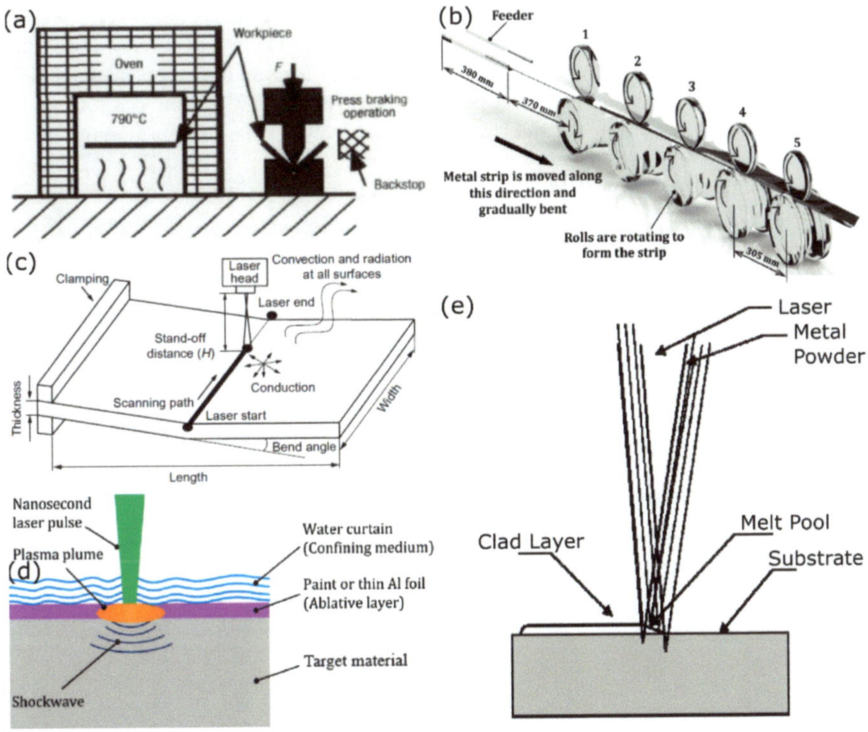

Figure 2. Common metal forming techniques include (**a**) press brake forming [27] over dies to produce sharp bends. Brittle materials, such as titanium, require a preheating step to exceed the ductile-brittle transition temperature, so they can be bent without breaking. Reprinted with permission of Elsevier, copyright 2000. Long sheets of metal can be (**b**) roll formed [31] to generate pieces with a constant cross-section. Reprinted with permission of Elsevier, copyright 2000. Laser forming is term that is commonly used to describe many processes, but is used in this review to refer to (**c**) the process by which a laser-induced thermal gradient generates plastic stresses in a workpiece that leads to a permanent deformation [47]. Reprinted with permission of Elsevier, copyright 2016 Some other process that are sometimes (erroneously) referred to as laser forming include (**d**) laser peen (shock) forming [44], where a laser-induced shockwave mechanically deforms a workpiece. Reprinted with permission of Elsevier, copyright 2018. Some author have also used laser forming to describe (**e**) laser metal cladding [46]. Reprinted with permission of Taylor and Francis, copyright 2000.

2. Laser Forming Mechanisms

Laser forming is a relatively broad term that refers to the plastic deformation of a workpiece resulting from laser-induced thermal stresses. From experimental studies and finite element modelling of laser forming, three main sub-mechanisms have been identified for understanding laser forming: the temperature gradient mechanism (TGM), the buckling mechanism (BM), and the upsetting (shortening) mechanism, (UM) [36–38]. All three mechanisms arise from plastic strains generated in the work piece as a result of the absorbed laser energy, but the dominance of one mechanism over the others depends on how that energy propagates in the work piece [51]. This energy propagation depends on the workpiece geometry and the lasing parameters.

2.1. Temperature Gradient Mechanism (TGM)

The temperature gradient mechanism is dominant when a thermal gradient is generated through the thickness of the work piece through laser heating [37]. This vertical gradient is achieved with a higher laser scan speed and a thicker substrate (or a thinner substrate with relatively poor thermal conductivity) [52]. The thickness of the material in the TGM case is typically on the order of the laser beam diameter [53,54]. For example, a researcher laser formed sheets between 0.5 and 4 mm thick, using a laser with a beam diameter of 5.2 mm travelling at 1.5 m/min [52]. Once the laser energy is absorbed by the surface of the metal, the temperature rises rapidly (Figure 3a). In most materials, the hotter areas expand, generating stresses on the cooler sections [55]. As the top of the workpiece is much hotter than the bottom, the top of the workpiece expands more than the bottom, leading to a small counter-bend (Figure 3b) away from the laser [38,52]. At these high temperatures, the mechanical properties, such as the Young's modulus, drop precipitously [56]. At these elevated temperatures, the thermal expansion stresses exceed the flow stress, which means the thermal stresses are large enough to maintain plastic deformation [36,39,40]. The work piece surrounding the thermally expanded portion is stiff and resists the expansion by exerting an equal compressive force [52,55]. Initially, the material bends away from the laser (the counter-bend), and is a consequence of the thermal expansion combined with the decreased yield stress of metals at higher temperatures [36]. Once the piece has time to cool, the material scanned by the laser returns to its normal volume, but the compressive stresses remain in the piece. Consequently, the laser scanned volume is under compression causing the work piece to develop a final bend angle, θ, toward the laser [36,50]. At the cooler temperatures, the mechanical properties return to their higher values which prevents the formation of new plastic stresses, so this bend angle is permanent [38,52,55]. The TGM mechanism, therefore, always results in a bend toward the laser source.

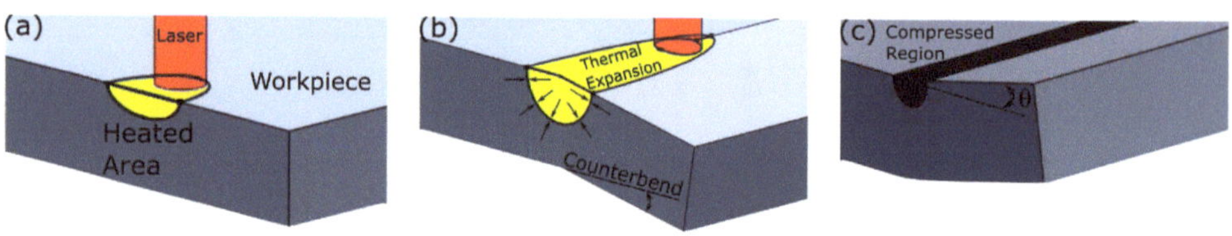

Figure 3. Schematic of the temperature gradient mechanism during the immediate laser exposure (**a**) showing the thermal gradient established through the thickness of the substrate, while (**b**) the thermal expansion causes a counter-bend that also generates plastic, compressive strains. After the laser has passed and the area locally cools, (**c**) the compressive forces remain, causing the substrate the bend toward the laser and generating a bend angle, θ.

2.2. Buckling Mechanism (BM)

The buckling mechanism also relies on a thermal gradient, but in this mechanism, the work piece is either thinner or has a high thermal conductivity relative to the laser scan speed [36]. The first report of laser forming using the buckling mechanism used a laser beam with a diameter of 0.12 mm traveling at 5 mm/s to laser form 0.1 mm thick steel foils [57]. In this case, there is essentially no temperature gradient through the thickness of the substrate, but rather, the thermal gradient spreads outward from the scan line (Figure 4a) [57]. This means the resulting compressive forces are pushing against each other, generating a buckling instability (Figure 4b) [57]. Consequently, the work piece can bend either toward or away from the laser (Figure 4c) [57]. As an instability, the bending direction should be random, but this assumes the sheet has no residual stresses prior to laser forming [57]. Commercially available materials have a complex internal stress state, because of the hot and cold working that the sheet experiences during manufacturing, and this stress state determines the buckling direction [58]. Complete knowledge of this stress state would allow the bending direction to be predicted [57,58], though this is usually unknown. Beyond predicting the bending direction, researchers have also developed ways to control the buckling direction. Such methods include pre-bending the metal sheet [52,59], or through judicious choice of the lasing parameters [60,61]. The ability to generate bidirectional bending expands the design space for laser forming [62,63], without the need for human input, i.e., flipping the work piece [50]. As bending with the buckling mechanism can occur both toward and away from the laser, there can be some ambiguity which mechanism is occurring. Downward bending currently remains the best confirmation that buckling is occurring, because the TGM only bends the workpiece toward the laser. It has been reported that buckling can lead to larger bend angles per pass [57,58], which suggests the bend angle can be another way to differentiate the mechanisms, though visual downward bending is the easier method.

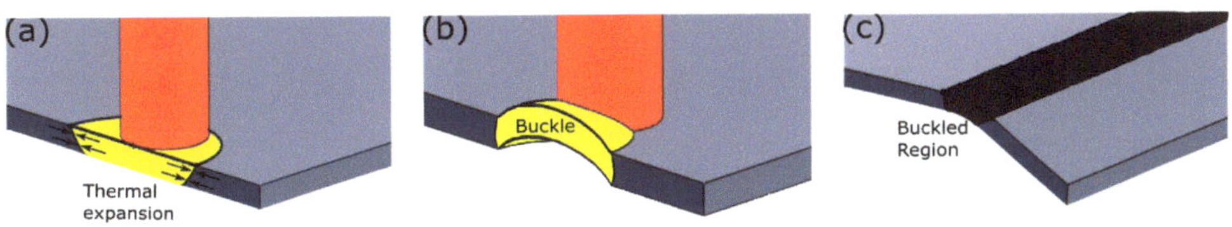

Figure 4. When laser forming thinner materials, the thermal gradient is unable to be established through the thickness of the material, so (**a**) the material expands outward. The compressive forces (**b**) are pushing opposite of each other, causing the workpiece to buckle. Once the buckling has formed, it (**c**) propagates and leads to bending in the direction opposite to the buckle. As the buckle is an instability, it can buckle in either direction.

2.3. Upsetting Mechanism (UM)

The third mechanism of laser forming is the upsetting mechanism [37,64]. The upsetting mechanism begins in a similar manner to the buckling mechanism. The laser scan speed is kept low to prevent a thermal gradient from developing through the thickness of the substrate, generating similar stresses to the buckling mechanism [54]. In the upsetting mechanism, however, the substrate is much stiffer along the scan path, preventing an out-of-plane bend [36,64] (Figure 5). This stiffness can be the result of using a thicker workpiece or one where the material has a higher Young's modulus [50]. Since the flow stress has been reached, but the substrate is unable to bend, the laser scan path becomes locally thicker and the substrate becomes, consequently, shorter [42]. One of the more comprehensive studies on the upsetting mechanisms reliably shortened 2 mm thick steel plates using 12 mm laser beams scanning at speeds around 1 mm/s [51]. The upsetting mechanism allows for in-plane substrate adjustments, which expands what shapes are laser formable by producing a change in the Gaussian curvature [53,65].

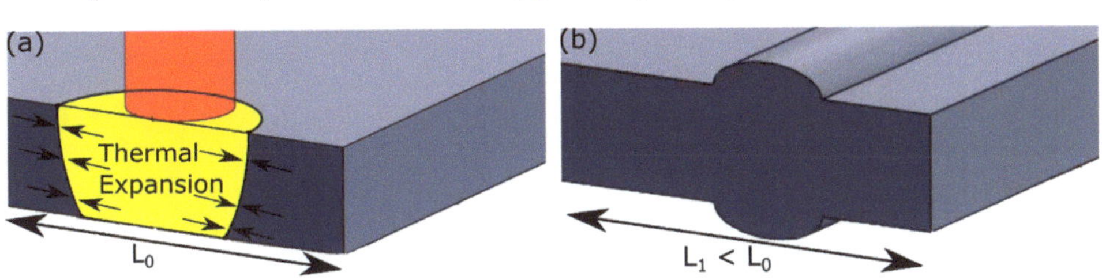

Figure 5. A slow laser scan speed (**a**) is used to minimize the thermal gradient through the thickness of the workpiece. Instead, the thermal gradient is established horizontally. The plastic compressive forces that resist the thermal expansion are insufficient to cause buckling, as the bending moment is too large. This results in the (**b**) scanned area locally thickening. Since volume is conserved, the workpiece shortens and changes its Gaussian curvature.

2.4. Coupling Mechanism

Some recent reports have suggested that the three mechanisms described above are not sufficient to capture the full range of experimental results, so they have proposed a coupling mechanism that combines both TGM and the upsetting mechanism [51,64,66]. This combination of forming mechanisms was already discussed [36,57] in early reports, but was not considered a separate mechanism. The proposed coupling mechanism is a consequence of the mechanisms above being idealized, limiting cases. As the laser forming parameters are adjusted, it is reasonable that the other mechanisms might start to play an increasingly important role, especially near the transition region between TGM and buckling [36]. For this reason, the proposed coupling mechanism will not be treated as a distinct mechanism of laser forming here, but it is still important to consider when designing a laser forming process, and is even useful for laser forming certain structures [66].

3. Design Considerations for Laser Forming

3.1. Laser and Substrate Selection

Since its first reports, laser forming has been used to bend sheets of common metals, such as stainless steel [67–69] and aluminum [70–72], out of plane without mechanical inputs [36,37,67]. As the understanding of the process developed, more varied substrates were explored such as titanium, [27,73] and copper alloys [74,75], hoping to develop new ways to form 3D structures for aerospace and electrical applications. Researchers have also explored laser forming on non-metallic substrates and have bent typically brittle materials such as silicon [76–78], ceramics [41,79], and glass [79,80]. More recently, there have also been demonstrations of the laser forming of more complex structures, such as metal foams [81,82] and laminates [83]. Despite the success of laser forming non-metals, metal bending has remained the primary application of laser forming, due to the use of metals as engineering materials in applications such as ship hulls [35,54,84]. There have also been some reports of laser forming of a limited number of polymers [85,86], although polymer laser forming remains relatively rare. Laser forming, therefore, is a general process reliant on controlled heating to generate plastic stresses, and appears possible for most materials. Large bending angles are more readily realized in metals as their ductility helps avoid crack formation at the bend line, [80,82] though experimental results suggest that the maximum bend angle is a strong function of material thickness with thinner samples being able to demonstrate larger bend angles [79,82,87]. Studies of many of the more well-studied substrates have been able to demonstrate deformation by all three mechanisms. Laser forming of the more exotic materials tends to be realized using the TGM, [76,80,82] though BM has been demonstrated in glass [79] and UM in silicon.

Critical to the success of the laser forming process is appropriate coupling of the laser energy to the material being formed. This coupling can be achieved by selecting the appropriate laser wavelength that corresponds to the absorption maximum of the substrate [75,88], by using a much higher power laser, so sufficient energy is absorbed by the substrate even with low absorptivity, or by using an absorbing coating layer that is matched with the laser wavelength being used (Figure 6) [85,89]. Metals thicker than 100 nm are optically opaque [90] and do not transmit appreciable amounts of light, so the metal substrates that have been used in laser forming will primarily either reflect or absorb the laser energy. The percentage of the incoming laser energy that is reflected is called the reflectance and these values have been measured as a function of wavelength [91]. The most common lasers [27] used for laser forming are Nd:YAG lasers that operate at 1.064 μm [57,58,76,78,85,86,92,93] and CO_2 lasers that emit at 10.6 μm [39,50,54,68,89,94–96]. CO_2 lasers are common in industrial setting, as they were one of the first gas lasers developed [97] and exhibit a high energy efficiency, while operating as a continuous-wave mode at high average powers (>1 kW); however, their absorption into metals is low and an absorbing coating is often required. Nd:YAG lasers are popular in industry as the 1.064 μm output wavelength is better absorbed by metals for cutting and welding, so absorbing coatings are not needed.

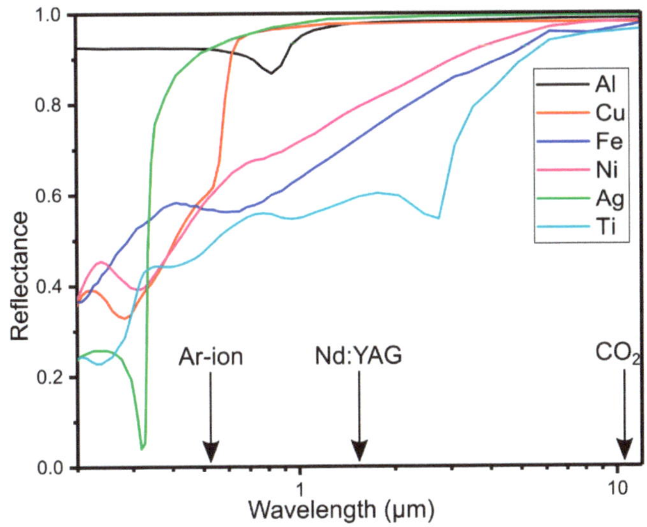

Figure 6. The spectral reflectance of metals, plotted from the data in [91], with the wavelength of some common lasers also identified. Almost all metals are entirely reflective to the 10.6 μm light of CO_2 lasers, while metals tend to be less reflective to the 1.064 μm light of the Nd:YAG laser, though copper, aluminum, and silver are still fairly reflective. Copper has a much higher absorbance to the 514 nm beam from an Ar-ion laser.

The early reports focused on using high power (>1 kW) lasers [40,60,61,70,71,98–103], as the intent was to bend large sheets as part of the ship building process [35]. The laser forming of thinner substrates enables the use of lower power (<100 W) lasers, such as those found in commercial metal marking laser systems [57,63,67,76,85,88,93,104].

Studies on the laser forming of plastics took advantage of the high transmissivity of high-density polyethylene (HDPE) to the wavelength of the Nd:YAG laser [85,86]. The laser energy was absorbed by a resinous black coating applied to the surface of the plastic. The laser power was kept low and the scan speed high, to ensure that the bending occurred through the temperature gradient mechanism, which reliably generates bending toward the laser. As expected, this was observed when the resin was on the side of the plastic exposed to the laser. With the same process parameters, but the coating placed on the opposite side, the plastic was reliably bent away from the laser. This downward bending should not be possible if using the TGM, but the optical transparency of HDPE to the laser made the system behave as if it was exposed to a laser on the underside and the TGM was causing the plastic to bend that direction. This same technique could be adopted for laser systems with multiple wavelengths, as glass absorbs the radiation from a CO_2 laser, but is transparent to the light from a Nd:YAG laser. Thus, sealed metal structures could still be bent if there is a glass window for the laser to pass through [105]. As seen in Figure 6, some metals, such as copper, are highly reflective to the fundamental wavelength of the Nd:YAG laser (1.064 μm). Consequently, laser forming copper with a Nd:YAG laser requires a substantially higher power or the use of a different wavelength. Recently, laser forming was demonstrated with other laser systems that might be commonly found in research environments, such as fiber lasers [106], exciplex lasers [74], and even Ar-ion lasers [67], which expand the substrate choice for laser forming.

Once the appropriate laser/substrate matching has been done, judicious selection of process parameters is essential to the laser forming process, as the laser power and scan speed control which mechanism is dominant [37]. Typically, laser power is kept low and speeds high to ensure that the substrate is being bent by the TGM, generating reliable bending toward the laser. As the TGM only generates a bend of one or two degrees per pass or less [38,74,101], many passes are needed to create structures with large bend angles, sometimes taking as many as 150 passes to produce a full 90 degree bend [88].

3.2. Cooling Effects in Laser Forming

To ensure that the same thermal gradient is established with each laser pass, an appropriate cooling time must also be built into the laser forming process. Consistent laser forming requires that the workpiece be cooled to the same thermal state in between each laser pass. The majority of laser forming setups use free convection with the surrounding air to cool the workpiece, which is relatively slow and leads to a pronounced increase in processing time (Figure 7a). In fact, cooling can be the longest part of a laser forming process [52,59,86,107]. To reduce the processing time, researchers have proposed multiple methods for forced cooling such as forced convection with compressed gas streams aimed at either side (Figure 7b) [92,108], passive water cooling with the bottom of the workpiece being placed in a water bath (Figure 7c) [109–111], and forced liquid cooling, such as a circulated cooling fluid placed in contact with the bottom of the substrate (Figure 7d) [112–115]. All these methods showed a pronounced reduction in the total processing time, as the workpieces cooled to room temperature in a matter of seconds, with active water cooling showing the largest reduction in processing time.

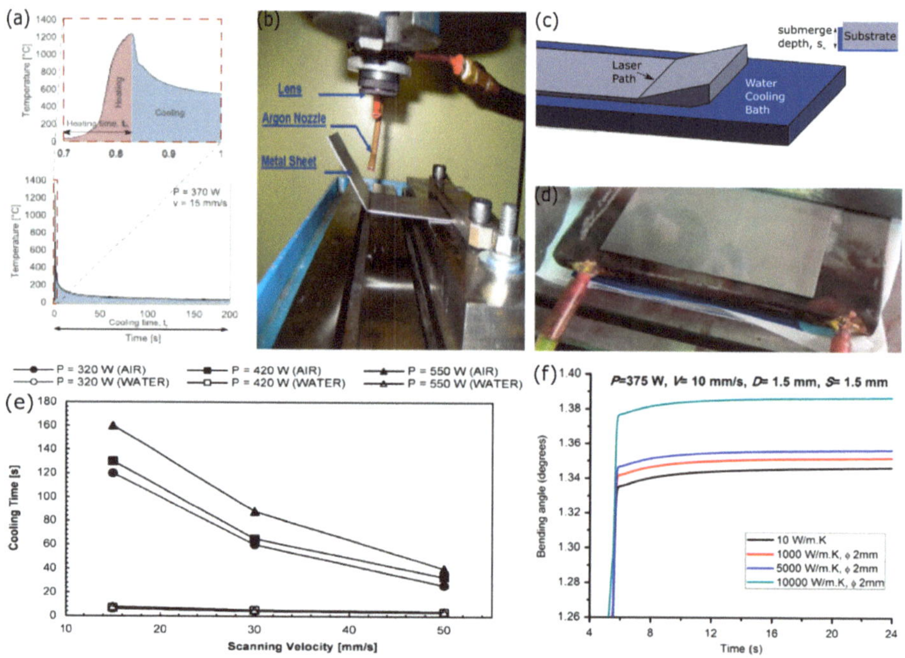

Figure 7. Most of the processing time (**a**) while laser forming is cooling the workpiece back to its initial state after each laser pass which is usually done by free convection [114]. Reprinted with permission from Springer Nature, copyright 2015. This time can be reduced by building in other cooling mechanisms, such as (**b**) forced air cooling [92], (**c**) passive water cooling [109] on the unexposed side, or (**d**) forced liquid cooling [115]. (**b**) Reprinted with permission from Elsevier, copyright 2013 (**d**). Reprinted with permission from Cambridge University Press, copyright 2017. Passive water cooling leads to a (**e**) dramatic reduction in cooling time for most processing conditions [109]. Reprinted with permission from Springer Nature, copyright 2012. Sometimes, cooling offers a small increase (**f**) in the bending angle achieved per pass [112]. Reprinted with permission from Springer Nature, copyright 2017.

Active cooling systems are not typically desirable when designing manufacturing processes, as they require pumps that increase both capital and operating costs of the process, but they are acceptable if the active cooling offers a substantial decrease in processing time or improvement in the reliability of a process. Fortunately, passive water cooling has also been demonstrated to provide sufficient reductions in processing time (Figure 7d) that active cooling may not be needed [109]. Some researchers have reported that forced cooling can lead to an increased bend angle per pass (Figure 7e) under the same lasing conditions, but reports differ on how pronounced this effect is, with some arguing there is no measurable effect [35,108,109,112,113]. Overall, integrated cooling systems offer a way to increase the throughput of laser forming by greatly reducing the time needed to establish thermal equilibrium in between laser passes for multi-pass forming.

The processing time can be further decreased by using the buckling mechanism as buckling is capable of generating larger bending angles per pass than the TGM, because more energy is put into the workpiece [56,57]. Typically, laser forming using the buckling mechanism is avoided as the mechanism is fundamentally an instability and so the workpiece can bend either toward the laser or away from it [57]. This instability is theoretically random but can be controlled by multiple factors, such as external loads [57,104], or the relaxation of internal stresses that exist because of the cold-working of common metal sheets [57]. The main reason to use the buckling mechanism is the downward bending, which greatly broadens the number of structures that can be laser formed [59,61].

3.3. Macro-Scale Laser Forming

Early research efforts were focused on macro-scale laser forming of sheet metals that are millimeters thick [35,50,103]. Among the macro-scale design targets were ship hulls [35,84], fuselage panels [70], and car doors (Figure 1g) [33]. These structures highlight different uses for laser forming in a manufacturing environment, as ship hulls and fuselage panels are low-volume parts, whereas car doors are high-volume components. Laser forming is considered less desirable for manufacturing high-volume metal parts, as it cannot compete with the speed of conventional methods, because the laser forming process is dominated by the cooling time needed between laser passes [33,50,52,114].

Both high-volume and low-volume products need to be joined to other parts, which is the second use for laser forming in manufacturing of macro-scale objects. Metal parts are often joined via welding, which can introduce distortions and lead to misalignment [35,116]. These distortions arise from two main contributions. First, the high heat of welding introduces thermal stresses similar to laser forming [116]. Second, the heat of welding releases stored plastic strains that result from mechanical forming [35]. While the distortions from welding are often small, they still need to be corrected, and laser forming offers a way to address these problems in a process known as hybrid laser forming [50,54,117,118]. Accurate manipulation of metals near weld lines is, however, challenging, because the local weld distortion is not uniform due to the complex stress state generated during welding [119].

The ability to shape large 3D objects using only a laser offers promising opportunities, such as remote deployment, the production of replacement parts where they are needed rather than at a centralized facility and shipped. In the 1980s, it was proposed that laser forming would be a valuable technology in space [103]. A laser system is more compact than a hydraulic press and the high energy efficiency of CO_2 and diode lasers lowers the energy consumption required for metal bending. Laser systems also offer the potential for cutting the workpiece [59] and joining [120] it with other pieces that traditional press brakes do not, making laser systems valuable for areas with minimal electricity generation or limited space.

3.4. Laser Forming Curved Surfaces

Ship hulls are an example of a doubly curved structure and so researchers needed to design methods of introducing curvature into laser formed parts [53]. Currently, there are two main methods for developing curvature in laser formed parts. The first is to make multiple bend lines close to each other [33,68,121], approximating a smooth curve as the limit of many bend lines close together (Figure 8d). By adjusting the distance between the laser passes, bends of varying curvature are able to be produced, as the heat affected zone is not limited to the laser pass line [68]. As this curvature is produced by simple bends, the resulting structures are considered developable surfaces [65]. Developable surfaces are the family of surfaces that can be produced by transforming a plane as long as the Gaussian curvature remains unchanged (Figure 8a) [65]. This means bending, rolling, and cutting are permitted, but stretching or compressing a region are forbidden [65]. As developable surfaces are produced from bending and folding, much of the knowledge gained in origami engineering is applicable to producing structures with laser forming [1,14,26,122,123].

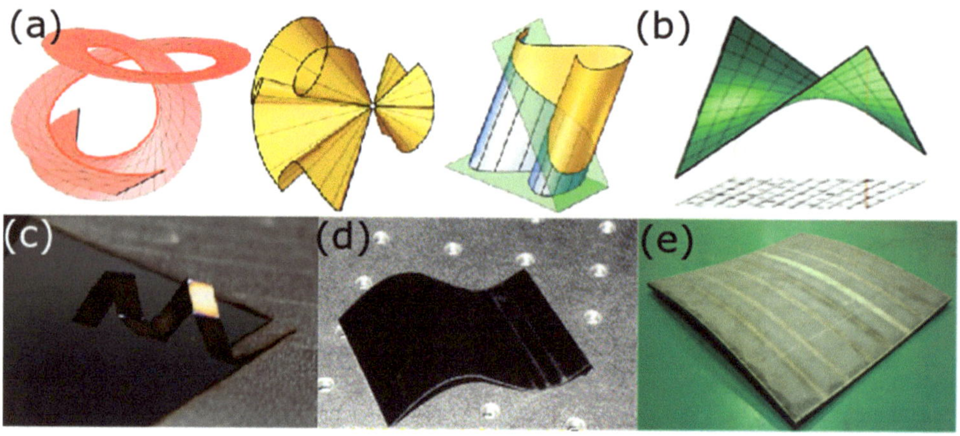

Figure 8. Some (**a**) developable surfaces [65] which are surfaces with zero Gaussian curvature, which means they can be produced from flat sheets, while non-developable surfaces, such as the (**b**) hyperbolic paraboloid [65] or "saddle shape", cannot be formed by bending and cutting inelastic sheets, as they have a non-zero Gaussian curvature. (**a**,**b**) Published under a CC BY License. Laser forming with the temperature gradient mechanism (TGM) or buckling mechanisms can produce developable surfaces, such as (**c**) a coil [59] or (**d**) a cubic spline curve [99], which only require simple bends to produce from a metal sheet. (**d**) Reproduced with permission from Elsevier, copyright 2003. The upsetting mechanism causes a shortening of the workpiece, which changes the Gaussian curvature, so (**e**) a doubly curved saddle shape can be successfully laser formed [84]. Reproduced with permission from Elsevier, copyright 2013.

The second method to produce curved structures relies on the upsetting mechanism that produces in-plane strains [53]. These planar strains cause local distance to be distorted, changing the Gaussian curvature of the workpiece [53,124], which simple bending does not. Since the strain changes the Gaussian curvature, the final workpiece is considered a non-developable surface,, as developable surfaces have zero Gaussian curvature [65]. Non-developable surfaces include hyperbolic paraboloids (Figure 8b) and hyperboloids, which are often called saddles (Figure 8e) [53,84] and pillows [53], respectively, in the laser forming literature. The ability to generate these surfaces from flat sheets using laser forming greatly expands the design space of 3D structures that can be rapidly prototyped.

While the majority of laser forming research has been done on planar substrates, some researchers have investigated laser forming as a means to bend metal tubes for heat exchangers and engines [40,125–127]. Laser formed tubes bend toward the laser, though researchers disagree about what mechanism is causing the bending. Some suggest the TGM is causing the bending [126], while others suggest that the stiff nature of metal pipes means that the upsetting mechanism is dominant, leading to a local shortening, which causes the tube to bend toward the laser without a spring-back effect [40,128]. Like the laser forming of sheets, laser tube bending is a highly flexible method that does not require specially designed dies. This makes laser tube bending valuable for rapid prototyping, as well as low volume, customized production [126]. When bending tubes, it is important to consider the distortion of the tube cross-section, or ovalization [40]. Multiple reports have confirmed that laser tube bending tends to produce less ovalization than mechanical bending, as the laser induced stresses are less than the mechanical forces used when cold bending the tubes [40,126].

Matching the optical absorbance of the substrate with the laser output allows the energy to couple more effectively, lowering the laser power required for successful laser forming. As lower powered (<100 W) laser cutting systems proliferated, researchers hoped to use these systems for laser forming as well as laser cutting. Laser cutting requires high laser fluences, so the beam size needs to be small to achieve clean cuts. Since the output power is lower, the fluence is kept high by decreasing the spot size. For successful laser forming, the laser spot size is typically the same order of magnitude as the substrate being bent which has led researchers to experiment with the laser forming of smaller and thinner substrates [67,72,129].

3.5. Micro-Laser Forming

Complex, 3D silicon microstructures are difficult to produce because silicon is a brittle material that requires high temperatures and specialized tools to produce the desired shape [130]. Laser forming has been applied to adjusting silicon microstructures [76]. The precise control of heating enables silicon microstructures to be bent out of plane, even with more thermally sensitive components, as long as the thermally sensitive components are not located near the laser scan path. Laser forming is not heavily used for the rapid prototyping of MEMS structures, but has been found tremendously successful as a quality control technique called laser micro-adjustment [64,131]. Laser micro-adjustment is a valuable application of laser forming, as evidenced by the industrial adoption of the technique [41,131,132].

Laser micro-adjustment uses a laser to make submicron final adjustments to microstructures [106,133]. Any of the mechanisms can be used for this adjustment, but the smaller bending angle per pass makes the TGM preferable to the buckling mechanism for out-of-plane bends [38,64]. The upsetting mechanism is useful for shortening the workpiece locally which has been used for aligning actuators [42,133]. The laser forming mechanism can be easily determined by adjusting the lasing parameters [36], but the size of the sheets being micro-adjusted makes edge effects more common [134], and increases the coupling between the TGM and the upsetting mechanism [64,101,106,135]. This coupling leads to both in-plane shortening and out-of-plane bending, which is especially common in actuators. Bridge actuators are micromechanical structures that hold functional components and allow fine adjustments to the final positioning to be made. Bridge actuators are produced by removing most of the structural material in a small area, so that they are connected by thin strips called bridges. When laser forming a two-bridge actuator, the scan path effectively creates two hot and two cold sides, the usual irradiated and unirradiated sides of the work piece, as well as a hot bridge and a cold bridge. The usual irradiated sides produce the out of plane bending, while the hot bridge causes an in-plane bend [42,135]. While actuators are one of the most common pieces laser micro-adjusted, the process is general and has been applied to multiple devices [136] and companies have filed for patents on using laser adjustments based on these reports [137–139]. There has also been a promising report of the laser forming of shape memory alloys, a material commonly used for MEMS actuators, although this forming has not yet been done on MEMS structures [140].

One application of laser micro-adjustment is the precise alignment of optical fibers to ensure optimal coupling with a photonic integrated circuit (PIC) [141]. While glass has been successfully laser formed [81,82], laser forming the optical fiber would only produce bends into the fiber, rather than aligning it. To align the optical fiber, the researchers sheathed the fiber into a thin metal tube and the tube was then laser formed [141,142]. The optical fiber is flexible, so the bend in the metal tube will cause a deflection in the fiber tip. In effect, the metal tube is being used as an alignment actuator with sub-micron precision, owing to the controllability of laser forming [141,142].

3.6. Laser Forming for Rapid Prototyping

The flexibility of laser forming makes it a promising technology for rapid prototyping, and researchers have identified rapid prototyping as one of the areas where laser forming is most likely to make meaningful contributions in the industrial product lifecycle [50]. This promise remains largely unfulfilled compared to more conventional 3D printing for various reasons. Despite the many different methods for 3D printing, such as fused filament fabrication [143,144] and stereolithography [145,146], 3D printing follows the same general workflow to produce a printed object from a computer aided design (CAD) file (Figure 9a). Once the engineer has designed the object they want to be 3D printed using a CAD software, they need to export it to a format that can be 3D printed [19]. The default file format for the additive manufacturing community is the STL file format, which approximates the surface of the CAD object as a collection of tessellated triangles [147]. Since 3D printers build structures in a layer-by-layer fashion, the STL file needs to be passed to a slicer, which converts the 3D object to the build layers. From this file, the scan path is developed, and support structures are calculated if the object needs them. For modern 3D printing, the conversion of the CAD file to printed object is entirely automated [19,147]. Critical to the broad adoption of laser forming for rapid prototyping is developing a similar software structure that can convert a CAD file into a path planning program, which also calculates the appropriate lasing setting to produce the desired 3D object without human intervention. Extensive research efforts have been undertaken to achieve this goal, with recent results suggesting that this goal might be realized soon [62].

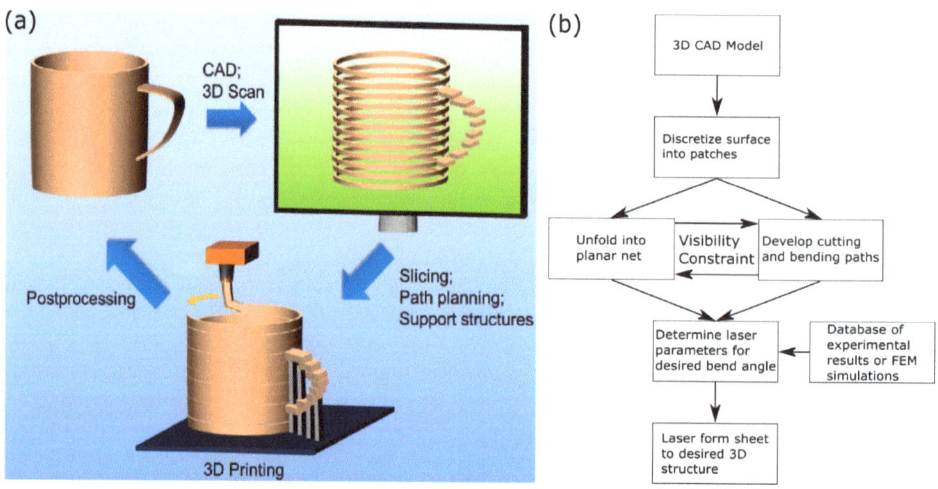

Figure 9. Comparison of workflows for (**a**) conventional 3D printing [19] showing the slicer and path planner, compared to (**b**) proposed workflow for the automated laser forming of arbitrary convex polyhedra. (**a**) Image originally published under a CC BY license. Unlike 3D printing, path planning for laser forming is strongly dependent on the material being formed, which requires a database to determine laser power and speed settings. For more advanced structures, laser forming algorithms need to consider the optical path of the laser beam, as this couples the unfolding algorithm and the path planning.

One of the first complex objects successfully prototyped using laser forming was a car door (Figure 1g) [33]. This demonstration is notable for many reasons, chiefly the entire production was done in the laser system. The researchers started from a blank sheet of metal that was laser formed to produce the desired bends, and the final structure was cut from the sheet using the same laser. As the buckling mechanism was only recently reported and control strategies were limited, the researchers were laser forming only using TGM. The complex shape of the car door required both concave and convex bending, so the workpiece needed to be manually flipped to produce the bi-directional bending needed for the car panel. While these experiments involved no prediction of laser settings, the researchers introduced a novel feedback system, where the scanning speed was adjusted to produce the desired bend angle. Additionally, a car panel might be considered far from an arbitrary design, so the scan pattern was relatively easy to design.

To produce more complex objects via laser forming, it is necessary to know which bend lines are needed to produce a given shape, a classic origami problem [1]. To this end, the inverse design of scan strategies to generate a desired laser formed structure has been a productive research topic [53,66,84,99,148–151]. The design of irradiation paths involves more than planning where the beam needs to be applied to generate a desired shape, but also the laser power and travel speed, to produce the desired degree of bending using the appropriate forming mechanism. These requirements remain a challenge, and have required researchers to design algorithms that plan a scan path and guesses appropriate lasing settings by consulting a database from experiments [99] or finite element simulations (Figure 9b) [53,121,150]. Despite the known disagreement between experimental results and simulations [38], these scan strategies are able to produce the final desired structures with a high degree of accuracy [53,121]. One limitation of these design systems is the limited degree of bending required in the validation structures. As the bend angles required per point are small to moderate, the relationships between bend angle and line energy (laser power divided by scan speed) is approximately linear [98,99]. As the laser spot size gets smaller and the required bending angle approaches 90 degrees, this linear relation fails to hold [88,152] and none of these design strategies account for this deviation. These limitations are more prominent, as engineers have started using laser forming to produce highly complex structures.

Realizing that laser forming was not limited to moderate bending, but could be used for larger folds (up to ninety degrees or higher), our group began envisioning what origami structures can be produced with laser forming. Laser forming with TGM is limited to ninety-degree bends, as further bending results in the workpiece blocking the laser path, but this limitation does not exist if using the buckling mechanism to bend away from the laser. Using both mechanisms, we were able to produce complex objects, such as cubes (Figure 10a) and airplanes, (Figure 10b), without the need for human intervention [59]. Similar to the car door forming [33], the outline of the shape was manufactured from metal sheets by using the laser to also cut the final structure, releasing it from the sheet. By using a Nd:YAG laser instead of a CO_2 laser, an absorbing coating was not needed, allowing for marking of the metal at low powers. Rapidly producing these structures from a blank metal sheet using multiple bending modes and laser cutting demonstrated the potential for laser forming to be a viable rapid prototyping strategy.

Soon after, we showed that laser forming could be used to produce electronic devices, such as antennas [153] and inductors [88]. When producing the antennas, a blank metal sheet was clamped on all sides, before laser cutting the slots for the array antenna and the perimeter of the waveguide was laser cut from the metal sheet, before the entire structure was bent to produce the final structure: a rectangular prism (Figure 10c) [153]. It was worth noting that the laser cutting made more precise cuts than electro-discharge machining, the usual technology used to produce the slots in the waveguide. In fact, the entire laser process of cutting and bending was faster than conventional machining that only produces the slots. Efficient waveguides require smooth surfaces to minimize losses [154], so new manufacturing techniques need to show that they do not greatly alter the metal surface. The impact of laser forming is limited to the laser scan paths and even after 100 passes only showed a modest increase of the surface roughness of 0.5 μm [155]. Similarly, the coils for the inductor were cut from a blank piece of copper before being bent out of plane to generate a toroidal inductor (Figure 10d) [88]. Laser forming can also be used to produce an inductor with an overpass or bending the inductor out of plane. Bending inductors out of plane offers a way to improve the Q-factor as eddy currents and skin effects are minimized [156], which is especially important for integrating these elements on semiconductor integrated circuits. Both reports demonstrated that laser forming could be used to rapidly prototype functional devices, as the designs can easily be iterated, as it only requires changing the location or size of lines in a 2D CAD drawing. This process, however, still requires human input to exchange the metal sheets between design iterations, which would limit the industrial adoption of laser forming for rapid prototyping or producing custom parts.

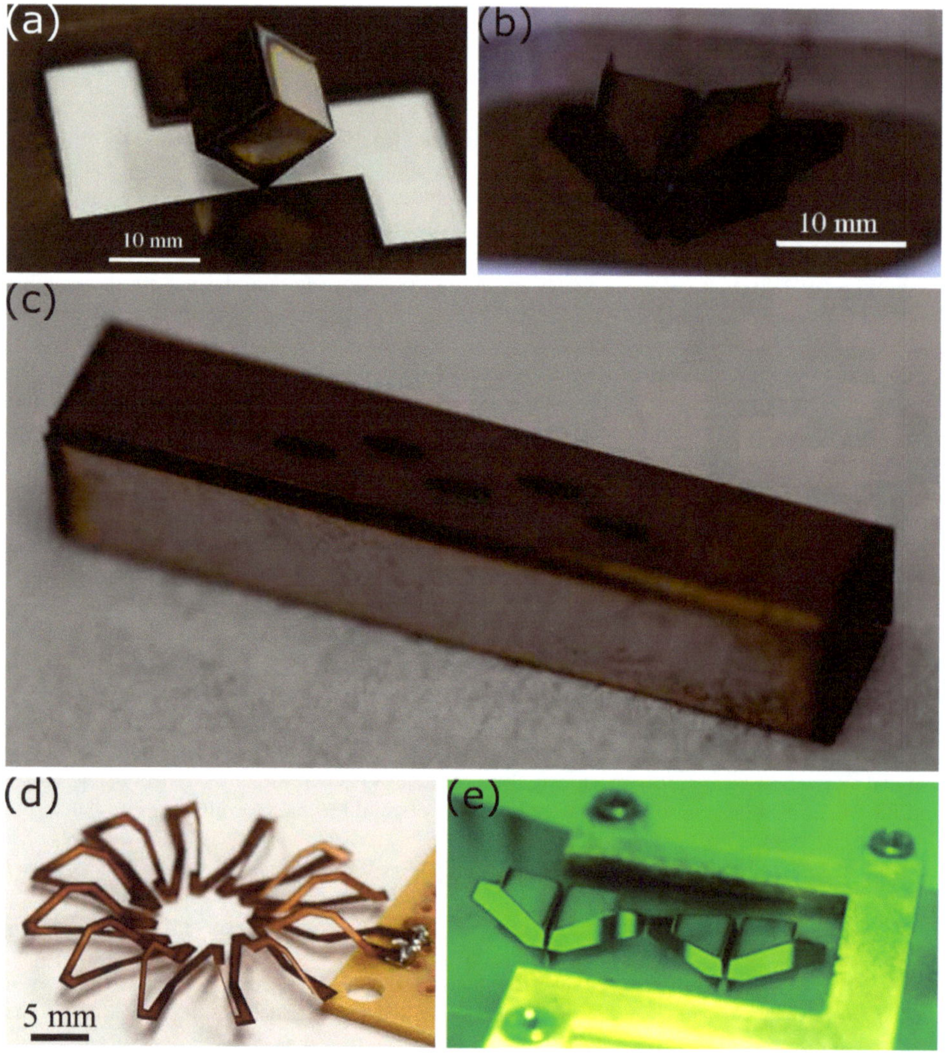

Figure 10. Laser forming can be used to produce complex and functional structures without the need for mechanical input. Three-dimensional structures that were cut and laser formed from nickel foil using a 20W Nd:YAG laser include (**a**) cubes and (**b**) airplanes [59]. (**a**,**b**) Reprinted with permission from John Wiley and Sons, copyright 2013. Laser forming can be used to produce functional structures as well, such as (**c**) a slotted waveguide for antennas from stainless steel [153] and even (**d**) toroidal inductors from copper [88]. (**c**) Reprinted with permission from IEEE, copyright 2018. (**d**) Reprinted with permission from IEEE, copyright 2018. New metal sheets are required between samples, but (**e**) continuous laser forming can be realized by combining it with roll-to-roll processing [63]. Reprinted with permission from Springer Nature, copyright 2018.

Working to automate the entire laser forming process, our group developed a roll-to-roll laser forming system, with the metal feedstock passing through the focal plane of the laser [63]. This set up allowed features to be readily cut and folded from the sheet metal using the TGM. Additionally, the metal sheet had a pre-strain from being wound onto a roll that was used to reliably generate downward bending using the buckling mechanism, producing the same complex shapes from our previous work in an automated process (Figure 10e). Once the piece was formed, it was released from the sheet and fell down a chute, before the rolls were spun to introduce a new working area. This was the first demonstration of a fully automated laser forming process to produce complex 3D structures. While impressive, producing these structures relied on our previously designed scan paths and laser settings. For many of the structures, we relied on the self-limiting nature of ninety-degree bends, so that precise control over the laser settings was not needed. Accurately determining the laser power, speed, and number of passes would be required, if the desired structures included intermediate bends.

Figuring out what scan path and what lasing setting are needed to produce a desired structure is known as the inverse design problem, and has been intensively studied [53,66,99,148–150]. Part of the difficulty of designing laser scan strategies is the highly-coupled and nonlinear thermo-mechanical nature of laser forming, so many of the previously proposed strategies are limited in the number of scan lines [66,99,150] or are computationally intensive, relying on full finite-element models [148,149]. Recently, researchers introduced an algorithm that takes a desired 3D structure as an input, and simultaneously unfolds the structure into a planar net and plans the cutting and bending paths for this net [62]. For normal origami, the planar net and the bending path can be solved for separately, because the craftsmen is able to access all needed fold lines at any given time [6]. As current laser forming setups rely on an unobstructed optical path between the laser and the fold line, this visibility constraint effectively couples the two problems.

Over the years, laser forming has emerged as a viable rapid prototyping strategy that is complementary to metal 3D printing. Understanding of the sub-mechanisms has allowed researchers to develop scan strategies for many 3D shapes, but the complex thermomechanical process makes it near mandatory to automate this process. This need becomes most pronounced when more complex 3D structures and devices are being laser formed, especially ones that require multiple forming mechanisms. Solutions to this inverse design problem are rapidly developing, and will hopefully make laser forming as accessible as 3D printing.

4. Conclusions and Outlook

Laser forming has developed dramatically over the past forty years, from a mechanistic understanding of the process to the successful laser origami of complex 3D shapes and the algorithms to design their laser scan patterns. As the field matures and laser forming is adopted as a viable rapid prototyping strategy, new research opportunities abound. Like any other prototyping technology, laser forming is valuable for certain structures, while not being preferable for others. Deciding if laser forming is the preferred fabrication methods requires design heuristics that have yet to be clarified. Continued research efforts should be focused on clarifying these heuristics, while expanding the capabilities of the laser forming by developing it as a robust technology that is able to reliably produce functional, near-arbitrary 3D structures from flat substrates in an automated manufacturing environment. To this end, researchers will need to address current gaps in the understanding of the laser forming process, which will inform the design and control algorithms.

Laser forming involves rapid heating and cooling cycles that can cause changes in the microstructure of the metal during the process. Microstructural control is very important for titanium pieces in the aerospace industry, as the mechanical properties and fatigue resistance of titanium and its alloys are highly dependent on having precise control over the grains. Preliminary reports suggest that laser forming leads to unfavorable grain structures in titanium [27,95,157]. Other industries and applications might not have as stringent requirements on the grain structure, but these reports suggest there may be some degradation in the mechanical properties of laser formed parts compared to mechanically bent structures, an area that needs further investigation.

The microstructure of a material influences more than mechanical properties, so these other properties need to be considered when deciding to laser form an object. Of particular concern to the shipbuilding industry might be corrosion resistance to the salty ocean water. The corrosion resistance of some laser formed metals has been briefly investigated [96,115,158,159], with many metals demonstrating a reduced corrosion resistance resulting from the disturbed microstructure. Interestingly, some alloys showed an increased corrosion resistance after being laser formed [159], though the role of the lasing parameters on this phenomenon was underexplored. There is a need to study systematically the suitability of a laser formed material for use in a corrosive environment as a function of the material's properties, the nature of the corrosive species, and the laser forming parameters. Applications could include ship hulls in salt water, or a laser bent tube in a chemical processing plant.

For laser forming to move from academic research to an industrial process, stronger control schemes and predictive modelling need to be developed. The state-of-the-art algorithms either develop the optimal laser settings for relatively simple shapes based on finite element modelling, or they use experimental data to develop a laser scan path to produce near-arbitrary 3D shapes. The next step would be to develop an algorithm that combines these methods to develop a scan path for near-arbitrary shapes and the optimal laser settings to produce this shape, as some regions might only need bending, while others require shortening. Combining these algorithms would enable additional constraints to be designed around, as the laser-substrate interaction does more than just bend the workpiece.

Most laser forming setups are run in a batch process with one sheet being bent at a time. A recent report demonstrated a way to transform laser forming into a continuous roll-to-roll process by combining laser cutting and bending [63]. Lasers are used to do much more, such as welding [120,160], marking [161,162], laser-induced chemistry [163–165], and are even used in analytical techniques [166,167]. Taken together, one could imagine a fully automated process wherein blank sheet metal is fed, then different lasers will cut, mark, chemically pattern, and then fold it into a desired 3D structure with inline quality control. Developing such a system will require developing further control schemes to know when and where to bend the structure in this complex process to yield the desired result.

Laser forming is a valuable technology that is poised to address two notable shortcomings of metal 3D printing—large structures and thin structures. Fully realizing this potential will require developing a detailed understanding of how the laser forming process impacts material properties to produce advanced planning and control schemes. With a completely automated process, laser forming will be available to make the rapid prototyping of metallic structures even lighter.

Author Contributions: A.L.B. performed the literature survey and wrote the initial draft of the paper. M.D.D. supervised the work and edited the paper. N.L. supervised the work and edited the paper. All authors have read and agreed to the published version of the manuscript.

Funding: The research was funded by the Army Research Laboratory and was accomplished under Cooperative Agreement Number W911NF-20-2-0243.

Acknowledgments: The views and conclusions contained in this document are those of the authors and should not be interpreted as representing the official policies, either expressed or implied, of the Army Research Laboratory or the U.S. Government. The U.S. Government is authorized to reproduce and distribute reprints for Government purposes notwithstanding any copyright notation herein.

Conflicts of Interest: The authors declare no conflict of interest.

References

1. Turner, N.; Goodwine, B.; Sen, M. A review of origami applications in mechanical engineering. *Proc. Inst. Mech. Eng. Part C J. Mech. Eng. Sci.* **2016**, *230*, 2345–2362. [CrossRef]
2. Hernandez, E.A.P.; Hartl, D.J.; Lagoudas, D.C. Introduction to Active Origami Structures. In *Active Origami*; Springer: Cham, Switzerland, 2019; pp. 1–53, ISBN 978-3-319-91865-5.

3. Felton, S.; Tolley, M.; Demain, E.; Rus, D.; Wood, R. A method for building self-folding machines. *Science* **2014**, *345*, 644–646. [CrossRef]
4. Taylor, A.; Miller, M.; Fok, M.; Nilsson, K.; Tsz Ho Tse, Z. Intracardiac Magnetic Resonance Imaging Catheter With Origami Deployable Mech. *Med. Devices* **2016**, *10*, 020957. [CrossRef]
5. Takano, T.; Miura, K.; Natori, M.; Hanayama, E.; Inoue, T.; Noguchi, T.; Miyahara, N.; Nakaguro, H. Deployable antenna with 10-m maximum diameter for space use. *IEEE Trans. Antennas Propag.* **2004**, *52*, 2–11. [CrossRef]
6. Tachi, T. Origamizing Polyhedral Surfaces. *IEEE Trans. Vis. Comput. Graph.* **2010**, *16*, 298–311. [CrossRef] [PubMed]
7. Zirbel, S.A.; Lang, R.J.; Thomson, M.W.; Sigel, D.A.; Walkemeyer, P.E.; Trease, B.P.; Magleby, S.P.; Howell, L.L. Accommodating Thickness in Origami-Based Deployable Arrays. *J. Mech. Des.* **2013**, 135. [CrossRef]
8. Lang, R.J.; Tolman, K.A.; Crampton, E.B.; Magleby, S.P.; Howell, L.L. A Review of Thickness-Accommodation Techniques in Origami-Inspired Engineering. *Appl. Mech. Rev.* **2018**, *70*, 010805. [CrossRef]
9. Tachi, T.; Hull, T.C. Self-Foldability of Rigid Origami. *J. Mech. Robot.* **2017**, *9*. [CrossRef]
10. Lang, R.J.; Howell, L. Rigidly Foldable Quadrilateral Meshes From Angle Arrays. *J. Mech. Robot.* **2018**, *10*, 021004. [CrossRef]
11. Zirbel, S.A.; Trease, B.P.; Magleby, S.P.; Howell, L.L. Deployment Methods for an Origami-Inspired Rigid-Foldable Array. In Proceedings of the 40th Aerospace Mechanisms Symposium, Baltimore, MD, USA, 14–16 May 2014; NASA Goddard Space Flight Center: Greenbelt, MD, USA, 2014.
12. Morgan, J.; Magleby, S.P.; Howell, L.L. An Approach to Designing Origami-Adapted Aerospace Mechanisms. *J. Mech. Des.* **2016**, *138*. [CrossRef]
13. Whitney, J.P.; Sreetharan, P.S.; Ma, K.Y.; Wood, R.J. Pop-up book MEMS. *J. Micromech. Microeng.* **2011**, *21*, 115021. [CrossRef]
14. Ahmed, S.; McGough, K.; Ounaies, Z.; Frecker, M. Origami-Inspired Folding and Unfolding of Structures: Fundamental Investigations of Dielectric Elastomer-Based Active Materials. In *Smart Materials, Adaptive Structures and Intelligent Systems*; American Society of Mechanical Engineers: Houston, TX, USA, 2013; p. V001T01A029/1-6.
15. Hayes, G.J.; Liu, Y.; Genzer, J.; Lazzi, G.; Dickey, M.D. Self-Folding Origami Microstrip Antennas. *IEEE Trans. Antennas Propag.* **2014**, *62*, 5416–5419. [CrossRef]
16. Tolley, M.T.; Felton, S.M.; Miyashita, S.; Aukes, D.; Rus, D.; Wood, R.J. Self-folding origami: Shape memory composites activated by uniform heating. *Smart Mater. Struct.* **2014**, *23*, 094006/1–9. [CrossRef]
17. Wang, D.H.; Tan, L.-S. Origami-Inspired Fabrication: Self-Folding or Self-Unfolding of Cross-Linked-Polyimide Objects in Extremely Hot Ambience. *ACS Macro Lett.* **2019**, *8*, 546–552. [CrossRef]
18. Upcraft, S.; Fletcher, R. The rapid prototyping technologies. *Assem. Autom.* **2003**, *23*, 318–330. [CrossRef]
19. Ligon, S.C.; Liska, R.; Stampfl, J.; Gurr, M.; Mülhaupt, R. Polymers for 3D Printing and Customized Additive Manufacturing. *Chem. Rev.* **2017**, *117*, 10212–10290. [CrossRef] [PubMed]
20. Das, S.; Bourell, D.L.; Babu, S.S. Metallic materials for 3D printing. *Mrs Bull.* **2016**, *41*, 729–741. [CrossRef]
21. Bak, D. Rapid prototyping or rapid production? 3D printing processes move industry towards the latter. *Assem. Autom.* **2003**, *23*, 340–345. [CrossRef]
22. Agarwala, M.; Bourell, D.; Beaman, J.; Marcus, H.; Barlow, J. Direct selective laser sintering of metals. *Rapid Prototyp. J.* **1995**, *1*, 26–36. [CrossRef]
23. Duda, T.; Raghavan, L.V. 3D Metal Printing Technology. *IFAC Pap.* **2016**, *49*, 103–110. [CrossRef]
24. Panchagnula, J.S.; Simhambhatla, S. Manufacture of complex thin-walled metallic objects using weld-deposition based additive manufacturing. *Robot. Comput. Integr. Manuf.* **2018**, *49*, 194–203. [CrossRef]
25. Hu, J.; Marciniak, Z.; Duncan, J. *Mechanics of Sheet Metal Forming*; Elsevier: Amsterdam, The Netherlands, 2002; ISBN 978-0-08-049651-1.
26. Qattawi, A.; Abdelhamid, M.; Mayyas, A.; Omar, M. Design Analysis for Origami-Based Folded Sheet Metal Parts. *SAE Int. J. Mater. Manf.* **2014**, *7*, 488–498. [CrossRef]
27. Walczyk, D.F.; Vittal, S. Bending of Titanium Sheet Using Laser Forming. *J. Manuf. Process.* **2000**, *2*, 258–269. [CrossRef]
28. Cleveland, R.M.; Ghosh, A.K. Inelastic effects on springback in metals. *Int. J. Plast.* **2002**, *18*, 769–785. [CrossRef]

29. Tseng, A.A.; Jen, K.P.; Chen, T.C.; Kondetimmamhalli, R.; Murty, Y.V. Forming properties and springback evaluation of copper beryllium sheets. *Met. Mater. Trans. A* **1995**, *26*, 2111–2121. [CrossRef]
30. Wagoner, R.H.; Lim, H.; Lee, M.-G. Advanced Issues in springback. *Int. J. Plast.* **2013**, *45*, 3–20. [CrossRef]
31. Abvabi, A.; Rolfe, B.; Hodgson, P.D.; Weiss, M. The influence of residual stress on a roll forming process. *Int. J. Mech. Sci.* **2015**, *101*, 124–136. [CrossRef]
32. Martin, J.H.; Yahata, B.D.; Hundley, J.M.; Mayer, J.A.; Schaedler, T.A.; Pollock, T.M. 3D printing of high-strength aluminium alloys. *Nature* **2017**, *549*, 365–369. [CrossRef]
33. Thomson, G.; Pridham, M.S. Controlled laser forming for rapid prototyping. *Rapid Prototyp. J.* **1997**, *3*, 137–143. [CrossRef]
34. Clausen, H.B. *DTU Plate Forming by Line Heating*; Department of Naval Architecture and Offshore Engineering, Technical University of Denmark: Lyngby, Denmark, 2000.
35. Scully, K. Laser Line Heating. *J. Ship Prod.* **1987**, *3*, 237–246.
36. Magee, J.; Watkins, K.G.; Steen, W.M. Advances in laser forming. *J. Laser Appl.* **1998**, *10*, 235–246. [CrossRef]
37. Geiger, M.; Vollertsen, F. The Mechanisms of Laser Forming. *Cirp Ann.* **1993**, *42*, 301–304. [CrossRef]
38. Shen, H.; Vollertsen, F. Modelling of laser forming—An review. *Comput. Mater. Sci.* **2009**, *46*, 834–840. [CrossRef]
39. Cheng, P.; Fan, Y.; Zhang, J.; Yao, Y.L.; Mika, D.P.; Zhang, W.; Graham, M.; Marte, J.; Jones, M. Laser Forming of Varying Thickness Plate—Part I: Process Analysis. *J. Manuf. Sci. Eng.* **2006**, *128*, 634–641. [CrossRef]
40. Li, W.; Yao, Y.L. Laser Bending of Tubes: Mechanism, Analysis, and Prediction. *J. Manuf. Sci. Eng.* **2001**, *123*, 674–681. [CrossRef]
41. Tam, A.C.; Poon, C.C.; Crawforth, L. Laser Bending of Ceramics and Application to Manufacture Magnetic Head Sliders in Disk Drives. *Anal. Sci. Suppl.* **2002**, *17*, s419–s421. [CrossRef]
42. Folkersma, G.; Römer, G.-W.; Brouwer, D.; in 't Veld, B.H. In-plane laser forming for high precision alignment. *Opt. Eng.* **2014**, *53*, 126105. [CrossRef]
43. Hu, Y.; Xu, X.; Yao, Z.; Hu, J. Laser peen forming induced two way bending of thin sheet metals and its mechanisms. *J. Appl. Phys.* **2010**, *108*, 073117. [CrossRef]
44. Yocom, C.J.; Zhang, X.; Liao, Y. Research and development status of laser peen forming: A review. *Opt. Laser Technol.* **2018**, *108*, 32–45. [CrossRef]
45. Arcella, F.G.; Froes, F.H. Producing titanium aerospace components from powder using laser forming. *JOM* **2000**, *52*, 28–30. [CrossRef]
46. Laeng, J.; Stewart, J.G.; Liou, F.W. Laser metal forming processes for rapid prototyping - A review. *Int. J. Prod. Res.* **2000**, *38*, 3973–3996. [CrossRef]
47. Kant, R.; Joshi, S.N.; Dixit, U.S. 4—Research issues in the laser sheet bending process. In *Materials Forming and Machining*; Woodhead Publishing Reviews: Mechanical Engineering Series; Davim, J.P., Ed.; Woodhead Publishing: Cambridge, UK, 2016; pp. 73–97, ISBN 978-0-85709-483-4.
48. Omidvar, M.; Fard, R.K.; Sohrabpoor, H.; Teimouri, R. Selection of laser bending process parameters for maximal deformation angle through neural network and teaching–learning-based optimization algorithm. *Soft Comput.* **2015**, *19*, 609–620. [CrossRef]
49. Lambiase, F. An Analytical Model for Evaluation of Bending Angle in Laser Forming of Metal Sheets. *J. Mater. Eng. Perform.* **2012**, *21*, 2044–2052. [CrossRef]
50. Dearden, G.; Edwardson, S.P. Some recent developments in two-and three-dimensional laser forming for macro and micro applications. *J. Opt. A Pure Appl. Opt.* **2003**, *5*, S8–S15. [CrossRef]
51. Shi, Y.; Yao, Z.; Shen, H.; Hu, J. Research on the mechanisms of laser forming for the metal plate. *Int. J. Mach. Tools Manuf.* **2006**, *46*, 1689–1697. [CrossRef]
52. Arnet, H.; Vollertsen, F. Extending Laser Bending for the Generation of Convex Shapes. *Proc. Inst. Mech. Eng. Part B J. Eng. Manuf.* **1995**, *209*, 433–442. [CrossRef]
53. Liu, C.; Yao, Y.L.; Srinivasan, V. Optimal Process Planning for Laser Forming of Doubly Curved Shapes. *J. Manuf. Sci. Eng.* **2004**, *126*, 1–9. [CrossRef]
54. Edwardson, S.P.; Dearden, G. *Laser Assisted Forming for Ship Building*; Sail: Williamsburg, VA, USA, 2003.
55. Steen, W.M.; Mazumder, J. Laser Bending or Forming. In *Laser Material Processing*; Steen, W.M., Mazumder, J., Eds.; Springer: London, UK, 2010; pp. 389–416, ISBN 978-1-84996-062-5.
56. Che Jamil, M.S.; Sheikh, M.A.; Li, L. A study of the effect of laser beam geometries on laser bending of sheet metal by buckling mechanism. *Opt. Laser Technol.* **2011**, *43*, 183–193. [CrossRef]

57. Vollertsen, F.; Komel, I.; Kals, R. The laser bending of steel foils for microparts by the buckling mechanism-a model. *Model. Simul. Mater. Sci. Eng.* **1995**, *3*, 107–119. [CrossRef]
58. Experimental and numerical modeling of buckling instability of laser sheet forming. *Int. J. Mach. Tools Manuf.* **2002**, *42*, 1427–1439. [CrossRef]
59. Lazarus, N.; Smith, G.L. Laser Forming for Complex 3D Folding. *Adv. Mater. Technol.* **2017**, *2*, 1700109. [CrossRef]
60. Shi, Y.; Liu, Y.; Yao, Z.; Shen, H. A study on bending direction of sheet metal in laser forming. *J. Appl. Phys.* **2008**, *103*, 053101. [CrossRef]
61. Li, W.; Yao, Y.L. Buckling based laser forming process: Concave or convex. In *International Congress on Applications of Lasers & Electro-Optics*; Laser Institute of America: Orlando, FL, USA, 2000; pp. D220–D229. [CrossRef]
62. Hao, Y.; Lien, J.-M. Computational laser forming origami of convex surfaces. In Proceedings of the ACM Symposium on Computational Fabrication—SCF '1, Pittsburgh, PA, USA, 16–18 June 2019; pp. 1–11.
63. Lazarus, N.; Smith, G.L. Laser Folding in a Roll-to-Roll Manufacturing Process. *Lasers Manuf. Mater. Process.* **2018**, *5*, 237–247. [CrossRef]
64. Shen, H. Mechanism of laser micro-adjustment. *J. Phys. D Appl. Phys.* **2008**, *41*, 245106. [CrossRef]
65. Lawrence, S. Developable Surfaces: Their History and Application. *Nexus Netw. J.* **2011**, *13*, 701–714. [CrossRef]
66. Maji, K.; Pratihar, D.K.; Nath, A.K. Forward and inverse predictions of deformations in laser forming of shaped surfaces under coupling mechanism. *J. Laser Appl.* **2018**, *30*, 032011. [CrossRef]
67. Chen, G.; Xu, X. Experimental and 3D Finite Element Studies of CW Laser Forming of Thin Stainless Steel Sheets. *J. Manuf. Sci. Eng.* **2000**, *123*, 66–73. [CrossRef]
68. Vásquez-Ojeda, C.; Ramos-Grez, J. Bending of stainless steel thin sheets by a raster scanned low power CO2 laser. *J. Mater. Process. Technol.* **2009**, *209*, 2641–2647. [CrossRef]
69. Paunoiu, V.; Squeo, E.A.; Quadrini, F.; Gheorghies, C.; Nicoara, D. Laser Bending of Stainless Steel Sheet Metals. *Int J. Mater.* **2008**, *1*, 1371–1374. [CrossRef]
70. Zaeh, M.F.; Hornfeck, T. Development of a robust laser beam bending process for aluminum fuselage structures. *Prod. Eng. Res. Devel.* **2008**, *2*, 149–155. [CrossRef]
71. Geiger, M.; Merklein, M.; Pitz, M. Laser and forming technology—An idea and the way of implementation. *J. Mater. Process. Technol.* **2004**, *151*, 3–11. [CrossRef]
72. Lubiano, G.; Ramos, J.A.; Magee, J. Laser Bending of Thin Metal Sheets by Means of a Low Power CO_2 Laser 537. In Proceedings of the 2000 International Solid Freeform Fabrication Symposium, Austin, TX, USA; 2000.
73. Magee, J.; Watkins, K.G.; Steen, W.M.; Calder, N.J.; Sidhu, J.; Kirby, J. Laser forming of aerospace alloys. In *International Congress on Applications of Lasers & Electro-Optics*; Laser Institute of America: Orlando, FL, USA, 1997; pp. E156–E165. [CrossRef]
74. Kitada, K.; Asahi, N. Laser adjustment of beryllium copper sheet using temperature gradient mechanism. In Proceedings of the Third International Symposium on Laser Precision Microfabrication; International Society for Optics and Photonics: Bellingham, WA, USA, 2003; Volume 4830, pp. 30–35.
75. Jiang, S.Q.; Liu, A.H.; Wang, X.X.; Chen, Z. The Bending Forming Mechanism of Copper Alloy by Different Lasers. *Adv. Mater. Res.* **2014**, *968*, 142–145. [CrossRef]
76. Gärtner, E.; Frühauf, J.; Löschner, U.; Exner, H. Laser bending of etched silicon microstructures. *Microsyst. Technol.* **2001**, *7*, 23–26. [CrossRef]
77. Xu, W.; Zhang, L.C.; Wang, X. Laser Bending of Silicon Sheet: Absorption Factor and Mechanisms. *J. Manuf. Sci. Eng.* **2013**, *135*. [CrossRef]
78. Wu, D.-J.; Ma, G.-Y.; Liu, S.; Wang, X.-Y.; Guo, D.-M. Experiments and simulation on laser bending of silicon sheet with different thicknesses. *Appl. Phys. A* **2010**, *101*, 517–521. [CrossRef]
79. Wu, D.; Zhang, Q.; Ma, G.; Guo, Y.; Guo, D. Laser bending of brittle materials. *Opt. Lasers Eng.* **2010**, *48*, 405–410. [CrossRef]
80. Wu, D.; Ma, G.; Niu, F.; Guo, D. Temperature Gradient Mechanism on Laser Bending of Borosilicate Glass Sheet. *J. Manuf. Sci. Eng.* **2010**, *132*. [CrossRef]
81. Bucher, T.; Cardenas, S.; Verma, R.; Li, W.; Lawrence Yao, Y. Laser Forming of Sandwich Panels With Metal Foam Cores. *J. Manuf. Sci. Eng.* **2018**, *140*, 111015. [CrossRef]

82. Guglielmotti, A.; Quadrini, F.; Squeo, E.A.; Tagliaferri, V. Laser Bending of Aluminum Foam Sandwich Panels. *Adv. Eng. Mater.* **2009**, *11*, 902–906. [CrossRef]
83. Gisario, A.; Barletta, M. Laser forming of glass laminate aluminium reinforced epoxy (GLARE): On the role of mechanical, physical and chemical interactions in the multi-layers material. *Opt. Lasers Eng.* **2018**, *110*, 364–376. [CrossRef]
84. Seong, W.-J.; Jeon, Y.-C.; Na, S.-J. Ship-hull plate forming of saddle shape by geometrical approach. *J. Mater. Process. Technol.* **2013**, *213*, 1885–1893. [CrossRef]
85. Okamoto, Y.; Uno, Y.; Ohta, K.; Shibata, T.; Kubota, S.; Namba, Y. Study on Precision Laser Forming of Plastic with YAG Laser. *J. Jpn. Soc. Precis. Eng.* **2000**, *66*, 891–895. [CrossRef]
86. Okamoto, Y.; Miyamoto, I.; Uno, Y.; Takenaka, T. Deformation characteristics of plastics in YAG laser forming. In Proceedings of the Fifth International Symposium on Laser Precision Microfabrication, Bellingham, WA, USA, 8 October 2004; International Society for Optics and Photonics: Bellingham, WA, USA, 2004; Volume 5662, pp. 576–581.
87. Cheng, P.; Fan, Y.; Zhang, J.; Yao, Y.L.; Mika, D.P.; Zhang, W.; Graham, M.; Marte, J.; Jones, M. Laser Forming of Varying Thickness Plate—Part II: Process Synthesis. *J. Manuf. Sci. Eng.* **2006**, *128*, 642–650. [CrossRef]
88. Lazarus, N.; Bedair, S.S.; Smith, G.L. Origami Inductors: Rapid Folding of 3-D Coils on a Laser Cutter. *IEEE Electron. Device Lett.* **2018**, *39*, 1046–1049. [CrossRef]
89. Gautam, S.S.; Singh, S.K.; Dixit, U.S. Laser Forming of Mild Steel Sheets Using Different Surface Coatings. In *Lasers Based Manufacturing: 5th International and 26th All India Manufacturing Technology, Design and Research Conference, AIMTDR 2014*; Joshi, S.N., Dixit, U.S., Eds.; Topics in Mining, Metallurgy and Materials Engineering; Springer: New Delhi, India, 2015; pp. 17–39, ISBN 978-81-322-2352-8.
90. Axelevitch, A.; Gorenstein, B.; Golan, G. Investigation of Optical Transmission in Thin Metal Films. *Phys. Procedia* **2012**, *32*, 1–13. [CrossRef]
91. Rumble, J. *CRC Handbook of Chemistry and Physics*, 101st ed.; CRC Press: Boca Raton, FL, USA, 2020; ISBN 978-0-367-41724-6.
92. Shidid, D.P.; Gollo, M.H.; Brandt, M.; Mahdavian, M. Study of effect of process parameters on titanium sheet metal bending using Nd: YAG laser. *Opt. Laser Technol.* **2013**, *47*, 242–247. [CrossRef]
93. Yau, C.L.; Chan, K.C.; Lee, W.B. Laser bending of leadframe materials. *J. Mater. Process. Technol.* **1998**, *82*, 117–121. [CrossRef]
94. Hennige, T.; Holzer, S.; Vollertsen, F.; Geiger, M. On the working accuracy of laser bending. *J. Mater. Process. Technol.* **1997**, *71*, 422–432. [CrossRef]
95. Fidder, H.; Ocelík, V.; Botes, A.; De Hosson, J.T.M. Response of Ti microstructure in mechanical and laser forming processes. *J. Mater. Sci.* **2018**, *53*, 14713–14728. [CrossRef]
96. Walczak, M.; Ramos-Grez, J.; Celentano, D.; Lima, E.B.F. Sensitization of AISI 302 stainless steel during low-power laser forming. *Opt. Lasers Eng.* **2010**, *48*, 906–914. [CrossRef]
97. Patel, C.K.N. Continuous-Wave Laser Action on Vibrational-Rotational Transitions of CO_2. *Phys. Rev.* **1964**, *136*, A1187–A1193. [CrossRef]
98. Lawrence, J. A comparative investigation of the efficacy of CO_2 and high-power diode lasers for the forming of EN3 mild steel sheets. *Proc. Inst. Mech. Eng. Part. B J. Eng. Manuf.* **2002**, *216*, 1481–1491. [CrossRef]
99. Kim, J.; Na, S.J. Development of irradiation strategies for free curve laser forming. *Opt. Laser Technol.* **2003**, *35*, 605–611. [CrossRef]
100. Silve, S.; Podschies, B.; Steen, W.M.; Watkins, K.G. Laser Forming —A New Vocabulary for Objects. In Proceedings of the ICALEO 1999, San Diego, FL, USA, 15–18 November 1999; Volume F, pp. 87–96.
101. Shi, Y.; Shen, H.; Yao, Z.; Hu, J. Temperature gradient mechanism in laser forming of thin plates. *Opt. Laser Technol.* **2007**, *39*, 858–863. [CrossRef]
102. Magee, J.; Sidhu, J.; Cooke, R.L. A Prototype laser forming system. *Opt. Lasers Eng.* **2000**, *34*, 339–353. [CrossRef]
103. Namba, Y. Laser Forming in Space. In Proceedings of the International Conference on Lasers '85, Las Vegas, NV, USA; 1985; pp. 403–407.
104. Liu, J.; Sun, S.; Guan, Y.; Ji, Z. Experimental study on negative laser bending process of steel foils. *Opt. Lasers Eng.* **2010**, *48*, 83–88. [CrossRef]
105. Yoshioka, S.; Miyazaki, T.; Misu, T.; Oba, R.; Saito, M. Laser forming of thin foil by a newly developed sample holding method. *J. Laser Appl.* **2003**, *15*, 6. [CrossRef]

106. Shen, H.; Peng, L.; Hu, J.; Yao, Z. Study on the mechanical behavior of laser micro-adjustment of two-bridge actuators. *J. Micromech. Microeng.* **2010**, *20*, 115010. [CrossRef]
107. Tetzel, H.; Grden, M.; Vollertsen, F. Stress analysis based on strain measurement in sheet metal laser bending. *Prod. Eng. Res. Devel.* **2013**, *7*, 647–655. [CrossRef]
108. Cheng, J.; Yao, Y.L. Cooling effects in multiscan laser forming. *J. Manuf. Process.* **2001**, *3*, 60–72. [CrossRef]
109. Lambiase, F.; Di Ilio, A.; Paoletti, A. An experimental investigation on passive water cooling in laser forming process. *Int. J. Adv. Manuf. Technol.* **2013**, *64*, 829–840. [CrossRef]
110. Seyedkashi, S.M.H.; Cho, J.R.; Lee, S.H.; Moon, Y.H. Feasibility of underwater laser forming of laminated metal composites. *Mater. Manuf. Process.* **2018**, *33*, 546–551. [CrossRef]
111. Shen, H.; Ran, M.; Hu, J.; Yao, Z. An experimental investigation of underwater pulsed laser forming. *Opt. Lasers Eng.* **2014**, *62*, 1–8. [CrossRef]
112. Paramasivan, K.; Das, S.; Marimuthu, S.; Misra, D. Increment in laser bending angle by forced bottom cooling. *Int. J. Adv. Manuf. Technol.* **2018**, *94*, 2137–2147. [CrossRef]
113. Shen, H.; Hu, J.; Yao, Z.Q. Cooling Effects in Laser Forming. *Mater. Sci. Forum* **2010**, *663–665*, 58–63. [CrossRef]
114. Lambiase, F.; Di Ilio, A.; Paoletti, A. Productivity in multi-pass laser forming of thin AISI 304 stainless steel sheets. *Int. J. Adv. Manuf. Technol.* **2016**, *86*, 259–268. [CrossRef]
115. Chinizadeh, M.; Kiahosseini, S.R. Deformation, microstructure, hardness, and pitting corrosion of 316 stainless steel after laser forming: A comparison between natural and forced cooling. *J. Mater. Res.* **2017**, *32*, 3046–3054. [CrossRef]
116. Arora, H.; Singh, R.; Brar, G.S. Thermal and structural modelling of arc welding processes: A literature review. *Meas. Control.* **2019**, *52*, 955–969. [CrossRef]
117. Geiger, M.; Vollertsen, F.; Deinzer, G. *Flexible Straightening of Car Body Shells by Laser Forming*; SAE: Warrendale, PA, USA, 1993; p. 930279.
118. Dearden, G.; Edwardson, S.P.; Abed, E.; Watkins, K.G. Laser forming for the correction of distortion and design shape in aluminium structures using laser forming. In *International Congress on Applications of Lasers & Electro-Optics*; Laser Institute of America: Orlando, FL, USA, 2006.
119. Gurova, T.; Estefen, S.F.; Leontiev, A.; de Oliveira, F.A.L. Welding residual stresses: A daily history. *Sci. Technol. Weld. Join.* **2015**, *20*, 616–621. [CrossRef]
120. Stavridis, J.; Papacharalampopoulos, A.; Stavropoulos, P. Quality assessment in laser welding: A critical review. *Int. J. Adv. Manuf. Technol.* **2018**, *94*, 1825–1847. [CrossRef]
121. Shi, Y.J.; Chen, J.; Qi, Y.G.; Yao, Z.Q. Processing strategy for laser forming of complicated singly curved shapes. *Mater. Sci. Technol.* **2009**, *25*, 925–930. [CrossRef]
122. Mehrpouya, M.; Huang, H.; Venettacci, S.; Gisario, A. LaserOrigami (LO) of three-dimensional (3D) components: Experimental analysis and numerical modeling-part II. *J. Manuf. Process.* **2019**, *39*. [CrossRef]
123. Castle, T.; Cho, Y.; Gong, X.; Jung, E.; Sussman, D.M.; Yang, S.; Kamien, R.D. Making the Cut: Lattice Kirigami Rules. *Phys. Rev. Lett.* **2014**, *113*, 245502. [CrossRef]
124. Cheng, J.; Yao, Y.L. Process Design of Laser Forming for Three-Dimensional Thin Plates. *J. Manuf. Sci. Eng.* **2004**, *126*, 217–225. [CrossRef]
125. Ibraheem Imhan, K.; Btht, B.; Zakaria, A.; Shah B Ismail, M.I.; Hadi Alsabti, N.M.; Ahmad, A.K. Features of Laser Tube Bending processing based on Laser Forming: A Review. *J. Laser Opt. Photonics* **2018**, *5*. [CrossRef]
126. Wang, X.Y.; Wang, J.; Xu, W.J.; Guo, D.M. Scanning path planning for laser bending of straight tube into curve tube. *Opt. Laser Technol.* **2014**, *56*, 43–51. [CrossRef]
127. Guglielmotti, A.; Quadrini, F.; Squeo, E.A.; Tagliaferri, V. Diode laser bending of tongues from slotted steel tubes. *Int. J. Mater.* **2009**, *2*, 107–111. [CrossRef]
128. Che Jamil, M.S.; Imam Fauzi, E.R.; Juinn, C.S.; Sheikh, M.A. Laser bending of pre-stressed thin-walled nickel micro-tubes. *Opt. Laser Technol.* **2015**, *73*, 105–117. [CrossRef]
129. Campbell, R.C.; Campbell, B.R.; Lehecka, T.M.; Palmer, J.A.; Knorovsky, G.A. Precision laser bending of thin precious metal alloys. In Proceedings of the Laser-Based Micro- and Nanopackaging and Assembly, Bellingham, WA, USA, 20 March 2007; Volume 6459, p. 64590U.
130. Frühauf, J.; Gärtner, E.; Jänsch, E. Silicon as a plastic material. *J. Micromech. Microeng.* **1999**, *9*, 305–312. [CrossRef]

131. Schmidt, M.; Dirscherl, M.; Rank, M.; Zimmermann, M. Laser micro adjustment—From new basic process knowledge to the application. *J. Laser Appl.* **2007**, *19*, 10. [CrossRef]
132. Widlaszewski, J. Applications of laser forming in micro technologies. In *Selected Problems of Modeling and Control in Mechanics*; Wydawnictwo: Kielce, Poland, 2011.
133. Hoving, W. *Accurate Manipulation Using Laser Technology*; Beckmann, L.H.J.F., Ed.; Proc. SPIE 3097: Munich, Germany, 1997; pp. 284–295.
134. Zhuang, Z.; Lu, Z.; Huang, Z.; Liu, C.; Qin, W. School of Mechanical Engineering, Shanghai Jiao Tong University, 200240, Shanghai, China Experimental study on edge effects in laser bending. *Math. Biosci. Eng.* **2019**, *16*, 4491–4505. [CrossRef] [PubMed]
135. Shen, H.; Wang, H.; Hu, J.; Yao, Z. Processing Optimization in Multiheating Positions for Laser Thermal Adjustment of Actuators. *J. Manuf. Sci. Eng.* **2016**, *138*. [CrossRef]
136. Zhang, X.R.; Xu, X. Laser bending for high-precision curvature adjustment of microcantilevers. *Appl. Phys. Lett.* **2005**, *86*, 021114. [CrossRef]
137. Inoue, M.; Kawamata, H.; Tanaka, H. Thin Plate Formation Method, Thin Plate and Suspension Correction Apparatus, and Correction Method. U.S. Patent 7,624,610, 1 December 2009.
138. Murata, A.; Mukae, H.; Maegawa, T.; Higashionji, M.; Okada, T. Rotary Head Adjuster. U.S. Patent 5,341,256, 1994.
139. Murata, A.; Mukae, H.; Maegawa, T.; Higashionji, M.; Okada, T. Rotary Magnetic Head Having Head Base Which is Bent Along Thermal Plastic Deformation Line. U.S. Patent 6,185,073, 2001.
140. Birnbaum, A.J.; Yao, Y.L. The Effects of Laser Forming on NiTi Superelastic Shape Memory Alloys. *J. Manuf. Sci. Eng.* **2010**, *132*, 41002. [CrossRef]
141. Folkersma, K.G.P.; Römer, G.R.B.E.; Brouwer, D.M.; Herder, J.L. High precision optical fiber alignment using tube laser bending. *Int. J. Adv. Manuf. Technol.* **2016**, *86*, 953–961. [CrossRef]
142. Folkersma, G.; Brouwer, D.; Römer, G.-W. Microtube Laser Forming for Precision Component Alignment. *J. Manuf. Sci. Eng.* **2016**, *138*. [CrossRef]
143. Thompson, Y.; Gonzalez-Gutierrez, J.; Kukla, C.; Felfer, P. Fused filament fabrication, debinding and sintering as a low cost additive manufacturing method of 316L stainless steel. *Addit. Manuf.* **2019**, *30*, 100861. [CrossRef]
144. Lathers, S.; Mousa, M.; La Belle, J. Additive Manufacturing Fused Filament Fabrication Three-Dimensional Printed Pressure Sensor for Prosthetics with Low Elastic Modulus and High Filler Ratio Filament Composites. *3D Print. Addit. Manuf.* **2017**, *4*, 30–40. [CrossRef]
145. Hegde, M.; Meenakshisundaram, V.; Chartrain, N.; Sekhar, S.; Tafti, D.; Williams, C.B.; Long, T.E. 3D Printing All-Aromatic Polyimides using Mask-Projection Stereolithography: Processing the Nonprocessable. *Adv. Mater.* **2017**, *29*, 1701240. [CrossRef]
146. Hull, C.W. Apparatus for Production of Three-Dimensional Objects by Stereolithography. U.S. Patent 6,027,324, 22 February 2000.
147. Negi, S.; Dhiman, S.; Sharma, R.K. Basics, Applications and Future of Additive Manufacturing Technologies: A review. *J. Manuf. Technol. Res.* **2013**, *5*, 75.
148. Gao, H.; Sheikholeslami, G.; Dearden, G.; Edwardson, S.P. Development of Scan Strategies for Controlled 3D Laser Forming of Sheet Metal Components. *Phys. Procedia* **2016**, *83*, 286–295. [CrossRef]
149. Gao, H.; Sheikholeslami, G.; Dearden, G.; Edwardson, S.P. Reverse Analysis of Scan Strategies for Controlled 3D Laser Forming of Sheet Metal. *Procedia Eng.* **2017**, *183*, 369–374. [CrossRef]
150. Kim, J.; Na, S.J. 3D laser-forming strategies for sheet metal by geometrical information. *Opt. Laser Technol.* **2009**, *41*, 843–852. [CrossRef]
151. Kim, J.; Na, S.J. Feedback control for 2D free curve laser forming. *Opt. Laser Technol.* **2005**, *37*, 139–146. [CrossRef]
152. Edwardson, S.P.; Abed, E.; Bartkowiak, K.; Dearden, G.; Watkins, K.G. Geometrical influences on multi-pass laser forming. *J. Phys. D Appl. Phys.* **2006**, *39*, 382–389. [CrossRef]
153. Smith, G.L.; Lazarus, N.; McCormick, S. Laser Folded Antenna. In Proceedings of the 2018 IEEE MTT-S International Microwave Workshop Series on Advanced Materials and Processes for RF and THz Applications (IMWS-AMP), Ann Arbor, MI, USA, 16–18 July 2018; pp. 1–3.
154. Morgan, S.P. Effect of Surface Roughness on Eddy Current Losses at Microwave Frequencies. *J. Appl. Phys.* **1949**, *20*, 352–362. [CrossRef]

155. Kügler, H.; Vollertsen, F. Determining Absorptivity Variations of Multiple Laser Beam Treatments of Stainless Steel Sheets. *J. Manuf. Mater. Process.* **2018**, *2*, 84. [CrossRef]
156. Chua, C.L.; Fork, D.K.; Schuylenbergh, K.V.; Lu, J.P. Out-of-plane high-Q inductors on low-resistance silicon. *J. Microelectromech. Syst.* **2003**, *12*, 989–995. [CrossRef]
157. Fidder, H.; Els-Botes, A.; Woudberg, S.; McGrath, P.J.; Ocelik, V.; de Hosson, J.T.M. A Study of Microstructural Fatigue and Residual Stress Evolution in Titanium Plates Deformed by Mechanical and Laser Bending. *WIT Trans. Eng. Sci. Southampt.* **2015**, *91*, 23–34.
158. Sami Yilbas, B.; Khaled, M.; Akhtar, S.; Karatas, C. Laser bending of steel sheets: Corrosion testing of bended sections. *Ind. Lubr. Tribol.* **2011**, *63*, 367–372. [CrossRef]
159. Liu, Z.; Guzmán, C.; Liu, H.; Anacleto, A.; Francisco, T.; Abdoalshafie, M.; Ma, L.; Abodunrin, O.; Skeldon, P. Corrosion performance and restoration of laser-formed metallic alloy sheets. *J. Laser Appl.* **2009**, *21*, 76–81. [CrossRef]
160. Olsen, F.O.; Alting, L. Pulsed Laser Materials Processing, ND-YAG versus CO_2 Lasers. *Cirp Ann.* **1995**, *44*, 141–145. [CrossRef]
161. Lazarus, N.; Wilson, A.A.; Smith, G.L. Contactless laser fabrication and propulsion of freely moving structures. *Extrem. Mech. Lett.* **2018**, *20*, 46–50. [CrossRef]
162. Noor, Y.M.D.; Tam, S.C.; Lim, L.E.N.; Jana, S. A review of the Nd: YAG laser marking of plastic and ceramic IC packages. *J. Mater. Process. Technol.* **1994**, *42*, 95–133. [CrossRef]
163. Ehrlich, D.J.; Tsao, J.Y. A review of laser–microchemical processing. *J. Vac. Sci. Technol. B: Microelectron. Process. Phenom.* **1983**, *1*, 969–984. [CrossRef]
164. Osgood, R.M.; Deutsch, T.F. Laser-Induced Chemistry for Microelectronics. *Science* **1985**, *227*, 709–714. [CrossRef]
165. Kindle, C.; Castonguay, A.; McGee, S.; Tomko, J.A.; Hopkins, P.E.; Zarzar, L.D. Direct Laser Writing from Aqueous Precursors for Nano to Microscale Topographical Control, Integration, and Synthesis of Nanocrystalline Mixed Metal Oxides. *ACS Appl. Nano Mater.* **2019**, *2*, 2581–2586. [CrossRef]
166. Wachs, I.E. Raman and IR studies of surface metal oxide species on oxide supports: Supported metal oxide catalysts. *Catal. Today* **1996**, *27*, 437–455. [CrossRef]
167. Kalinushkin, V.P.; Uvarov, O.V.; Gladilin, A.A. Photoluminescent Tomography of Semiconductors by Two-Photon Confocal Microscopy Technique. *J. Electron. Mater.* **2018**, *47*, 5087–5091. [CrossRef]